Walter D. and Deella Toms
Endowed Library Fund

Established
in loving memory
by

Dr. Esther C. Toms,
Class of 1943

THE NETTER COLLECTION OF MEDICAL ILLUSTRATIONS

VOLUME 4

A Compilation of Paintings Depicting
Anatomy and Pathophysiology of the

ENDOCRINE SYSTEM
AND
SELECTED METABOLIC DISEASES

Prepared by

FRANK H. NETTER, M.D.

Guest Editor

PETER H. FORSHAM, M.D., M.A. (Cantab)

Commissioned and published by

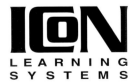

LEARNING
SYSTEMS

The Netter Collection of Medical Illustrations
Endocrine System & Selected Metabolic Diseases: Volume 4
Prepared by
Frank H. Netter, M.D.

See page 289 for a complete list of The Netter Collection of Medical Illustrations

Published by Icon Learning Systems, LLC, a subsidiary of MediMedia USA, Inc.
All rights reserved.
©Copyright 1962 MediMedia USA, Inc.

Copies of NETTER COLLECTION books, ATLAS of HUMAN ANATOMY and CLINICAL SYMPOSIA
are available from Icon Learning Systems, 295 North Street, Teterboro, N.J. 07608 or call 1-201-727-9123.

FIRST PRINTING, 1965
SECOND PRINTING, 1970
THIRD PRINTING, 1974
FOURTH PRINTING, 1977
FIFTH PRINTING, 1981
SIXTH PRINTING, 1992
SEVENTH PRINTING, 1999
EIGHTH PRINTING, 2001

ISBN 0-914168-87-8
LIBRARY OF CONGRESS CATALOG NO.: 97-76569
PRINTED IN U.S.A.

ORIGINAL PRINTING BY COLORPRESS, NEW YORK, NY

COLOR ENGRAVINGS BY EMBASSY PHOTO ENGRAVING CO., INC., NEW YORK, NY

OFFSET CONVERSION BY R.R. DONNELLEY & SONS COMPANY

FILM PREP BY PAGE IMAGING, INC., PITTSBURGH, PA

EIGHTH PRINTING BY HOECHSTETTER PRINTING, INC.

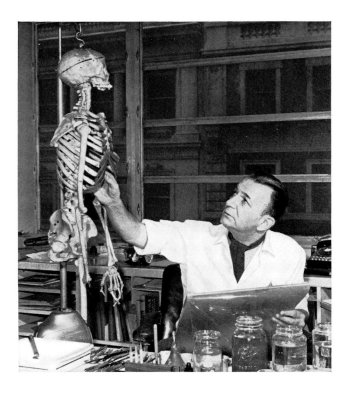

THE ARTIST

Many readers of the NETTER COLLECTION have expressed a desire to know more about Dr. Netter. In response to these requests this summary of Dr. Netter's career has been prepared.

Frank Henry Netter, born in 1906 in Brooklyn, New York, received his M.D. degree from New York University in 1931. To help pay his way through medical school and internship at Bellevue, he worked as a commercial artist and as an illustrator of medical books and articles for his professors and other physicians, perfecting his natural talent by studying at the National Academy of Design and attending courses at the Art Students' League.

In 1933 Dr. Netter entered the private practice of surgery in New York City. But it was the depth of the depression, and the recently married physician continued to accept art assignments to supplement his income. Soon he was spending more and more time at the drawing board and finally, realizing that his career lay in medical illustration, he decided to give up practicing and become a full-time artist.

Soon, Dr. Netter was receiving requests to develop many unusual projects. One of the most arduous of these was building the "transparent woman" for the San Francisco Golden Gate Exposition. This 7-foot-high transparent figure depicted the menstrual process, the development and birth of a baby, and the physical and sexual development of a woman, while a synchronized voice told the story of the female endocrine system. Dr. Netter labored on this project night and day for 7 months. Another interesting assignment involved a series of paintings of incidents in the life of a physician. Among others, the pictures showed a medical student sitting up the night before the osteology examination, studying away to the point of exhaustion; an emergency ward; an ambulance call; a class reunion; and a night call made by a country doctor.

During World War II, Dr. Netter was an officer in the Army, stationed first at the Army Institute of Pathology, later at the Surgeon General's Office, in charge of graphic training aids for the Medical Department. Numerous manuals were produced under his direction, among them first aid for combat troops, roentgenology for technicians, sanitation in the field, and survival in the tropics.

After the war, Dr. Netter began work on several major projects for CIBA Pharmaceutical Company, culminating in THE CIBA COLLECTION OF MEDICAL ILLUSTRATIONS. To date, five volumes have been published and work is in progress on the sixth, dealing with the urinary tract.

Dr. Netter goes about planning and executing his illustrations in a very exacting way. First comes the study, unquestionably the most important and most difficult part of the entire undertaking. No drawing is ever started until Dr. Netter has acquired a complete understanding of the subject matter, either through reading or by consultation with leading authorities in the field. Often he visits hospitals to observe clinical cases, pathologic or surgical specimens, or operative procedures. Sometimes an original dissection is necessary.

When all his questions have been answered and the problem is thoroughly understood, Dr. Netter makes a pencil sketch on a tissue or tracing pad. Always, the subject must be visualized from the standpoint of the physician; is it to be viewed from above or below, from the side, the rear, or the front? What area is to be covered, the entire body or just certain segments? What plane provides the clearest understanding? In some pictures two, three, or four planes of dissection may be necessary.

When the sketch is at last satisfactory, Dr. Netter transfers it to a piece of illustration board for the finished drawing. This is done by blocking the back of the picture with a soft pencil, taping the tissue down on the board with Scotch tape, then going over the lines with a hard pencil. Over the years, our physician-artist has used many media to finish his illustrations, but now he works almost exclusively in transparent water colors mixed with white paint.

In spite of the tremendously productive life Dr. Netter has led, he has been able to enjoy his family, first in a handsome country home in East Norwich, Long Island, and, after the five children had grown up, in a penthouse overlooking the East River in Manhattan.

ALFRED W. CUSTER

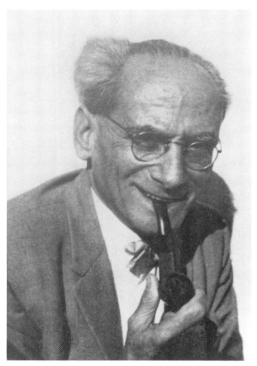

Dedicated

to

ERNST OPPENHEIMER, M.D.

I first met Dr. Oppenheimer many years ago, when he was Chief Pharmacologist for CIBA Pharmaceutical Company. I remember him, from those days, as a vociferous, energetic individual who always insisted on seeing every new group of pictures which I had made, and on going over them in detail. At first I looked upon this as interference, and even resented it a little. As time went on, however, I came to realize that this man's interest in my work was sincere and genuine and that any criticisms or suggestions he made were always in a spirit of helpfulness. His comments were forceful, sometimes even stinging in their directness, but, whenever I was able to prove him wrong, he was always ready to change his viewpoint. Little by little, I came to feel that here was a man who understood what I was trying to do, who grasped the difficulties and the multitudinous problems with which I was confronted in my efforts to pictorialize medicine, a man deeply interested and wanting to help.

When the day came for him to retire as Vice President in Charge of Research at CIBA, I was very glad indeed that he agreed to join me in this project and to take over the editorship of the volumes upon which I was at work. As we worked together through the years, our alliance grew into a very warm friendship. His understanding of my efforts, his appreciation of my accomplishments, and his encouragement in the face of difficulties meant a great deal. Even his criticisms were stimulating, for I knew they were sincere. I like to feel also that my acceptance of his aid and regard for his judgment were rewarding to him.

Upon his retirement "Oppy", as I called him, and his wife, Emma, went to live in a charming house on the mountainside in Mill Valley, Calif. Here he became truly absorbed in the work we were doing together. His patience and perseverance in searching out details of scientific information often aroused my admiration. His wide acquaintance and friendship with

men in the forefront of medical knowledge frequently proved most useful. More significantly, however, these friendships demonstrated to me the character of the man: beneath the brusque surface were a warm personality that had won the love of men of science throughout the world, and a devotion to scientific truth that had won their respect.

Once he was settled in his mountainside home and I in New York, our contacts were largely by mail. Recently, in a sentimental mood, I reread some of our correspondence. In doing so, I ran across a phrase which is very revealing of the relationship that existed between us. He wrote plaintively, "Frank what is wrong, you have not insulted me in your last three letters?" Here, then, was the true nature of this friendship; one could say to the other what he thought and felt, without regard to petty proprieties. We never pulled any punches in expressing our opinions to each other, but sincerity was never lessened by disagreement.

Some of the best times in both our lives were those when I would go to visit him, and we would sit on his terrace in the warm California sun, reviewing pictures and discussing problems. On these occasions I could feel his enthusiasm for the whole project, and I am sure that he sensed the same devotion in me. Between us, then, there was a sort of communion, a common interest never spoken but clearly understood.

"Dr. Oppy" was well versed in all fields of medical science, but his strongest interest was endocrinology. Accordingly, I looked forward eagerly to having his aid and counsel in producing this atlas on the endocrine system and metabolism. But scarcely had I started, when word came that he had only a short time to live. He was never to have the satisfaction of seeing the completion of this volume. When his death came, a great and important influence had gone out of my life. The dedication of this volume to the memory of Dr. Oppenheimer is thus most appropriate.

FRANK H. NETTER, M.D.

Dr. Ernst Oppenheimer, the son of a physician, was born in 1888 in Frankfurt, Germany, and received his medical education in a number of European institutions, culminating in his M.D. at the University of Freiburg in 1913. Through association with some of the best medical minds of that era, and steeped in the tradition of liberal yet critical thought, he early recognized the importance of research in the development of the field of medicine. After receiving training in pharmacology, he became an instructor at the University of Freiburg, from 1918 to 1922, and then assumed a number of research positions in the pharmaceutical industry. The political upheavals throughout Europe during the late 1930's fortunately led him, in 1937, to become Chief Pharmacologist with the newly formed CIBA Pharmaceutical Company, in Summit, N.J. This was followed, in 1943, by his appointment as Vice President in Charge of Research at CIBA. At the end of 1952, he retired from that position and became the first editor of THE CIBA COLLECTION OF MEDICAL ILLUSTRATIONS.

In all his endeavors there was one outstanding feature which endeared him to the hearts of men in clinical and pharmacological research throughout the world, and that was his determination to pursue the truth logically at all times, often with considerable disregard for any commercial considerations that might have entered into the picture. Because of this he had the complete confidence of the medical academicians of that day. This, together with the good fortune that Dr. Frank Netter consented to devote his talents so unstintingly to the CIBA COLLECTION, accounts for its continued excellence.

I first met Dr. Oppenheimer when I was a research fellow at the Peter Bent Brigham Hospital in 1945, during one of his frequent visits to discuss matters with Professor George W. Thorn. Soon a friendship developed, which eventually culminated in his decision to spend his years of retirement in Mill Valley, Calif., after visiting with us there. At the Metabolic Research Unit of The University of California Medical Center in San Francisco, we had Dr. Oppenheimer spend every Friday afternoon with us to take part in our scientific and medical discussions. He acted as an emeritus

Mill Valley, Calif., 1965

consultant and, above all, as a healthy critic of our work. These were delightful and exciting periods, enjoyed equally by my associates and by Dr. Oppenheimer.

He spent much of his working hours in directing the preparation of the CIBA COLLECTION from his lovely home perched high on a wooded hillside. In the spring of 1960, this happy era came to a sudden halt, with the chance discovery of a bronchogenic carcinoma in the right lung field.

X-ray therapy led to a brief remission, during which plans were laid for the present volume. At this point I was asked by Dr. Netter and the CIBA organization to act as an associate in editing Volume 4. On February 6, 1962, the increasingly anoxic state of the patient led to his peaceful demise at the age of 73. Then I was asked to assure the completion of Volume 4 as guest editor, in keeping with the expressed wish of Dr. Oppenheimer. In this atlas the particular challenge lay in the need to supplement the morphological illustrations with the necessary biochemistry and biophysics to explain the underlying mechanisms. The influence of the keen mind of Dr. Oppenheimer pervades this volume; this is so because he was responsible for the selection of many of the contributors and had set high standards of excellence in the previous editorial management of the CIBA COLLECTION.

As a friend and collaborator one could not ask for any better, since he combined an extensive, enthusiastic, and relentless quest for knowledge with a most hardy rejection of mediocrity. I shall always cherish the thought that my work with him, as his physician, allowed me to alleviate some of the anxiety and discomfort of his declining state of health and to share the load with his dear wife, Emma, as well as their two daughters, Mrs. Walter N. Holmstrom and Mrs. Donald R. McVittie. My only regret is that it will not be possible for Ernst Oppenheimer to see the fruits of his last endeavor in the field of endocrinology, which was his favorite subject.

This volume thus constitutes a monument to him. It represents the work of a great artist and many others of his friends, united in offering for future generations, in his memory, this atlas in the health sciences.

PETER H. FORSHAM, M.D.

CONTRIBUTORS AND CONSULTANTS

The artist, editor, and publishers express their appreciation
to the following authorities for their generous collaboration:

ALEXANDER G. BEARN, M.D.

Professor, The Rockefeller Institute and Senior Physician to the Hospital of The Rockefeller Institute, New York, N. Y.

EDWARD G. BIGLIERI, M.D., F.A.C.P.

Assistant Professor of Medicine, The University of California School of Medicine, San Francisco; Chief, Endocrine-Metabolic Service, and Director, Clinical Study Center, San Francisco General Hospital, San Francisco, Calif.

JOSEPH J. BUNIM, M.D., F.A.C.P. (Deceased)

Formerly Clinical Director and Chief of the Arthritis Branch, National Institute of Arthritis and Metabolic Diseases, Bethesda, Md.; Associate Professor of Medicine, Johns Hopkins University, Baltimore, Md.; Clinical Professor of Medicine, Georgetown University School of Medicine, Washington, D. C.

OLIVER COPE, M.D., F.A.C.S.

Professor of Surgery, Harvard Medical School, Boston; Visiting Surgeon, Massachusetts General Hospital, Boston, Mass.

E. S. CRELIN, Ph.D.

Associate Professor of Anatomy, Yale University School of Medicine, New Haven, Conn.

CALVIN EZRIN, M.D., F.R.C.P. (C)

Physician, Toronto General Hospital; Consultant in Medicine, Sunnybrook Hospital (Department of Veterans' Affairs), Toronto; Associate, Department of Medicine, and Research Associate, Department of Pathology, Division of Neuropathology, University of Toronto, Toronto, Canada.

PETER H. FORSHAM, M.D., M.A. (Cantab), F.A.C.P.

Professor of Medicine and Pediatrics; Director, Metabolic Research Unit; Chief of Endocrinology, Department of Medicine, University of California School of Medicine, San Francisco; Physician, University of California Hospitals, San Francisco, Calif.

DONALD S. FREDRICKSON, M.D.

Clinical Director and Head, Section on Molecular Diseases, National Heart Institute, National Institutes of Health, Bethesda, Md.

MAURICE GALANTE, M.D., F.A.C.S.

Assistant Professor of Surgery, Associate Professor of Oncology, University of California School of Medicine, San Francisco, Calif.

WALTER GILBERT, D.Phil.

Associate Professor of Biophysics, Physics Department, Harvard University, Cambridge, Mass.

ROY O. GREEP, Ph.D.

Dean and Professor of Anatomy in the School of Dental Medicine, Harvard University, Boston, Mass.

ALEXANDER B. GUTMAN, M.D., Ph.D., F.A.C.P.

Director, Department of Medicine, The Mount Sinai Hospital, New York; Professor of Medicine, Columbia University College of Physicians and Surgeons, New York, N. Y.

KURT J. ISSELBACHER, M.D.

Associate Professor of Medicine, Harvard Medical School, Boston; Chief, Gastrointestinal Unit, Massachusetts General Hospital, Boston, Mass.

BENJAMIN M. KAGAN, M.D., F.A.C.P., F.A.A.P.

Professor of Pediatrics, University of California at Los Angeles; Director and Chairman, Department of Pediatrics, Cedars of Lebanon Hospital, Division of Cedars-Sinai Medical Center, Los Angeles, Calif.

FELIX O. KOLB, M.D., F.A.C.P.

Associate Clinical Professor of Medicine and Assistant Director, Metabolic Research Unit, The University of California School of Medicine, San Francisco; Associate Physician, University of California Hospitals, San Francisco, Calif.

AARON B. LERNER, M.D., Ph.D.

Professor of Dermatology, Yale University School of Medicine, New Haven, Conn.

RACHMIEL LEVINE, M.D., F.A.C.P.

Professor and Chairman, Department of Medicine, New York Medical College, New York; Director of Medical Services, Flower and Fifth Avenue Hospitals, Metropolitan Hospital, and Bird S. Coler Hospital, New York, N. Y.

G. A. G. MITCHELL, O.B.E., T.D., M.B., Ch.M., D.Sc.

Professor of Anatomy and Director of the Anatomical Laboratories, University of Manchester, England.

ROBERT E. OLSON, Ph.D., M.D.

Doisy Professor of Biochemistry and Director, Department of Biochemistry, Saint Louis University School of Medicine, St. Louis, Mo. — as of September 1, 1965.

RULON W. RAWSON, M.D., F.A.C.P.

Chairman, Department of Medicine, Memorial Hospital, New York; Chief, Division of Clinical Investigation, Sloan-Kettering Institute, New York; Professor of Medicine, Cornell University Medical College, New York, N. Y.

SANFORD I. ROTH, M.D.

Associate in Pathology at the Massachusetts General Hospital, Harvard Medical School; Assistant Pathologist, Massachusetts General Hospital, Boston, Mass.

ALBERT SEGALOFF, M.D., F.A.C.P.

Director of Endocrine Research, The Alton Ochsner Medical Foundation, New Orleans; Department of Medicine, Ochsner Clinic, New Orleans; Professor of Clinical Medicine, Tulane University School of Medicine, New Orleans, La.

LLOYD H. SMITH, M.D.

Professor and Chairman, Department of Medicine, The University of California School of Medicine, San Francisco; Physician, University of California Hospitals, San Francisco, Calif.

ARTHUR R. SOHVAL, M.D., F.A.C.P.

Associate Attending Physician, Member of Endocrine Research Laboratory and Clinic, The Mount Sinai Hospital, New York, N. Y.

HOWARD L. STEINBACH, M.D., F.A.C.R.

Professor of Radiology and Vice-Chairman, Department of Radiology; Chief, Section of Diagnostic Radiology, The University of California School of Medicine, San Francisco, Calif.

DAVID H. P. STREETEN, M.B., D.Phil., M.R.C.P.

Professor of Medicine, State University of New York Upstate Medical Center, Syracuse; Attending Physician, State University Hospital, Syracuse, N. Y.

SOMERS H. STURGIS, M.D., F.A.C.O.G.

Clinical Professor, Gynecology, Harvard Medical School, Boston; Surgeon, Gynecology, Peter Bent Brigham Hospital, Boston, Mass.

S. J. THANNHAUSER, M.D., Ph.D. (Deceased)

Formerly Clinical Professor of Medicine Emeritus, Tufts College Medical School, Boston; Consulting Physician, Pratt Diagnostic Hospital, New England Medical Center, Boston, Mass.

FRANK H. TYLER, M.D., F.A.C.P.

Professor of Medicine, University of Utah College of Medicine, Salt Lake City, Utah.

JUDSON J. VAN WYK, M.D., F.A.A.P.

Professor of Pediatrics, The University of North Carolina School of Medicine, Chapel Hill, N. C.; U. S. Public Health Service Career Research Awardee.

INTRODUCTION

In the early days the endocrine glands were looked upon as an isolated group of structures, secreting substances which, in some strange way, influenced the human organism. The thyroid gland was known to be an organ of considerable significance. The clinical syndromes of hyper- and hypothyroidism and the therapeutic effects of thyroid administration and thyroidectomy were recognized. Insulin had become available, and its use in controlling diabetes was being explored. It was known generally that the pituitary gland exerted some influence over the growth and sex life of mankind. Nonetheless, the endocrine glands were still considered as a system apart, secreting mysterious and potent substances. In the light of modern knowledge, however, this is not an isolated system at all but, rather, an essential and controlling mechanism of all the other systems; indeed, together with the nervous system, the integrator of biochemistry and physiology in the living organism.

Thus, although this volume was originally planned as an atlas on the endocrine glands, it was impossible to execute it intelligently without becoming involved in such basic and related subjects as carbohydrate, protein, and fat metabolism; the major vitamins; enzyme chemistry; genetics; and inborn metabolic errors. As a matter of fact, as I now survey the entire subject, it seems to me that the growth of our understanding of the function of the endocrine glands has come about as much or more from study of the basic physiology of the glandular secretions as from study of the morphological effects of the endocrine system itself. I have also been tremendously impressed and awed by the painstaking, patient, and unrelenting work of the men and women who have, bit by bit, unraveled and correlated the mysteries of these various fields. It has been my great pleasure, in creating this volume, to have worked with some of these pioneers or with their disciples. No words of appreciation for the help and encouragement I received from all my collaborators can completely convey the satisfaction I obtained from getting to know each of them and becoming their friend.

In finding my way through the uncharted space of the endocrine universe, I sorely needed a guide — one who could plot a course among the biochemical constellations, yet at all times would know his way back to earthly clinical considerations. Such a one I found in Dr. Peter H. Forsham, who took over the editorship of this volume upon the death of Dr. Ernst Oppenheimer, about whom I have written in the preceding pages. I shall always cherish the stimulating hours Dr. Forsham and I spent together in work and, occasionally, in play.

A creative effort such as that which this volume has demanded absorbs a great deal of one's time, effort, and dreams. In short, it tends to detach the artist from his surroundings and personal relationships and to make him difficult to live with! For these reasons I must express special appreciation to my wife, Vera, for patiently bearing with me through these tribulations. She always managed to return me to reality when I became too detached, bring a smile to my face when I was distressed, and help me in so many other ways during this challenging but rather awesome assignment.

FRANK H. NETTER, M.D.

The unforeseen privilege and opportunity to work closely with Dr. Frank H. Netter will forever remain an indelible experience. Here is a man who combines the genius of a great artist with the curiosity, knowledge, and attitudes that one would wish to see in every physician, presumably because he himself was once in active practice. To see dry anatomical descriptions and metabolic schemes suddenly jump into live reality under the bold strokes of his pencil, as he inquires about the necessary details, is exhilarating and impressive; I am certain that this moved many of the consultants, and especially me, to make a maximal effort in providing the necessary material for Dr. Netter. The by-products of our association may be even more lasting than the atlas, for, during the many hours of work and delightful play together, we developed a sincere friendship.

I wish to express my lasting gratitude to all our consultants for their splendid cooperation and meticulous care in preparing and supplying their texts. In addition to the official contributors, all of whom are listed on pages viii to x, many other physicians and scientists indirectly contributed greatly to this book by their advice and suggestions. Only a few can be mentioned here:

The contribution in Section I, Plate 10, on gonadotropin assay, supplied by Dr. Allan Dyer, Chief of the Bioassay Division of the Connaught Medical Research Laboratories, University of Toronto, Canada, is gratefully acknowledged.

In connection with the two plates on the pineal gland in Section I, Dr. Netter obtained valuable advice from Dr. Richard Wurtman of the National Institutes of Health, Bethesda, Md.; Dr. David Wolf and Dr. Willard Roth of Harvard College, Cambridge, Mass.; Dr. K. Scharenberg, University of Michigan, Ann Arbor; and Dr. Douglas Kelly, University of Washington, Seattle.

Dr. Luis Vallecillo, an outstanding surgeon of Santurce, Puerto Rico, gave expert advice to Dr. Netter on the structure of the thyroid and parathyroid glands.

The invaluable help of Professor A. Prader, Head of the Pediatric Clinic, Zurich University, and of Dr. R. E. Seibenmann of the Pathological Institute, Zurich University, Switzerland, in providing special photomicrographs in Section III, Plate 14, was much appreciated.

In Section VI, Plate 10, valuable dental information was supplied by Dr. Sol Silverman, Jr., Associate Professor of Oral Biology and Chairman of the Division, The University of California School of Dentistry, San Francisco.

In the same section, Plate 19, Dr. E. R. Schottstaedt, Chief of the Orthopedic Service, Shriner's Hospital, San Francisco, contributed some of the illustrations on neurofibromatosis, and Dr. R. Arkoff of the Children's Hospital, San Francisco, made available to us the splendid X-rays on polyostotic fibrous dysplasia.

In Section VIII, Plate 7, Hormonal Effects on Protein Anabolism and Catabolism, was inspired by earlier discussion with Dr. H. N. Munro of the Department of Biochemistry, The University, Glasgow, Scotland.

The preparation of a pictorial atlas that will have an initial printing of 45,000 copies, the supply of which (based on CIBA's experience with the previous CIBA COLLECTION volumes) will probably be exhausted in a matter of a few years, could not possibly be undertaken without a key figure acting as the anchor man, coordinating the numerous problems involved in the over-all management of a nonprofit educational enterprise to which a great artist and many prominent physicians and scientists have contributed. I was fortunate to have such a man in Mr. A. W. Custer of the CIBA staff. His excellent understanding of medical problems was most impressive. His patience and good humor were never exhausted, even when inevitable delays slowed the progress and heightened the shadow under which any modern book in the health sciences is created today, namely, that of becoming out of date while it is still being written. Fortunately, because of the superior quality of Dr. Netter's art and the most advanced contributions of all the expert consultants, there is, with the present volume, little danger of this for the time being.

Members of the "inside" organization deserve the greatest credit for having seen the volume through to its completion at a time when they were suddenly deprived of their trusted and tried leader by the premature demise of the editor, Dr. Ernst Oppenheimer. To mention only a few: Wallace and Anne Clark, of Buttzville, N.J., did a superb job as our literary consultants in copy editing all of the material, so as to introduce some uniformity and style in the language of the numerous articles that make up this volume, thereby contributing greatly to clarity and preciseness. Without the watchdog rôle of Harold B. Davison of Embassy Photo Engraving Company, Inc., this volume, with its many intricate illustrations, could never have been brought to fruition; this was also largely due to the excellence of the staff of Colorpress, who have kept up the high standard of workmanship they developed over the years in the production of the preceding books.

Finally, last but not least, I wish to mention the one person who was always at the center of the occasionally tumultuous events that arise in making up a volume such as this: Mrs. L. A. Oppenheim, assistant to the editor under Dr. Oppenheimer, carried on in making available to me her most valuable, long-time experience and gave unstintingly of time, effort, and advice to assure the completion of this volume just before her well-deserved retirement.

PETER H. FORSHAM, M.D.

Mill Valley, Calif., 1965

CONTENTS

Section I

THE HYPOPHYSIS (PITUITARY GLAND)
THE PINEAL GLAND

by

FRANK H. NETTER, M.D.

in collaboration with

CALVIN EZRIN, M.D.
Plates 1-33

AARON B. LERNER, M.D., Ph.D.
Plates 34 and 35

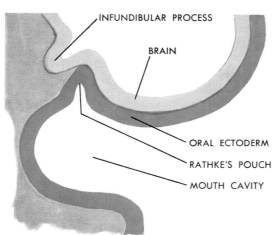

1. BEGINNING FORMATION OF RATHKE'S POUCH AND INFUNDIBULAR PROCESS

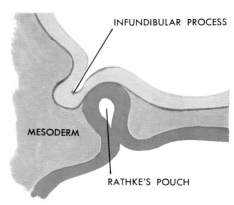

2. NECK OF RATHKE'S POUCH CONSTRICTED BY GROWTH OF MESODERM

DEVELOPMENT OF THE PITUITARY GLAND

The anterior lobe, or adenohypophysis, is derived from the ectoderm of the stomodeum; the posterior, or neural, lobe is derived from the neural ectoderm of the floor of the forebrain.

Prior to the rupture of the oral membrane, a pouchlike recess is present in the ectodermal lining of the roof of the stomodeum. This *pouch of Rathke* is destined to form the anterior lobe of the hypophysis. It lies immediately ventral to the cephalic border of the stomodeal membrane, and it extends upward in front of the rostral end of the notochord, in contact with the undersurface of the forebrain.

It is then *constricted* by the surrounding *mesoderm* to form a closed cavity. Its margin retains temporarily a connection to the ectoderm of the stomodeum by a solid cord of cells, which can be found at the posterior edge of the nasal septum. Epithelial cells grow on each side and in the ventral wall of the cavity; the stroma of the anterior lobe develops from the mesenchyme. The original stalk connecting Rathke's pouch with the stomodeum, known as the craniopharyngeal canal, runs from the anterior part of the pituitary fossa to the undersurface of the skull. Although it usually is largely obliterated, a remnant may persist in adult life as a "pharyngeal pituitary", embedded in the mucosa on the dorsal wall of the pharynx.

Behind Rathke's pouch a hollow neural outgrowth extends toward the mouth from the floor of the diencephalon. This neural process forms a funnel-shaped sac, the *infundibular process,* which becomes a solid body, except at its upper end where the cavity persists as the infundibular recess of the third ventricle.

The solid posterior lobe of the hypophysis (pars nervosa) becomes invested by the dorsal extension of the anterior lobe on each side of it. The anterior lobe also gives off two processes from its ventral wall, which extend along the infundibulum as the *pars tuberalis* and fuse to surround the upper end of the stalk in relation with the tuber cinereum.

The *cleft,* which can also be identified in sagittal sections through the adult gland, is the remains of the original cavity of the stomodeal diverticulum. The

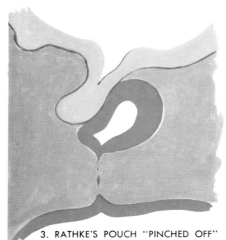

3. RATHKE'S POUCH "PINCHED OFF"

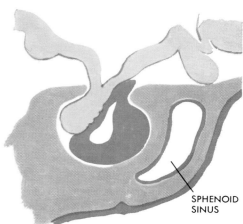

4. "PINCHED OFF" SEGMENT CONFORMS TO NEURAL PROCESS, FORMING PARS DISTALIS, PARS INTERMEDIA AND PARS TUBERALIS

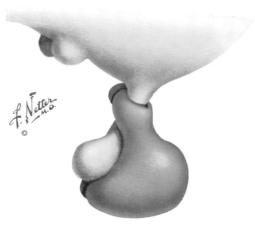

5. PARS TUBERALIS ENCIRCLES INFUNDIBULAR STALK (LATERAL SURFACE VIEW)

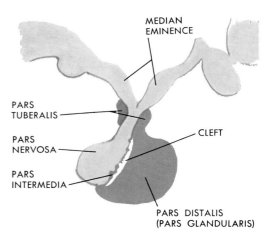

6. MATURE FORM

dorsal wall of this cleft remains thin and fuses with the adjoining part of the posterior lobe to constitute the *pars intermedia.* On horizontal section of the adult gland, this portion can be identified by its content of colloid-filled follicles. The part of the tuber cinereum which lies immediately above the pars tuberalis of the hypophysis is termed the *median eminence.* Both the adenohypophysis and the neurohypophysis are subdivided into three parts. The adenohypophysis consists of the *pars tuberalis,* a thin strip of tissue surrounding the median eminence and the upper part of the neural stalk; the *pars intermedia,* that portion posterior to the cleft and in contact with the neural lobe; and the *pars distalis (pars glandularis),* the major secretory part of the gland lying exterior to the cleft. The neurohypophysis is composed of an expanded distal portion termed the *infundibular process,* or neural lobe; the nervous part

of the stalk, known as the *infundibular* stem, or neural *stalk;* and the expanded upper end of the stalk, which is the *median eminence* of the tuber cinereum. An important anatomical and functional relationship, common to all vertebrates, is the *encirclement of the median eminence by the pars tuberalis,* which forms the bed of a vascular path linking the median eminence of the neurohypophysis and the pars distalis.

Tumors arising from Rathke's pouch rests show characteristics reflecting their origin in the stomodeum. They contain cells resembling those of the buccal epithelium of the embryo, including the adamantoblast of the embryonic enamel organ. These tumors are very liable to undergo calcification and may even develop bone. They usually arise above the sellar diaphragm but may sometimes occur within the sella itself.

DIVISIONS OF THE PITUITARY GLAND AND RELATIONSHIP TO HYPOTHALAMUS

In the standardized nomenclature of the major divisions and subdivisions of the human hypophysis, the *neurohypophysis* (posterior lobe) is described as consisting of three parts: the *median eminence* of the tuber cinereum, the *infundibular stem,* and the *infundibular process* (neural lobe). The *adenohypophysis* (anterior lobe) is likewise divided into three parts: the *pars tuberalis,* the *pars intermedia,* and the *pars distalis* (glandularis). The infundibular stem, together with portions of the adenohypophysis that form a sheath around it, is designated as the *hypophysial stalk.* In man, the extension of neurohypophysial tissue up the stalk and into the median eminence of the tuber cinereum may constitute 15 per cent of the total gland tissue. A low stalk section may leave enough of the gland still in contact with its higher connections in the *paraventricular* and *supra-optic nuclei* to prevent the onset of diabetes insipidus.

Atrophy and disappearance of cell bodies in the supra-optic and paraventricular nuclei follow damage to their axons in the supra-opticohypophysial tract. If the tract is cut at the level of the diaphragma sellae, only 70 per cent of these cells are affected; if the tract is severed above the median eminence, about 85 to 90 per cent of the cells will atrophy. Thus, approximately 15 per cent of the axons terminate between these levels.

The main nerve supply, both functionally and anatomically, of the neurohypophysis is the *hypothalamo-hypophysial tract* in the pituitary stalk. It consists of two main parts: the *supra-opticohypophysial tract,* running in the anterior or ventral wall of the stalk, and the *tuberohypophysial tract* in the posterior, or dorsal, wall of the stalk. The tuberohypophysial tract originates in the central and posterior parts of the hypothalamus, possibly from the *paraventricular nucleus* and from scattered cells and nuclei in the tuberal region and *mamillary bodies.* The supra-opticohypophysial tract arises from the supra-optic and paraventricular nuclei. On entering the median eminence, it occupies a very superficial position, where it is liable to be affected by basal infections of the brain and granulomatous inflammatory processes. There is little decussation of fibers from opposite sides. The tuberohypophysial tract in the dorsal region of the median eminence is smaller and consists of finer fibers. In the *neural stalk,* all the fibers congregate into a dense bundle lying in

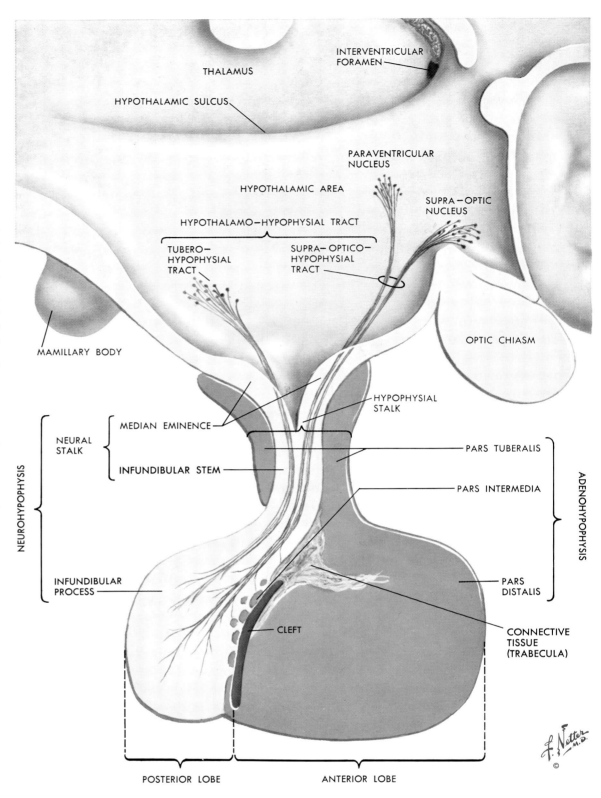

a central position, leaving a peripheral zone in contact with the pars tuberalis, which is relatively free of nerve elements. The hypothalamo-hypophysial tract terminates mainly in the neurohypophysis, probably in all three parts.

The *hypothalamus* has ill-defined boundaries. Antero-inferiorly, it is limited by the *optic chiasm* and optic tracts; passing posteriorly, it is bounded by the posterior perforated substance and the cerebral peduncles. On sagittal section it can be seen to be separated from the *thalamus* by the *hypothalamic sulcus* on the wall of the third ventricle. Anteriorly, it merges with the preoptic septal region, and posteriorly with the tegmental area of the midbrain. Its lateral relations are the subthalamus and the internal capsule.

A *connective tissue trabecula* separates the neural lobe from the pars distalis; it also extends out into

the pars distalis for a variable distance as a vascular bed for the large-lumened artery of the trabecula. The embryonic *cleft,* that marks the site of Rathke's pouch within the gland, may be contained, in part, in this trabecula. It is easier to see in the newborn and tends to disappear in later life. *Colloid-filled follicles* in the adult gland mark the site of the pars intermedia at the junction between the pars distalis and the neurohypophysis. This boundary may be quite irregular, as fingerlike projections of adenohypophysial tissue are frequently found in the substance of the neurohypophysis.

Purves has suggested recently that the pars intermedia, in man, is represented by certain adenohypophysial basophils in the anteromedial portion of the gland that produce melanocyte-stimulating hormone (MSH), or intermedin, and develop Crooke's hyaline change in response to a sustained excess of cortisol.

BLOOD SUPPLY OF THE PITUITARY GLAND

The pituitary gland of man receives its arterial blood supply from two paired systems of vessels; from above come the right and left *superior hypophysial arteries* and from below arise the right and left *inferior hypophysial arteries*. Each superior hypophysial artery divides into two main branches—the *anterior* and *posterior hypophysial arteries* passing to the hypophysial stalk. Communicating branches between these anterior and posterior superior hypophysial arteries run on the lateral aspects of the hypophysial stalk; numerous branches arise from this arterial circle. Some pass upward to supply the optic chiasm and the *hypothalamus*. Other branches, called infundibular arteries, pass either superiorly to penetrate the stalk in its upper part or inferiorly to enter the stalk at a lower level. Another important branch of the anterior superior hypophysial artery of each side is the *artery of the trabecula*, which passes downward to enter the pars distalis. The *trabecula* is a prominent, compact band of connective tissue and blood vessels lying within the pars distalis on either side of the midline. At its central end the trabecula is contiguous with the mass of connective tissue which is interposed between the pars distalis and the lower infundibular stem. Peripherally, the components of the trabecula spread out to form a fibrovascular tuft. On approaching the lower infundibular stem, the artery of the trabecula gives off numerous straight parallel vessels to the superior portion of this area and thus constitutes the "superior artery of the lower infundibular stem". The "inferior artery of the lower infundibular stem" is derived from the inferior hypophysial arterial system. The artery of the trabecula is of large caliber throughout its course; it gives off no branches to the epithelial tissue through which it passes. It is markedly tortuous and is always surrounded by connective tissue.

The inferior hypophysial arteries arise as a single branch from each internal carotid artery in its intracavernous segment. Near the junction of the anterior and posterior lobes, the artery gives off one or more tortuous vessels to the dural covering of the pars distalis and finally divides into two main branches—a *medial* and a *lateral inferior hypophysial artery*. The infundibular process is surrounded by an arterial ring formed by the medial and lateral branches of the paired inferior hypophysial arteries. From this arterial ring, branches are given off to the posterior lobe and to the lower infundibular stem. Components of the superior and inferior hypophysial arterial systems anastomose freely.

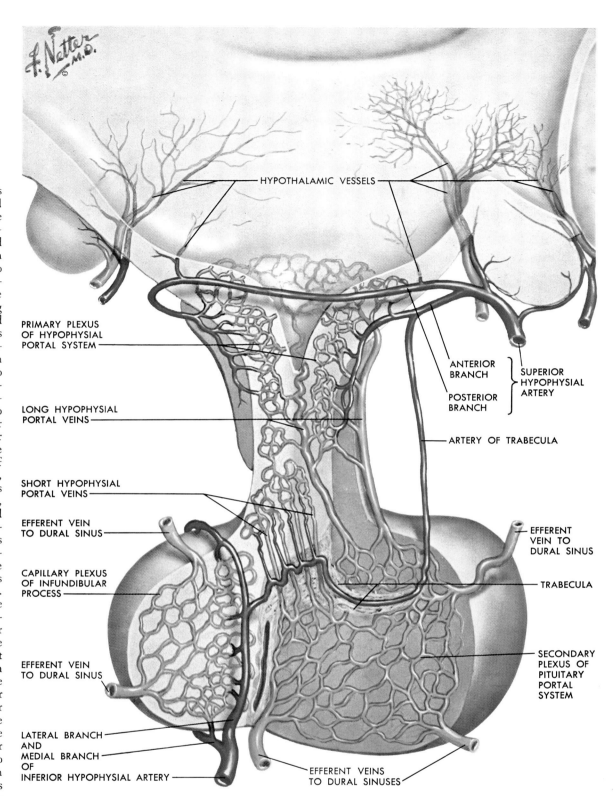

HYPOTHALAMIC VESSELS

PRIMARY PLEXUS OF HYPOPHYSIAL PORTAL SYSTEM

ANTERIOR BRANCH

POSTERIOR BRANCH

SUPERIOR HYPOPHYSIAL ARTERY

ARTERY OF TRABECULA

LONG HYPOPHYSIAL PORTAL VEINS

SHORT HYPOPHYSIAL PORTAL VEINS

EFFERENT VEIN TO DURAL SINUS

EFFERENT VEIN TO DURAL SINUS

CAPILLARY PLEXUS OF INFUNDIBULAR PROCESS

TRABECULA

SECONDARY PLEXUS OF PITUITARY PORTAL SYSTEM

EFFERENT VEIN TO DURAL SINUS

LATERAL BRANCH AND MEDIAL BRANCH OF INFERIOR HYPOPHYSIAL ARTERY

EFFERENT VEINS TO DURAL SINUSES

The epithelial tissue of the pars distalis receives no direct arterial blood. The sinusoids of the anterior lobe receive their blood supply from the hypophysial portal vessels, which arise from the capillary beds within the median eminence and the upper and lower portions of the infundibular stem. Blood is conveyed from this primary capillary network through hypophysial portal veins to the epithelial tissue of the anterior lobe. Here, a *secondary plexus of the pituitary portal system* is formed, leading to the venous *dural sinuses,* which surround the pituitary, and to the general circulation. Some of the *long hypophysial portal veins* run along the surface of the stalk, chiefly on its anterior and lateral aspects. Most of the long hypophysial portal vessels leave the neural tissue to run down within the pars tuberalis, but a few remain deep within the stalk until they reach the pars distalis. The *short hypophysial portal veins* are embedded in the tissue surrounding the lower infundibular stem. They supply the sinusoidal bed of the posterior part of the pars distalis, whereas the long portal veins supply its anterior and lateral regions.

Vascular tufts, comprising the primary capillary network in the median eminence and infundibular stem, are intimately related to the great mass of nerve fibers of the hypothalamo-hypophysial tract running in this region. On excitation, these nerve fibers liberate into the portal vessels specific substances which, being conveyed to the sinusoids of the pars distalis, act as releasing factors for specific pituitary hormones. Extensive occlusion of the hypophysial portal vessels or of the capillary beds of the hypophysial stalk may lead to ischemic necrosis of the anterior pituitary, since these hypophysial portal vessels are the only afferent channels to the sinusoids of the pars distalis.

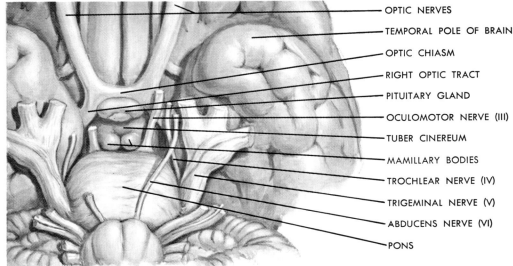

- OPTIC NERVES
- TEMPORAL POLE OF BRAIN
- OPTIC CHIASM
- RIGHT OPTIC TRACT
- PITUITARY GLAND
- OCULOMOTOR NERVE (III)
- TUBER CINEREUM
- MAMILLARY BODIES
- TROCHLEAR NERVE (IV)
- TRIGEMINAL NERVE (V)
- ABDUCENS NERVE (VI)
- PONS

ANATOMY AND RELATIONS OF THE PITUITARY GLAND

The *pituitary gland* is a reddish-gray, rather ovoid body, measuring about 12 mm transversely, 8 mm in its anteroposterior diameter, and 6 mm in its vertical dimension. In the adult male it weighs about 500 mg; in the adult female it is slightly heavier—about 600 mg. In multiparas the average weight is closer to 700 mg. It is contiguous with the end of the infundibulum and is situated in the hypophysial fossa of the *sphenoid bone*. A circular fold of dura mater, termed the *diaphragma sellae,* forms the roof of this fossa. In turn, the floor of the hypophysial fossa forms part of the roof of the *sphenoidal sinus*. The diaphragma sellae is pierced by a small central aperture through which the pituitary stalk passes, and it separates the anterior part of the upper surface of the gland from the *optic chiasm*. The hypophysis is bounded on each side by the cavernous sinus and the structures which it contains. Inferiorly, it is separated from the floor of the fossa by a large, partially vacuolated venous sinus, which communicates freely with the circular sinus. The meninges blend with the capsule of the gland and cannot be identified as separate layers of the fossa. However, the subarachnoid space often extends a variable distance into the sella, particularly anteriorly. In some cases of subarachnoid hemorrhage, the dorsal one third of the gland may be covered with blood that has extended down into this space.

The hypothalamus is in important relation to the pituitary gland, both anatomically and functionally. This designation refers to the structures contained in the anterior part of the floor of the third ventricle and to those comprising the lateral wall of the third ventricle below and in front of the *hypothalamic sulcus*. The *mamillary bodies* are two round, white, pea-sized masses placed side by side below the gray matter of the floor of the third ventricle, in front of the posterior perforated substance. They form the posterior limits of the hypothalamus. Introduction of air into

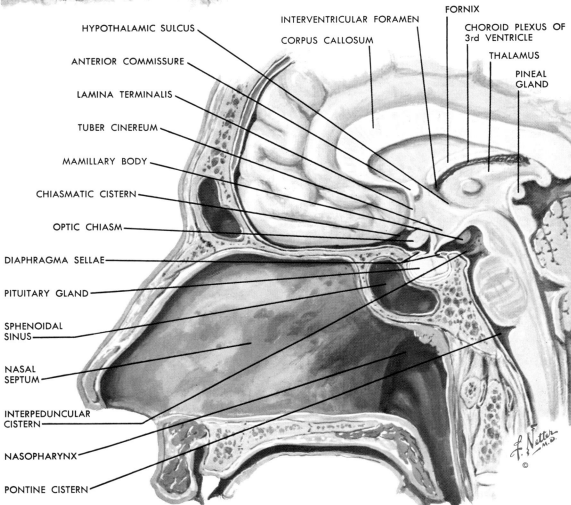

- HYPOTHALAMIC SULCUS
- ANTERIOR COMMISSURE
- LAMINA TERMINALIS
- TUBER CINEREUM
- MAMILLARY BODY
- CHIASMATIC CISTERN
- OPTIC CHIASM
- DIAPHRAGMA SELLAE
- PITUITARY GLAND
- SPHENOIDAL SINUS
- NASAL SEPTUM
- INTERPEDUNCULAR CISTERN
- NASOPHARYNX
- PONTINE CISTERN
- INTERVENTRICULAR FORAMEN
- CORPUS CALLOSUM
- FORNIX
- CHOROID PLEXUS OF 3rd VENTRICLE
- THALAMUS
- PINEAL GLAND

the subarachnoid space shows that, at certain sites at the base of the brain, the arachnoid is separated from the pia mater by wide intervals which communicate freely with one another; these are called subarachnoid cisterns. As the arachnoid extends across between the two temporal lobes, it is separated from the cerebral peduncles by the *interpeduncular cistern*. Anteriorly, this space is continued in front of the optic chiasm as the *chiasmatic cistern*. Space-occupying lesions distort these cisterns.

The *optic chiasm* is an extremely important superior relation of the pituitary gland. It is a flat, somewhat quadrilateral, bundle of optic nerve fibers, situated at the junction of the anterior wall of the third ventricle with its floor. Its anterolateral angles are contiguous with the *optic nerves*, and its posterolateral angles, with the *optic tracts*. The *lamina terminalis,* which represents the cephalic end of the primitive neural

tube, forms a thin layer of gray matter stretching from the upper surface of the chiasm to the rostrum of the *corpus callosum*. Inferiorly, the chiasm rests on the diaphragma sellae just behind the optic groove of the sphenoid bone. A small recess of the third ventricle, called the optic recess, passes downward and forward over its upper surface as far as the lamina terminalis. A more distant relationship is the *pineal gland*, which is a small, conical, reddish-gray body lying below the splenium of the corpus callosum. Rarely, ectopic pineal tissue occurs in the floor of the third ventricle and gives rise to tumors of that region. Compression of neighboring cranial nerves, other than the optic nerves, rarely occurs with pituitary enlargement unless malignant invasion is present. The anterior end of the temporal lobe, the *temporal pole*, may be compressed by a large pituitary tumor extending laterally through the cavernous sinus.

RELATIONSHIP OF THE PITUITARY GLAND TO THE CAVERNOUS SINUS

The *sinuses of the dura mater* are venous channels which drain the blood from the brain. The *cavernous sinuses* are so named because of their reticulated structure, being traversed by numerous interlacing filaments that radiate out from the *internal carotid artery* extending anteroposteriorly in the center of the sinuses. They are placed astride and on either side of the body of the *sphenoid bone* and thus come into intimate relation with the *pituitary gland*. Each opens behind into the superior and inferior petrosal sinuses. On the medial wall of each cavernous sinus, the internal carotid artery is in close contact with the *abducens nerve (VI)*. On the lateral wall are the *oculomotor (III)* and *trochlear nerves (IV)* and the *ophthalmic* and *maxillary divisions* of the *trigeminal nerve (V)*. These structures are separated from the blood flowing along the sinus by the endothelial lining membrane. The two cavernous sinuses communicate with each other by means of two intercavernous sinuses. The anterior sinus passes in front of the pituitary gland and the posterior behind it. Together, they form a *circular sinus* around the hypophysis. These channels are found between the two layers of dura mater that comprise the *diaphragma sellae* and are responsible for copious bleeding when this structure is incised to expose the pituitary gland lying below. Sometimes, profuse bleeding from an inferior circular sinus is encountered in the transsphenoidal approach to the pituitary gland.

The *superior petrosal sinus* is a small and narrow channel that connects the cavernous with the transverse sinus. It runs backward and laterally from the posterior end of the cavernous sinus over the trigeminal nerve (V) and lies in the attached margin of the tentorium cerebelli and in the superior petrosal sulcus of the temporal bone. The cavernous sinus also receives the small *sphenoparietal sinus,* which runs anteriorly along the undersurface of the lesser wing of the sphenoid.

The intercavernous portion of the internal carotid artery runs a complicated course. At first, it ascends toward the posterior clinoid process; then it passes forward, alongside the body of the sphenoid bone, and again curves upward on the medial side of the anterior clinoid process. It perforates the dura mater that forms the roof of the sinus. This por-

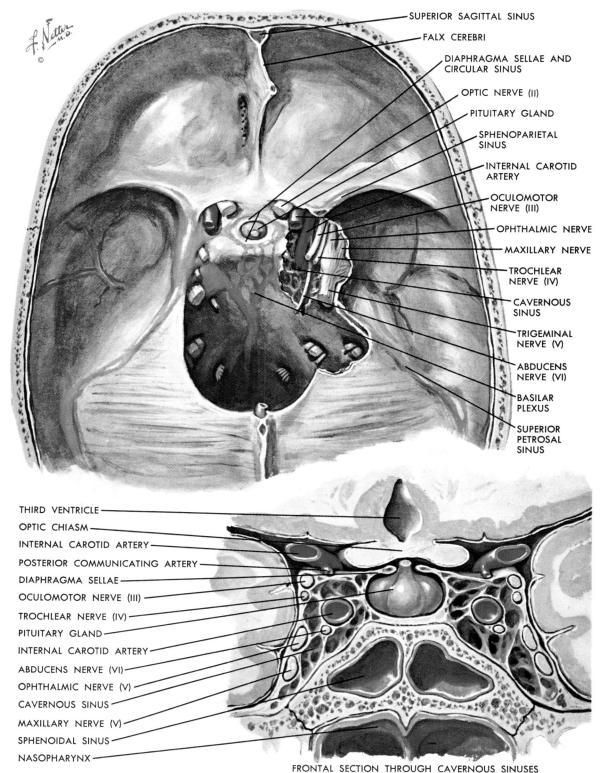

SUPERIOR SAGITTAL SINUS
FALX CEREBRI
DIAPHRAGMA SELLAE AND CIRCULAR SINUS
OPTIC NERVE (II)
PITUITARY GLAND
SPHENOPARIETAL SINUS
INTERNAL CAROTID ARTERY
OCULOMOTOR NERVE (III)
OPHTHALMIC NERVE
MAXILLARY NERVE
TROCHLEAR NERVE (IV)
CAVERNOUS SINUS
TRIGEMINAL NERVE (V)
ABDUCENS NERVE (VI)
BASILAR PLEXUS
SUPERIOR PETROSAL SINUS

THIRD VENTRICLE
OPTIC CHIASM
INTERNAL CAROTID ARTERY
POSTERIOR COMMUNICATING ARTERY
DIAPHRAGMA SELLAE
OCULOMOTOR NERVE (III)
TROCHLEAR NERVE (IV)
PITUITARY GLAND
INTERNAL CAROTID ARTERY
ABDUCENS NERVE (VI)
OPHTHALMIC NERVE (V)
CAVERNOUS SINUS
MAXILLARY NERVE (V)
SPHENOIDAL SINUS
NASOPHARYNX

FRONTAL SECTION THROUGH CAVERNOUS SINUSES

tion of the artery is surrounded by filaments of sympathetic nerves as it passes between the optic and oculomotor nerves. The hypophysial arteries are branches of the intercavernous segment of the internal carotid. The inferior branch supplies the posterior lobe, whereas the superior branch leads into the median eminence to start the hypophysial portal system to the anterior lobe.

The surgical approaches to the pituitary gland are designed to circumvent the major vascular channels and to avoid injury to the *optic nerves* and to the *optic chiasm*. The "frontal approach" involves lifting the frontal lobe, preferably on the nondominant side, to enter the fossa between the two optic nerves from above. Although an excellent exposure is obtained, the lifting of the frontal lobe apparently tends to traumatize the vasculature, in most diabetic patients, sufficiently to lead to a postoperative tend-

ency to seizures. Also, the filaments of the olfactory nerve penetrating the cribriform plate are destroyed by this approach, and the sense of smell is significantly diminished. In spite of these limitations, however, this is still the preferred approach. Another is the transsphenoidal technique, in which the pituitary fossa is entered from below through an intranasal approach. In this instance the central nervous system is not disturbed, and mortality is at a minimum. However, frequent sepsis, postoperative rhinorrhea, and a somewhat blind removal of the pituitary are disadvantages. A combined transantral and then a transsphenoidal approach, in which the pituitary is viewed laterally suspended from its stalk, facilitates easier and more nearly total removal of the gland. However, in the presence of a tumor reaching above the tegmentum sellae, this technique is inferior to the frontal approach.

RELATIONSHIP OF THE SELLA TURCICA

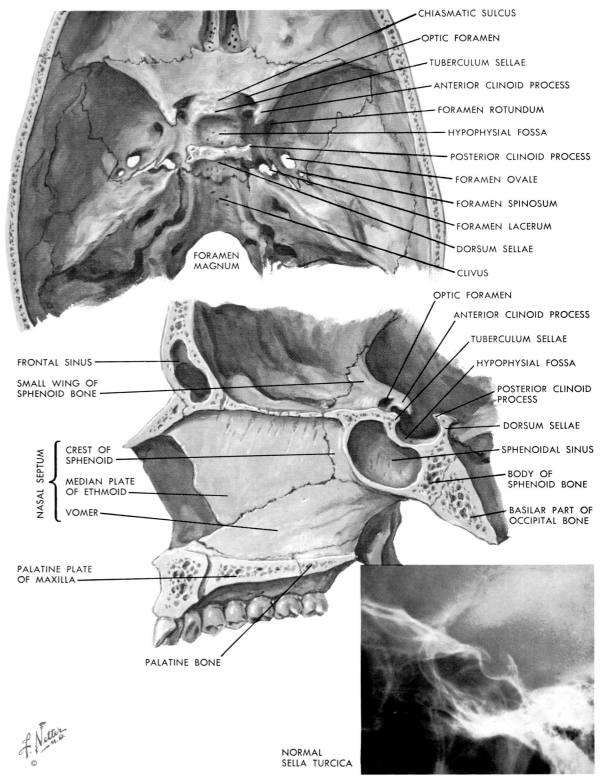

CHIASMATIC SULCUS
OPTIC FORAMEN
TUBERCULUM SELLAE
ANTERIOR CLINOID PROCESS
FORAMEN ROTUNDUM
HYPOPHYSIAL FOSSA
POSTERIOR CLINOID PROCESS
FORAMEN OVALE
FORAMEN SPINOSUM
FORAMEN LACERUM
DORSUM SELLAE
CLIVUS
FORAMEN MAGNUM

OPTIC FORAMEN
ANTERIOR CLINOID PROCESS
TUBERCULUM SELLAE
HYPOPHYSIAL FOSSA
POSTERIOR CLINOID PROCESS
DORSUM SELLAE
SPHENOIDAL SINUS
BODY OF SPHENOID BONE
BASILAR PART OF OCCIPITAL BONE

FRONTAL SINUS
SMALL WING OF SPHENOID BONE
NASAL SEPTUM
CREST OF SPHENOID
MEDIAN PLATE OF ETHMOID
VOMER
PALATINE PLATE OF MAXILLA
PALATINE BONE

NORMAL SELLA TURCICA

The *sella turcica* is the deep depression, in the body of the sphenoid bone, which lodges the pituitary gland. In the adult the normal mean A-P length is less than 14 mm, and the height from the floor to a line between the *tuberculum sellae* and the tip of the *posterior clinoid* is less than 12 mm. The dimension varies with the size of the subject, yet the figures allow one to diagnose quickly, by X-ray, an enlargement of the sella.

To understand its relations, a more general description of the sphenoid bone is in order. Situated at the base of the skull in front of the *temporal bones* and the *basilar part of the occipital bone,* the *sphenoid bone* somewhat resembles a bat, with its wings extended; it is divided into a median portion, or *body,* two great and *two small wings* extending outward from the sides of the body, and two pterygoid processes projecting below. The cubical body is hollowed out to form two large cavities, the *sphenoidal air sinuses,* which are separated from each other by a septum, which is often oblique. The superior surface of the body articulates anteriorly with the cribriform plate of the *ethmoid* and laterally with the frontal bones. Most of the frontal articulation is with the small wing of the sphenoid bone, however. Behind the ethmoidal articulation is a smooth surface, slightly raised in the midline and grooved on either side, for the olfactory lobes of the brain. This surface is bounded behind by a ridge, which forms the anterior border of a narrow transverse groove, the *chiasmatic sulcus,* above and behind which lies the optic chiasm. The groove

ends on either side in the *optic foramen,* through which the optic nerve and ophthalmic artery enter into the orbital cavity.

Behind the chiasmatic sulcus is an elevation, the *tuberculum sellae.* Immediately posteriorly there is a deep depression, the sella turcica, the deepest part of which is called the *hypophysial fossa.* The anterior boundary of the sella turcica is completed by two small prominences, one on each side, called the middle *clinoid processes.* The posterior boundary of the sella is formed by an elongated plate of bone, the *dorsum sellae,* which ends at its superior angles as two tubercles, the posterior clinoid processes.

Behind the dorsum sellae is a shallow depression, the *clivus,* which slopes obliquely backward to continue as a groove on the basilar portion of the *occipital bone.* The lateral surfaces of the body of the sphenoid are united with the great wings and the medial

pterygoid plates. Above the attachment of each great wing is a broad groove that lodges the internal carotid artery and the cavernous sinus. The superior surface of each great wing forms part of the middle fossa of the skull. The internal carotid artery passes through the *foramen lacerum,* a large somewhat triangular aperture bounded in front by the great wing of the sphenoid, behind by the apex of the petrous portion of the temporal bone, and medially by the body of the sphenoid and the basilar portion of the occipital bone. The nasal relations of the pituitary fossa are the *crest* of the *sphenoid bone* and the *median,* or *perpendicular, plate of the ethmoid.*

Because of the availability of antibiotic protection against meningitis, there has been a recent resurgence of interest in the surgical *transsphenoidal approach* to the pituitary fossa. This operation may be done, through an orbital incision, with relative ease.

ANTERIOR PITUITARY HORMONES

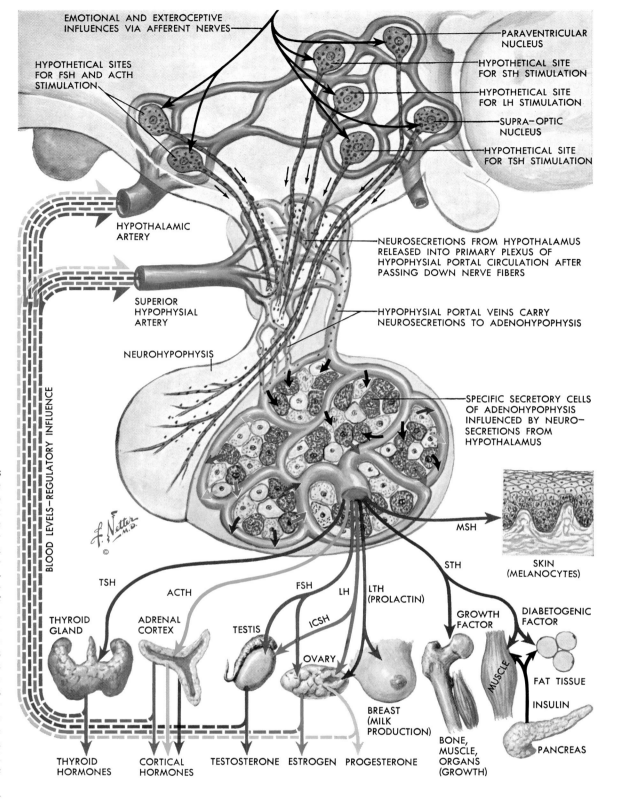

There is much evidence that nervous influences affect the function of the *anterior hypophysis,* although it has no direct innervation. It would appear that the regulatory *neurohumors from the hypothalamus* reach the pituitary by way of the *hypophysial portal circulation* (see page 5). This neurovascular hypothesis of adenohypophysial regulation suggests that the anterior pituitary is governed by a reflex arc comprised of a neural segment ending in the median eminence and a vascular segment formed by the hypophysial portal system. The portal trunks in man are of two varieties —"long" and "short". The "long" vessels originate mainly on the median eminence and upper portion of the stalk, whereas the "short" portal vessels arise mainly from the lower stalk. Some of these short portal vessels arise below the level of the diaphragma sellae; thus, stalk sections may not transect the entire portal blood supply, which probably accounts for the sparing of a variable portion of the adenohypophysis from infarction following this procedure.

The sites of origin of hypophysiotropic factors in the hypothalamus are indefinite. An attractive possibility is that certain areas of the hypothalamus may influence specific regions of the adenohypophysis by secreting specific releasing factors which are carried to the anterior pituitary via the portal circulation. Many attempts have been made to link the known posterior lobe hormones or the *neurosecretory material* of the hypothalamo-neurohypophysial tract with the synthesis and release of anterior lobe hormones; a number of releasing factors have been isolated, and some synthesized, representing relatively short-chain polypeptides. The relationship between the

primary capillary plexus of the portal system and the nerve endings suggests that the chemotransmitters passing from nerve to capillary would have to be small peptides of low molecular weight in the order of that of the well-characterized posterior lobe hormones.

There are now enough specific cell types demonstrable in the human adenohypophysis to suggest that each cell is responsible for the secretion of only one, or at most two, closely related pituitary hormones. The acidophil seems to be the site of production of *prolactin,* or luteotropic hormone (*LTH*), and *somatotropic hormone* (*STH*). All the other hormones — *thyrotropin* (*TSH*), *adrenocorticotropin* (*ACTH*), *follicle-stimulating hormone* (*FSH*), *luteinizing hormone* (*LH*) or *interstitial-cell-stimulating hormone* (*ICSH*), and *melanocyte-stimulating hormone* (*MSH*) — come from subtypes of the *basophil series.*

These anterior pituitary hormones, with the excep-

tion of STH and MSH, act primarily on *target glands,* in which they stimulate the secretion of specific hormones. These, in turn, check the stimulatory action of the pituitary by a so-called *"negative feedback" control.*

"Feedback" control of adenohypophysial secretions is complex, and the details have not been established for all the hormones. In general, the hypothalamus is sensitive to the influence of secretions from the target glands, which block the messages from the hypothalamus to the pituitary cells. However, a direct effect of *thyroid hormone* and *estrogen* on pituitary cells has been demonstrated following intrapituitary injection of minute amounts of these substances. The hypothalamus appears to have a tonic-inhibiting effect on the secretion of prolactin, which, when reduced by a surgical lesion or a tumor in the hypothalamus, allows for the secretion of prolactin.

FUNCTIONAL HISTOLOGY OF THE ANTERIOR LOBE OF THE PITUITARY GLAND

The cells of the adenohypophysis are divided into red-staining *acidophils,* blue-colored *basophils,* and unstained *chromophobes* by staining procedures such as the Mallory and *Mann techniques,* which use *eosin* and *methyl blue.* Hematoxylin and eosin staining of the pituitary often gives poor differentiation of the acidophils and basophils; even for routine work, it is advisable to use an eosin–methyl blue stain for the pituitary gland. The description that follows will attempt to link the newer, more complicated special stains of the pituitary gland to the eosin–methyl blue routine procedure.

The *periodic acid Schiff technique* (*PAS*) has been extremely important in the development of our newer knowledge of pituitary histology. The PAS procedure was originally introduced as a stain for carbohydrates in fixed tissues; subsequent work has shown that it is not specific for carbohydrates, so it can no longer be regarded as a histochemical procedure. The PAS stain affects only the *basophil series* and some related *chromophobes,* producing a *red color.* If eosin were used as a counterstain, there would be confusion between acidophil and basophil; therefore, *orange-G* is employed, along with PAS, as a yellow-orange counterstain for acidophils. Three of the seven generally recognized adenohypophysial hormones contain carbohydrates and could, therefore, be expected to stain with the periodic acid Schiff procedure. These glycoproteins or mucoproteins are *TSH, FSH,* and *LH.* It seemed reasonable to search for additional subtypes of PAS-positive cells that might be responsible for the manufacture of these different glycoprotein hormones. A methyl blue counterstain was added to the PAS–orange-G procedure. This disclosed another basophil subtype, which stained blue-purple because of the combined effect of PAS and methyl blue, in contrast to the other type of basophil, which took on only the PAS red color. Subsequently, this Δ-cell, as it came to be known, was more easily disclosed by the addition of a dialyzed iron procedure to the PAS technique. The large polyhedral red-staining basophil in the *iron-PAS procedure* was called the β-cell.

There are two types of chromophobes, large and small. Some of the larger chromophobes have a slight

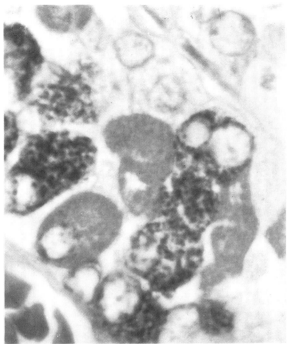

NORMAL ADENOHYPOPHYSIS: EOSIN–METHYL BLUE (MANN) STAIN, X 900–RED ACIDOPHILS AND BLUE BASOPHILS

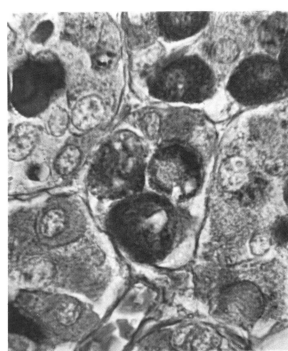

ADULT ADENOHYPOPHYSIS: IRON–PAS STAIN, X 900–TWO TYPES OF BASOPHILS: RED BETA CELLS AND BLUE DELTA CELL

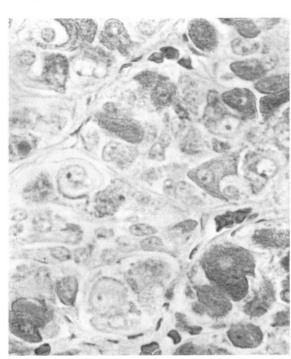

ADENOHYPOPHYSIS IN CUSHING'S SYNDROME: MANN STAIN, X 450–CROOKE'S HYALINE CHANGE AFFECTING BASOPHILS

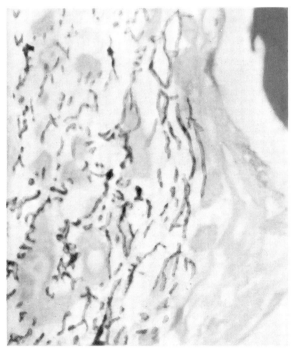

NEUROHYPOPHYSIS: ALDEHYDE THIONIN–PAS STAIN, X 450–NEUROSECRETION AND PART OF COLLOID FOLLICLE (UPPER RIGHT)

granulation that stains more readily with the PAS technique than with the eosin–methyl blue procedure. These large, slightly granulated chromophobes at first were called γ-cells. They were regarded as actively secreting, degranulated forms of the other chromophilic cell types. In cell counts we wish to separate them from the *smaller chromophobes,* which are regarded as *primordial cells,* or the *resting stage* of previously granulated cells. The *cell* labeled Δ¹ is not present in pituitaries of children under the age of 10 years and is virtually absent in the last two trimesters of pregnancy. It appears to be very sensitive to the duration of final illness. The greatest numbers of Δ¹-cells were found in the pituitaries of patients who had died suddenly. In chronic illness the number of Δ¹-cells decreases significantly. It was felt that the Δ¹-cell made one or more gonadotropins. In our earlier studies we did not recognize the Δ²-cell.

This subtype was split off later when we had occasion to study more material and found that another kind of cell could be distinguished with the iron-PAS procedure. Like the Δ¹-cell, it is often scattered singly throughout the gland, but, instead of staining blue-purple, it stains red like the β-cell. Our working hypothesis is that it makes FSH and the Δ¹-cell makes LH.

The most recent modification of the human pituitary special stains is a combined *aldehyde thionin–PAS procedure.* Aldehyde thionin resembles aldehyde fuchsin in that it selectively stains some types of basophils. When combined with the PAS technique, it discloses an additional cell type in the human adenohypophysis, which has been tentatively designated the β²-cell. The β¹-cell and the Δ²-cell are PAS-positive and reject aldehyde thionin; their final

(Continued on page 11)

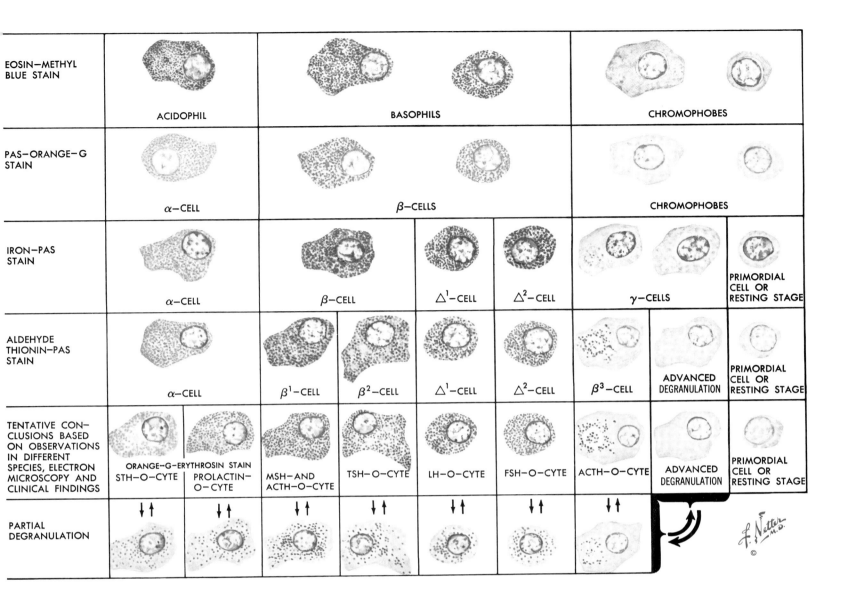

FUNCTIONAL HISTOLOGY OF THE ANTERIOR LOBE OF THE PITUITARY GLAND

(Continued from page 10)

color is red. The β^2-cell and the Δ^1-cell are positive for both PAS and aldehyde thionin stains. Their final color is blue-purple. The α-cell, or the conventional acidophil, is stained only with the orange-G and not with any of the other stains; its final color is yellow-orange.

There is another cell type found in some human pituitaries stained with the aldehyde thionin–PAS technique. It has been called the β^3-cell, because it appears to have a close relationship to the β^1- and β^2-cells. It is found most often in untreated Addison's disease and in conditions of sudden death or acute illness, where one might expect an increased secretion of ACTH. With the eosin–methyl blue procedure, it has been called a Crooke-Russell cell.

The γ-cell nomenclature has been changed to eliminate this designation for a separate cell type. If possible, the partially degranulated cells are assigned to the group of heavily granulated cells from which they are thought to be derived. The term "chromophobe" is reserved for the primordial, or resting, cell stage. Cell counts based on these premises result in a much smaller

number of chromophobes than have usually been reported.

Clinical evidence has been used to decide about the function of these separate cell types. Evidence that the β^1-cell is the source of *ACTH* and possibly the closely related *MSH* (melanocyte-stimulating hormone) will now be presented.

Cortisol, or hydrocortisone, is the physiological inhibitor of ACTH secretion. Prolonged high levels of circulating cortisol, induced either by ACTH therapy, by high doses of cortisol or its analogues, or by endogenous secretion under the influence of spontaneous Cushing's syndrome, selectively affect the β^1-cell to produce *Crooke's hyaline change;* this is a wiping out of part of the basophil granulation, eventually going on to a complete loss of stainable granules and their replacement by a steel-gray hyalinelike material. This change is a regressive phenomenon induced by cortisol; it is reasonable to suspect that the one cell in the pituitary gland thus affected, the β^1-cell, is a source of *ACTH*. Purves has suggested that, in man, the β^1-cells are the counterpart of the pars intermedia of lower animals and, as such, are responsible for the production of intermedin, or MSH.

The β^2-cell has been linked with *TSH,* because, in cases of primary myxedema, this cell undergoes extreme hyperplastic changes. In myxedema the β^2-cell often appears quite degranulated, presumably because of excessive secretion of its stored hormone. We have speculated that there may be a rapidly released source

of ACTH, the β^3-cell, and a more slowly degranulating form, the β^1-cell. If *animal evidence* is also accepted, seven cell types can be designated as the source of seven different anterior pituitary hormones, bearing in mind a relative uncertainty as to the origin of ACTH. In the rat there are *two types of acidophils* — one that makes *prolactin* and another that makes *somatotropin*. In man, these two hormones are immunologically identical. Azocarmine–orange-G staining can sometimes differentiate two types of acidophils in the human gland, but the results are difficult to reproduce. The best stain for differentiating two types of acidophils in the human gland appears to be that of Herlant, employing *erythrosin and orange-G*. The erythrosinophils are prominent at the time of lactation and appear to make prolactin. There appear to be two types of gonadotropin in the rat, one of which makes FSH and the other LH. They have staining properties similar to those of the Δ^2- and Δ^1-cells in the human gland.

The Greek-letter terminology has been employed because it seemed premature to assign specific functions to all these different cell types in the absence of more direct evidence. A functional nomenclature will evolve gradually as this evidence accumulates. There is no general agreement as to the proper functional terminology. Such terms as "thyrotroph" and "somatotroph" will likely be retained. For interim use, we have set down a uniform tentative scheme linking each hormone with a separate cell, *e.g.,* TSH-o-cyte.

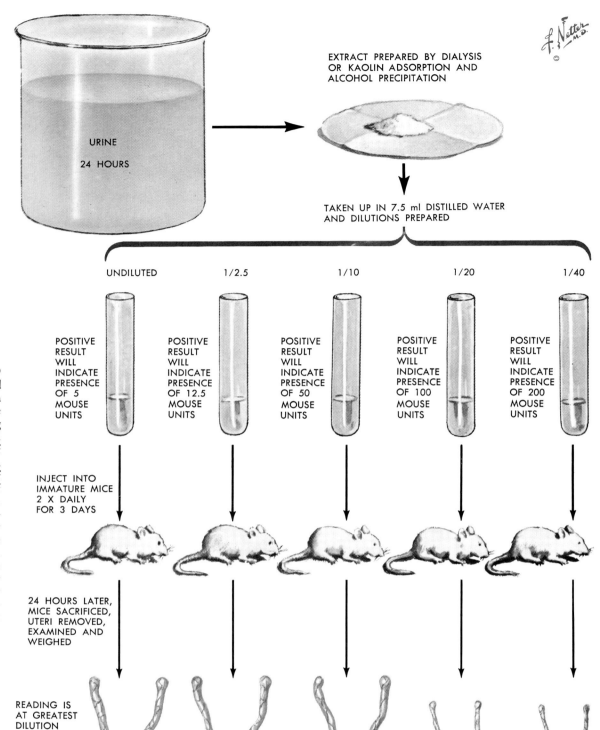

URINE

24 HOURS

EXTRACT PREPARED BY DIALYSIS
OR KAOLIN ADSORPTION AND
ALCOHOL PRECIPITATION

TAKEN UP IN 7.5 ml DISTILLED WATER
AND DILUTIONS PREPARED

UNDILUTED   1/2.5   1/10   1/20   1/40

POSITIVE RESULT WILL INDICATE PRESENCE OF 5 MOUSE UNITS

POSITIVE RESULT WILL INDICATE PRESENCE OF 12.5 MOUSE UNITS

POSITIVE RESULT WILL INDICATE PRESENCE OF 50 MOUSE UNITS

POSITIVE RESULT WILL INDICATE PRESENCE OF 100 MOUSE UNITS

POSITIVE RESULT WILL INDICATE PRESENCE OF 200 MOUSE UNITS

INJECT INTO IMMATURE MICE 2 X DAILY FOR 3 DAYS

24 HOURS LATER, MICE SACRIFICED, UTERI REMOVED, EXAMINED AND WEIGHED

READING IS AT GREATEST DILUTION WHICH CAUSES DOUBLING OF UTERINE SIZE AND WEIGHT

READING

GONADOTROPIN ASSAY

Follicle-stimulating hormone (FSH) by itself stimulates the growth and maturation of ovarian follicles; although it causes some estrogen secretion, more estrogen is produced if some luteinizing hormone (LH) is secreted or injected along with the FSH. The ovaries of mice, when injected with gonadotropin, enlarge and increase their secretion of estrogen. A readily measurable effect of estrogen is an increase in uterine weight. Thus, pituitary gonadotropins are determined by *bioassay of urinary extracts* by either the *uterine weight method* in the *mouse* or the ovarian weight method in the rat. Although the latter is a more direct method, the former still has wider use. A definite identification of FSH or LH is not possible in the clinical laboratory. The usual assay method is most sensitive to FSH. Despite the fact that it is often described as a test for FSH, it really measures the combined estrogen-stimulating activity of the various gonadotropic components—FSH, LH, and LTH.

The assay is carried out on an aliquot of a freshly collected *24-hour urine specimen*. The gonadotropins, which are proteins, are either *precipitated by alcohol* or tannic acid or are separated by dialysis through cellophane membranes or by *kaolin adsorption*, the latter being the most useful method at this time. Many of the toxic substances, that otherwise might kill the mice, may be removed by subsequent dialysis or by alcohol precipitation. After drying and partial purification of the precipitate, the gonadotropins are obtained by leaching out with water. A series of *dilutions* are prepared and are injected into *immature mice* twice daily for 3 days. At the end of the fourth day, the animals are sacrificed, and their *uterine weights* are compared with controls. A mouse unit represents that quantity of gonadotropic hormone which will produce a 100 per cent increase in the weight of the uterus of an immature mouse.

There is, as yet, no completely satisfactory assay for determining the LH

content of the urine. The most specific assay method appears to be the one which measures the enlargement of the prostate in hypophysectomized immature male rats. Two new assays for LH that deserve mention are (1) immunologic determination by the inhibition of hemagglutination, in which the LH crossreacts with antiserums prepared against human chorionic gonadotropin; and (2) the ovarian ascorbic acid depletion method of Parlow.

Gonadotropins are not demonstrable in the urine of children before puberty. In girls, positive tests are found from 11 years, but, in boys, a positive response is not often obtained before the age of probably 13 years. During the reproductive years of females, the daily gonadotropin excretion fluctuates in relationship to the menstrual cycle. Small amounts are found during the early follicular phase, with a rather abrupt rise in the preovulatory and ovulatory phases. In

some cycles, more than one such spurt may be noted. In the corpus luteum phase the gonadotropin titer is low, as measured by the mouse uterine method. At the menopause there is usually a rise in gonadotropins that may persist for many years, with titers of 100 to 200 mouse units being commonly observed. No such rise in gonadotropin titers occurs in men, and thus many investigators are reluctant to speak of a male menopause. In old age (above 70 years) in both sexes, the gonadotropins eventually fall to nondemonstrable levels.

The assay of pituitary gonadotropins is of enormous help in determining whether hypogonadism is primary, owing to an abnormality in the gonad, or secondary to a pituitary insufficiency. In primary gonadal failure, gonadotropins are present in high titer, whereas in pituitary underfunction they are usually not demonstrable.

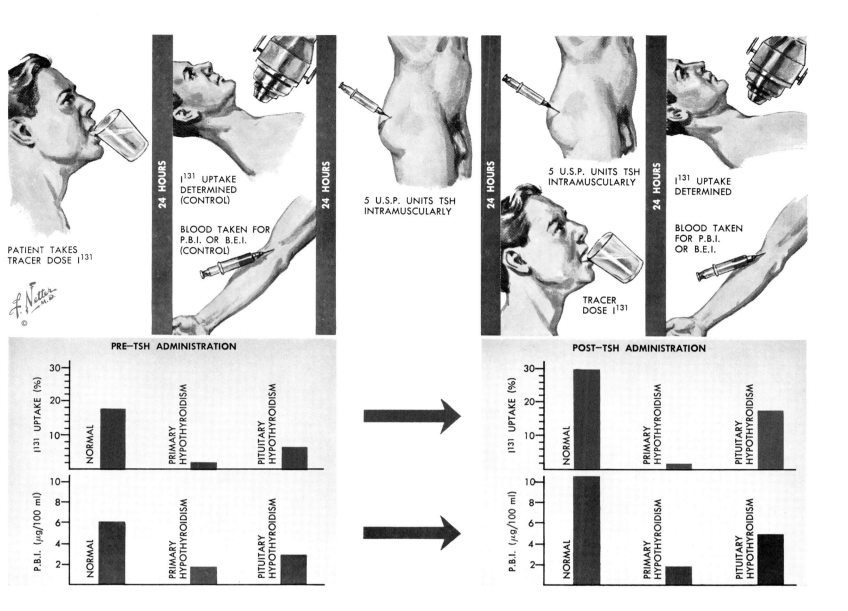

PATIENT TAKES
TRACER DOSE I¹³¹

24 HOURS

I¹³¹ UPTAKE
DETERMINED
(CONTROL)

BLOOD TAKEN FOR
P.B.I. OR B.E.I.
(CONTROL)

24 HOURS

5 U.S.P. UNITS TSH
INTRAMUSCULARLY

24 HOURS

5 U.S.P. UNITS TSH
INTRAMUSCULARLY

TRACER
DOSE I¹³¹

24 HOURS

I¹³¹ UPTAKE
DETERMINED

BLOOD TAKEN
FOR P.B.I.
OR B.E.I.

PRE–TSH ADMINISTRATION

I131 UPTAKE (%) — NORMAL / PRIMARY HYPOTHYROIDISM / PITUITARY HYPOTHYROIDISM

P.B.I. (µg/100 ml) — NORMAL / PRIMARY HYPOTHYROIDISM / PITUITARY HYPOTHYROIDISM

POST–TSH ADMINISTRATION

I131 UPTAKE (%) — NORMAL / PRIMARY HYPOTHYROIDISM / PITUITARY HYPOTHYROIDISM

P.B.I. (µg/100 ml) — NORMAL / PRIMARY HYPOTHYROIDISM / PITUITARY HYPOTHYROIDISM

TEST FOR
THYROID-STIMULATING
HORMONE DEFICIENCY

The thyroid-stimulating hormone (*TSH,* also called thyrotropin and thyrotropic hormone) increases the size of the thyroid, its vascularity, and its metabolic activity, and leads to the secretion of the thyroid hormone. A deficiency of this hormone can produce all of the characteristic features of primary thyroidal myxedema.

The term "pituitary myxedema" has been employed to designate such unusual cases of severe anterior pituitary insufficiency in which the manifestations of a secondary thyroid deficiency dominate the clinical picture and obscure the deficiency of the other pituitary and target gland hormones. If such a patient is given only thyroid treatment, the coexistent latent adrenal cortical insufficiency may progress to adrenal crisis from the over-all stimulation of metabolism by thyroid therapy. A much rarer condition has been termed "monotropic thyrotropin deficiency"; in these cases, meticulous study has failed to reveal any deficiency other than that of TSH; presumably, only the cells that make thyrotropin are defective or absent. These two types of pituitary, or "secondary", hypothyroidism can most readily be distinguished from "primary" thyroid deficiency by their response to TSH administration. *Base-line studies of 24-hour I*¹³¹ *thyroid uptake* and serum protein-bound iodine (*P.B.I.*), or, more accurately, serum butanol extractable iodine (*B.E.I.*), are performed, and then the patient receives *TSH by the intramuscular route.* The *normal range of serum P.B.I.,* in most laboratories, extends from 4 to 8 µg per 100 ml. The usual dose employed is 5 to 10 units, and two or three daily injections may be given; then the I¹³¹ uptake and P.B.I. are again determined within 24 to 48 hours. In *normal subjects* TSH produces a substantial rise in the serum P.B.I. This is due to the discharge of stored hormone from colloid-filled follicles. There is also an appreciable rise of radioactive uptake. In *primary hypothyroidism* P.B.I. and uptake remain low, even after TSH administration. In *pituitary hypothyroidism,* in which control values of uptake and P.B.I. are usually not as greatly reduced as in primary myxedema, a significant rise of I¹³¹ uptake and a somewhat slower rise in P.B.I. occur because of the relative lack of stored hormone available for quick release.

In highly specialized laboratories, confirmatory evidence may be obtained from bioassays of circulating TSH in the serum. In primary myxedema the level is usually high, unless the pituitary itself is impaired by myxedema. In such cases, repeat testing, after small doses of thyroid, will show the elevation of TSH.

In some patients with moderate anterior pituitary insufficiency involving gonadotropins, TSH, and ACTH, the administration of replacement doses of cortisone or its analogues has been shown to increase thyroid function, as evidenced by a return of the P.B.I. and I¹³¹ uptake to levels in the normal range. In such cases, the TSH production by the pituitary remnant presumably had been impaired somewhat by the mild associated adrenal cortical insufficiency.

TEST FOR ADRENAL CORTICAL HORMONE RESERVE

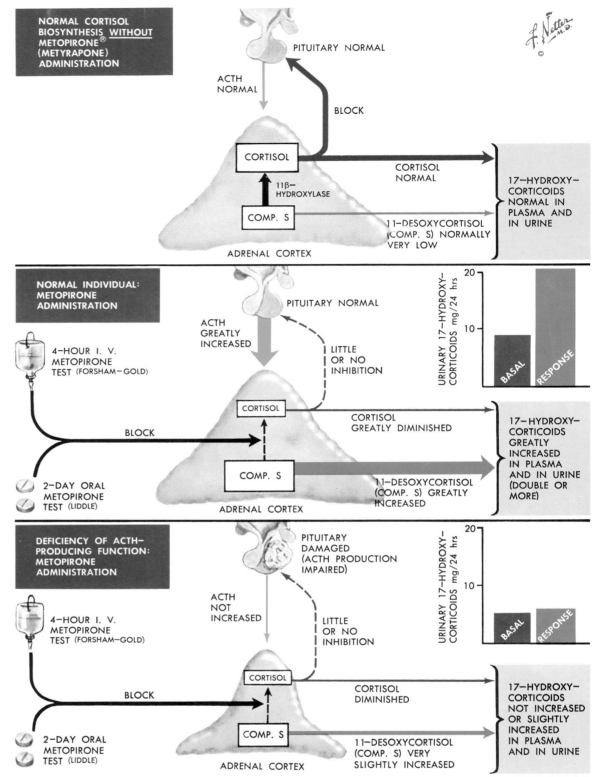

NORMAL CORTISOL BIOSYNTHESIS WITHOUT METOPIRONE® (METYRAPONE) ADMINISTRATION

PITUITARY NORMAL

ACTH NORMAL

BLOCK

CORTISOL

11β—HYDROXYLASE

COMP. S

ADRENAL CORTEX

CORTISOL NORMAL

11—DESOXYCORTISOL (COMP. S) NORMALLY VERY LOW

17—HYDROXY—CORTICOIDS NORMAL IN PLASMA AND IN URINE

NORMAL INDIVIDUAL: METOPIRONE ADMINISTRATION

4—HOUR I. V. METOPIRONE TEST (FORSHAM—GOLD)

2—DAY ORAL METOPIRONE TEST (LIDDLE)

PITUITARY NORMAL

ACTH GREATLY INCREASED

LITTLE OR NO INHIBITION

BLOCK

CORTISOL

COMP. S

ADRENAL CORTEX

CORTISOL GREATLY DIMINISHED

11—DESOXYCORTISOL (COMP. S) GREATLY INCREASED

17—HYDROXY—CORTICOIDS GREATLY INCREASED IN PLASMA AND IN URINE (DOUBLE OR MORE)

URINARY 17—HYDROXY—CORTICOIDS mg/24 hrs

20

10

BASAL RESPONSE

DEFICIENCY OF ACTH—PRODUCING FUNCTION: METOPIRONE ADMINISTRATION

4—HOUR I. V. METOPIRONE TEST (FORSHAM—GOLD)

2—DAY ORAL METOPIRONE TEST (LIDDLE)

PITUITARY DAMAGED (ACTH PRODUCTION IMPAIRED)

ACTH NOT INCREASED

LITTLE OR NO INHIBITION

BLOCK

CORTISOL

COMP. S

ADRENAL CORTEX

CORTISOL DIMINISHED

11—DESOXYCORTISOL (COMP. S) VERY SLIGHTLY INCREASED

17—HYDROXY—CORTICOIDS NOT INCREASED OR SLIGHTLY INCREASED IN PLASMA AND IN URINE

URINARY 17—HYDROXY—CORTICOIDS mg/24 hrs

20

10

BASAL RESPONSE

Cortisol is the physiologic inhibitor of ACTH secretion in the usual feedback mechanism. A rising level of this substance in the blood will shut off the output of ACTH by acting on centers in the hypothalamus. Cortisol is produced from *11-desoxycortisol* by an enzyme *11 β-hydroxylase. Normally,* in man, very little *11-desoxycortisol* circulates in the *plasma* or is found either free or as its tetrahydro derivative in the urine. Most of the *urinary 17-hydroxycorticoids* are normally derived from cortisol. *Metyrapone (Metopirone®),* in appropriate dosage, selectively inhibits 11 β-hydroxylase. The fall in cortisol levels then normally causes a pituitary discharge of ACTH which then stimulates the *adrenal cortex* to secrete large amounts of 11-desoxycortisol, or compound S, which is also measurable in the urine by the Porter-Silber method as either 17-hydroxycorticoids or 17-ketogenic steroids. *Compound S has little or no inhibitory effect on ACTH output and has relatively weak glucocorticoid biological activity.*

Metyrapone has found wide use as a test of ACTH reserve in evaluating pituitary disorders. It may be given *intravenously* in a dose of 30 to 60 mg per kilogram administered over 4 hours (*Forsham-Gold*) and *orally* for 1 or 2 days in a dose of 750 mg every 4 hours (*Liddle*). *Normal subjects* show a significant *rise* in 6-hour *plasma* levels or 24-hour *urinary 17-hydroxycorticoids* during and shortly after the administration of metyrapone. No significant increase occurs in severe, spontaneous pituitary insufficiency, or in subjects who have recently been on a potent ACTH suppressant, such as dexamethasone, when metyrapone is given. Lesions involving the hypothalamus inhibit the response. Some patients, with poorly defined central nervous system disease but with apparently intact pituitaries and normal adrenal function, fail to respond to metyrapone with the expected increase

in urinary 17-hydroxycorticoids and, conversely, fail to demonstrate the anticipated suppression of endogenous ACTH secretion by rather large doses of dexamethasone. In these patients there appears to be a disturbance of the central nervous system mechanisms responsible for adjusting the secretion of ACTH by the pituitary to varying levels of circulating glucocorticoids.

The test is most useful in the investigation of cases of pituitary disease with apparently normal adrenal function under base-line conditions. *Impaired ACTH production,* under the stimulus of a falling level of cortisol, strongly suggests that stressful stimuli would also fail to increase ACTH output. Thus, it is an indirect aid in assessing pituitary ACTH reserve. Perhaps the greatest use of metyrapone is in proving ACTH inhibition in the presence of a cortisol-secreting adrenal cortical tumor in the differential

diagnosis between adrenal neoplasia and hyperplasia. In cases of hyperplasia, there is normal or elevated ACTH secretion. With functional adrenal cortical tumors, there is no rise in 17-hydroxycorticoids following metyrapone administration.

Prolonged administration of metyrapone in the normal subject leads to greatly increased ACTH production, which eventually overcomes the block to cortisol manufacture, and, by the second day, usually appreciable amounts of cortisol can be found in the plasma. Such a compensatory effect is not observed with the *damaged pituitary,* and, in these cases, prolonged metyrapone administration is both hazardous and unnecessary. The use of metyrapone intravenously, along with newly developed column methods for the rapid determination of plasma and urinary corticoids, allows the estimation of pituitary ACTH reserve within a few hours.

MANIFESTATIONS OF SUPRASELLAR DISEASE

Suprasellar lesions, resulting from *craniopharyngioma, dermoid cysts, trauma, encephalitis,* etc., often produce disturbances of sleep, as well as hunger, thirst, and *sex malfunctions.*

Hypersomnia and *somnolence* have frequently been associated with *damage* to the posterior *hypothalamus.* This part of the midbrain forms the rostral portion of the ascending reticular formation of the brain stem; sustained activity within this ascending system accounts for wakefulness. Narcolepsy and cataplexy are sometimes associated with abnormal hypothalamic somnolence. Rarely, a sustained hyperkinetic state is observed in children with diencephalic tumors.

Much experimental evidence suggests the presence of dual mechanisms in the hypothalamus for the regulation of food intake. These are paired "feeding" centers in the lateral hypothalamus and "satiety" centers in the medial hypothalamus. The activity of the "feeding" center determines the state of hunger. The "satiety" center is activated by feeding. Certain bodily changes, resulting from food intake, influence the activity of this center. The nature of these effects is still uncertain; leading suggestions include the availability of glucose for utilization by the center; the concentration of various circulating metabolites, including serum amino acids; the specific dynamic action of food; and sensory impulses arriving from the alimentary tract, leading to a feeling of satiety. Destructive lesions involving the "satiety" center bilaterally lead to obesity because of hyperphagia. Conversely, more laterally placed lesions have been shown, in rats, cats, and monkeys, to lead to food refusal and death from starvation. In humans, such paired lesions arise very rarely because of the wider separation of the two "feeding" centers as compared to the relatively contiguous "satiety" centers. Thus, hypothalamic *obesity* occurs far more frequently than does *emaciation.*

The thirst that follows hypothalamic injury is usually the result of *diabetes insipidus.* However, primary thirst centers have been described in experiments involving electrical stimulation of the hypothalamus in goats. Irritative stimulation of these areas could be expected to lead to primary polydipsia; destruction of this region is followed by hypodipsia.

The hypophysial portal vessels are responsible for the transport of circulating chemical substances termed neurohumors or releasing factors and originating in the

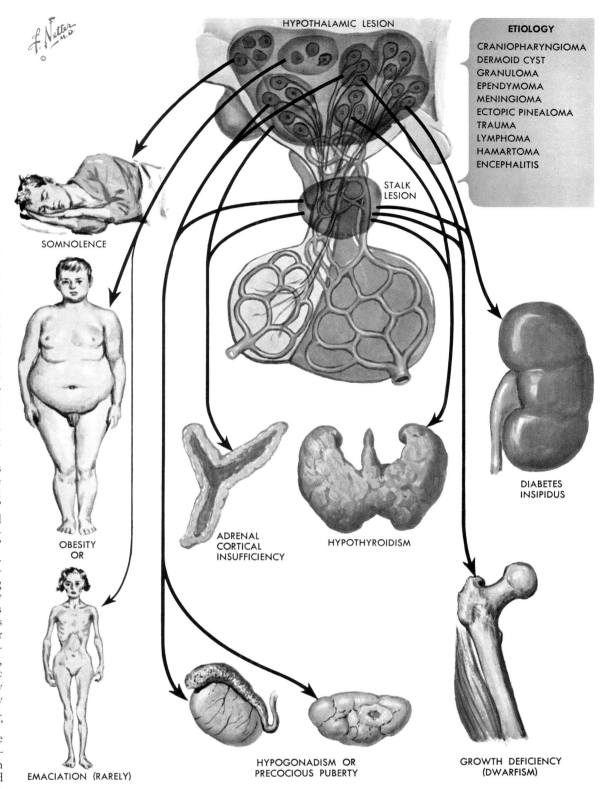

ETIOLOGY
CRANIOPHARYNGIOMA
DERMOID CYST
GRANULOMA
EPENDYMOMA
MENINGIOMA
ECTOPIC PINEALOMA
TRAUMA
LYMPHOMA
HAMARTOMA
ENCEPHALITIS

HYPOTHALAMIC LESION

STALK LESION

SOMNOLENCE

OBESITY OR

EMACIATION (RARELY)

ADRENAL CORTICAL INSUFFICIENCY

HYPOTHYROIDISM

DIABETES INSIPIDUS

HYPOGONADISM OR PRECOCIOUS PUBERTY

GROWTH DEFICIENCY (DWARFISM)

hypothalamus, which are delivered to the median eminence for transmission to the adenohypophysis. It would appear, at present, that there is a specific chemotransmitter for each hormone of the anterior lobe. Some preliminary evidence suggests the presence of four such substances: corticotropin-releasing factor, thyrotropin-influencing factor, prolactin-inhibiting factor, and luteinizing-hormone-releasing factor. Recently, it has been shown that damage to the medial aspect of the hypothalamus inhibits secretion of somatotropic hormone normally evoked by induction of hypoglycemia.

The consequences of severing the *pituitary stalk* vary with the level of severance and the extent of interruption of portal circulation. Low stalk section, frequently performed in palliative treatment of metastatic breast cancer and severe diabetic retinopathy, usually produces severe necrosis and extreme pituitary

insufficiency if the procedure included insertion of a polyethylene plate between the cut ends, to prevent regeneration of the portal circulation. In some patients persistent lactation followed transection of the stalk, presumably the result of excessive prolactin secretion by the uninhibited pituitary remnant.

Slowly growing suprasellar lesions may produce pituitary insufficiency, without direct involvement of the gland itself, by interrupting the portal circulation, because virtually all the blood reaching the pars distalis is of portal venous origin. Posttraumatic diabetes insipidus is often the result of a shearing injury that tears the stalk away from the brain in such a fashion as to leave the portal circulation in the stalk intact, while cutting the axons, transporting antidiuretic hormone to the posterior pituitary and its vascular channels. In these cases there is no interference with adenohypophysial function.

Adiposogenital Dystrophy

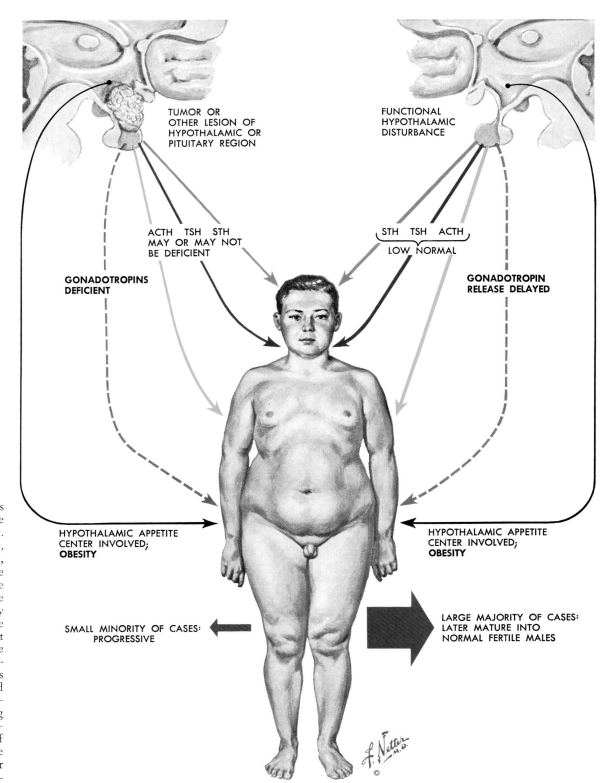

TUMOR OR OTHER LESION OF HYPOTHALAMIC OR PITUITARY REGION

FUNCTIONAL HYPOTHALAMIC DISTURBANCE

ACTH TSH STH MAY OR MAY NOT BE DEFICIENT

STH TSH ACTH LOW NORMAL

GONADOTROPINS DEFICIENT

GONADOTROPIN RELEASE DELAYED

HYPOTHALAMIC APPETITE CENTER INVOLVED; OBESITY

HYPOTHALAMIC APPETITE CENTER INVOLVED; OBESITY

SMALL MINORITY OF CASES: PROGRESSIVE

LARGE MAJORITY OF CASES: LATER MATURE INTO NORMAL FERTILE MALES

In 1901 Alfred Fröhlich published his memorable case report of a tumor of the hypophysis cerebri without acromegaly. The patient had *hypogonadism, obesity,* and encroachment on the optic chiasm, resulting in complete blindness on the left and a temporal hemianopsia on the right. Fröhlich attributed the whole syndrome to destruction of the pituitary gland; he did not, at that time, appreciate that the symptom complex itself might be due, in part, to *involvement of the hypothalamus.* With the benefit of hindsight, we can now state that, in Fröhlich's case, the *pituitary tumor* evidently caused hypogonadism by destruction or compression of the gonadotropin-producing cells of the anterior pituitary. By extension upward through the diaphragm of the sella, the tumor encroached on the chiasm, causing blindness. With further upward extension, it involved the hypothalamus, causing obesity. It has taken a long time to eradicate the idea that destruction of the pituitary causes obesity. We now know that hypothalamic lesions, in experimental animals and in rare clinical cases, cause obesity, whether or not the pituitary is intact. True Fröhlich's syndrome (*i.e.,* tumor of or in the neighborhood of the pituitary gland, causing hypogonadism and extending into the hypothalamus to cause obesity) occurs rarely.

The term adiposogenital dystrophy has been used to refer both to true Fröhlich's syndrome and to the much more common type of case, occurring usually in prepuberal boys, showing obesity and, in some instances, moderately delayed puberty. In these patients the genitalia often seem unduly small, because the phallus is partly hidden in suprapubic fat. This condition probably represents some *functional upset* in the complex mechanisms that govern the onset of puberty (see page 117). These reside in the *hypothalamus,* as evidenced by cases of delayed and precocious puberty associated with hypothalamic lesions. The obesity, in the usual case of adiposogenital dystrophy, is not due to any organic hypothalamic lesion or to any endocrinopathy but is based, usually, on severe psychological maladjustment. Nearly always, an oversolicitous protective mother figure is part of the clinical picture, and often a lengthy period of confinement to bed, because of an intercurrent illness, has started the excessive weight gain. Such boys require no hormone treatment. They and their parents need reassurance that they will eventually go through a normal puberty. Treatment of obesity by caloric restriction and, if necessary, an appetite depressant is usually all that is required. These patients tend to be inactive, so they should be encouraged to increase their participation in sports. Unfortunately, they often are objects of derision by their more athletic comrades, and, therefore, it may be necessary to suggest some activity not requiring group involvement. Follow-up studies have shown that the *large majority* of these cases later *mature into normal fertile males.*

In the differential diagnosis between these two types of adiposogenital dystrophy, evidence of *thyroid* or *adrenal deficiency* is strongly suggestive of some organic etiology rather than the more common functional disturbance. The other tropic hormones of the pituitary are secreted in adequate amounts, although measure of thyroid function usually shows it to be in the low-normal range. Enlargement of the testes often precedes other signs of puberty by several months and is a favorable prognostic sign.

CRANIOPHARYNGIOMA

Craniopharyngioma is the most common tumor found in the region of the pituitary of children and adolescents. Being slow-growing, it may not give rise to symptoms until late in life, but, in most instances, symptoms occur before the age of 40 years. These tumors do not elaborate any hormone but produce symptoms by pressing on, and damaging, the adjacent structures. The clinical picture depends on their direction of growth. They may press on the *optic chiasm* and cause visual disturbances. *Suprasellar craniopharyngiomas* may compress the infundibulum and cause diabetes insipidus. *Pressure on the hypothalamus* may give rise to various hypothalamic syndromes such as obesity, somnolence, and, rarely, extreme emaciation, or even precocious puberty. Those cases in which the *tumor is intrasellar* may present with manifestations of pituitary insufficiency, which, in the young, include failure of growth and delayed puberty; in adults, hypogonadism; and, at all ages, thyroid and adrenal insufficiency. Symptoms of increased intracranial pressure, such as headache, vomiting, and papilledema, may occur with suprasellar craniopharyngioma, whereas they are rarely associated with pituitary adenomas. Nausea and vomiting may also be due to adrenal cortical insufficiency in both suprasellar and intrasellar tumors.

The most important diagnostic sign of a craniopharyngioma is the *radiologic evidence of irregular calcification* in the tumor. This is usually seen in parts of the tumor above the sella, but, occasionally, it is observed within the sella itself. The sella may be wider in its dorsal part, where the tumor has forced its way through the diaphragma from above. A generalized ballooning, which is usually produced by intrasellar tumors, is not commonly seen. There may be erosion of the dorsum sellae and of both anterior

CRANIOPHARYNGIOMA

LARGE CYSTIC CRANIOPHARYNGIOMA OF SUPRASELLAR ORIGIN COMPRESSING OPTIC CHIASM AND HYPOTHALAMUS AND INVADING THIRD VENTRICLE

ASPIRATION OF OILY FLUID CONTENTS

CYSTIC CRANIOPHARYNGIOMA OF INTRASELLAR ORIGIN

CRANIOPHARYNGIOMA (H. AND E., X 125)

INTRA— AND SUPRASELLAR CRANIOPHARYNGIOMA (AIR STUDY)

FLOCCULENT CALCIFICATION IN CRANIOPHARYNGIOMA

VARIABLE DEGREE OF HYPOPITUITARISM AND/OR HYPOTHALAMIC MANIFESTATIONS

and posterior clinoid processes.

An epidermoid cyst is rare but simulates the craniopharyngioma in its time of origin and clinical features. Radiologically, it may be seen to encroach on only one side of the sella, and, if calcification is present, it usually affects only the wall of the tumor and is seen as a ring rather than as diffuse specks of calcification.

Pathologically, craniopharyngiomas have been referred to as adamantinomas, Rathke's pouch tumors, and suprasellar cysts; their structure suggests an origin from cells related to Rathke's pouch, an embryonic cavity lined by ectoderm, which separates the adenohypophysis from the neurohypophysis (see page 3). These tumors vary greatly—from simple cystic structures, containing dark, *oily fluid*, to solid tumors composed of columnar cells on a basement membrane in a pattern which resembles adamanti-

nomas. Sometimes, squamous cells with masses of cornified tissue are found within the tumor (see *photomicrograph*). Calcification may occur in these cornified areas.

Attempting total removal of a suprasellar craniopharyngioma may cause hypothalamic damage, with resultant disturbances in temperature regulation, water and electrolyte balance, appetite control, and wakefulness. Steroid coverage, during and after operation, will compensate for the failure of the pituitary to release ACTH because of interruption of the hypothalamic pathways or of their vascular link with the adenohypophysis. Craniopharyngiomas are compatible with long survival, even, as is often the case, when the tumor cannot be entirely removed surgically because of its adherence to the floor of the third ventricle. Recurrences are common, and cysts may have to be *aspirated* several times.

EFFECTS OF PITUITARY TUMORS ON THE VISUAL APPARATUS

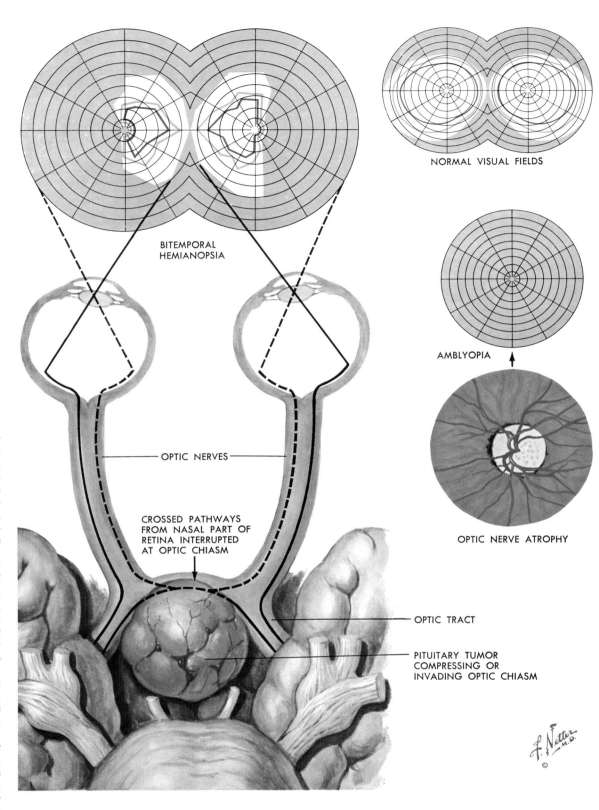

BITEMPORAL
HEMIANOPSIA

NORMAL VISUAL FIELDS

AMBLYOPIA

OPTIC NERVES

OPTIC NERVE ATROPHY

CROSSED PATHWAYS
FROM NASAL PART OF
RETINA INTERRUPTED
AT OPTIC CHIASM

OPTIC TRACT

PITUITARY TUMOR
COMPRESSING OR
INVADING OPTIC CHIASM

The *optic chiasm* lies above the diaphragma sellae. The most common sign of extension of a *pituitary tumor* beyond the confines of the sella turcica is a visual defect caused by the *growth pressing on the optic chiasm*. The most frequent disturbance is a *bitemporal hemianopsia*, which is produced by the tumor pressing on the *crossing* central fibers of the chiasm and sparing the uncrossed lateral fibers. The earliest changes are usually enlargement of the blind spot, loss of color vision, especially for *red*, and a wedge-shaped area of defective vision in the upper temporal quadrants, which gradually enlarges to occupy the *whole* of the *quadrant* and subsequently extends to include the *lower quadrant* as well.

The type of visual defect produced depends on the position of the chiasm, in relation to the pituitary body, and the direction of growth of the tumor. In about 10 per cent of the cases, the chiasm may be found almost entirely anterior or posterior to the diaphragma instead of in its usual position, which is directly above the diaphragma. There are also lateral displacements of the chiasm, which may cause either its right or its left branch to come to lie above the diaphragma. If the chiasm is abnormally fixed, the adenoma may grow upward for a long time before it seriously disturbs sight. Bilateral central scotomas are caused by damage to the posterior part of the chiasm, and their occurrence suggests that the chiasm is prefixed and that the tumor is large. In other cases of prefixed chiasm, the tumor may extend in such a direction as to compress the optic tract rather than the chiasm, thus producing a homonymous hemianopsia. However, homonymous defects do not always indicate a prefixed chiasm, as they may also be produced by lateral extension into the temporal lobe below a normally placed chiasm. Other visual defects which may occur are

unilateral central scotoma, dimness of vision (*amblyopia*) in one eye, caused by compression of one optic nerve, and an inferior quadrantal hemianopsia, presumably resulting from a large tumor causing the anterior cerebral arteries to cut into the dorsal surface of a normally placed chiasm.

Primary *optic atrophy* is present in most cases, but it may be absent when the lesion is behind the chiasm. Although papilledema is rare, it may occur with large tumors that cause increased intracranial pressure. If pressure on the visual pathway is relieved soon enough, the visual fields are usually restored to normal.

Field defects can be detected on gross examination by observing the angle at which an object, such as the examiner's finger, becomes visible when the patient looks straight ahead. Tangent screen and perimetry are necessary for exact plotting of the size and shape of the field defect. Tests should be done

with red, green, and white objects, because defects in color vision may occur earlier than do defects of black and white vision.

In some cases of pituitary tumor showing expansive growth sufficient to enlarge the sella, the visual pathway escapes damage because the sellar diaphragm is tough and prevents expansion toward the chiasm. This structure shows considerable variation, from a dense, closely knit membrane to a small rim with a wide infundibular opening. In most cases the diaphragm does yield to pressure from below. Usually, the chiasm lies directly on the diaphragm and is separated from it by only a potential cleft. In a few instances, particularly where there is a well-developed chiasmatic cistern, the optic chiasm may be as high as 1 cm above the diaphragm, which allows an invading tumor considerable room for expansion before it presses on the visual pathway.

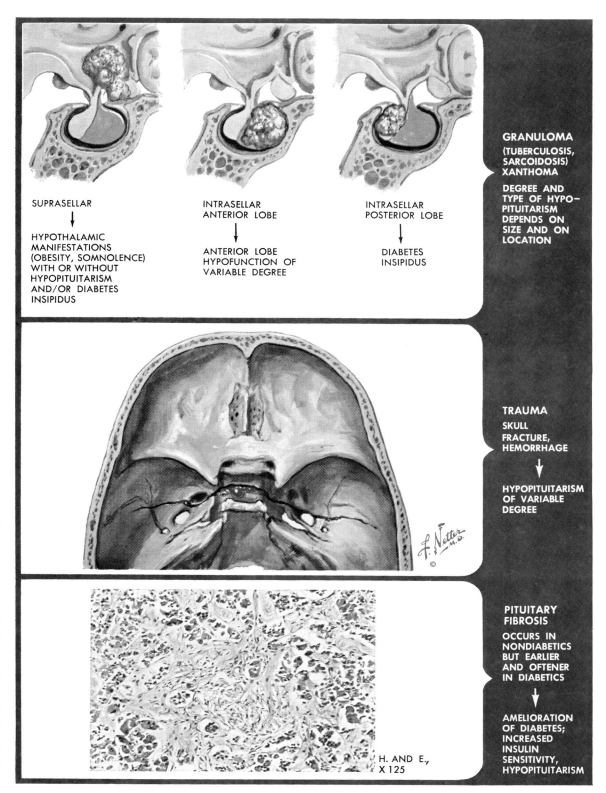

SUPRASELLAR
↓
HYPOTHALAMIC MANIFESTATIONS (OBESITY, SOMNOLENCE) WITH OR WITHOUT HYPOPITUITARISM AND/OR DIABETES INSIPIDUS

INTRASELLAR ANTERIOR LOBE
↓
ANTERIOR LOBE HYPOFUNCTION OF VARIABLE DEGREE

INTRASELLAR POSTERIOR LOBE
↓
DIABETES INSIPIDUS

GRANULOMA (TUBERCULOSIS, SARCOIDOSIS) XANTHOMA

DEGREE AND TYPE OF HYPO-PITUITARISM DEPENDS ON SIZE AND ON LOCATION

TRAUMA SKULL FRACTURE, HEMORRHAGE
↓
HYPOPITUITARISM OF VARIABLE DEGREE

H. AND E., X 125

PITUITARY FIBROSIS OCCURS IN NONDIABETICS BUT EARLIER AND OFTENER IN DIABETICS
↓
AMELIORATION OF DIABETES; INCREASED INSULIN SENSITIVITY, HYPOPITUITARISM

NONTUMOROUS LESIONS OF THE PITUITARY GLAND

Granulomatous lesions are rarely the cause of severe *pituitary insufficiency;* milder degrees of involvement have been reported more often. *Sarcoidosis, tuberculosis,* syphilis, Hand-Schüller-Christian syndrome or *lipoid granuloma,* and actinomycosis have, at times, involved the hypophysis and neighboring suprasellar region in a destructive granulomatous process, with subsequent fibrosis. Giant cell granuloma, involving the pituitary gland as well as the adrenals, appears to be a distinct disease entity. *Suprasellar* disease often presents with symptoms of *hypothalamic disturbance* such as *weight gain,* increased thirst, and polyuria, followed sooner or later by mild to moderate symptoms of pituitary insufficiency. The *adenohypophysis* is affected by a combination of ischemic atrophy induced by interruption of the portal circulation and the cutting off of neural impulses or neuro-endocrine substances that help to regulate anterior pituitary activity, particularly in the gonadotropin sphere. With the development of an increasing degree of *anterior pituitary insufficiency, diabetes insipidus,* which was present at the outset, may disappear. This is due to the *ameliorating* effect of secondary adrenal cortical underfunction on excessive water excretion, chiefly by a moderate decrease in glomerular filtration rate and by reduction in the antagonism of corticosteroids to antidiuretic hormone at the tubular level. Treatment with glucocorticoids brings a prompt return of the

polyuria of diabetes insipidus.

In some cases of *fracture of the base of the skull,* the *pituitary stalk* is *torn.* Depending on the level of severance, diabetes insipidus may result. Sometimes, a shearing injury will cause stalk section without the production of any fracture. Occasionally, the anterior pituitary gland is destroyed as a result of *hemorrhage* associated with cranial *trauma.* At post-mortem examination of such a case, a shrunken anterior lobe, with very few glandular cells, is found. There is no gross fibrosis, as is sometimes found in another group of cases characterized by *pituitary destruction with fibrosis.* In some of these cases, the fibrous tissue is a scar of a former active syphilitic lesion; however, any other granuloma may have such an end result. Scattered remnants of glandular cells, at post mortem, are

found to be enmeshed in and surrounded by coarse, fibrous tissue. Sometimes, collections of leukocytes and plasma cells are found. Severe amyloid infiltration is a very rare cause of pituitary insufficiency. Destruction of the adenohypophysis also may occur by an increase in fibrous connective tissue, which gradually replaces the glandular cells. This appears to be the result of slowly increasing ischemia. It is found mainly in *diabetics,* but a less-advanced picture is not uncommon in old age. In diabetes the occurrence of *increased insulin sensitivity* should suggest the development of such anterior pituitary insufficiency. Usually, such cases will show evidences of thyroid and adrenal cortical underfunction as well. It is known that a deficiency of growth hormone contributes to the increased tendency to hypoglycemia.

PITUITARY ANTERIOR LOBE DEFICIENCY

Juvenile Onset

The commonest cause of hypofunction of the testes is a selective *failure of gonadotropic production* by the pituitary gland, with or without some associated organic lesion. In the absence of a pituitary stimulus to testicular maturation, puberal development does not take place, and secondary sex characteristics do not develop (see CIBA COLLECTION, Vol. 2, page 75). The *penis* remains *small,* with *infantile proportions;* the scrotum fails to develop mature rugae, and the prostate does not grow to adult size. The larynx fails to enlarge, and the voice maintains the high pitch of childhood. Some *pubic hair* appears, but it is usually *sparse* and fine, in contradistinction to the coarse, mature pubic hair; also it does not extend upward along the linea alba (male escutcheon). *Axillary hair* either fails to appear or is also sparse. Beard growth is completely absent. Frontal baldness fails to develop, and *head hair* is *abundant.*

Owing to the prolonged persistence of open epiphysial lines, growth in length continues for a longer period than normal, particularly in the extremities, provided somatotropic (growth) hormone secretion is adequate. *Arms* and *legs* become disproportionately *long. Eunuchoid proportions* are seen in the following measurements: The *lower length* of the body (from soles to symphysis pubis) *exceeds* the *upper length* (from symphysis to top of cranium), and the *span exceeds* the standing height, whereas they should normally be equal. Eventually, but generally not until the third decade of life, the epiphysial lines do close, even in untreated eunuchoid patients. Usually, the administration of sex hormones leads to prompt epiphysial closure. Excessive growth is not found in anterior pituitary insufficiency of adult onset (see page 22). Osteoporosis is sometimes observed in these eunuchoid patients, presumably because of the absence of the protein anabolic effect of testicular androgens. These patients do not develop libido or potency; they are usually shy and introverted—characteristics which can often be considerably ameliorated by adequate replacement therapy.

In more *severe* cases of *anterior pituitary insufficiency* of juvenile onset, caused by tumors of the pituitary gland or extrapituitary lesions, such as craniopharyngiomas, encroaching on the gland, the clinical picture usually includes symptoms, signs, and laboratory features of *hypothyroidism* and *adrenal cortical insufficiency.* Such a patient maintains *normal body proportions* because of low somatotropic hormone secretion. Hypothyroidism may be an additional cause for *dwarfism,* either because of the lack of the usual direct effect of thyroid hormone on skeletal maturation or because

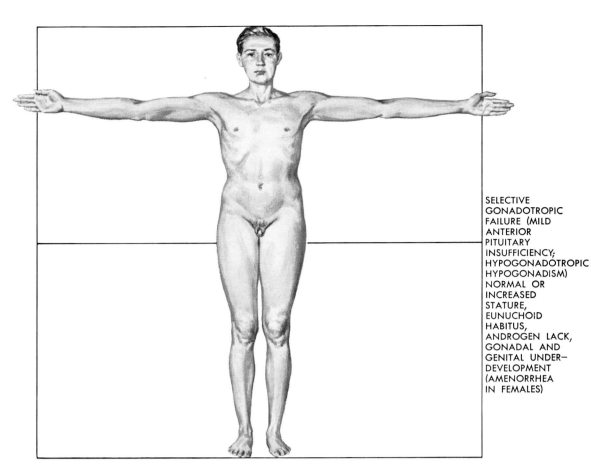

SELECTIVE GONADOTROPIC FAILURE (MILD ANTERIOR PITUITARY INSUFFICIENCY; HYPOGONADOTROPIC HYPOGONADISM) NORMAL OR INCREASED STATURE, EUNUCHOID HABITUS, ANDROGEN LACK, GONADAL AND GENITAL UNDER—DEVELOPMENT (AMENORRHEA IN FEMALES)

FAILURE OF MOST ANTERIOR PITUITARY HORMONES, INCLUDING STH (SEVERE ANTERIOR PITUITARY INSUFFICIENCY; PITUITARY DWARFISM) NORMAL BODY PROPORTIONS, GONADAL AND GENITAL UNDERDEVELOPMENT, VARIABLE DEGREES OF HYPOTHYROIDISM AND ADRENOCORTICAL INSUFFICIENCY, WITH OR WITHOUT DIABETES INSIPIDUS

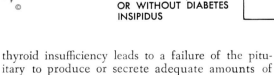

thyroid insufficiency leads to a failure of the pituitary to produce or secrete adequate amounts of somatotropic hormone (see page 23). In adults no changes in body proportions result (see page 23).

Treatment of eunuchoidism due to pituitary insufficiency is the same as for that due to primary testicular failure; it consists of the replacement of testicular hormone by either parenteral injection of testosterone or its esters or by oral administration of methyltestosterone. In cases of pituitary *hypogonadotropism,* it has been possible to induce testicular growth and androgenic function by administration of gonadotropic hormones. Under the stimulus of human urinary chorionic gonadotropin, with its almost exclusive action as LH (ICSH), the testes grow in size and begin to secrete testosterone, which, in turn, leads to the development of secondary sex characteristics. The usual dose schedule is from 500 to 2000

I.U. three times a week, intramuscularly. However, the chief purpose of treatment with gonadotropins is to induce spermatogenesis as well as function of the Leydig cells. Because human pituitary gonadotropins are species-specific, antibodies develop against animal preparations. However, human pituitary gonadotropins with a high titer of FSH, isolated from female urine, are becoming available, and spermatogenesis may be induced and fertility established by their use.

Hypogonadotropic hypogonadism is rarer in the female. In a young girl the most frequent lesion is a craniopharyngioma, usually of suprasellar location. Sometimes, diabetes insipidus accompanies gonadotropin failure when the other endocrine functions are normal. Cyclic administration of human gonadotropic hormones will induce ovulation, and several pregnancies have now been reported following such treatment of hypopituitary women.

PITUITARY ANTERIOR LOBE DEFICIENCY IN THE ADULT

In 1914 Simmonds first described cases of cachexia of hypophysial origin, the fatal termination being associated with septic *infarction of the anterior lobe* of the pituitary at puerperium. Also observed was *atrophy of the gonads,* thyroid, and adrenal glands. This was an important advance in our understanding of pituitary target organ interrelations. Later, it was recognized that cachexia was not an essential feature of this disease. Because of the importance of puerperal infarction in the etiology of pituitary insufficiency, in any series females are more often affected. The term "Sheehan's syndrome" is sometimes used to refer to the type of extreme pituitary insufficiency associated with postpartum necrosis, because Sheehan collected a large series in which pregnancy was associated with onset (see page 25). Milder degrees of insufficiency have been produced by a *pituitary tumor* compressing the remaining normal rim of the gland.

The clinical picture sometimes shows a degree of *wasting* of the body, precocious senility, and *wrinkled, dry skin,* yielding a typical "crow's-feet" configuration of wrinkles around the mouth and up the cheeks. Pigment is absent, and pallor, out of proportion to the moderate anemia usually present, is observed. A peculiar fawnlike color is common. There is loss of *axillary* and *pubic* hair and sometimes of the teeth. In women, *amenorrhea,* sterility, and loss of libido are found; the latter is found also in men, with *impotence* as a rule. Thyroid deficiency produces a subnormal temperature, increased sensitivity to cold, a low metabolic rate, dry skin, and constipation. Also, the combined decrease of thyroid hormone and testosterone results in loss of the lateral third of the eyebrows. Adrenal insufficiency is responsible for *low blood pressure, asthenia,* and crises of nausea and vomiting, which may be associated with spontaneous *hypoglycemia.* Prolonged reduction in blood sugar may lead to permanent intellectual impairment. A few patients with incomplete pituitary insufficiency have become pregnant, with some apparent improvement in pituitary function resulting from the hyperplasia associated with pregnancy.

The dangerous mistake, in these cases, is to confuse primary *myxedema* with hypothyroidism of pituitary origin,

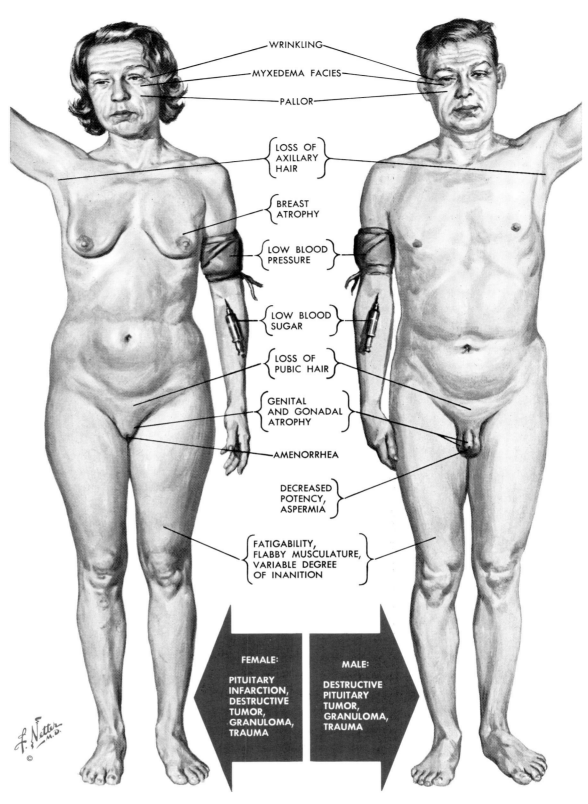

WRINKLING

MYXEDEMA FACIES

PALLOR

LOSS OF AXILLARY HAIR

BREAST ATROPHY

LOW BLOOD PRESSURE

LOW BLOOD SUGAR

LOSS OF PUBIC HAIR

GENITAL AND GONADAL ATROPHY

AMENORRHEA

DECREASED POTENCY, ASPERMIA

FATIGABILITY, FLABBY MUSCULATURE, VARIABLE DEGREE OF INANITION

FEMALE: PITUITARY INFARCTION, DESTRUCTIVE TUMOR, GRANULOMA, TRAUMA

MALE: DESTRUCTIVE PITUITARY TUMOR, GRANULOMA, TRAUMA

which may sometimes closely *resemble* it. The administration of thyroid therapy to patients with underlying latent adrenal cortical insufficiency may precipitate adrenal crisis that is sometimes fatal. If the suspicion of pituitary insufficiency is strong, cortisone should be added to thyroid therapy. The response of the thyroid gland to administration of thyrotropin, by an increase in radio-iodine uptake and serum P.B.I., is very helpful in ruling out primary thyroidal myxedema. This response does not eliminate the diagnosis of unihormonal insufficiency involving only TSH secretion.

Besides the clinical and laboratory evidences of hormonal deficiency, some diagnostic help may be obtained by X-rays of the sella turcica and by determination of the visual fields. In those cases secondary to space-occupying lesions of this region, severe encroachment on the visual pathway is an indication

for surgical interference. Surgery usually further impairs adenohypophysial function and, in many cases, may produce associated diabetes insipidus.

Hypophysectomy is being performed commonly as a palliative measure in metastatic breast cancer and in certain cases of diabetes with progressive retinopathy. In metastatic breast cancer, pituitary resection may act, in part, by abolishing secretion of sex steroids from the ovary and the adrenal cortex. Abolishing growth hormone and prolactin secretion may also be helpful. An improvement of the ocular complications of diabetes has followed hypophysectomy in some patients. The pituitary insufficiency thus produced usually does not lead to the clinical picture of spontaneous cases, because replacement therapy is given straightaway. Hypopituitarism following hypophysectomy is more often complicated by diabetes insipidus than is that which occurs spontaneously.

MILD AND MODERATE HYPOPITUITARISM

The clinical picture resulting from loss of anterior pituitary function may be due to a variety of lesions. The term panhypopituitarism is reserved for the syndrome resulting from the loss of all the hormonal functions of the pituitary, including those of the neurohypophysis; some authors use it in a less-restricted sense to apply to severe anterior pituitary insufficiency, involving the loss of all hormonal functions of the pars distalis. The *gonadotropic function* of the pituitary is usually the first to fail, probably because the delta cells responsible for these secretions are more sensitive to adverse conditions than are the other anterior pituitary cells. Congenital isolated deficiencies of gonadotropic secretion are not uncommon.

In *mild anterior pituitary deficiency,* the symptoms due to loss of gonadotropic function are prominent. *Loss of libido* and testicular atrophy, with flabby, soft testes, often reduced in size and devoid of rugae, are found *in the male. In women, amenorrhea* is an early and constant finding. Urinary gonadotropins are absent, indicating pituitary failure, in contrast with primary gonadal failure in which the urinary gonadotropins are higher than normal. The vaginal mucosa is atrophic, as revealed both by inspection and by vaginal cytology. In men there is usually some *loss of hair* on the *chest* and extremities and some decrease in or *loss of facial hair.* In women the pubic and axillary hair appears to be mainly under the control of adrenal cortical androgen, and loss of hair in these regions does not occur except in more severe cases. *In the child* with mild pituitary destruction or *congenital lack* of gonadotropin function, due presumably to failure *of delta cells* to appear, puberty is delayed or does not occur. If *somatotropic hormone* is present in normal quantities and the other functions of the pituitary are not impaired, then *overgrowth of the long bones* will occur, and a *eunuchoid habitus* will develop.

Moderate anterior pituitary deficiency leads, first, to decrease in gonadotropic function; next, it usually involves *thyroid function;* and, last and least commonly, in a more insidious way, a loss of ACTH reserve. In some instances the secondary hypothyroidism may dominate the clinical picture. Such cases are called pituitary myxedema. Treatment with desiccated thyroid may throw an additional metabolic strain on the patient and bring out latent *adrenal cortical insufficiency.* Similar crises may be precipitated by *infections or operations. Partial deficiency of ACTH* may be detected by the metyrapone test (see page 14). *Pallor,* out of proportion to the moderate anemia sometimes seen, may be present. This is due to a loss of

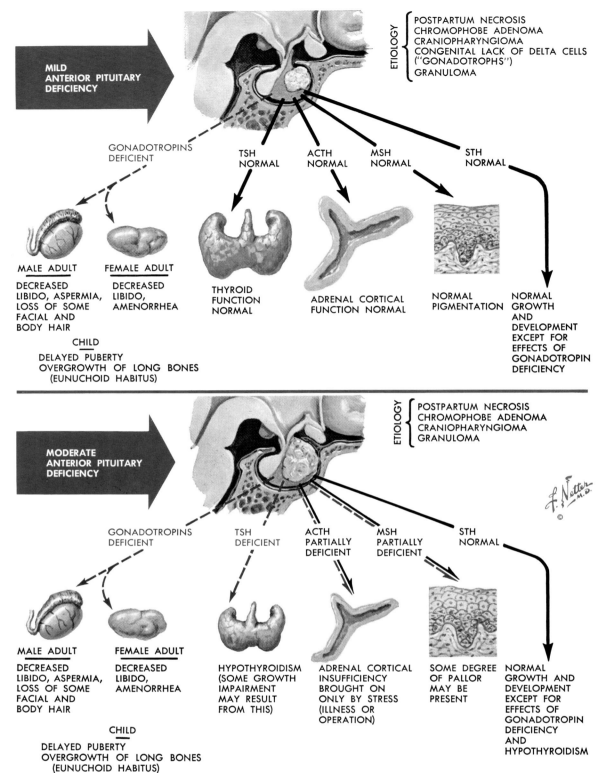

ETIOLOGY
POSTPARTUM NECROSIS
CHROMOPHOBE ADENOMA
CRANIOPHARYNGIOMA
CONGENITAL LACK OF DELTA CELLS ("GONADOTROPHS")
GRANULOMA

MILD ANTERIOR PITUITARY DEFICIENCY

GONADOTROPINS DEFICIENT — TSH NORMAL — ACTH NORMAL — MSH NORMAL — STH NORMAL

MALE ADULT
DECREASED LIBIDO, ASPERMIA, LOSS OF SOME FACIAL AND BODY HAIR

FEMALE ADULT
DECREASED LIBIDO, AMENORRHEA

CHILD
DELAYED PUBERTY OVERGROWTH OF LONG BONES (EUNUCHOID HABITUS)

THYROID FUNCTION NORMAL

ADRENAL CORTICAL FUNCTION NORMAL

NORMAL PIGMENTATION

NORMAL GROWTH AND DEVELOPMENT EXCEPT FOR EFFECTS OF GONADOTROPIN DEFICIENCY

ETIOLOGY
POSTPARTUM NECROSIS
CHROMOPHOBE ADENOMA
CRANIOPHARYNGIOMA
GRANULOMA

MODERATE ANTERIOR PITUITARY DEFICIENCY

GONADOTROPINS DEFICIENT — TSH DEFICIENT — ACTH PARTIALLY DEFICIENT — MSH PARTIALLY DEFICIENT — STH NORMAL

MALE ADULT
DECREASED LIBIDO, ASPERMIA, LOSS OF SOME FACIAL AND BODY HAIR

FEMALE ADULT
DECREASED LIBIDO, AMENORRHEA

CHILD
DELAYED PUBERTY OVERGROWTH OF LONG BONES (EUNUCHOID HABITUS)

HYPOTHYROIDISM (SOME GROWTH IMPAIRMENT MAY RESULT FROM THIS)

ADRENAL CORTICAL INSUFFICIENCY BROUGHT ON ONLY BY STRESS (ILLNESS OR OPERATION)

SOME DEGREE OF PALLOR MAY BE PRESENT

NORMAL GROWTH AND DEVELOPMENT EXCEPT FOR EFFECTS OF GONADOTROPIN DEFICIENCY AND HYPOTHYROIDISM

melanocyte-stimulating hormone (MSH). In addition to isolated *gonadotropin lack,* the occurrence of myxedema or of adrenal insufficiency of pituitary origin as single hormone deficiencies has been reported. In these cases only the response to TSH or ACTH will differentiate with certainty the primary thyroid and adrenal deficiencies from those secondary to a tropic hormone deficiency. In primary Addison's disease, the increased pigmentation usually present helps with the differential diagnosis.

In *children* with moderate pituitary insufficiency, *growth may be impaired* because of *hypothyroidism.* However, growth failure which occurs in other conditions of recognized etiology, such as cretinism or malnutrition, may also be mediated, in part, by effects on growth hormone secretion. Better measurements of circulating growth hormone levels will eventually allow the recognition of unihormonal or partial deficiencies of growth hormone in many cases presently classified as constitutional dwarfs.

The explanation for the development of secretory failure of only a single pituitary hormone follows easily from the premise that each pituitary hormone comes from a separate and distinct cell (see page 11). It should be remembered, however, that anterior pituitary deficiency can also result from damage to the hypothalamic centers which regulate the secretion of individual pituitary hormones.

It is surprising and gratifying how well patients with damage of several pituitary functions respond to replacement therapy with corticosteroids, thyroid hormone, and sex steroids, if indicated. Provision should be made for increased amounts of adrenal glucocorticoids during periods of metabolic stress. If the causative lesion is not progressive, the prognosis for a long and active life is excellent.

SEVERE ANTERIOR HYPOPITUITARISM AND PANHYPOPITUITARISM

Severe symptoms of *anterior pituitary insufficiency* appear only when *destruction* of the *adenohypophysis* is nearly complete. Lesions affecting the adenohypophysis without any extrasellar effect cause only *hypogonadism* until approximately three quarters of the anterior lobe has been destroyed. With progressive destruction, mild hypogonadism becomes more severe, and general symptoms attributable to *thyroid* and *adrenal cortical underfunction* such as asthenia, fatigue, loss of appetite, and cold intolerance appear and progress. The lesion in the pituitary is often an infarction, the result of an ischemic *postpartum necrosis* following postpartum hemorrhage. In a large proportion of cases, there is a history of retention of the placenta, afibrinogenemia, or other causes of severe postpartum bleeding. In fibrosis of the pituitary gland, there is some evidence to incriminate syphilis in a few reported cases. *Trauma* rarely destroys the pituitary. *Tumors* and *granulomas* seldom completely destroy the anterior lobe, and often the symptoms of pituitary underfunction are relatively mild even when the tumor is large enough to cause serious symptoms from compression of adjacent structures. However, *surgical intervention* in these cases is often enough to convert them to a state of complete pituitary insufficiency.

An extreme atrophy of the gonads is a constant finding in this disease. There also occurs a *regression of secondary sexual characteristics.* The *ovaries* become small and fibrous; the uterus regresses to infantile proportions, with an extremely thin layer of endometrium; the external genitalia shrink, as does the vagina, which develops a smooth atrophic epithelium. The breasts regress, and the areolae lose pigmentation. In better-nourished patients the gland may contain an appreciable amount of fat. In the male the penis is small, the *testes* are greatly shrunken and devoid of rugae, and the prostate is markedly atrophied. In all cases the *thyroid gland* is small, with follicles lined with low cuboidal epithelium. The general architecture of the gland persists, however. Shrinkage of the *adrenal cortex* is most obvious in the zona fasciculata and zona reticularis; the zona glomerulosa, which is the site of aldosterone production, appears not to depend very much on ACTH secretion, in contrast to the other two layers. The general architectural pattern of the adrenal cortex is maintained, but the cells are poor in lipid content.

Pallor, out of proportion to the moderate anemia present, is a striking feature of most cases. It is probably

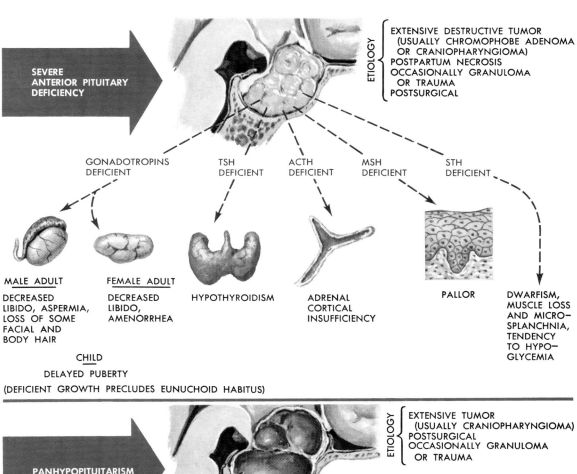

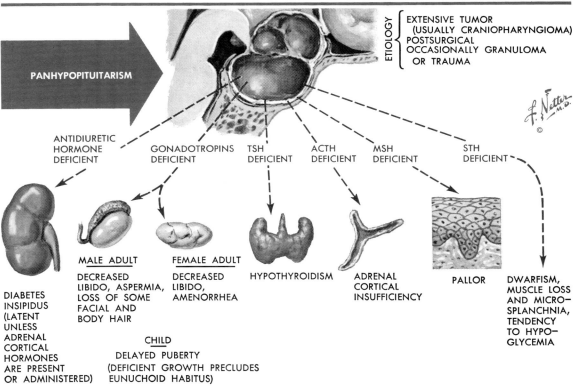

due to a *deficiency of melanocyte-stimulating hormone.* Next to the atrophy of the endocrine glands, the smallness of the viscera is the most striking general pathological change in severe anterior pituitary insufficiency. This *microsplanchnia,* particularly of the heart, liver, and kidneys, has been noted almost universally in published reports of this condition, whether the patient has been emaciated, normally nourished, or even slightly overweight. It is greater than that generally found in patients dying in a more-emaciated condition from various wasting diseases. The *muscles lose bulk,* apparently because of reduction in the size and number of muscle fibers. The *lack of somatotropin* presumably is responsible. These patients have a *tendency to hypoglycemia,* which may cause attacks of coma and convulsions. Deficiency of adrenal glucocorticoids as well as lack of somatotropic hormone, together with poor food

intake, contribute to these crises of hypoglycemia.

The term *panhypopituitarism* should be reserved for cases in which *all the functions of the adenohypophysis* are affected and there is, as well, a deficiency of neurohypophysial function, namely, *diabetes insipidus.* Patients with slowly progressive destructive lesions of this region may first manifest diabetes insipidus, which disappears when involvement of the adenohypophysis becomes extreme enough to cause secondary adrenal cortical insufficiency. This antagonism between vasopressin and glucocorticoids is further demonstrated by the reappearance of diabetes insipidus when these patients are treated with replacement doses of cortisol. In recent years the most common *cause* of panhypopituitarism has been *surgical* hypophysectomy, which is performed frequently on patients with metastatic breast cancer and, less often, in cases of progressive diabetic retinopathy.

CHROMOPHOBE ADENOMA

Pituitary adenomas are comparatively common. They have been estimated to comprise about 15 per cent of all intracranial tumors, and, in that group, the chromophobe adenoma is much the commonest pituitary neoplasm. Such tumors may be found in 15 per cent of all pituitary glands on routine examination, with a greater incidence being obtained if the gland is sectioned serially. Most of these tumors are microscopic in size. They occur equally in the two sexes, with the *greatest frequency* in the *sixth decade of life.*

The usual nonfunctioning chromophobe adenomas cause neighborhood symptoms by pressure on the optic pathway, *compressing the optic chiasm,* with typical bitemporal hemianopsia presenting (see page 18). The constitutional symptoms of pituitary insufficiency are produced by compressing the surrounding normal gland, but these tumors may reach a considerable size, thus compressing the optic chiasm and impairing vision, before much evidence of pituitary insufficiency appears. Hypogonadism, with amenorrhea in females, loss of libido and potency, and a decrease in facial, pubic, and axillary hair in males, is common in these cases. Thyroid and adrenal underfunction are slower to appear. *Radiologic examination* of the *sella turcica* in a lateral skull film shows that its cavity is *enlarged* in all directions. Atrophy of the clinoid processes is a frequent finding. By the use of a small amount of air introduced into the spinal canal, one may visualize the cisternal system and thus outline the soft tissue mass as it rises above the tegmentum sellae, as shown in the X-ray in the accompanying plate.

In some instances of chromophobe adenoma, the tumor appears to have been elaborating one or more hormones, as evidenced by their presence in cases of Cushing's syndrome, active acromegaly, virilizing adrenal hyperplasia, and galactorrhea. Sometimes these tumors, though predominantly chromophobic, have small numbers of either basophil or acidophil cells, which would justify the term "mixed adenoma". In these patients the features of hyperpituitarism and hypopituitarism may be present at the same time. The chromophobes in the adenoma can be regarded as cells that secrete

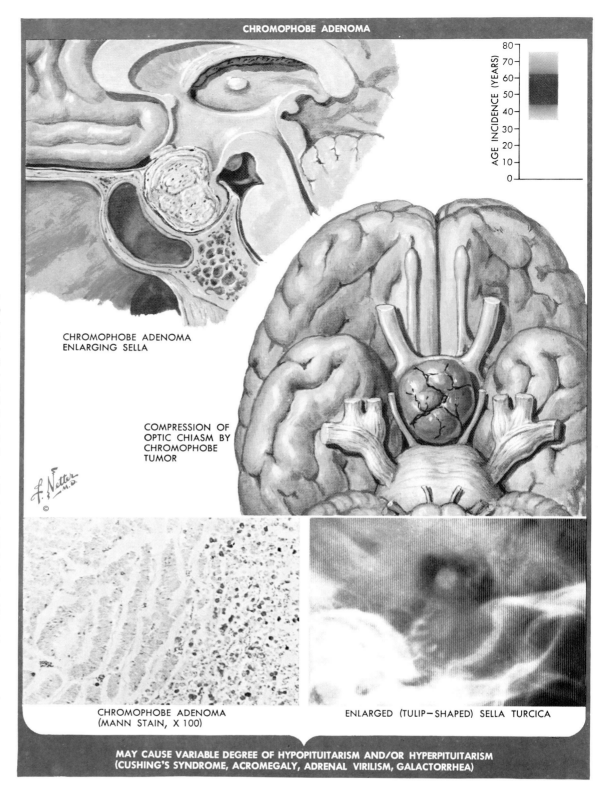

CHROMOPHOBE ADENOMA

CHROMOPHOBE ADENOMA ENLARGING SELLA

COMPRESSION OF OPTIC CHIASM BY CHROMOPHOBE TUMOR

CHROMOPHOBE ADENOMA (MANN STAIN, X 100)

ENLARGED (TULIP-SHAPED) SELLA TURCICA

MAY CAUSE VARIABLE DEGREE OF HYPOPITUITARISM AND/OR HYPERPITUITARISM (CUSHING'S SYNDROME, ACROMEGALY, ADRENAL VIRILISM, GALACTORRHEA)

excessive quantities of hormonal product without storing much of it in a recognizable granular form. Most of the postadrenalectomy pituitary tumors that occur in cases of Cushing's syndrome are composed entirely of chromophobes; occasionally, some basophilic or PAS-positive granules are also found. Similarly, some cases of active acromegaly have very little acidophil granulation in the cells of the pituitary tumor. Isolated galactorrhea has been noted in chromophobe adenoma; such tumors are presumed to produce prolactin.

Treatment of chromophobe adenoma is determined by the presence of visual impairment. Surgery is directed to the preservation or recovery of vision. It is not likely to help pituitary insufficiency, except in rare situations where removal of a soft adenoma seems to lead to some functional recovery of the surrounding gland. In such a case, the menses may return

postoperatively. Radiotherapy may help reduce the pituitary overactivity of a functioning chromophobe adenoma but should not be used when vision is markedly impaired. It is prescribed often, following surgical relief of pressure on the visual pathway. There is reason to believe that it will also limit further growth of the nonfunctioning pituitary, so that its use postoperatively seems justified.

Hemorrhage into a pituitary containing a chromophobe adenoma is a rare case of acute pituitary insufficiency. It may also cause a sudden failure of vision. Spontaneous diabetes insipidus rarely develops, even with large chromophobe adenomas, which, despite their size, usually spare the neurohypophysial remnant in the stalk and the tuber cinereum. However, operative removal of the tumor is sometimes complicated by diabetes insipidus, which may be permanent.

POSTPARTUM PITUITARY NECROSIS

Among the earliest cases of severe *pituitary insufficiency* were those described by Simmonds from 1914 to 1918. He reported cases of cachexia of hypophysial origin, with a fatal termination, associated with what he believed was septic puerperal infarction of the anterior lobe of the pituitary gland. It was soon recognized that cachexia was not an essential feature of the disease.

Twenty-five years after Simmonds' original description, Sheehan reemphasized the importance of a preceding pregnancy in the pathogenesis of many cases of anterior pituitary insufficiency. Postpartum necrosis appears to be due to spasm and associated thrombosis of the nutrient vessels to the adenohypophysis. The most common cause of this is severe general circulatory collapse associated with *postpartum hemorrhage*. In most animal species, including man, all the blood reaching the adenohypophysis is of portal venous origin. The *pituitary gland* is markedly *hyperplastic* at the end of *pregnancy* and thus is more vulnerable to a sudden falloff in blood supply. Sheehan suggests that the primary vascular disturbance is a spasm of the infundibular arteries, which are drained by the hypophysial portal vessels. If the spasm continues for several hours, most of the tissues in the anterior lobe die; when blood finally starts to flow, stasis and *thrombosis* occur in the stalk and in the adenohypophysis.

In Sheehan's opinion, variations in the extent and duration of the spasm account for variations in the extent of the necrosis. In about half of the cases of postpartum necrosis, the lesion involves about 97 per cent of the anterior lobe, but the pars tuberalis and a small portion of tissue on the superior surface of

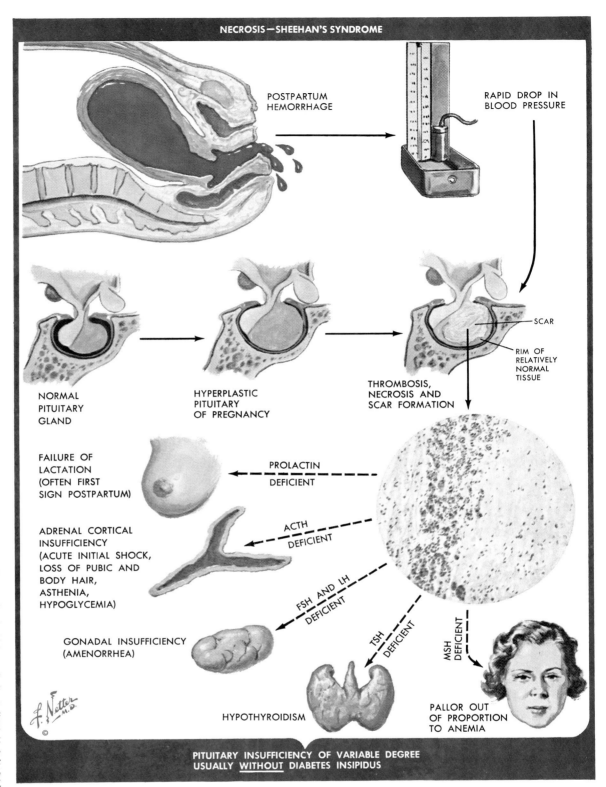

NECROSIS—SHEEHAN'S SYNDROME

POSTPARTUM HEMORRHAGE

RAPID DROP IN BLOOD PRESSURE

NORMAL PITUITARY GLAND

HYPERPLASTIC PITUITARY OF PREGNANCY

THROMBOSIS, NECROSIS AND SCAR FORMATION

SCAR

RIM OF RELATIVELY NORMAL TISSUE

FAILURE OF LACTATION (OFTEN FIRST SIGN POSTPARTUM)

PROLACTIN DEFICIENT

ADRENAL CORTICAL INSUFFICIENCY (ACUTE INITIAL SHOCK, LOSS OF PUBIC AND BODY HAIR, ASTHENIA, HYPOGLYCEMIA)

ACTH DEFICIENT

FSH AND LH DEFICIENT

GONADAL INSUFFICIENCY (AMENORRHEA)

TSH DEFICIENT

MSH DEFICIENT

HYPOTHYROIDISM

PALLOR OUT OF PROPORTION TO ANEMIA

PITUITARY INSUFFICIENCY OF VARIABLE DEGREE USUALLY WITHOUT DIABETES INSIPIDUS

the adenohypophysis usually are preserved. This remnant retains its structural connections with the hypothalamus and receives a portal blood supply from the neural portion of the stalk. Another type of anterior lobe remnant, sometimes found in these cases, is a small area of parenchyma at the lateral pole of the gland, without vascular or neural connections with the stalk and hypothalamus. It is unlikely that such tissue is capable of normal function. In other instances a thin layer of parenchyma remains up against the wall of the sella under the capsule. Presumably, these peripheral remnants are nourished by a small capsular blood supply.

If more than 30 per cent of the gland is preserved, there is usually sufficient function to forestall the development of pituitary insufficiency. If more of the gland is destroyed, these patients *fail to lactate* following delivery, and the pubic hair that was shaved

does not grow back. Although *amenorrhea* is usual, there have been some reports of irregular but true menstruation in patients following postpartum necrosis. In some instances this has occurred in the presence of well-marked *thyroid* and *adrenal insufficiency*. Hence, it must be concluded that some gonadotropin was produced. Rarely, such patients become pregnant and seem to improve because of the hypertrophy of the pituitary remnant that accompanies pregnancy. In the absence of the stimulus of pregnancy, there is little tendency for regeneration of the remnant after the initial damage to the pituitary.

Very rarely, the normal nonparturient pituitary may become infarcted in association with hemorrhagic shock. Severe pituitary insufficiency of this type has been observed by the author, following shock from a bleeding peptic ulcer in a middle-aged male.

ANOREXIA NERVOSA

This syndrome occurs chiefly in adolescent girls of psychoneurotic constitution. It is characterized by *extreme emaciation* and *amenorrhea* in the absence of any demonstrable structural disease. The loss of appetite results from a morbid *psychogenic aversion to eating* rather than a physiological loss of desire for food because of tension, worry, or fatigue. Sir William Gull, in 1873, pointed out: "These willful patients are often allowed to drift their way into a state of extreme exhaustion, when it might have been prevented by placing them under different moral conditions". Generally, there is an underlying discontent owing to failure of adaptation to the environment. There may be an abnormal desire to become thin or a fear of gastro-intestinal symptoms believed to be produced by the ingestion of food. Many patients admit later that the compulsion to avoid food had been stronger than the hunger they sometimes experienced. Emaciation increases because of a slowly progressive, self-induced starvation. The patient remains quick, *alert,* active, and restless, denying ill health until wasted to a degree not seen in patients with organic disease who are still able to get about. When emaciation is greatest, edema of the lower extremities may develop, especially on refeeding. Amenorrhea may appear early but sometimes does not occur until after considerable weight loss. In the well-developed syndrome, body temperature is often subnormal, and the pulse rate and *blood pressure* are *low*. The blood sugar and *basal metabolic rate* are usually *decreased*. Because of these metabolic consequences of undernutrition, this disease has sometimes been considered a form of severe pituitary insufficiency, but the only pituitary function consistently affected is *gonadotropic hormone production* or release. Thyroid function is only moderately decreased, since *radio-iodine uptake* and *P.B.I.* are usually in the *lower part of the normal* range. Adrenal function appears to be normal until death from *inanition*.

Anorexia nervosa was often diagnosed and reported as Simmonds' disease (extreme insufficiency of the adenohypophysis). Superficially, the syndromes resemble each other; in both are found amenorrhea, emaciation, lowered blood sugar values, reduced basal metabolic rate, and changes in mental outlook. Their fundamental differences, however, make separation easy in most cases: Simmonds' disease occurs most typically in adult women who have had several children, the disease often dating from the last puerperium. The anorexia of Simmonds' disease is a physiological lack of

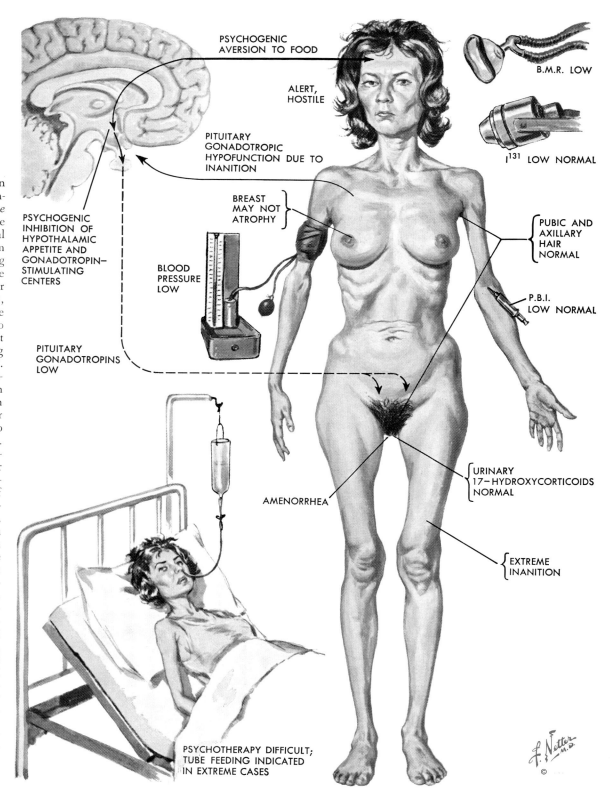

desire for food in patients with rather prominent adrenal insufficiency. Most patients with Simmonds' disease have little or no emaciation. The amenorrhea is associated with loss of sexual function and secondary sexual characteristics (falling out of axillary and pubic hair) and with atrophy of sex organs. In anorexia nervosa, amenorrhea occurs as a single symptom and is usually not associated with evidence of gross failure of sexual function. The *breasts* remain fairly *well developed* in spite of emaciation, and *axillary* and *pubic hair persist*. There is no atrophy of external genitalia. In pituitary insufficiency the P.B.I. and radio-iodine uptake are usually much further below the normal range. Whereas *urinary 17-hydroxycorticoids* are *normal* in anorexia nervosa, they are typically very low in hypopituitarism. In pituitary insufficiency the patient is dull and apathetic; in anorexia nervosa she is characteristically

quick, alert, active, stubborn, obsessive, and resentful.

The aims of treatment are to change the patient's attitude toward food and to eradicate the underlying mental conflict. In some cases, even prolonged and repeated explanation and encouragement fail to bring the patient to an understanding of the nature of her illness. *Tube feeding,* gradually increased to 3000 or 4000 calories daily, may be required to begin the weight gain that seems to be necessary before the obsession about eating is overcome. Thus, confidence is engendered, and improvement in the sense of well-being aids in the essential and active psychotherapy that must be maintained after tube feeding has been discontinued. Once the patient learns to understand her problem, her mental attitude toward food changes, and recovery often results, but a certain number prove incurable, dying of inanition or intercurrent infection.

ACIDOPHIL ADENOMA

RELATIVELY SMALL, SLOW—GROWING ADENOMA, CAUSING ENDOCRINE SYMPTOMS (ACROMEGALY) WITH LITTLE MECHANICAL DISTURBANCE

LARGE ACIDOPHIL ADENOMA; EXTENSIVE DESTRUCTION OF PITUITARY SUBSTANCE, COMPRESSION OF OPTIC CHIASM, INVASION OF THIRD VENTRICLE AND FLOOR OF SELLA

INVASIVE (MALIGNANT) ADENOMA; EXTENSION INTO RIGHT CAVERNOUS SINUS

ACIDOPHIL ADENOMA (MANN STAIN, X 125)

MIXED ACIDOPHIL—CHROMOPHOBE ADENOMA (MANN STAIN, X 250)

ENLARGED SELLA TURCICA

GIGANTISM, ACROMEGALY (MAY BE ASYMPTOMATIC IF VERY SMALL)

ACIDOPHIL ADENOMA

Hyperfunction of the *acidophilic cells* of the *adenohypophysis* results in the well-recognized clinical pictures of *acromegaly* and gigantism. The most conspicuous results are those referable to excessive secretion of growth, or somatotropic, hormone. This causes overgrowth in length in young individuals with epiphysial lines still open, producing gigantism. In older individuals after closure of the epiphysial lines precludes further growth in length, only appositional growth is possible, and the result is acromegaly. Hyperpituitary giants sometimes develop, even in childhood. Although cases of acromegaly have been reported showing only hyperplasia of the gland, involving chiefly the acidophilic elements, by far the most common finding in this condition is an *acidophil adenoma*. The size of the tumor varies considerably; in some instances it is small and embedded within a normal or small anterior lobe. Occasionally, a *small* asymptomatic *acidophil adenoma* may be found, on routine examination, without any features of acromegaly being noted. Presumably, such a tumor is not putting out excessive quantities of growth hormone.

Usually, the tumor in acromegaly is large enough to erode and *enlarge* the walls of the *sella turcica*, so that most cases show an *enlarged sella turcica* on X-ray examination of the skull. Extension upward into the cranial cavity and downward into the sphenoidal sinuses is common. Lateral extension of the tumor through the wall of the *cavernous sinus* occasionally occurs, producing a syndrome of paralysis of one or more of the third, fourth, fifth, and sixth cranial nerves that traverse the sinus. Lateral spread may extend to involve the temporal lobe. Extension upward to the diaphragma sellae usually affects the *optic chiasm*. Occasionally, the position of the chiasm may be sufficiently anterior or posterior to the diaphragma so that the optic pathway may not be compressed by the growing tumor. Forward progression sometimes involves the frontal lobe. Upward extension may fill the *third ventricle* with tumor and may obstruct the foramen of Monro on one or both sides, as well as the aqueduct of Sylvius, leading to marked dilatation of the ventricle.

The condition of the nonadenomatous portion of the gland is important. If the adenoma is small, the remaining tissue may not be compressed and thus will be able to function normally. Larger adenomas may press on the remaining glandular tissue to produce complete atrophy and loss of function.

Most of the tumors reported are predominantly acidophilic, but some cases of "active" acromegaly have presented with tumors that were found to be chromophobic. It is likely that these chromophobes resulted from excessive secretion without much storage of hormone. Thus, it is not possible to assess the activity of acromegaly by the intensity of the staining reaction of the tumor cells. Cases of *mixed acidophil-chromophobe adenoma* may contain some acidophilic cells capable of both storage of hormone granules and excessive secretion. Large chromophobe cells with copious cytoplasm are considered to have secreted

their hormone product soon after its manufacture. Some of the smaller chromophobes, without much obvious cytoplasm, may be functionless. When such cells form the majority, the tumor is on its way to the "burned-out" stage. That is the end result of most adenomas, in the long run. Radiation therapy will induce degenerative changes in the acidophil adenoma. Mixed chromophobe and acidophil adenomas may be associated with only mild acromegalic features, such as tufting of the terminal phalanges. Such cases have been called "fugitive" acromegaly. Rarely, acidophil adenomas may cause isolated galactorrhea; such tumors are held to be the source of excessive quantities of prolactin, which, in man, is closely related, if not identical with, growth hormone. More commonly, galactorrhea may be an associated finding in florid acromegaly. Other causes of galactorrhea are discussed on page 140.

GIGANTISM

FEET AND INCHES

X-RAY OF TUMOR PROTRUDING ABOVE TUBERCULUM SELLAE OUTLINED BY AIR

PITUITARY GIANT CONTRASTED WITH NORMAL MAN (ACROMEGALY AND SIGNS OF SECONDARY PITUITARY INSUFFICIENCY MAY OR MAY NOT BE PRESENT)

Gigantism is defined as excessive growth in height, greatly exceeding the average for the person's race. Earlier authors concluded that gigantism was due to hyperpituitarism during the period of growth before the epiphyses had united and that the same disturbance caused acromegaly in the adult. Patients with gigantism often have manifestations of acromegaly also, if the excessive growth stimulus was continued beyond the period of epiphysial closure, and occasional patients develop both acromegaly and gigantism before the closure of the epiphyses, presumably owing to stimulation of both appositional and longitudinal bony growth.

Gigantism may occur in eunuchoidism, in which condition a normal amount of pituitary growth hormone is able to exert its action over a longer period than usual, because epiphysial closure is delayed through a deficiency of androgen. Extreme height is often familial or genetic. Gigantism usually is found in men, but several cases in females have been reported. It is true, however, that the tallest giants have been men.

In gigantism due to hyperpituitarism, the pituitary gland is usually enlarged sufficiently to distort the sella turcica, as revealed by X-ray of the *skull*. As in acromegaly, the tumor may extend beyond the sella, *e.g.,* into the sphenoid sinus.

Because growth in the length of the bones is possible, they may retain their normal proportions, unlike the disproportion that is produced in acromegaly. The increased growth is gradual and insidious; it may begin in infancy and usually proceeds at a fairly constant rate, ceasing with sexual maturity, when epiphysial closure takes place. *Final height* is usually *between 7 and 8 ft.* The changes in the endocrine glands and in the viscera are similar to those found in acromegaly (see page 29). The skeletal muscles may be powerfully developed, but, later, pituitary insufficiency may occur, with associated muscular weakness. If, however, sufficient normally functioning gland is spared, pituitary insufficiency does not develop. Goiter and hyper-metabolism occur as in acromegaly, but diabetes is rare. There may be hypertension, with or without cardiac hypertrophy. The life of giants is shorter than normal because of their increased susceptibility to injury, infection, and adrenal crisis in association with moderate pituitary insufficiency.

The treatment of gigantism due to an acidophil adenoma is similar to that for acromegaly. Compression of the visual pathway is an indication for immediate surgery. Operation, or radiation by implantation of radioactive materials into the pituitary fossa, would appear to be the most certain means of halting the excessive disfiguring growth of young people with this condition. Unfortunately, most cases usually present when it is too late for treatment to control their height.

ACROMEGALY

Acromegaly was the first pituitary syndrome to be recognized. It was described clearly and named by Pierre Marie in 1886. Soon after, it was generally accepted that the clinical picture of somatic overgrowth was usually associated with a pituitary adenoma and that the syndrome was due to overproduction of hormone by pituitary tumor cells.

Acromegalic manifestations result from the effects of pituitary hypersecretion and from pressure by an expanding tumor on neighboring structures. The disease usually develops gradually, and the patient may not seek medical advice until the condition has become well marked. The skeleton and the viscera tend to be enlarged. By then, *bigness of the features* and *enlargement* of the *hands* and *feet* are obvious. The facial features coarsen, the *lips* and *nose* becoming particularly *large*. The skin of the whole body thickens, with corrugated furrows, sometimes being well marked on the forehead and the soles of the feet. Hair follicles, sebaceous glands, and sweat glands increase in size. The tongue becomes big, and the *nasal sinuses* often *enlarge* greatly. Overgrowth of bone (*hyperostosis*) is associated with osteoporosis, and these deform the *spine* and render the joints more susceptible to degenerative lesions. Arthritis is common. Paresthesia of the thumb, with thenar atrophy, may result from compression of the carpal tunnel due to bony overgrowth.

The effect of the disease on gonadal function varies. In the early stages the gonads may be large; later, they shrink because of compression by the expanding tumor on the surrounding rim of normal gland that is responsible for production of gonadotropic hormones. As the syndrome progresses, sexual function tends to fail; women cease to menstruate, and men lose libido and potency.

Approximately one quarter of acromegalics become diabetic, and about a third exhibit some decrease in sugar tolerance if this is tested. Occasionally, diabetes may cause the presenting symptoms of polyuria and polydipsia. Often, some insulin resistance is present because excessive amounts of growth hormone act as an insulin antagonist. Serum insulin levels are usually elevated.

Among other symptoms, heat intolerance and excessive malodorous perspiration occur frequently. Sometimes headache (bifrontal, bitemporal, or occipital) may become troublesome. Hyperthyroidism occurs in only a small proportion of patients — probably less than 5

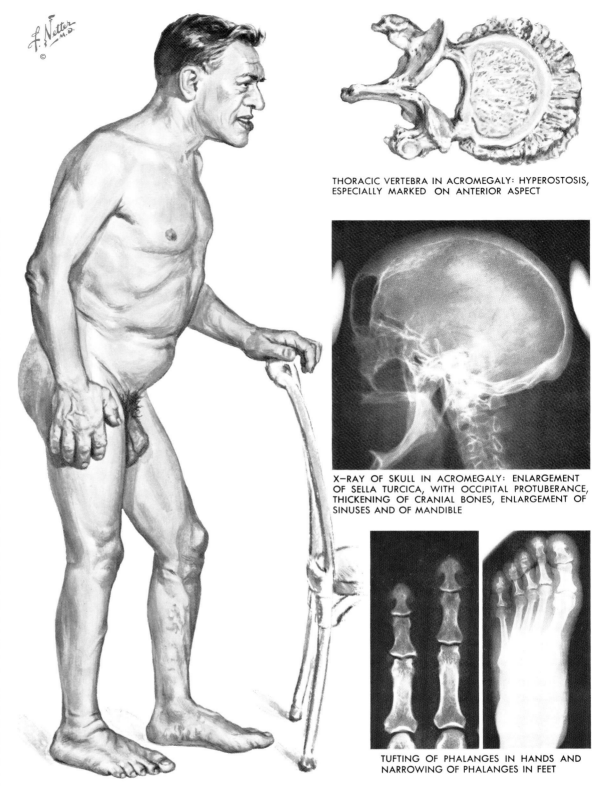

THORACIC VERTEBRA IN ACROMEGALY: HYPEROSTOSIS, ESPECIALLY MARKED ON ANTERIOR ASPECT

X-RAY OF SKULL IN ACROMEGALY: ENLARGEMENT OF SELLA TURCICA, WITH OCCIPITAL PROTUBERANCE, THICKENING OF CRANIAL BONES, ENLARGEMENT OF SINUSES AND OF MANDIBLE

TUFTING OF PHALANGES IN HANDS AND NARROWING OF PHALANGES IN FEET

per cent. Adrenal cortical function is usually normal, although some female acromegalics may have rather marked virilism along with increased urinary excretion of 17-ketosteroids, presumably of adrenal origin. Stein-Leventhal ovaries have been reported, presenting with menstrual irregularities. Renal calculi, sometimes resulting from coexistent hyperparathyroidism, may complicate acromegaly. The course of acromegaly, the number of complicating disorders (such as emphysema), and the cause of death vary greatly.

Skull films reveal the disease, as do films of the *hands* and *feet*. The diagnosis is confirmed by finding an elevated level of serum growth hormone (>5 mμg per ml), an elevated phosphorus (>4.5 mg per 100 ml) in two thirds of the patients, and, more importantly, by the absence of the normal diurnal variation in serum phosphorus levels, which are normally higher in the morning than in the after-

noon; also, by X-ray, a heel pad thicker than 22 mm.

Shrinkage of the visual fields is an indication for resection of the pituitary tumor, and progressive disfiguring growth, with or without headache, calls for radiation therapy. If growth continues in spite of radiation, surgery should be performed. The soft tissue overgrowth may regress somewhat after resection or ablation of the hormone-producing tumor, but the bony disfigurement is permanent. Since surgery offers more certain control of hormone production, it should be considered in treating young women with early acromegaly (even those with normal visual fields) before irreversible ugliness supervenes. Excellent cosmetic results have been observed following hypophysectomy or implantation of radioactive pellets into the pituitary substance, when the coarsening of the countenance was caused chiefly by hypertrophy of soft tissue and edema.

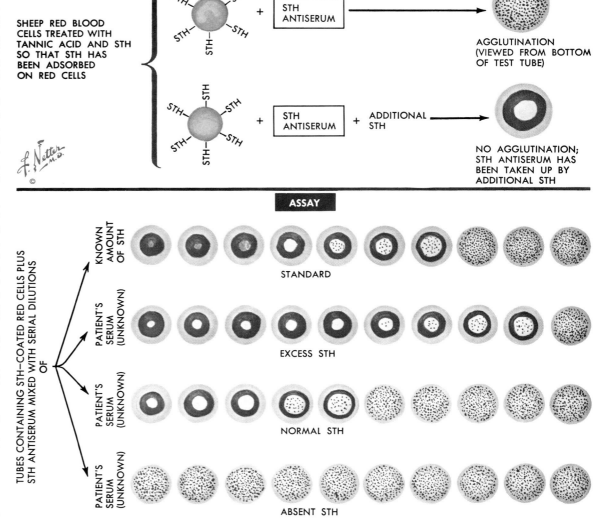

THEORY

REPEATED INJECTIONS OF PURIFIED HUMAN SOMATOTROPIC HORMONE (STH) INTO RABBIT

5 TO 6 WEEKS

BLOOD WITHDRAWN

STH ANTISERUM

SHEEP RED BLOOD CELLS TREATED WITH TANNIC ACID AND STH SO THAT STH HAS BEEN ADSORBED ON RED CELLS

STH ANTISERUM

AGGLUTINATION (VIEWED FROM BOTTOM OF TEST TUBE)

STH ANTISERUM + ADDITIONAL STH

NO AGGLUTINATION; STH ANTISERUM HAS BEEN TAKEN UP BY ADDITIONAL STH

ASSAY

TUBES CONTAINING STH–COATED RED CELLS PLUS STH ANTISERUM MIXED WITH SERIAL DILUTIONS OF

KNOWN AMOUNT OF STH — STANDARD

PATIENT'S SERUM (UNKNOWN) — EXCESS STH

PATIENT'S SERUM (UNKNOWN) — NORMAL STH

PATIENT'S SERUM (UNKNOWN) — ABSENT STH

GROWTH HORMONE ASSAY

An early immunologic method for the assay of growth hormone was the hemagglutination inhibition technique of Boyden. This immuno-assay provides a reliable method of measurement of human somatotropin when applied to purified preparations of the hormone and to crude anterior pituitary extract. However, the method has been found to be unreliable when applied to human serum, because of nonspecific factors, present in the serum, which induce hemagglutination inhibition. This nonspecific effect is apparently due to serum globulins which cannot easily be removed.

The species specificity of growth hormone makes it necessary to employ human growth, or *somatotropic, hormone* (*STH*) in the preparation of serum with a high antibody titer. Growth hormone mixed with Freund's adjuvant is administered subcutaneously to *rabbits* in three divided doses at 2-week intervals, and the animals are bled 6 weeks after the first injection. Hemagglutination titers of antibody sera from 1 in 32,000 to 1 in 64,000 are usually obtained. *Sheep red blood cells* are formalized and then treated with *tannic acid* before being coated with somatotropic hormone prior to use in the hemagglutination reaction. The mechanism of the *hemagglutination inhibition assay* involves the reaction of additional somatotropic hormone with the specific antiserum; thus, insufficient antiserum is left to react with the antigen coating the red blood cells, and *agglutination does not occur*.

It is possible to extract human growth hormone from acromegalic sera and thus separate it from the major portion of the serum proteins. In acromegaly the level of growth hormone ranges from 3.5 to 30 mμg per ml of serum. In normal extracted sera no growth hormone can be detected, which indicates that the normal level is below the lower limit of the range of sensitivity of the method, viz., 2 mμg per ml. Human somatotropin has been recovered by acid acetone extract of serum following intravenous administration of a single 5-mg. dose. The exogenous hormone was measurable in the serum for periods up to 2 hours. The half-life of exogenous somatotropin in the serum was approximately 40 minutes.

There is immunologic similarity between purified human somatotropin, obtained from normal pituitary glands,

and the hemagglutination-inhibiting activity present in the acid acetone fraction of the sera of acromegalics. Both exhibit the same quantitative relationship with antiserum to somatotropin, when varying concentrations of serum are used in the hemagglutination reaction. Unextracted human serum usually fails to show a similar quantitative relationship, indicating that the hemagglutination inhibition, produced by most human sera, is not due to growth hormone. Earlier workers in this field failed to take these factors into account and reported rather high levels, ranging from 10 to 30 mμg per ml in normal adult serum, with somewhat lower values in patients with pituitary insufficiency. The first clue to the unreliability of these earlier methods came from the finding of hemagglutination inhibition in moderately high titers in sera of hypophysectomized patients. Incomplete removal of the pituitary was eliminated as an expla-

nation, by careful histologic examination of the contents of the sella turcica in some of these cases. Nonspecific inhibition was the most reasonable explanation and has proved to be the case.

At this time the most reliable technique for estimating small quantities of STH in human serum appears to be the radio-immuno-assay developed by Roth, Glick, Yalow, and Berson (using the same technique as for the immuno-assay of insulin [see page 172]), based on the preparation of pure I[131] somatotropin by Greenwood and Hunter. Normal levels are from 1 to 5 mμg per ml, with rises from 10 to 50 mμg per ml in active acromegaly. Roth et al. have clearly shown that hypoglycemia leads to an acute rise in serum STH (up to twenty times normal levels), whereas starvation will raise it only three- to fivefold, and exercise variably. Thus, conditions must be carefully defined when reporting on levels.

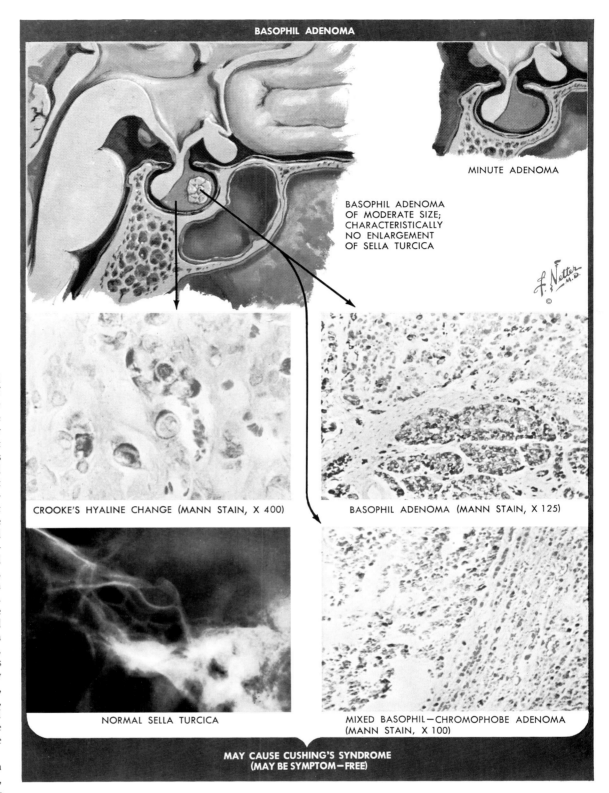

BASOPHIL ADENOMA

MINUTE ADENOMA

BASOPHIL ADENOMA
OF MODERATE SIZE;
CHARACTERISTICALLY
NO ENLARGEMENT
OF SELLA TURCICA

CROOKE'S HYALINE CHANGE (MANN STAIN, X 400)

BASOPHIL ADENOMA (MANN STAIN, X 125)

NORMAL SELLA TURCICA

MIXED BASOPHIL—CHROMOPHOBE ADENOMA
(MANN STAIN, X 100)

MAY CAUSE CUSHING'S SYNDROME
(MAY BE SYMPTOM—FREE)

BASOPHIL ADENOMA

Basophil adenomas are usually small tumors embedded in the parenchyma of the gland. They are uncommon but may be found in about 1 per cent of routine necropsies, particularly if the anterior lobe is sectioned at several levels. In most of these cases there are no symptoms referable to the pituitary or adrenal glands. The basophil adenoma is most frequently associated with Cushing's syndrome, although it is now agreed that the clinical features of the syndrome result from hyperfunction of the adrenal cortex. Cushing considered that the disorder was due primarily to a basophil adenoma of the anterior pituitary gland, although he recognized the contribution of the adrenal cortices in its expression. Many cases of Cushing's syndrome associated with bilateral adrenal cortical hyperplasia have been studied, in which there was no evidence of pituitary tumor, even at necropsy when the gland was serially sectioned. The recent discovery that certain nonendocrine neoplasms, such as carcinoma of the lung, pancreas, and ovary, may produce a type of ACTH explains the absence of a pituitary source for excessive ACTH in some of these cases.

In Cushing's syndrome, when an adenoma is present, it is usually small, and the *sella turcica* is *normal*. Sometimes, the adenoma is *minute* — not more than a few millimeters in diameter. Occasionally, it is sufficiently large to expand the sella turcica and even to give rise to defects of the visual pathway. The pituitary adenoma found in Cushing's syndrome is not always composed of basophilic cells. In some cases a *mixed basophil-chromophobe adenoma* has been reported; in others, a predominantly chromophobe tumor has been found. Rarely, sufficient nuclear pleomorphism and the invasive qualities of the tumor have justified the diagnosis of pituitary carcinoma.

Crooke observed a constant *change* in pituitary basophils, in cases of Cushing's syndrome, even when pituitary adenoma was absent. This consisted of the replace-

ment of most of the cytoplasmic granules by a homogeneous *hyaline* material. When an adenoma is present, the hyaline change tends to spare the basophils in the tumor and to involve, in varying degrees, most of the basophil cells of the rest of the gland. The earliest change is a crescentic loss of granularity separating a peripheral rim of granules from the juxtanuclear zone, which is the last place to become degranulated. Crooke's hyaline change has been found in Cushing's syndrome associated with adrenal tumor and also in patients treated with prolonged courses of ACTH or of cortisol and its analogues. It appears to be a regressive phenomenon induced in the subtype of basophil responsible for the production of ACTH or MSH by excessive prolonged circulating levels of cortisol.

Absence of Crooke's hyaline change should lead to serious doubt as to the diagnosis of Cushing's

syndrome. Recent experience with patients who have had total adrenalectomy for Cushing's syndrome, and who have subsequently developed an obvious progressive pituitary tumor, favors the pituitary origin of the disease in most of these cases. Also in keeping with this concept is the remission or improvement of symptoms which sometimes takes place after irradiation of the pituitary gland in previously untreated patients.

The rarity of basophil adenomas should be stressed. Small areas of basophil hyperplasia that do not compress the surrounding gland are sometimes considered basophil adenomas, but such a concept increases the incidence of these "tumors" to as high as 5 to 10 per cent of normal subjects. It would appear justifiable to reserve the diagnosis of basophil adenoma for a group of cells that show some evidence of compression of the surrounding gland.

PSYCHOGENIC STIMULI

PARAVENTRICULAR NUCLEUS OF HYPOTHALAMUS (SITE OF OXYTOCIN PRODUCTION)

OXYTOCIN MIGRATES ALONG NERVE FIBERS

OXYTOCIN PICKED UP BY PRIMARY PLEXUS OF PORTAL SYSTEM AND CARRIED BY PORTAL VEINS TO ADENOHYPOPHYSIS

OXYTOCIN STIMULATES OUTPUT OF PROLACTIN

OXYTOCIN PICKED UP BY CAPILLARIES OF POSTERIOR LOBE

PROLACTIN STIMULATES MILK PRODUCTION IN ENDOCRINOLOGICALLY PREPARED BREAST

OXYTOCIN CAUSES MILK EXPULSION

AFFERENT IMPULSES FROM NIPPLE

OXYTOCIN CAUSES UTERINE CONTRACTION

AFFERENT IMPULSES FROM CERVICAL DILATATION OR VAGINAL STIMULATION

SECRETION AND ACTION OF OXYTOCIN

Oxytocin is structurally very similar to vasopressin. Both contain 8 amino acid residues, but the amino acid sequence of oxytocin differs from that of vasopressin in two locations. Their structural similarities explain the overlapping biological properties. Vasopressin has considerable oxytocic potency, and oxytocin has a mild antidiuretic effect. Oxytocin exerts its physiological effect in an obstetrical setting. It is still a matter of controversy as to whether oxytocin has any physiological rôle in the control of renal hemodynamics and electrolyte excretion.

There is some circumstantial evidence supporting the suggestion that oxytocin is a humoral mediator which stimulates the *secretion* of *prolactin* in the *adenohypophysis;* under normal conditions, prolactin output is kept somewhat depressed by an inhibiting factor also of hypothalamic origin. When the *breast has been developed* as the result of the effects of estrogen, progesterone, prolactin, and growth hormone, the *secretion of milk* appears to be dependent on an additional increased pituitary secretion of *prolactin.* Emotional disturbances may adversely affect milk ejection, probably by a combination of a central nervous inhibition of the release of oxytocin, and by a peripheral effect of epinephrine, causing vasoconstriction of the mammary blood vessels and so preventing access of oxytocic hormone to the contractile myoepithelial tissue (see page 140).

A *neurohormonal reflex* is responsible for *milk ejection.* On the *afferent* side the stimuli travel from *sensory nerve endings* in the *nipple;* the *efferent* side is formed by *oxytocic hormone* in the blood stream. The *paraventricular nucleus* appears to be associated with the secretion of oxytocin, whereas the *supra-optic nucleus* is related mainly to vasopressin production. It is still unclear whether the neurohypophysis can release oxytocin independently from vasopressin. There is a latent period of about 30 seconds between the onset of active suckling and the commencement of milk flow. This latent period, which is much longer than the time required for a purely nervous reflex, is taken up by the release and transport

of oxytocin to the myo-epithelial cells of the breast, which form basketlike networks around individual alveoli and around the ducts. Stimulation of these contractile elements causes milk ejection.

Oxytocin appears to have a rôle in parturition, reinforcing uterine contractions. The mechanism of oxytocin's action on the uterus has been studied intensively. It appears to act on the membrane of the myometrial cell and not on the contractile myoplasm. Oxytocin increases membrane permeability to potassium, lowering the membrane potential and, thus, the excitability threshold. These observations suggest that, under the influence of oxytocin, a greater number of fibers respond to each spontaneous stimulus originating in any "pacemaker" of the intact uterus. In experimental animals, progesterone decreases the uterine response to oxytocin. In a study conducted on rabbits 8 to 48 hours after parturition,

Ferguson showed that mechanical *dilatation* of the body of the uterus, *cervix,* or *vagina stimulates* a nervous *reflex* release of oxytocic hormone and an increase in contractions of the body of the uterus. He suggested that the mechanism of labor involves a reflex stimulation of oxytocic secretion, probably in amounts varying with the part of the reproductive canal undergoing dilatation. There is a case report of expulsion of milk from the nipples of a woman in labor who was lactating from a previous pregnancy. The expulsion of milk coincided with the labor pains and was duplicated when posterior lobe extract was injected at the end of the second stage of labor.

Afferent impulses from vaginal stimulation during coitus may activate the release of oxytocin, which may have a rôle in the transport of sperm in the female genital tract after mating. Abnormal causes of galactorrhea are discussed on page 140.

SECRETION AND ACTION OF VASOPRESSIN

Vasopressin is antidiuretic and hypertensive by favoring arteriolar constriction. Increase of the osmotic pressure of the plasma stimulates *osmoreceptors* in the *anterior hypothalamus*. From such osmoreceptors or other cells stimulated by emotions or drugs such as nicotine, stimuli pass to the cells and fibers of the supraopticohypophysial tract. *Vasopressin*, or *antidiuretic hormone (ADH)*, appears to be formed in the neuronal cell bodies of the supra-optic nuclei of the *hypothalamus* and to be passed along the length of the axons in combination with a stainable carrier substance. Vasopressin is released at and stored near nerve endings in the median eminence, pituitary stalk, or neural lobe. These nerve fibers end in close relation to capillaries of the *neurohypophysis*. The released hormone thus enters the blood stream and reaches the kidney to exert its antidiuretic action.

The urinary changes produced by vasopressin are due solely to its action on the *renal tubules,* in which it increases reabsorption of water by reducing the intrinsic impermeability of the lower nephron to water without any effect on the tubular handling of solutes. In 24 hours *glomerular filtration* presents from 70 to 100 liters of fluid that is iso-osmotic with plasma to the *proximal convoluted tubule*. A deficiency of *adrenal glucocorticoids* (as in Addison's disease) will reduce glomeruler filtration and thereby produce a more concentrated urine. Other factors decreasing arterial blood pressure may produce a similar effect, thereby simulating the action of the antidiuretic hormone. Eighty-five per cent of the filtered water is *reabsorbed in the proximal tubule* without the help of vasopressin. This *passive* "obligatory" transfer of water is determined by the active reabsorption of solutes, particularly sodium and chloride taking along water by osmotic forces. Thus, proximal tubular urine remains iso-osmotic with plasma. In contrast, the distal tubular reabsorption of water is termed "active" or "facultative" and is controlled by the antidiuretic hormone. The *loop of Henle* has an important rôle in urine formation. These long, U-shaped loops form a hairpin-countercurrent concentrating system. The ascending, or *distal, limb* of Henle's loop actively transports sodium without water from the tubular urine to the interstitial fluid of the *renal medulla*, making it very hypertonic. The *impermeability* of this limb of Henle's loop to water

OSMORECEPTORS IN ANTERIOR PART OF HYPOTHALAMUS RESPOND TO BLOOD OSMOLALITY AND REGULATE PRODUCTION AND RELEASE OF ANTIDIURETIC HORMONE (VASOPRESSIN)

ANTIDIURETIC HORMONE DESCENDS NERVE FIBERS AND IS PICKED UP BY CAPILLARIES OF NEUROHYPOPHYSIS

WATER AND ELECTROLYTE EXCHANGE BETWEEN BLOOD AND TISSUES: NORMAL OR PATHOLOGICAL (EDEMA)

FLUID INTAKE (ORAL OR PARENTERAL)

WATER AND ELECTROLYTE LOSS VIA GUT (VOMITING, DIARRHEA); VIA CAVITIES (ASCITES, EFFUSION); OR EXTERNALLY (SWEAT, HEMORRHAGE)

ACTH

ADRENAL CORTICAL HORMONES

ANTIDIURETIC HORMONE (ADH OR VASOPRESSIN)

CIRCULATING BLOOD

80 TO 85% OF FILTERED WATER PASSIVELY REABSORBED IN PROXIMAL CONVOLUTED TUBULE DUE TO ACTIVE REABSORPTION OF SALTS, LEAVING 15 TO 20 LITERS PER DAY

APPROXIMATELY 70 TO 100 LITERS OF FLUID FILTERED FROM BLOOD PLASMA BY GLOMERULI IN 24 HOURS (FILTRATION PROMOTED BY ADRENAL CORTICAL HORMONES)

ANTIDIURETIC HORMONE MAKES DISTAL CONVOLUTED TUBULE PERMEABLE TO WATER AND THUS PERMITS IT TO BE REABSORBED ALONG WITH ACTIVELY REABSORBED SALT

ANTIDIURETIC HORMONE MAKES COLLECTING TUBULE PERMEABLE TO WATER, PERMITTING ITS REABSORPTION DUE TO HIGH OSMOLALITY OF RENAL MEDULLA

DISTAL LIMB OF HENLE'S LOOP IMPERMEABLE TO WATER; ACTIVELY REABSORBS SALT, CREATING HIGH OSMOLALITY OF RENAL MEDULLA

14 TO 18 LITERS REABSORBED DAILY UNDER INFLUENCE OF ANTIDIURETIC HORMONE, RESULTING IN 1 TO 2 LITERS OF URINE IN 24 HOURS

renders the urine entering the *distal tubule* hypotonic with respect to plasma. In the absence of vasopressin, the distal tubule and *collecting duct* remain largely impermeable to water, and very dilute urine leaves the kidney. Vasopressin renders these portions of the tubule permeable to water, which can thus pass from the tubular urine into interstitial fluid surrounding the distal segments of the nephron, producing a concentrated urine. Tissue experiments have suggested that vasopressin increases their permeability to water by increasing the size or number of cellular pores through which water traverses the epithelial cells. *Glucocorticoids* directly counteract the action of antidiuretic hormone on the collecting tubule and in the toad bladder, its experimental analogue, and are thus diuretic.

Excessive and "inappropriate" elaboration of antidiuretic hormone is sometimes found in the presence of certain carcinomas, notably bronchogenic ones. In such instances, or when too much ADH is administered chronically, an increased urinary sodium excretion results and hyponatremia ensues. There is no evidence that vasopressin acts directly to increase renal electrolyte loss. Increased blood volume, induced by the water-retaining effect of vasopressin, would tend to increase sodium excretion by inhibiting aldosterone secretion and also by increasing glomerular filtration.

Exogenous vasopressin has its greatest effect in diabetes insipidus and in water diuresis, which are circumstances of insufficient release of endogenous hormone. If endogenous release is already sufficient, *e.g.,* during the diuresis from hypertonic sodium chloride, then administration of vasopressin has little effect. There would appear to be a limited number of receptor sites with which the hormone can react.

DIABETES INSIPIDUS

Diabetes insipidus is a clinical condition characterized by *uncontrolled water diuresis, polyuria,* and polydipsia. However, it is frequently associated with other signs of hypothalamic and adenohypophysial diseases. The polyuria may occur abruptly or gradually. *Outputs* of 4 or 5 liters in 24 hours are more common than are the more severe 10- to 15-liter volumes. The specific gravity of the urine is usually 1.004 or less. Concentration, after withholding fluids, fails to occur, except in mild cases. A reduction in polyuria suggests combined adenohypophysial and neurohypophysial deficiency, since deficiency of *adrenal cortical hormones* (glucocorticoids) leads to a *decreased glomerular filtration* and to reduction in the tubular antagonism to vasopressin, which may still be secreted in small amounts.

The polyuria is primary, and thirst is essentially a compensatory symptom. Patients with diabetes insipidus often prefer ice-cold drinks, which is a distinguishing feature from other types of polyuria. Depression of the thirst mechanism, however, may follow administration of anesthetic or narcotic drugs or may be the result of a central nervous system disease. In these circumstances serious dehydration may develop quickly.

Interruption of the *hypothalamic* or *neurohypophysial tracts* frequently gives rise to a characteristic pattern of disturbed function, seen best in experimental animals. A "transient phase" of polyuria appears in a matter of hours and lasts for 1 to 6 days, followed by a so-called "normal interphase" with normal urine output, lasting about 5 days, and leading to the "permanent phase". The normal interphase is a period when the denervated neurohypophysis is undergoing atrophy, with resorption of the hormonal content in the gland, sufficient to maintain a normal urine volume.

Destruction of the neurohypophysial system may have a number of causes. *Craniopharyngioma,* especially of the suprasellar type, is a particularly common cause. Many patients develop diabetes insipidus only after surgical attempts to remove a pituitary tumor. Destruction of the osmoreceptor center by *metastatic carcinoma* may lead to a loss of vasopressin secretion in response to hyperosmolality, but with retention of the response to nicotine, which acts to release vasopressin by a different mechanism. *Syphilis* may cause diabetes insipidus, either in the secondary stage, with basal syphilitic meningitis, or late, by gummas

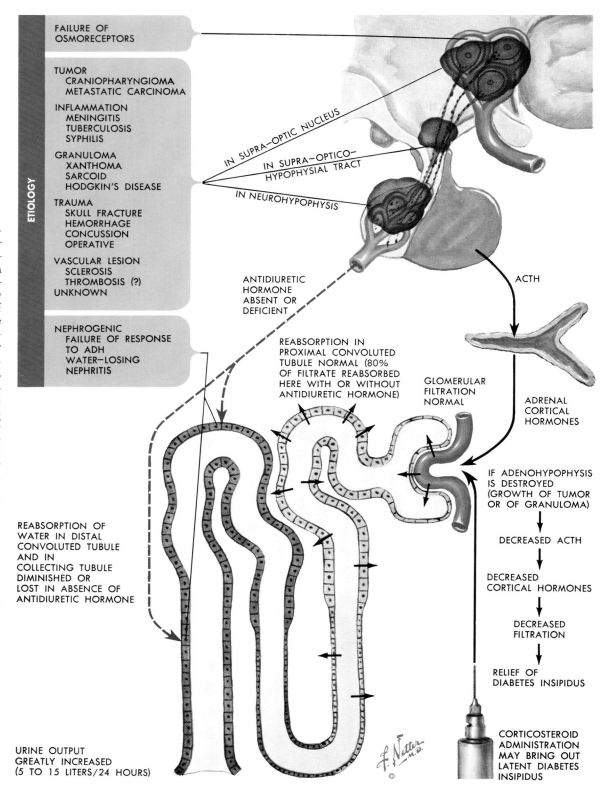

ETIOLOGY

FAILURE OF OSMORECEPTORS

TUMOR
CRANIOPHARYNGIOMA
METASTATIC CARCINOMA

INFLAMMATION
MENINGITIS
TUBERCULOSIS
SYPHILIS

GRANULOMA
XANTHOMA
SARCOID
HODGKIN'S DISEASE

TRAUMA
SKULL FRACTURE
HEMORRHAGE
CONCUSSION
OPERATIVE

VASCULAR LESION
SCLEROSIS
THROMBOSIS (?)
UNKNOWN

NEPHROGENIC
FAILURE OF RESPONSE TO ADH
WATER-LOSING NEPHRITIS

IN SUPRA-OPTIC NUCLEUS
IN SUPRA-OPTICO-HYPOPHYSIAL TRACT
IN NEUROHYPOPHYSIS

ANTIDIURETIC HORMONE ABSENT OR DEFICIENT

ACTH

REABSORPTION IN PROXIMAL CONVOLUTED TUBULE NORMAL (80% OF FILTRATE REABSORBED HERE WITH OR WITHOUT ANTIDIURETIC HORMONE)

GLOMERULAR FILTRATION NORMAL

ADRENAL CORTICAL HORMONES

IF ADENOHYPOPHYSIS IS DESTROYED (GROWTH OF TUMOR OR OF GRANULOMA)

DECREASED ACTH

DECREASED CORTICAL HORMONES

DECREASED FILTRATION

RELIEF OF DIABETES INSIPIDUS

REABSORPTION OF WATER IN DISTAL CONVOLUTED TUBULE AND IN COLLECTING TUBULE DIMINISHED OR LOST IN ABSENCE OF ANTIDIURETIC HORMONE

URINE OUTPUT GREATLY INCREASED (5 TO 15 LITERS/24 HOURS)

CORTICOSTEROID ADMINISTRATION MAY BRING OUT LATENT DIABETES INSIPIDUS

in or near the neural lobe. Lipoid *granulomas* of the Hand-Schüller-Christian variety are a cause of the disease in infancy, whereas *sarcoidosis* and *Hodgkin's disease* occur in adults. With *trauma,* the most common site of the lesion is a tear in the stalk. A rather large number of cases are relegated to the *idiopathic* category, many being presumably the result of subclinical encephalitis. Rarely, true diabetes insipidus due to vasopressin deficiency may be congenital and familial. In *nephrogenic diabetes insipidus,* a rare hereditary disorder which occurs in males and is transmitted as a sex-linked recessive gene, the child may not survive the critical period of infancy if sufficient water is not provided. In the recovery phase of acute tubular necrosis, after the sudden relief of ureteral obstruction, in hypercalcemia, and in hypokalemic nephropathy, damaged renal tubular cells show an inadequate response to antidiuretic hormone.

Whereas lack of vasopressin reduces urinary specific gravity to 1.004 or below, chronic renal failure usually fixes it at 1.010.

Treatment of diabetes insipidus is most satisfactorily achieved by the administration of a slowly absorbed form of posterior pituitary extract, such as vasopressin tannate in oil, yielding adequate hormone levels for about 36 to 48 hours following a single intramuscular injection of 0.5 to 1 ml. Posterior pituitary powder may be administered as a snuff at 4- to 6-hour intervals. Synthetic lysine vasopressin has been used successfully in a nasal spray for short-term control, especially in patients who are allergic to pituitary powder. The polyuria of nephrogenic diabetes insipidus and that of true diabetes insipidus due to lack of vasopressin may be decreased by the administration of chlorothiazide, which appears to act in this condition by reducing free water clearance.

TESTS FOR DIABETES INSIPIDUS

In patients with marked polydipsia and polyuria without glycosuria, the differential diagnosis usually lies between *diabetes insipidus* and *psychogenic polydipsia*. Most cases of diabetes insipidus are caused by a lack of *antidiuretic hormone (vasopressin)*, although, rarely, a congenital unresponsiveness of the renal tubule to vasopressin may be present. Psychogenic polydipsia in *compulsive water drinkers* is usually observed in emotionally disturbed persons, the cause being in the control of thirst rather than in secretion of vasopressin. In some cases of prolonged compulsive water drinking, the renal tubules become secondarily resistant to the effects of vasopressin, which complicates interpretation of diagnostic tests.

The neurohormonal unit responsible for vasopressin production and secretion includes the *supra-optic nuclei*, the *supra-opticohypophysial tract*, and the *neurohypophysis itself*. There are at least two routes of stimulation of vasopressin secretion by the neurohypophysis. One is through neuronal pathways leading to activation of hypothalamic nuclei by noxious agents, psychic stress, and drugs such as acetylcholine or nicotine. The other mechanism is by way of stimulation of "osmoreceptors" somewhere within the distribution of the internal carotid arteries by alterations in the osmotic pressure of the plasma.

The functional state of the neurohypophysial-renal system in patients with polyuria may be evaluated by serial *tests*, including the *intravenous administration of hypertonic saline* solution, *nicotine*, or *vasopressin* under constant water-loading conditions. Prior to carrying out the test, all antidiuretic therapy is discontinued until there is full return of the polydipsia and polyuria. Free access to water may be allowed. Thirty minutes after hydration has started with 20 ml of water per kilogram, urine specimens are collected at 15-minute intervals, measuring *urine flow* in milliliters per minute. After urine flow is greater than 15 ml per minute, the infusion of 3 *per cent sodium chloride* is given at the rate of

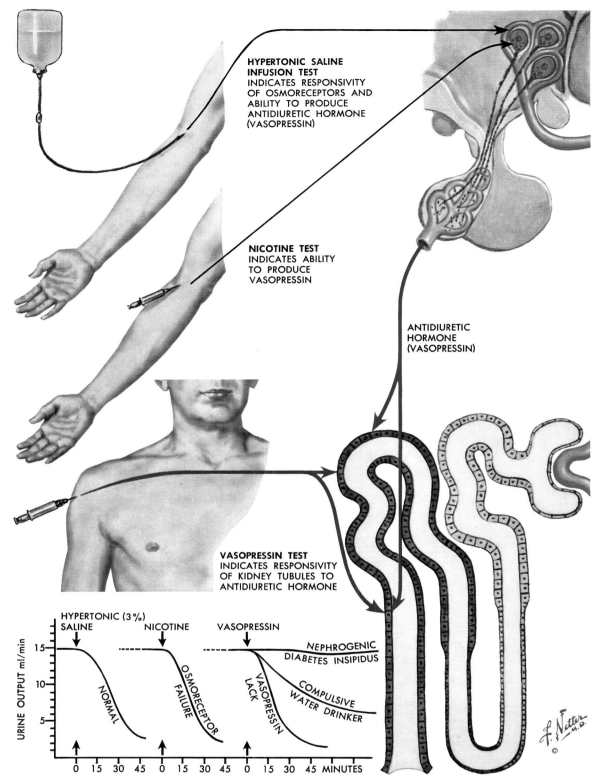

0.25 ml per kilogram per minute for 45 minutes. If no decrease in urine flow occurs during the infusion or in the first two postinfusion periods of 15 minutes each, *nicotine salicylate* solution is injected intravenously over a 3- to 5-minute period. It may be prepared by dissolving 185 mg of nicotine salicylate in 500 ml of 5 per cent dextrose in water, acidifying with 1 drop of 50 per cent sulfuric acid, and autoclaving it. Five milliliters of solution contain 1 mg of nicotine base. Usually, the dose is 1 mg of nicotine base for nonsmokers and 3 mg for smokers. Nicotine frequently causes nausea and vomiting in this test, and it should be used with caution. If nicotine causes no fall in the urine flow, then 0.1 *unit of vasopressin* is given intravenously. In normal individuals there is a decrease in urine volume during and following the administration of the hypertonic salt solution. This also occurs, but to a lesser extent, in patients

with psychogenic polydipsia. There is no response in true diabetes insipidus; in fact, there usually is a rise in urine flow. In patients with *osmoreceptor failure*, vasopressin may still be released in the circulation under the stimulus of nicotine, with a consequent fall in urine volume. Chronic water excess may decrease the response to both hypertonic saline and nicotine, and the urine volume may fail to decrease much on vasopressin injection. In nephrogenic diabetes insipidus no decrease whatever follows the injection of vasopressin.

More accurate information can be obtained by including determinations of total solute concentrations (osmolality) of urine and plasma measured by the freezing-point-depression technique. From these data, free water clearance can be calculated. A sharp decrease in free water clearance is an absolute indication of vasopressin action.

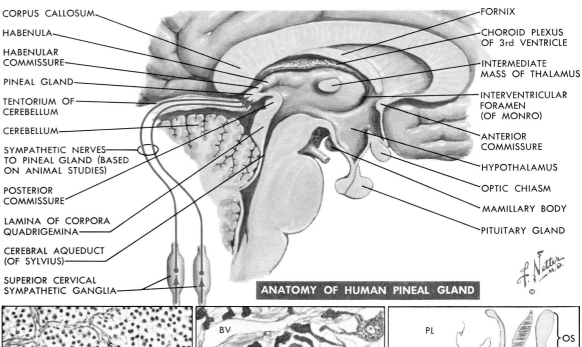

CORPUS CALLOSUM
HABENULA
HABENULAR COMMISSURE
PINEAL GLAND
TENTORIUM OF CEREBELLUM
CEREBELLUM
SYMPATHETIC NERVES TO PINEAL GLAND (BASED ON ANIMAL STUDIES)
POSTERIOR COMMISSURE
LAMINA OF CORPORA QUADRIGEMINA
CEREBRAL AQUEDUCT (OF SYLVIUS)
SUPERIOR CERVICAL SYMPATHETIC GANGLIA

FORNIX
CHOROID PLEXUS OF 3rd VENTRICLE
INTERMEDIATE MASS OF THALAMUS
INTERVENTRICULAR FORAMEN (OF MONRO)
ANTERIOR COMMISSURE
HYPOTHALAMUS
OPTIC CHIASM
MAMILLARY BODY
PITUITARY GLAND

ANATOMY OF HUMAN PINEAL GLAND

THE PINEAL GLAND

The mystery of the pineal body, or gland, resembles that of the thymus. Although anatomic details of both organs have been known for a long time, their physiologic rôles, until the past few years, have been obscure. Yet, the intensity of interest in these structures has been very great.

Mammals, birds, many fishes, and amphibians have a single *pineal*, or *epiphysis* cerebri, which is derived embryologically from the roof of the posterior portion of the diencephalon and is located deep in the brain as part of the epithalamus. However, in lower vertebrates it is necessary to think in terms of pineal organs or pineal systems instead of a single, discrete unit. In lizards the embryonic pineal structure is made up of two parts, which originate from the lateral edge of the anterior neural plate and, later, fuse into a single pineal mass. Subsequently, a second doubling may take place to form a dual pineal system. One part lies on the diencephalic roof and is the pineal. The second part is parapineal and may be derived as an outpouching from the pineal. It is very superficial, lying just beneath the *epidermis* of the head. In some *lizards* this pineal structure is highly differentiated into a small, eyelike organ, with *lens* and *retina*, and is called the *parietal*, or "third, *eye*". Thus, it is not surprising to find that, in various species, the two parts of the pineal system are made up of different kinds of cells. In mammals and birds the pineal gland is composed largely of *parenchymal cells* which may be secretory. In other forms many cells are photoreactive units. Soon after puberty, a diffuse calcification of the pineal commences. The *corpora arenacea*, or "brain sand", appear on histological sections. Sooner or later, the pineal becomes visible on a flat film and is an important X-ray landmark; any space-

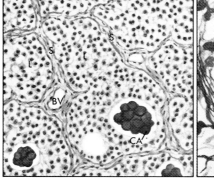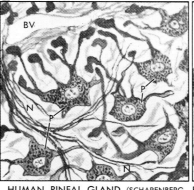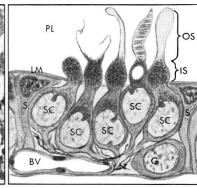

HUMAN PINEAL GLAND (H.+ E., X 50) L=LOBULE; S=SEPTUM; BV=BLOOD VESSEL; CA=CORPORA ARENACEA (CALCIFIED BODIES, "BRAIN SAND")

HUMAN PINEAL GLAND (SCHARENBERG MODIFICATION OF del RIO HORTEGA PREPARATION) P=PARENCHYMAL CELLS WITH CLUBLIKE PROCESSES AND (SECRETORY?) GRANULES; N=NERVE FIBRILS

FROG PINEAL GLAND (SCHEMATIC, AFTER KELLY AND van de KAMER) PL=PINEAL RECESS (LUMEN); OS= OUTER SEGMENTS; IS=INNER SEGMENTS OF PROTUBERANCES OF SC=SENSORY CELLS; S=SUPPORTIVE CELL; G= GANGLION CELL; N=NERVE FIBRILS; LM=LIMITING MEMBRANE

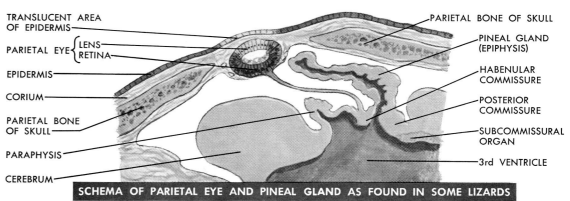

TRANSLUCENT AREA OF EPIDERMIS
PARIETAL EYE { LENS RETINA
EPIDERMIS
CORIUM
PARIETAL BONE OF SKULL
PARAPHYSIS
CEREBRUM

PARIETAL BONE OF SKULL
PINEAL GLAND (EPIPHYSIS)
HABENULAR COMMISSURE
POSTERIOR COMMISSURE
SUBCOMMISSURAL ORGAN
3rd VENTRICLE

SCHEMA OF PARIETAL EYE AND PINEAL GLAND AS FOUND IN SOME LIZARDS

occupying lesion of the central nervous system will displace the pineal image from the customary normal midline position in the anteroposterior view.

Because of the location of the pineal, its nerve supply was formerly thought to be that of the epithalamus, with afferents from the *habenular* and *posterior commissures*. It is now clear that the rat pineal receives its sole innervation from two large, *sympathetic nerve tracts* originating in the *superior cervical ganglia* and terminating directly on parenchymal cells.

In man the pineal gland is 8 mm long. Its fresh weight varies from 100 to 200 mg, its dry weight from 20 to 40 mg.

If it expands in size because of tumor formation, it may impinge on the *corpora quadrigemina* and compress the *cerebral aqueduct* (of Sylvius), thereby leading, relatively early, to internal hydrocephalus.

From a biochemical standpoint the pineal gland has unique features. It appears to be the only organ in which *melatonin* is made. The formation of melatonin from *serotonin* through N-acetyl serotonin and subsequent O-methylation takes place in the presence of *hydroxyindole-O-methyl transferase* (HIOMT). Like melatonin, HIOMT is made only in the pineal gland. This enzyme differs from catechol-O-methyl transferase (COMT) in that it is found only in or near the pineal gland; and it catalyzes the methylation of hydroxyindoles, whereas COMT is present in most cells and brings about methylation of epinephrine and norepinephrine. It is of interest that both enzymes catalyze the O-methylation of 5,6-dihydroxyindole, but HIOMT does this primarily at the 5 position and COMT at the 6 position. The presence of melatonin in peripheral nerves, where no HIOMT is found,

(Continued on page 37)

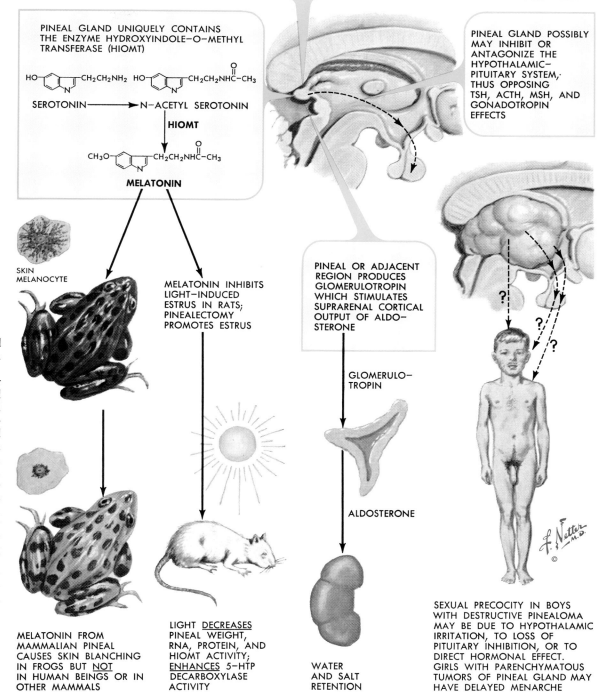

INTENSE METABOLIC ACTIVITY OF PINEAL GLAND INDICATED BY HIGH LEVELS OF NOREPINEPHRINE, SEROTONIN, MELATONIN, HISTAMINE, ACETYLCHOLINE, 5–METHOXYINDOLE AND 5–HYDROXYINDOLE ACETIC ACIDS, HIGH I^{131} UPTAKE, HIGH AMINO ACID PEPTIDASE AND SUCCINIC DEHYDROGENASE ACTIVITIES: THESE ARE NOT DECREASED BY PINEAL CALCIFICATION. BLOOD FLOW THROUGH PINEAL GLAND IS VERY GREAT (SECOND ONLY TO KIDNEY ON WEIGHT FOR WEIGHT BASIS)

PINEAL GLAND UNIQUELY CONTAINS THE ENZYME HYDROXYINDOLE–O–METHYL TRANSFERASE (HIOMT)

SEROTONIN ⟶ N–ACETYL SEROTONIN

HIOMT

MELATONIN

PINEAL GLAND POSSIBLY MAY INHIBIT OR ANTAGONIZE THE HYPOTHALAMIC–PITUITARY SYSTEM, THUS OPPOSING TSH, ACTH, MSH, AND GONADOTROPIN EFFECTS

SKIN MELANOCYTE

MELATONIN INHIBITS LIGHT–INDUCED ESTRUS IN RATS; PINEALECTOMY PROMOTES ESTRUS

PINEAL OR ADJACENT REGION PRODUCES GLOMERULOTROPIN WHICH STIMULATES SUPRARENAL CORTICAL OUTPUT OF ALDO-STERONE

GLOMERULO-TROPIN

ALDOSTERONE

MELATONIN FROM MAMMALIAN PINEAL CAUSES SKIN BLANCHING IN FROGS BUT NOT IN HUMAN BEINGS OR IN OTHER MAMMALS

LIGHT DECREASES PINEAL WEIGHT, RNA, PROTEIN, AND HIOMT ACTIVITY; ENHANCES 5–HTP DECARBOXYLASE ACTIVITY

WATER AND SALT RETENTION

SEXUAL PRECOCITY IN BOYS WITH DESTRUCTIVE PINEALOMA MAY BE DUE TO HYPOTHALAMIC IRRITATION, TO LOSS OF PITUITARY INHIBITION, OR TO DIRECT HORMONAL EFFECT. GIRLS WITH PARENCHYMATOUS TUMORS OF PINEAL GLAND MAY HAVE DELAYED MENARCHE

THE PINEAL GLAND

(Continued from page 36)

suggests that it is a neurohormone released by the pineal into the general circulation and subsequently taken up by nerves.

In addition to melatonin, many other biologically active substances are found in relatively large amounts in the pineal gland, including *norepinephrine, serotonin, 5-methoxyindole acetic acid* and *5-hydroxyindole acetic acid.* Even when the pineal undergoes partial *calcification,* these substances seem to be present in unchanged amounts. There is some evidence to support the view that tissues in or near the pineal structure contain *glomerulotropin*—a factor which may stimulate *aldosterone* release from the *suprarenal cortex,* thereby affecting *water and salt retention* (see page 95).

Blood flow through the pineal is very great, being second only to the kidney on a weight-for-weight basis. Radioiodine (I^{131}) and radiophosphorus (P^{32}) are taken up faster by the pineal gland than by any other part of the brain. The iodine uptake, on a per-gram basis, is second only to that of the thyroid gland, and in hypophysectomized animals it is greater than that of any other organ, including the thyroid.

A great amount of investigative work is being carried out on the relationship of the pineal and light exposure to neuroendocrine systems. When male or female *rats* are exposed to *increased light,* the following changes occur in the pineal: (1) decrease in *pineal weight, HIOMT, serotonin, RNA synthesis,* glycogen, and succinic dehydrogenase activity; (2) no change in ATP, P^{32} uptake, and monamine oxidase activity; and (3) increase in *5-hydroxytryptophan decarboxylase activity.* Light also produces other changes in the female rat: (1) decrease in adrenal size and melatonin uptake by the ovaries, and (2) increase in ovarian weight and incidence of estrus. *Pinealectomy* appears to produce the same effect

as exposing the animals to light. In addition, pinealectomy in the rat fetus results in marked changes in the lower ileum, the epithelial cells becoming filled with distinct acidophilic inclusions.

Melatonin is the most potent *skin-lightening agent* known for *frogs,* tadpoles, and some other animals. However, melatonin seems to have *no effect on human* or guinea-pig *melanocytes.* The blanching effect is opposite to the melanin-dispersing, pigmentary effect of melanocyte-stimulating hormone and ACTH, both of pituitary origin. Thus, in frogs, pigmentation is affected in opposite fashion by the epiphysis and the hypophysis.

Administration of melatonin to rats produces some changes opposite those following exposure to light or pinealectomy; that is, *melatonin inhibits ovarian growth and the incidence of estrus.* It is not known if melatonin or increased light exposure produces

similar changes in human beings treated the same.

Consistent with these findings is the observation that *girls with parenchymatous pineal tumors* have a significant *delay* in the onset of their *menarche.* On the other hand, *boys* with *destructive pinealomas* may have *precocious sexual development.* Not all pineal tumors associated with endocrine symptoms are large. Cases have been described of precocity with small tumors. Thus, it would appear that secretions from the pineal could inhibit the elaboration or secretion of anterior pituitary gonadotropins. How many of these phenomena may be ascribed to this mechanism, as opposed to the effects of an irritation of neighboring centers by pineal tumors, remains to be established.

From all these studies, much evidence has emerged to suggest that the pineal gland plays an important rôle in neuro-endocrine control in mammals.

Section II

THE THYROID GLAND
THE PARATHYROID GLANDS

by

FRANK H. NETTER, M.D.

in collaboration with

OLIVER COPE, M.D.
Plates 1 and 2

E. S. CRELIN, Ph.D.
Plates 3 and 4

RULON W. RAWSON, M.D.
Plates 5-33

ANATOMY OF THE THYROID AND PARATHYROID GLANDS

The therapy of thyroid disease, in general, is in transition from surgical to medical, and the internist must be able to determine with great certainty the type of presenting lesion before he can decide which therapy to apply. Parathyroid disease is more common than was anticipated 25 years ago, and it behooves both internist and surgeon to be alert to the most intimate aspects of neck anatomy.

In the upper drawing (Plate 1) the skin, subcutaneous fat, and *platysma muscle* have been excised, exposing, on the right half of the neck, the anterior or first cervical fascia. This fascia envelops the *external* and *anterior jugular veins* and the *transverse cervical nerves.* The subcutaneous fat and platysma muscle contain a rich blood supply, so that wide surgical exposures may be obtained, without sacrificing skin, by raising flaps of skin, subcutaneous fat, and platysma. The veins and nerves thus exposed are left initially in situ, to be moved later with the muscles beneath.

On the left side of the neck (upper drawing), the first cervical fascia, the external jugular vein, the transverse nerves, and the *sternocleidomastoid muscle* have been excised. This excision shows the positions of the *omohyoid muscle,* the *ansa hypoglossal nerve,* the important limiting insertion of the shorter inner pretracheal muscle, the *sternothyroid muscle,* and the entire course of the longer *thyrohyoid muscle.* The same fascial layer has been incised down the midline, exposing the medial borders of the *sternohyoid muscle.* These muscles, normally meeting together in the midline, have been partially retracted to expose the *thyroid* and *cricoid cartilages,* the *isthmus of the thyroid,* and the *upper trachea* lying beneath. The anterior jugular veins supplement the external jugular vein in returning the blood from the mouth and upper neck. They also receive tributaries throughout their length: first, from the platysma superficial to them; second, from the pretracheal muscles (sternohyoid, sternothyroid, and omohyoid) deep to them; and third, at the level of the larynx, particularly at the notch, from several fine tributaries from the upper larynx near the midline. In exposing the thyroid and parathyroid glands and the trachea, it is important to save as many of these vessels as possible by retracting them rather than dividing them, in order to avoid unnecessary edema of the upper neck and larynx. These anterior veins may be greatly dilated when tumors of the thyroid or other organs deep in the neck have pressed on one or another of the internal jugular veins.

The transverse cervical nerves may be severed with impunity, since they are sensory only and will regenerate. Not so the two *lower branches of the facial nerve.* Transection of the marginal man-

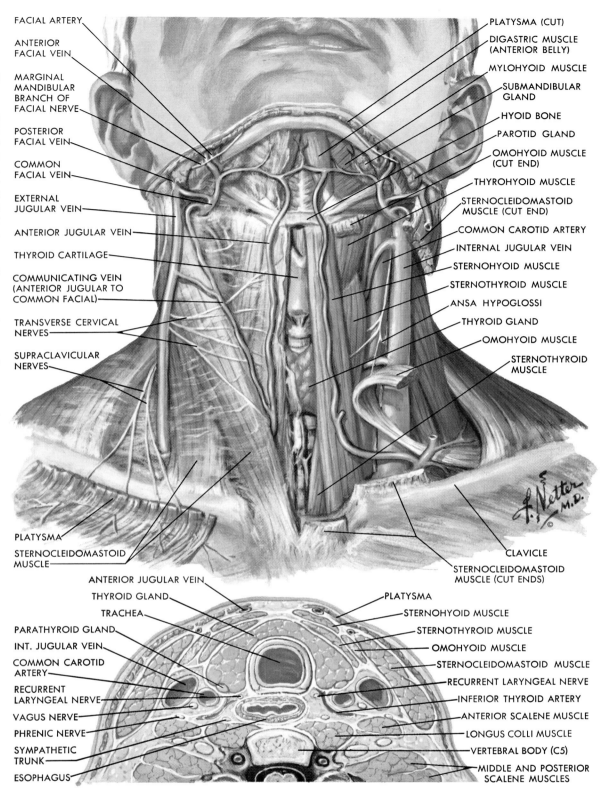

dibular branch is followed by drooping of the lower lip on the paralyzed side. The ansa hypoglossal nerve, lying along the anterior medial aspect of the carotid sheath, is to be preserved. In exposing the nerve, it is helpful to remember that a small branch of the superior thyroid artery comes down just in front of the nerve, delivering branches to the posterior edge of the muscle as well as supplying the nerve. Division of this nerve renders swallowing more difficult after operation.

The lymphatic vessels in the superficial fascia, anterior to the prethyroid muscles, are not prominent. Lymph nodes are rare; the first one consistently encountered lies immediately in front of the thyroid isthmus in the midline between the pretracheal muscles, deep to the anterior fascia and superficial to the second or middle cervical fascia, the false capsule of the thyroid. This node drains the pharynx or

larynx but not the thyroid gland or deeper tissues beneath. It is thus enlarged in patients with acute pharyngitis and laryngitis but not in thyroiditis or tracheitis.

Exposure of the *thyroid, parathyroids,* and *thymus glands* is achieved by retracting the pretracheal or prethyroid muscles. Widest exposure is obtained if the muscles are cut transversely and the ends retracted up and down. A good view of the upper thyroid pole often requires transection of the inner muscle.

The position of the esophagus, shown slightly to the left of the midline, is occasioned by the usually somewhat larger right lobe of the thyroid.

The upper drawing (Plate 2) depicts the organs of the neck and anterior superior mediastinum with the anterior neck muscles and the bones of the upper thorax removed.

(Continued on page 42)

ANATOMY OF THE THYROID AND PARATHYROID GLANDS

(Continued from page 41)

When the *thyroid,* parathyroid, and thymus glands are first exposed, they lie enveloped on their anterior, lateral, and posterior surfaces by an ill-defined loose areolar fascia (also called the false capsule of the thyroid) which permits the glands, larynx, and trachea to rise and fall with swallowing.

The normal thyroid gland is nearly always asymmetric. The *right lobe* may be even twice as large as the *left.* The right upper pole extends higher up in the neck, and the lower pole lower. In a patient with dextrocardia, lobe size is reversed.

Four developmental anomalies are to be noted. A *pyramidal lobe* persists, in at least 15 per cent of the population, becoming enlarged if the thyroid is enlarged by a diffuse process. It is occasionally the site or origin of a malignant tumor. The second anomaly is the failure of globs of thyroid tissue to be contained within the main thyroid mass posteriorly, in at least 5 per cent of the people. Their separateness may, on physical examination, give rise to suspicion of a tumor. The third and fourth anomalies are the failure of the isthmus to fuse in the midline and the absence of a significant part of the lateral lobe, notably the lower half of the left lobe. These are rare, occurring in less than 1 per cent of the population. When the isthmus fails to fuse, the medial aspects of the lateral lobes may feel like tumors, but palpating the tracheal rings where the isthmus should be will give the clue. Similarly, absence of the lower half of a lateral lobe may lead to the mistaken impression that the upper half is a tumor.

The lower drawing is a lateral view of the organs of the right side of the neck, with the neck muscles, right clavicle, and sternum removed.

The position and size of the normal *parathyroids* are variable. Usually, there are four — two upper and two lower. Rarely, there is a fifth, which the surgeon may need to find if it is the seat of an adenoma or is involved in hyperplasia.

The *upper glands* are more constant and circumscribed in position than the lower, often significantly larger, and, therefore, easier to find. They lie in the plane behind the thyroid, from the upper thyroid pole to the lower branches of the *inferior thyroid artery.* When enlarged by disease, they may be displaced downward into the posterior mediastinum.

The *lower glands,* arising from a branchial cleft higher than the upper glands and associated, in their embryologic descent, with the thymus, are found over a much wider extent — above or behind the thyroid, and down into the anterior mediastinum as far as thymic tissue is found.

The lymphatic vessels and *nodes,* in the upper drawing, follow a consistent pattern. The most readily felt and the first encountered are those in the midline

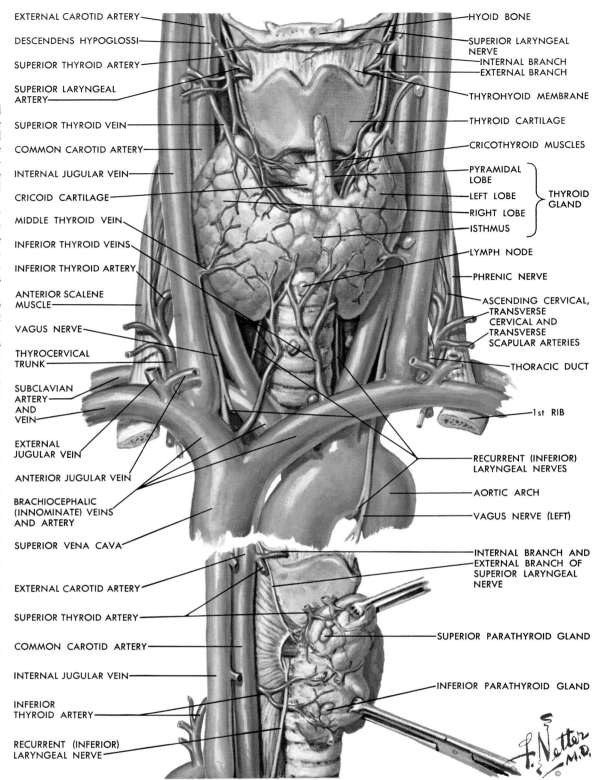

in front. The uppermost, just above the *thyroid isthmus,* in front of the *cricoid cartilage,* and medial to a pyramidal lobe, if present, is a constant node group of one to five nodes, which has been dubbed the Delphian node. If involved in cancer or Hashimoto thyroiditis, it may be felt preoperatively. The pretracheal nodes below the thyroid isthmus are harder to identify, because they are embedded in fat and not so constant in position as the Delphian. The other node groups, in the order of operative importance, are those on the lateral thyroid surface along the lateral thyroid vein, the nodes along the upper stretch of the *recurrent laryngeal nerve* behind the thyroid lobe, those at the angle of the jaw, those along the carotid sheath (jugular chain), and the more lateral nodes in the supraclavicular fossa. The sentinel nodes of Virchow are the lowermost of the jugular chain at the upper end of the *thoracic duct.*

These nodes may be involved with thyroid and parathyroid carcinoma as well as with abdominal cancers.

The *laryngeal* motor *nerves* are well depicted in both drawings. The *superior* nerve carries the motor branch to the *cricothyroid muscle.* This muscle tenses the vocal cord by drawing the front of the *thyroid cartilage* down on the cricoid. Fuzziness of the voice follows section of the nerve, particularly if the injury is bilateral.

The different sites of origin of the two *inferior* or *recurrent laryngeal nerves* induce a different course for the nerve on either side. The *right nerve* passes diagonally from lateral to medial on its upward course, but the *left* is thrown by the *aortic arch,* at its inception, against the trachea and esophagus and comes straight up in the tracheo-esophageal groove. This constant course makes it the easier of the two to find.

DEVELOPMENT OF THE THYROID AND PARATHYROID GLANDS

Pharynx By the beginning of the second month of embryonic development, the portion of the originally tubular entodermal foregut caudal to the *buccopharyngeal* (oral) *membrane* has differentiated into the *pharynx* (see CIBA COLLECTION, Vol. 3/II, pages 2, 3, 4, and 5). At this time, the pharynx is relatively wide, is compressed dorsoventrally, and has, on each side, a series of four lateral outpocketings, the *pharyngeal pouches* (A and B). Each pouch is in close relationship to an *aortic arch* and is situated opposite a *branchial cleft* (gill furrow) (A).

In certain aquatic forms, the tissue, in the depths of the branchial clefts and at the extremities of the pharyngeal pouches, disintegrates to produce communications (the gill slits) between the pharyngeal cavity and the surface of the body. Even though gill slit formation is slurred over in man, persistent gill slits can occur. The anomaly may be a slender, epithelially lined tract (*branchial* or cervical *fistula*) that extends from the pharyngeal cavity to an opening near the *auricle* (first pouch) or onto the *neck* (second and third pouches) (see Plate 4). When the anomaly is less extensive, it is either a cervical diverticulum or an epithelially lined cervical cyst. A blind diverticulum may extend either outward from the pharynx, for a variable distance, or inward from the neck. A cyst may be located at one site or another in the depths of the neck, causing no trouble unless it becomes infected or filled with fluid, in postnatal life.

The central lumen of the embryonic pharynx gives rise to the *adult pharynx* (see Plate 4). The first, or most cephalic, pair of pharyngeal pouches gives rise to the *auditory* (Eustachian) *tubes*, to the *tympanic* (middle ear) *cavities*, and to the mucous membrane lining the inner surface of each *tympanum*. The first branchial clefts, located opposite the first pouches, give rise to the *external acoustic* (auditory) *meatuses* and to the outer epithelial lining of each eardrum. The second pouches give rise to the *epithelium lining the palatine tonsils*. The latter pouches are, for the most part, absorbed into the pharyngeal wall, persisting only as pharyngeal outpocketings by contributing to the formation of the *supratonsillar fossae* (see Plate 4).

Thyroid Gland At a level between the first and second pharyngeal pouches, a saclike entodermal diverticulum (the thyroid sac) appears in the midline of the ventral surface of the pharynx. This sac, destined to give rise to the parenchyma of the *thyroid gland* (A), is the first glandular derivative of the pharynx. When it appears, near the end of the fourth week, it almost immediately becomes bilobated, and a narrow, hollow neck connects the two lobes. This neck is known as the

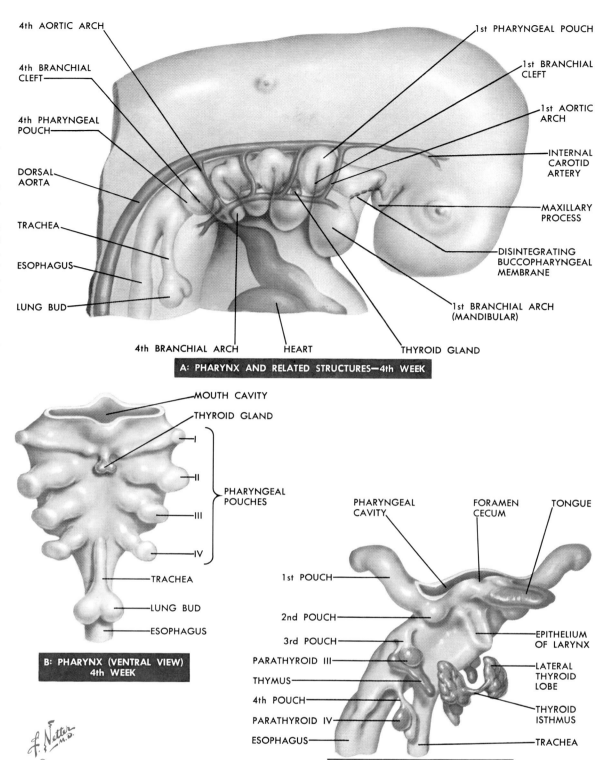

4th AORTIC ARCH
4th BRANCHIAL CLEFT
4th PHARYNGEAL POUCH
DORSAL AORTA
TRACHEA
ESOPHAGUS
LUNG BUD
1st PHARYNGEAL POUCH
1st BRANCHIAL CLEFT
1st AORTIC ARCH
INTERNAL CAROTID ARTERY
MAXILLARY PROCESS
DISINTEGRATING BUCCOPHARYNGEAL MEMBRANE
1st BRANCHIAL ARCH (MANDIBULAR)
4th BRANCHIAL ARCH   HEART   THYROID GLAND

A: PHARYNX AND RELATED STRUCTURES—4th WEEK

MOUTH CAVITY
THYROID GLAND
I
II
PHARYNGEAL POUCHES
III
IV
TRACHEA
LUNG BUD
ESOPHAGUS

B: PHARYNX (VENTRAL VIEW) 4th WEEK

PHARYNGEAL CAVITY   FORAMEN CECUM   TONGUE
1st POUCH
2nd POUCH
3rd POUCH
PARATHYROID III
THYMUS
4th POUCH
PARATHYROID IV
ESOPHAGUS
EPITHELIUM OF LARYNX
LATERAL THYROID LOBE
THYROID ISTHMUS
TRACHEA

C: PHARYNX AND DERIVATIVES (BETWEEN 6th AND 7th WEEKS)

thyroglossal duct, because its pharyngeal attachment is located where the ventral floor of the pharynx contributes to the formation of the tongue. The duct becomes a solid stalk and begins to atrophy by the sixth week; however, its pharyngeal connection results in a permanent pit, the *foramen cecum,* at the apex of the V-shaped sulcus terminalis on the dorsum of the *tongue* (see C and Plate 4).

The thyroid sac is converted into a solid mass of cells by the time the thyroglossal stalk disappears. By the end of the seventh week, the developing thyroid becomes crescentic in shape and is relocated to a position at the level of the developing *trachea* (C). This relocation occurs because the thyroid is left behind as the pharynx grows forward. At this time the thyroid's *two* (lateral) *lobes,* one on each side of the trachea, are connected in the midline by a very narrow *isthmus* of developing thyroid tissue (C).

The formation of thyroid follicles begins during the eighth week of development. They acquire colloid by the third month. By the end of the fourth month, new follicles arise only by the budding and subdivision of those already present. The mesenchyma, surrounding the thyroid primordium, differentiates into the stroma of the gland and its thin proper fibro-elastic capsule.

The thyroglossal duct may persist either as an epithelial tract, which is open from the foramen cecum of the tongue to the level of the larynx, or as a series of blind pockets (thyroglossal duct cysts) (see Plate 4). Persistent portions of the duct or stalk may give rise to accessory thyroids or to a median fistula which opens onto the neck. When a portion of the *thyroglossal duct persists* at the level of the *hyoid bone,* it passes through the body of the bone (see Plate 4).

(*Continued on page 44*)

DEVELOPMENT OF THE THYROID AND PARATHYROID GLANDS

(*Continued from page 43*)

The variably occurring *pyramidal lobe* of the thyroid results from the retention and growth of the lower end of the stalk. A ligament or a band of muscle, usually located to the left of the midline, may connect the pyramidal lobe either to the thyroid cartilage or to the hyoid bone. The pyramidal lobe undergoes gradual atrophy; therefore, it is found more often in children than in adults.

Other variations of the thyroid gland are as follows: The isthmus may be voluminous, rudimentary, or absent. The lateral lobes may be of different sizes, or both may be absent, with only the isthmic portion present. The shape of the gland may be more like that of an **H** than that of a horseshoe **U**. Rarely, the gland may be located at the base of the tongue or deep to the sternum. Complete absence of the gland or failure of the gland to function is seldom noticed until a few weeks after birth, because the fetus is supplied, through the placenta, with sufficient maternal thyroid hormone to permit normal development. If proper hormonal treatment is not instituted after birth, the result is cretinism (see page 61).

Parathyroid and Thymus Glands

During the fifth and sixth weeks of development, the entodermal epithelium of the dorsal portions of the distal ends of the *third* and *fourth pharyngeal pouches* differentiates into the *primordia* of the *parathyroid glands*. At the same time, the ventral portions of the distal ends of the *third pouches* differentiate into the *primordia* of the *thymus gland* (see Plate 3, C). The ventral portions of the distal ends of the fourth pouches may give rise to thymic primordia, which soon disappear without contributing to the adult thymus.

Usually, two pairs of parathyroid glands are formed. Because of their origin, those arising from the third pouches are designated as *parathyroids III*, and those from the fourth pouches as *parathyroids IV* (see Plate 3, C). By the end of the sixth week, the primordia of the parathyroids and thymus lose their connection with the pouches. At this time, the lumen of the third and fourth pouches becomes obliterated. Parathyroids III and the thymic primordia migrate, during the seventh week, in a caudomedial direction. During the eighth week, the lower ends of the thymic primordia enlarge and become superficially fused together in the midline. This bilobated lower end continues to descend, to be located in the superior mediastinum of the thorax, posterior to the *manubrium*. During this descent the upper ends of the thymic primordia are drawn out into taillike extensions which usually disappear. Occasionally, they *persist* as fragments embedded in the thyroid gland or as isolated *thymic* nests or *cords*.

Parathyroids III migrate with the thy-

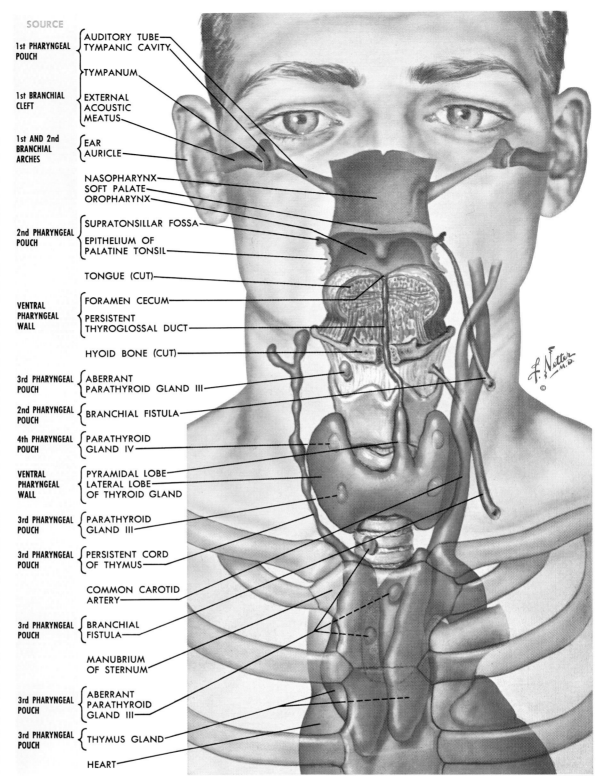

SOURCE	
1st PHARYNGEAL POUCH	AUDITORY TUBE, TYMPANIC CAVITY
	TYMPANUM
1st BRANCHIAL CLEFT	EXTERNAL ACOUSTIC MEATUS
1st AND 2nd BRANCHIAL ARCHES	EAR AURICLE
	NASOPHARYNX, SOFT PALATE, OROPHARYNX
2nd PHARYNGEAL POUCH	SUPRATONSILLAR FOSSA
	EPITHELIUM OF PALATINE TONSIL
	TONGUE (CUT)
VENTRAL PHARYNGEAL WALL	FORAMEN CECUM
	PERSISTENT THYROGLOSSAL DUCT
	HYOID BONE (CUT)
3rd PHARYNGEAL POUCH	ABERRANT PARATHYROID GLAND III
2nd PHARYNGEAL POUCH	BRANCHIAL FISTULA
4th PHARYNGEAL POUCH	PARATHYROID GLAND IV
VENTRAL PHARYNGEAL WALL	PYRAMIDAL LOBE, LATERAL LOBE OF THYROID GLAND
3rd PHARYNGEAL POUCH	PARATHYROID GLAND III
3rd PHARYNGEAL POUCH	PERSISTENT CORD OF THYMUS
	COMMON CAROTID ARTERY
3rd PHARYNGEAL POUCH	BRANCHIAL FISTULA
	MANUBRIUM OF STERNUM
3rd PHARYNGEAL POUCH	ABERRANT PARATHYROID GLAND III
3rd PHARYNGEAL POUCH	THYMUS GLAND
	HEART

mic primordia and, usually, come to rest at the caudal level of the thyroid gland, to become the *inferior parathyroid glands* of the adult. Situated within the cervical fascial sheath of the thyroid, they are attached to the back of the proper capsule of each lateral thyroid lobe; however, each has its own proper capsule. Occasionally, parathyroids III descend with the thymic primordia to a lower level, being *located in the thorax, close to the thymus*.

Parathyroids IV do not shift their position appreciably; therefore, parathyroids III pass them in their caudal migration to a lower level. Thus, parathyroids IV become the *superior parathyroid glands* of the adult, located within the fascial sheath of the thyroid, attached to the back of the proper capsule of each lateral thyroid lobe at the level of the lower border of the cricoid cartilage. Variations in the number, size, and location of the parathyroids are common.

Both the regularly occurring and accessory glands may be situated at some distance from the thyroid.

The parathyroids produce parathyroid hormone, which maintains the normal relation between the blood and the skeletal calcium (see page 178).

The thymus is a conspicuous organ in the infant. At about 2 years of age, it attains its largest relative size, continuing to grow until puberty. It undergoes a gradual involution after puberty, as the thymic tissue is replaced by fat. Therefore, in the adult the thymus is of approximately the same form and size as during the earlier years, but it now consists chiefly of adipose tissue. Since thymic tissue, in the young child, consists primarily of lymphocytes, previously its only established function was that of lymphocyte production; however, it recently has been shown to play an essential rôle in the development of the immunological, antibody-producing system of the body.

ABERRANT AND
NORMAL LOCATIONS
OF THYROID TISSUE

LINGUAL
INTRALINGUAL
THYROGLOSSAL TRACT
SUBLINGUAL
THYROGLOSSAL CYST
PRELARYNGEAL
NORMAL
INTRATRACHEAL
SUBSTERNAL

CONGENITAL ANOMALIES OF THE THYROID GLAND

Aberrant, or abnormal, *locations of thyroid tissue* in man may be explained on the basis of abnormal embryological migration of the thyroid and of its close association with lateral thyroid anlagen. These abnormal settings of thyroid tissue can better be understood if one considers the embryology of the thyroid gland, which, in the human being, arises about the seventeenth day of gestation and is derived from the alimentary tract (see page 43). The median part of the thyroid is formed from the ventral evagination of the floor of the pharynx, at the level of the first and second pharyngeal pouches. Although some controversy exists, most investigations indicate that the lateral thyroid anlage, from the area of the fourth pouch, becomes incorporated into the median thyroid anlage to contribute a small proportion of the final thyroid parenchyma. The thyroid anlage becomes elongated and enlarges laterally, with the pharyngeal region contracting to become a narrow stalk, the *thyroglossal tract* or duct. This subsequently atrophies, leaving, at its point of origin on the tongue, a depression known as the foramen cecum. Normally, the thyroid continues to grow and simultaneously migrates caudally.

The anatomical sites for the location of anomalously formed thyroid tissue range from the posterior tongue down into the region of the heart, within the mediastinum. Persistence of thyroid tissue on the posterior tongue is a fairly uncommon anomaly known as *lingual thyroid.* This may be the only source of thyroid tissue in the individual. It can often be demonstrated with radioactive iodine techniques and *scintigrams,* revealing the localization of radio-iodine only within the lingual thyroid, without any being demonstrated in the neck.

LINGUAL THYROID

SCINTIGRAM; LINGUAL THYROID

Intralingual and *sublingual rests* of thyroid tissue have been described, but these are quite uncommon.

In the adult form of some species, the thyroglossal tract persists, but in man it usually atrophies completely. Not infrequently, however, it may fail to atrophy, remaining as a cystic mass in the midline of the neck, somewhere between the base of the tongue and the hyoid bone. A *thyroglossal cyst* should, therefore, be considered in any individual presenting an enlarging cystic mass immediately beneath the chin in the midline. Occasionally, such cysts may be associated with thyroid tissue capable of concentrating radioactive iodine.

Substernal aberrant thyroid tissue in the mediastinum is rarely the consequence of abnormal development, representing glandular rests remaining from the time of the caudal descent of the thyroid. Most often, it results from a downward growth of a nodular

goiter. *Prelaryngeal thyroid tissue* may exist, being attached to a very long pyramidal lobe or to a thyroglossal cyst. *Intratracheal thyroid rests* have also been reported, though infrequently. The "lateral aberrant thyroid" may represent original branchial tissue which did not fuse with the median thyroid. However, the demonstration of microscopic carcinoma, in the thyroids of some patients with so-called lateral aberrant thyroid tissue, suggests that, in most instances, these may actually be metastases from a low-grade, well-differentiated thyroid carcinoma.

The medical significance of aberrant thyroid tissue is quite limited. Occasionally, an inflammatory change or, rarely, enlargement and consequent thyrotoxicity will call for surgical or radiotherapeutic intervention. The exact interpretation of these lesions necessitates an understanding of their embryological derivation.

EFFECTS OF THYROTROPIC HORMONE ON THE THYROID GLAND

The anterior pituitary gland plays an indispensable rôle in the regulation of thyroid function. Removal of the pituitary leads to *diminished thyroid mass* and *decreased production* and *secretion* of *thyroid hormones,* but administration of adequate amounts of pituitary extracts to hypophysectomized animals restores the structure and function of the thyroid to a *normal* state. Administration of *excessive* amounts of *pituitary extracts* to hypophysectomized or intact animals results in an *increased thyroid mass* with hypertrophied and hyperplastic thyroids, which *synthesize* and *secrete* thyroid hormones in excess.

The pituitary hormone, which has the thyroid as its target, is known variously as the *thyrotropic,* thyrotrophic, or thyroid-stimulating hormone (TSH). Notwithstanding the efforts of many investigators, attempts to clarify the actions and mechanisms of action of TSH are hampered by the fact that the work is still being conducted with an impure or nonhomogeneous protein complex, which probably is contaminated with many other pituitary hormones. The administration of TSH to responsive animals, *e.g.,* day-old chicks, results in a series of changes which occur in the following order: *loss of thyroid hormonal iodine,* increase in thyroid mean cell height, as they become *columnar; increased uptake of* I^{131}; and, then, an increased thyroid mass, in spite of marked *loss of colloid.* It has been suggested that the first and, possibly, primary actions of TSH are to activate proteolytic enzymes (which hydrolyze thyroglobulin and thus promote the secretion of thyroxine and of 3,5,3'-tri-iodo-L-thyronine into the circulation) and to stimulate or activate the thyroid iodide trap. The increased growth of the thyroid cell may be due to a primary effect of the hormone molecule on the thyroid cell, or it may be secondary to the secretory effects of the hormone. Efforts to demonstrate, with in vitro systems, the direct effects of TSH on the proteolytic systems or on the iodide trap have been unrewarding. Thus, it has been postulated that TSH activates one or more oxidative enzyme systems necessary to the functions of the thyroid cell. Studies done with very crude pituitary extracts, rich in thyroid-stimulating activity, have demonstrated that such preparations are also capable

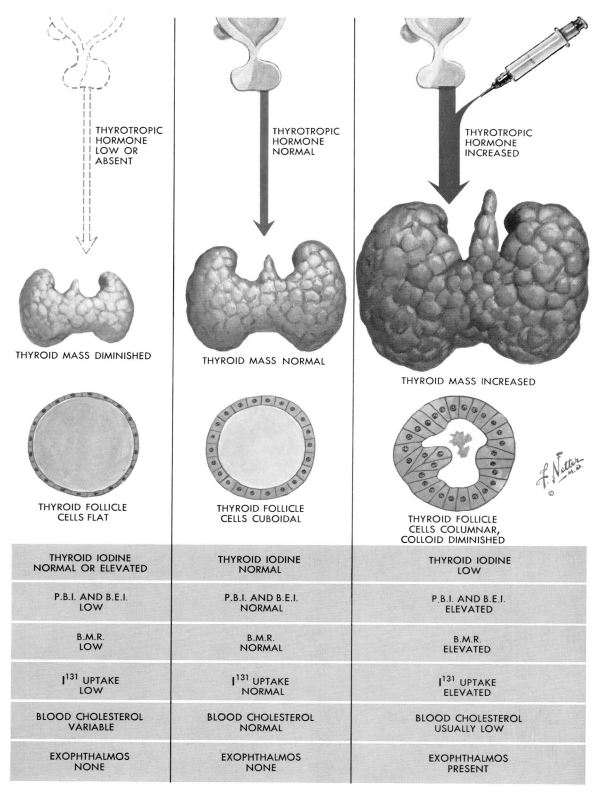

THYROTROPIC HORMONE LOW OR ABSENT	THYROTROPIC HORMONE NORMAL	THYROTROPIC HORMONE INCREASED
THYROID MASS DIMINISHED	THYROID MASS NORMAL	THYROID MASS INCREASED
THYROID FOLLICLE CELLS FLAT	THYROID FOLLICLE CELLS CUBOIDAL	THYROID FOLLICLE CELLS COLUMNAR, COLLOID DIMINISHED
THYROID IODINE NORMAL OR ELEVATED	THYROID IODINE NORMAL	THYROID IODINE LOW
P.B.I. AND B.E.I. LOW	P.B.I. AND B.E.I. NORMAL	P.B.I. AND B.E.I. ELEVATED
B.M.R. LOW	B.M.R. NORMAL	B.M.R. ELEVATED
I^{131} UPTAKE LOW	I^{131} UPTAKE NORMAL	I^{131} UPTAKE ELEVATED
BLOOD CHOLESTEROL VARIABLE	BLOOD CHOLESTEROL NORMAL	BLOOD CHOLESTEROL USUALLY LOW
EXOPHTHALMOS NONE	EXOPHTHALMOS NONE	EXOPHTHALMOS PRESENT

of producing *exophthalmos* in intact and thyroidectomized guinea pigs and Atlantic minnows. More recently, it has been possible to separate the thyroid-stimulating factor from the exophthalmos-producing factor of the pituitary. Notwithstanding, both the exophthalmos-producing substance and the thyroid-stimulating factor of the pituitary (but not the gonadotropic factor of the pituitary) can be inactivated by exposure to explanted thyroid tissue.

It is commonly recognized that, between the pituitary and the thyroid, a fine balance exists, which has been compared to a very sensitive thermostat, and that any increase in the level of circulating thyroid hormone will shut off the synthesis or secretion of TSH, whereas any decreased level of circulating thyroid hormone will be followed by an increased production and secretion of TSH by the anterior pituitary gland. Instances of decreased production of

thyroid hormone are associated with the development of large hyperplastic goiters only in the presence of functional pituitaries. Extensive studies by neuroendocrinologists have demonstrated an area within the hypothalamus which is necessary to the production of TSH by the anterior pituitary. Electrostimulation of this area may cause increased production of thyrotropic hormone and thyroid stimulation. Local microperfusion of the area of the hypothalamus with tri-iodothyronine results in a decreased production of TSH by the anterior pituitary. Thus, it would appear that this fine balance between the thyroid and the pituitary is mediated via the hypothalamus. Present evidence indicates that the hypothalamic control of the pituitary is mediated via neurohormones which are carried from the median eminence of the hypothalamus to the anterior pituitary via a hypophysial portal circulatory system.

PHYSIOLOGY OF THE THYROID HORMONES

The rôle of the thyroid gland in the total body economy comprises the synthesis, storage, and secretion of thyroid hormones, which are necessary to growth, development, and normal body metabolism. These thyroid functions can be considered almost synonymous with iodine metabolism. *Inorganic iodine* (I^-) is absorbed in the *gastro-intestinal tract* and circulated as *iodide,* until it is either trapped by the *thyroid* or salivary glands or excreted by the *urinary tract.* The thyroid extracts iodine from the plasma, against a 25-fold concentration, by virtue of its *iodide trap,* which can be enhanced by *thyrotropic hormone* or blocked by agents such as *perchlorate* or *thiocyanate.* Iodide ($2I^-$) is oxidized by an *oxidative enzyme* to iodine (I_2). This is inhibited by *thiouracil* and imidazole derivatives. The oxidized iodine is rapidly utilized in the iodination of tyrosine to *mono-iodotyrosine* and *di-iodotyrosine.* *Sulfonamide* derivatives interfere with iodination of tyrosine. A de-iodinase has been demonstrated in the thyroid, which is capable of de-iodinating mono-iodotyrosine and di-iodotyrosine, but not of de-iodinating *thyroxine* or *tri-iodothyronine.* The iodine removed from the tyrosine molecules by this de-iodinase is available again in the total body iodide pool and for reutilization in the thyroid.

Iodination of the tyrosine molecule leads to a synthesis of L-thyroxine (T_4) and of 3,5,3'-tri-iodo-L-thyronine (T_3). It is generally accepted that this step results from the action of a *coupling enzyme* uniting 2 di-iodotyrosine molecules to form tetra-iodothyronine, or thyroxine, or to couple 1 molecule of mono-iodotyrosine with 1 of di-iodotyrosine to form T_3. It has been suggested that 1 molecule of 3,3',5'-tri-iodothyronine may result from a coupling of 1 molecule of mono-iodotyrosine and one of di-iodotyrosine, or that, from a coupling of 2 molecules of mono-iodotyrosine, 1 molecule of 3,3'-di-iodothyronine may result. The ratio of T_4 to T_3 in human thyroids is 4 to 1 but because of greater dissociation of T_3 from carrier proteins in the blood stream, it accounts for 50 per cent or more of the calorigenic action.

The organic compounds of iodine are stored in the thyroid as a part of a large molecule known as *thyroglobulin* (molecular weight, 650,000). Histological examination of thyroid with light microscopy reveals that this thyroglobulin is stored within the *follicle,* surrounded by an acinar wall of closely packed cuboidal cells. The thyroglobulin is too large a molecule to be transported across the acinar cell wall; it has been demonstrated in the serum only after acute damage to the cellular structure of the thyroid by the acute inflammation of

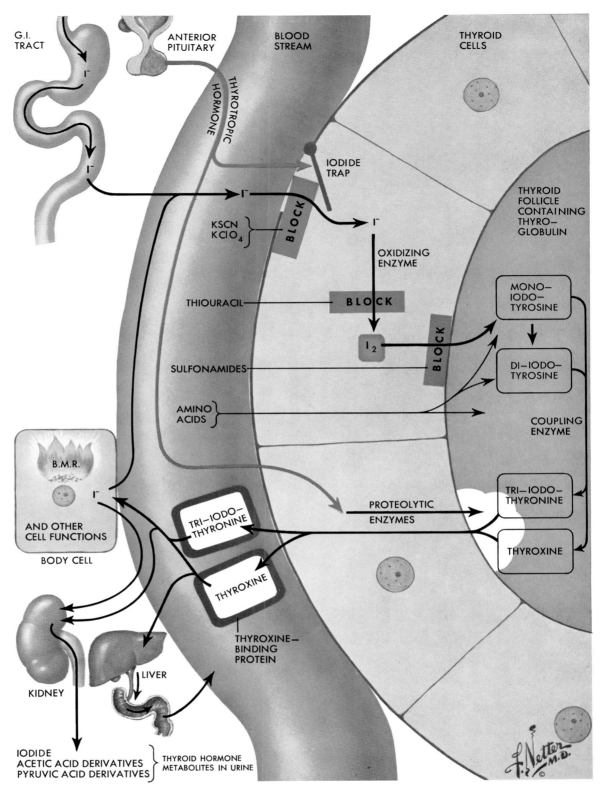

subacute thyroiditis or following intensive intrathyroidal irradiation with radioactive iodine.

The thyroid hormones T_3 and T_4, released by *proteolytic enzymes* from thyroglobulin following the activation of these enzymes by the thyrotropic hormone, are transported across the acinar cell wall into the circulation. This action is inhibited by large amounts of iodine, as in the treatment of hyperthyroidism.

The thyroid hormones are transported from the thyroid to peripheral tissues by thyroxine-binding proteins in the serum. The major *thyroxine-binding protein* is a globulin located between the α_1- and α_2-globulins. It is known as an interalpha globulin or as the thyroxine-binding globulin (TBG). It carries most of the thyroxine. Both thyroid hormones have also been localized in the pre-albumin area, and T_3 travels largely in albumin. Thyroid hormone, bound

to pre-albumin or to the thyroxine-binding globulin, is presumed to be metabolically inactive. The active hormone is the small, free fraction, albeit in equilibrium with the bound hormone. The thyroxine-binding globulin is increased during pregnancy and following the administration of estrogens; it is decreased by the administration of androgen.

From thyroxine-binding proteins, the thyroid hormones enter the *body cells,* where they exert their metabolic actions which are, predominantly, calorigenic (raising B.M.R.). Both T_4 and T_3 have been found to be metabolized by *kidney* and by *liver* tissue to their *pyruvic acid* and *acetic acid derivatives* and, eventually, to *iodide.* The rôles played by these metabolites in cellular metabolism are not known. These thyroid hormones are concentrated and conjugated in the liver to glucuronic acid, excreted with the bile, hydrolyzed in the small bowel, and reabsorbed.

COMMON TESTS FOR THYROID FUNCTION

Common tests for thyroid function are directed at measuring either the function of the thyroid gland or the effects of the thyroid hormone on the organism.

The *24-hour uptake of radioactive iodine* (I^{131}) tests the avidity of the thyroid gland for iodine and thereby measures, secondarily, the production rate of the thyroid hormones. By following the conversion of I^{131} to the protein-bound (*P.B.I.*) or the butanol-extractable radioactive iodine (*B.E.I.*), one can also determine directly the rate at which the gland is secreting *thyroid hormones* into the *circulation*. Most commonly, one determines the uptake by the thyroid of the smallest measurable dose of radioactive iodine at the end of a given period of time, *i.e.*, usually at 5 and 24 hours. The *normal* thyroid gland concentrates between 12 and 16 per cent of a standard dose of I^{131} in 5 hours, and between 20 and 45 per cent in 24 hours. In the normal individual this uptake can be suppressed by the administration of 3,5,3'-tri-iodo-L-thyronine (T_3) in a dose of 50 to 100 µg daily for 3 to 5 days. In *hypothyroidism* or myxedema the uptake of I^{131} is less than 20 per cent of the dose. In *Graves' disease* the uptake of I^{131} is usually well over 30 per cent in 5 hours and over 45 per cent of the dose in 24 hours. The earlier measurement will reveal hyperthyroidism where the labeled thyroid hormones are discharged within 24 hours. This increased avidity of the thyroid for I^{131} in Graves' disease is not suppressed by the administration of T_3. Uptake of I^{131} by a *hyperfunctioning adenoma* may be within the normal range; however, the radio-iodine is *localized in the functioning tumor* (see scintigram on page 53), and this is not suppressed by T_3. An *iodine-deficiency goiter,* or one following goitrogenic treatment, may show a marked increase in avidity for radioactive iodine (up to 90 per cent of the tracer dose), but the P.B.I. or B.E.I. is not raised. A patient receiving *thiouracil, perchlorate,* or *iodine* will not readily concentrate radioactive iodine. If iodinated radiopaque dyes have recently been administered to the patient, a significant suppression of I^{131} uptake results.

The T_3 red cell uptake test is used increasingly on the patient's serum. This test relies on the competitive binding capacity for radioactively labeled T_3 between the thyroxine-binding globulin and the red cells. Normally, 10 to 20 per cent of the radioactivity is bound by red cells. In hyperthyroidism the thyroxine-binding globulin is nearly saturated with thyroxine (T_4), and the red cells bind more than 20 per cent of the added T_3. The test is not useful in hypothyroidism, and it gives falsely high values in respiratory acidosis. There is relative non-interference by iodine-containing dyes and inorganic iodides.

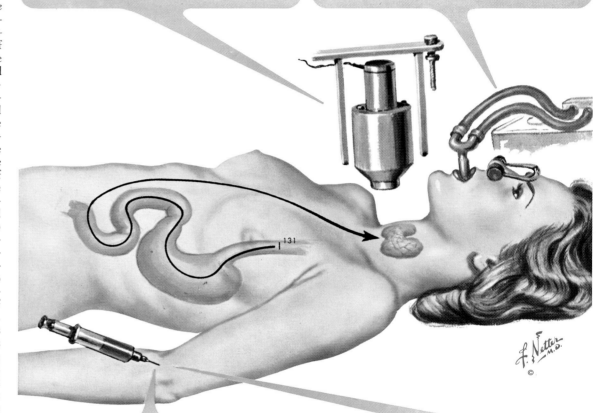

24-HOUR I¹³¹ UPTAKE

MEASURES AVIDITY OF THYROID GLAND FOR IODINE

NORMAL	20 to 45% (SUPPRESSED BY T₃)
HYPOTHYROIDISM	0 to 20%
GRAVES' DISEASE	45 to 90% (NOT SUPPRESSED BY T₃)
HYPERFUNCTIONING ADENOMA	40 to 45% (LOCALIZED IN TUMOR; NOT SUPPRESSED BY T₃)
IODINE DEFICIENCY GOITER	50 to 90%
UNDER THIOURACIL, KSCN OR LARGE DOSES OF IODINE	0 to 20%

BASAL METABOLIC RATE (B.M.R.)

MEASURES EFFECT OF CIRCULATING THYROID HORMONE ON OXYGEN CONSUMPTION

NORMAL	−10% to +10%
HYPOTHYROIDISM	−15% to −40%
GRAVES' DISEASE	+35% to +60%
HYPERFUNCTIONING ADENOMA	+20% to +30%

ELEVATED IN PATIENTS NOT RELAXED, IN ACROMEGALY, ESSENTIAL HYPERTENSION, PHEOCHROMOCYTOMA, HEART FAILURE, LEUKEMIA LOW IN ADDISON'S DISEASE AND PANHYPOPITUITARISM

P.B.I. AND B.E.I.

MEASURES LEVEL OF CIRCULATING THYROID HORMONE

	P.B.I.	B.E.I.
NORMAL	3.5 to 8.5 µg/100 ml	3.2 to 6.5 µg/100 ml
HYPOTHYROIDISM	0.5 to 3.0 µg/100 ml	0.5 to 3.0 µg/100 ml
GRAVES' DISEASE	9.0 to 20.0 µg/100 ml	7.0 UP µg/100 ml
HYPERFUNCTIONING ADENOMA	8.0 to 10.0 µg/100 ml	7.0 to 10.0 µg/100 ml

FALSE HIGH AFTER IODIDE INGESTION, RADIOPAQUE MEDIA (GALLBLADDER DYE MAY LAST MONTHS; RENAL DYE, A FEW DAYS)
FALSE LOW AFTER MERCURIAL DIURETICS (LASTS A FEW DAYS)

SERUM CHOLESTEROL

MEASURES ONE PERIPHERAL ACTION OF THYROID HORMONE

NORMAL	150 to 250 mg/100 ml
HYPOTHYROIDISM	ELEVATED (IF ON NORMAL DIET)
HYPERTHYROIDISM	NORMAL TO LOW

Circulating thyroid hormone may be estimated by determining the *P.B.I.* or the *B.E.I.,* which is closer to the true hormonal value. In *normal* individuals the P.B.I. varies between 3.5 and 8.5 µg per 100 ml, and the B.E.I. between 3.2 and 6.5 µg per 100 ml; in *hypothyroidism* both are below 3.0 µg per 100 ml, and in *Graves' disease* they are above 7 µg per 100 ml. In patients with *hyperfunctioning adenomas,* both the P.B.I. and B.E.I. are raised only to levels between 7 and 10 µg per 100 ml. Falsely high levels may be obtained in patients on large doses of *iodides* or after *radiopaque media.* The *kidney dyes* produce increased levels for a few days or up to a week, the *gallbladder dye* and bronchograms for many months; myelograms interfere for years. Blood drawn shortly after administering a *mercurial diuretic* will show falsely low results.

The *basal metabolic rate* (B.M.R.) test measures the rate of *oxygen consumption* and simply reflects the level at which the thyroid hormone is maintaining metabolism. In *normal* individuals the range is between −10 and +10 per cent; in *hypothyroidism,* between −15 and −40 per cent; and, in *Graves' disease,* between +35 and +60 per cent. With *hyperfunctioning adenomas,* the B.M.R. ranges only between +20 and +30 per cent.

The first B.M.R. may be falsely elevated, if the patient is *not relaxed.* It is high in *acromegaly, essential hypertension* with *heart failure, pheochromocytoma,* leukemia, and polycythemia. The B.M.R. is low in patients suffering from *Addison's disease,* malnutrition, or *panhypopituitarism.*

Serum cholesterol in *hypothyroidism* is usually elevated, though hypothyroid individuals on a low caloric intake may have a low serum cholesterol. In *hyperthyroidism* it is usually decreased. The cholesterol is also low in leukemic states.

DIFFUSE HYPERTHYROIDISM (GRAVES' DISEASE)

Clinical Manifestations

Graves' disease, an eponym used in English-speaking countries to describe a clinical syndrome characterized by hyperthyroidism and exophthalmos, is found in females more commonly than in males (8:1) and more frequently during the childbearing years, though it may occur as early as infancy and in extreme old age. Although this malady's primary signs are an enlarged thyroid and prominent eyes, along with cardiovascular symptoms, it actually involves most systems of the body and is thus a systemic disease.

The thyroid is diffusely enlarged (*goiter*) and is anywhere from two to several times its normal size. Some asymmetry may be observed, the right lobe being somewhat larger than the left. The pyramidal lobe is usually enlarged. In a rare patient with Graves' disease, there is no palpable enlargement of the thyroid gland. The gland has an increased vascularity, as evidenced by a *bruit* and sometimes by a *thrill* which may be demonstrated over the upper poles. Histologically (see pages 54 and 55), the gland shows a marked loss of colloid from the follicles and an increased cell height, with high columnar acinar cells which may demonstrate papillary infolding into the follicles. Late in the disease there may occur a significant lymphocytic infiltration throughout the thyroid, and, occasionally, even lymph follicles may be seen within the thyroid parenchyma. There is also generalized *lymphadenopathy* and a *relative lymphocytosis* which may be quite marked.

This hyperplastic thyroid functions at a markedly accelerated pace, evidenced by an *increased uptake* and turnover of *radioactive iodine* and increased levels of thyroid hormone, as shown by a *rise* in protein-bound iodine (*P.B.I.*) and butanol-extractable iodine (*B.E.I.*), which cause an increased rate of oxygen consumption or basal metabolic rate (*B.M.R.*), a fall in *serum cholesterol* and *phospholipids*, and an increased *urinary nitrogen, phosphorus, calcium,* and *creatine. Serum uric acid* is low. Occasionally, *glycosuria* is found.

The increased levels of thyroid hormone cause a variety of physical and physiological changes. Patients with this malady are usually *nervous, excitable, restless,* suffering from *insomnia* and being *emotionally unstable.* On physical examination they present a *tremor* of the extended fingers. The increased levels of thyroid hormone and, possibly, the increased levels of oxygen consumption, with concomitant generalized vasodilatation, result in increased cardiac output,

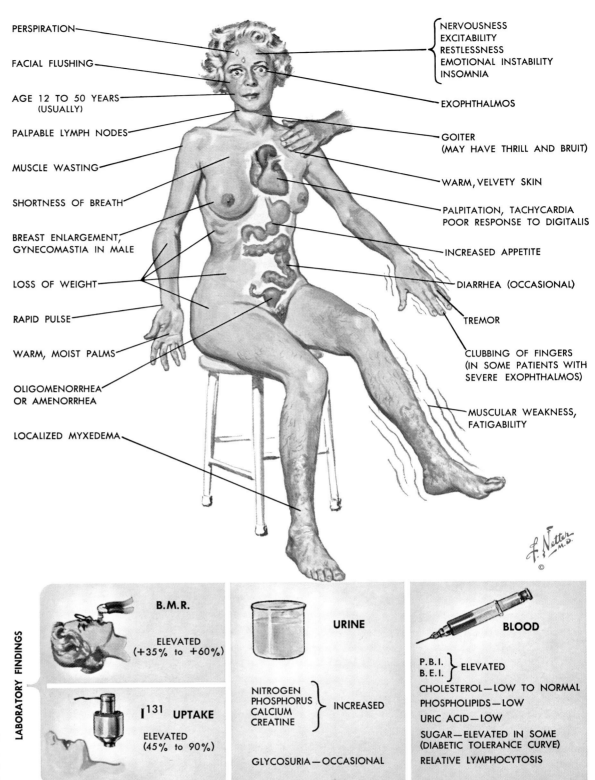

PERSPIRATION

FACIAL FLUSHING

AGE 12 TO 50 YEARS (USUALLY)

PALPABLE LYMPH NODES

MUSCLE WASTING

SHORTNESS OF BREATH

BREAST ENLARGEMENT, GYNECOMASTIA IN MALE

LOSS OF WEIGHT

RAPID PULSE

WARM, MOIST PALMS

OLIGOMENORRHEA OR AMENORRHEA

LOCALIZED MYXEDEMA

NERVOUSNESS EXCITABILITY RESTLESSNESS EMOTIONAL INSTABILITY INSOMNIA

EXOPHTHALMOS

GOITER (MAY HAVE THRILL AND BRUIT)

WARM, VELVETY SKIN

PALPITATION, TACHYCARDIA POOR RESPONSE TO DIGITALIS

INCREASED APPETITE

DIARRHEA (OCCASIONAL)

TREMOR

CLUBBING OF FINGERS (IN SOME PATIENTS WITH SEVERE EXOPHTHALMOS)

MUSCULAR WEAKNESS, FATIGABILITY

LABORATORY FINDINGS

B.M.R. ELEVATED (+35% to +60%)

I^{131} **UPTAKE** ELEVATED (45% to 90%)

URINE
NITROGEN PHOSPHORUS CALCIUM CREATINE } INCREASED

GLYCOSURIA—OCCASIONAL

BLOOD
P.B.I. B.E.I. } ELEVATED
CHOLESTEROL—LOW TO NORMAL
PHOSPHOLIPIDS—LOW
URIC ACID—LOW
SUGAR—ELEVATED IN SOME (DIABETIC TOLERANCE CURVE)
RELATIVE LYMPHOCYTOSIS

with *palpitation* and *tachycardia.* Some *shortness of breath* may also be associated with the palpitation. The increased stimulus to the heart action may result in fibrillation and heart failure, which *responds poorly to digitalis* in the customary dosage but larger doses will have a better effect. The *skin* of patients with this disease is *warm* and *velvety;* it may also be *flushed* and is often associated with a rather marked *perspiration.* Occasionally, *vitiligo* on the exposed skin is observed. Patients with this condition, however, generally state that the vitiligo has been of long duration, having developed first at the time of puberty, of a pregnancy, or of the menopause. The increased metabolic rate of these patients leads to a *loss of weight,* in spite of a good-to-*increased appetite,* and to a *wasting of certain muscles,* which is associated with *muscular weakness.* Severe hyperthyroidism may be associated with *diarrhea,* and, quite characteristically,

women of the childbearing years report an *oligomenorrhea* or even an *amenorrhea,* which may be corrected by restoring the patient to a euthyroid state. *Localized myxedema* is the term given to a skin change which sometimes occurs in the lower extremities, or on the forearms, of patients having severe progressive exophthalmos. This is associated with a brawny, nonpitting thickening of the skin, as a rule in the lower third of the leg. It has been demonstrated that this tissue contains mucinlike substances, which disappear on local injection of tri-iodothyronine.

Extrathyroid Pathology
(Plates 10 and 11, pages 50 and 51)

Patients with Graves' disease manifest the symptoms and signs of profound muscle changes known
(*Continued on page 50*)

DIFFUSE HYPERTHYROIDISM (GRAVES' DISEASE)

(Continued from page 49)

as thyroid myopathy. *Atrophy of the temporal muscles* and of the *muscles of the shoulder girdle,* as well as those of the lower extremities—notably the quadriceps femoris group—is typical. Muscular weakness is present, and these patients often are unable to climb steps or to lift their own weight from a chair. Characteristically, they have a *tremor,* and, when asked to extend a leg, they manifest a marked trembling and are usually unable to hold the leg in the extended position more than 1 minute. The muscles have been described as showing fatty infiltration, Zenker's degeneration, and round cell infiltration. It is thought that these anatomical changes may explain the muscular weakness as well as the marked creatinuria and the intolerance to creatine seen in these patients.

"Localized myxedema" is shown here as it commonly presents itself—a rubbery, nonpitting swelling of the cutaneous and subcutaneous tissues, with a violaceous discoloration of the skin in the lower third of the legs. Usually, it is predominant in the outer half of the leg. Nodules (as large as 1 cm in diameter) over the tibia, extending up as high as the knees, may be associated with classical localized myxedema. This lesion may also occur in the forearms, and it has been known to involve the foot and even the toes. Characteristically, hair does not grow in such myxedematous sites, but the occasional presence of hair follicles, producing hair at the site, does not rule out the diagnosis. When localized myxedema occurs, it is practically always in patients who have severe and progressive exophthalmos. It may be worsened by a thyroidectomy. It may also be associated with *clubbing of the fingers* and of the toes (see Plate 9).

The earliest descriptions of Graves' disease concerned patients who had goiters as well as some degree of heart failure. Characteristically, patients with hyperthyroidism complain of a variety of cardiac symptoms and signs. An *increased heart rate* is always present, though this may be less marked in the male than in the female. *Cardiac output is increased,* and those who develop *heart failure* present the manifestations of high-output failure characterized by a shorter-than-normal circulation time in spite of an elevated venous pressure. *Enlargement of the heart* is unusual, except in a case of frank heart failure or in a patient with previous heart disease. The heart does not show any characteristic anatomical or microscopic changes which can be attributed to the

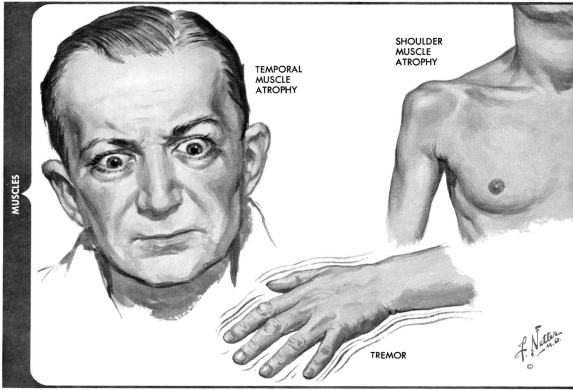

TEMPORAL MUSCLE ATROPHY

SHOULDER MUSCLE ATROPHY

MUSCLES

TREMOR

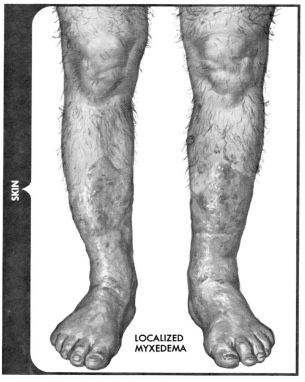

SKIN

LOCALIZED MYXEDEMA

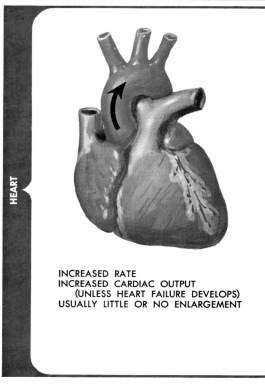

HEART

INCREASED RATE
INCREASED CARDIAC OUTPUT
(UNLESS HEART FAILURE DEVELOPS)
USUALLY LITTLE OR NO ENLARGEMENT

hyperthyroidism. The stimulus to cardiac output has been attributed to the elevated B.M.R. and the increased oxygen demands of the body. Also, it has recently been established that thyroid hormones may produce changes in the heart which are independent of changes in the total body oxygen consumption. Thus, it has been demonstrated that the administration of rapidly acting analogues of thyroxine cause an increase in the metabolism of heart muscle before affecting other tissues of the body. Another possible mechanism for the increased cardiac output in patients with Graves' disease might be attributed to an arteriovenous shunt through the extremely vascular thyroids and the dilated peripheral vessels. The usual cardio-accelerator effect of the catecholamines is accentuated by thyroid hormones, and, in fact, all sympathetic activity is exaggerated in hyperthyroidism. Thus, a central blocker (reserpine) or a

peripheral blocker (guanethidine) will control all circulatory manifestations, will reduce sweating, and will diminish lid retraction without in any way interfering with the oversecretion of thyroid hormones. Hemic murmurs are frequently heard (including typical presystolic ones), suggesting the presence of mitral stenosis on an anatomical basis. However, once circulatory overactivity has been brought under control, either by the administration of reserpine or by arresting the hyperthyroid state, purely functional murmurs will disappear. Patients with heart failure of hyperthyroidism usually are moderately or markedly resistant to treatment with digitalis. However, as the hyperthyroidism is reduced, the heart failure is usually very satisfactorily controlled, and, in a large percentage of patients who had been fibrillating, the rhythm is converted to normal.

(Continued on page 51)

DIFFUSE HYPERTHYROIDISM (GRAVES' DISEASE)

(Continued from page 50)

In the female, functions of the *reproductive system* may be significantly altered in the hyperthyroid state. As a rule, these patients, during the child-bearing years, report increasing intervals between menstrual periods, as well as a decreasing amount of menstrual flow (oligomenorrhea) or an absolute amenorrhea, all of which is rectified after correction of the hyperthyroidism. The mechanism of these manifestations has not been clarified.

The male patient with hyperthyroidism does not, as a rule, describe any significant changes in the reproductive system. Usually, no loss of potentia is experienced, except when a profound weakness accompanies the disease. However, examination often reveals *gynecomastia*. This may be localized entirely to the subareolar tissue, or a significant enlargement of the breasts, comparable to that observed in an adolescent girl, may be evident. This is not necessarily associated with any change in testicular size or function. It may occur in patients with or without exophthalmos. The gynecomastia in patients who do not have severe exophthalmos usually regresses after correction of the hyperthyroidism. However, recurrence may be noted if the patient becomes myxedematous, but, once more, the enlargement disappears with restoration to a euthyroid state after the administration of adequate replacement therapy. In those patients with severe exophthalmos in whom gynecomastia has appeared, no significant regression is observed as the hyperthyroidism is brought under control. An occasional *female* patient, with severe exophthalmos, will describe an *enlargement of the breasts*, appearing at about the time when the eye abnormality developed.

Marine and Warthin and Kocher were all impressed by the incidence of *enlarged thymus glands* and of *enlarged lymph nodes* in patients succumbing to this malady. Kocher was the first to call attention to a *relative lymphocytosis* and *monocytosis* in the blood of individuals with this disease. No characteristic histological pattern of the lymph nodes or of the thymus has been found in these patients.

It is known that administration of excess thyroid hormone to rats will lead to a depletion of muscle tissue, with a concurrent hyperplasia of the lymphoid tissue. In contrast, adrenal glucocorticoids favor atrophy of both muscle and lymphoid tissue. Autopsy has revealed that the *adrenal glands* of patients with

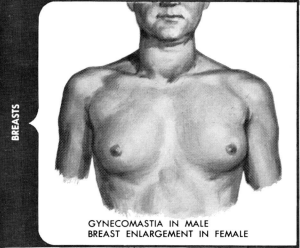

GYNECOMASTIA IN MALE
BREAST ENLARGEMENT IN FEMALE

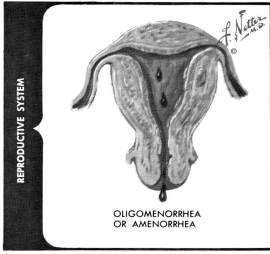

OLIGOMENORRHEA
OR AMENORRHEA

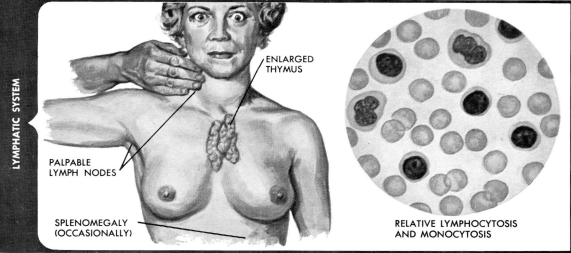

ENLARGED THYMUS

PALPABLE LYMPH NODES

SPLENOMEGALY (OCCASIONALLY)

RELATIVE LYMPHOCYTOSIS AND MONOCYTOSIS

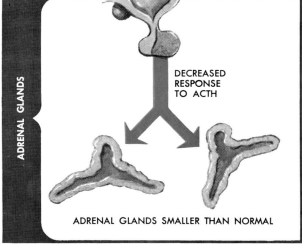

DECREASED RESPONSE TO ACTH

ADRENAL GLANDS SMALLER THAN NORMAL

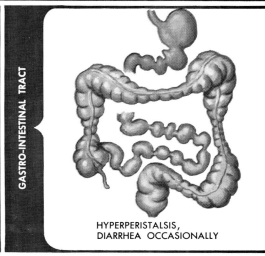

HYPERPERISTALSIS, DIARRHEA OCCASIONALLY

Graves' disease have *smaller cortices* than do the adrenals of patients whose death was caused by other maladies. A *decreased response to adrenocorticotropic hormone (ACTH)* has also been reported. Thus, either excess thyroid or a decrease in active glucocorticoids (both known to exist in severe hyperthyroidism) may contribute to lymphoid hyperplasia. It has also been suggested that since the thymic tissue, lymphoid tissue, and thyroid tissue are the only three tissues which inactivate thyrotropic hormone, all three of these organs may be target organs of the thyrotropic hormone.

The *gastro-intestinal tract* does not present any classical anatomical changes, although *hyperperistalsis* is common. However, patients with extreme hyperthyroidism may complain of severe *diarrhea*, and, indeed, it may be the diarrhea which brings the patient to the doctor.

Exophthalmos (Plate 12, page 52)

Parry, in his private writings around the beginning of the nineteenth century; Graves, in 1835, and Basedow, in 1845, in their published writings described patients with hyperthyroidism, heart symptoms, and eye signs which they called "prominence of the eyes".

The eye signs of *exophthalmos* vary in degree from mild to extremely severe and progressive. If the distance from the canthus to the front of the cornea exceeds 18 mm in an adult, exophthalmos is present. Fortunately, in most patients the eye signs are mild, being characterized by a retraction of the lids which leads to widened palpebral fissures and a stare. Dilatation of the pupils is frequently seen. Other signs may be infrequent blinking, tremor of the closed

(Continued on page 52)

DIFFUSE HYPERTHYROIDISM (GRAVES' DISEASE)

(Continued from page 51)

lids, difficulty in elevating the upper lid, absence of forehead wrinkling on upward gaze, weakness of convergence, and palsy of one or more extra-ocular muscles. Frequently, a lid lag can be demonstrated. This is simply a failure of the upper lid to maintain its position relative to the globe as the gaze is directed downward. There also may be globe lag; *i.e.,* the lid moves upward more rapidly than does the globe as the patient looks upward. The eye symptoms usually regress after correction of the hyperthyroidism; the pupillary dilatation disappears, and a significant decrease in lid retraction and lid lag is usual. However, the eye signs of some patients become markedly worse following correction of the hyperthyroidism, especially if corrected suddenly, as with thyroidectomy.

Most patients manifest more severe eye symptoms when they first present themselves to the clinic. The danger signals of *progressive exophthalmos* include an excessive ocular proptosis, some edema of the upper and lower lids, and, frequently, chemosis (conjunctival edema). Patients often complain of increased lacrimation and a sandy feeling in the eyes, as well as an uncomfortable sense of fullness in the orbits. When the patient is requested to look in one direction or another, a very significant weakness of one or more of the extra-ocular muscles may be noted. The patient may complain of blurred vision, or even of diplopia, on looking either upward or to the side.

Testing the eye and the orbital contents *for resiliency to pressure* is most useful. This is done by applying the fingers to the eyeball, over the closed eyelid, and attempting to move the eyeball backward. Normally, the eyeball can be pushed back easily and without resistance; in severe exophthalmos, however, a significant decrease in resiliency is evident, and in some patients it is impossible to push the eyeball back at all. This is looked upon by many as a serious prognostic sign of progressive exophthalmos.

The exophthalmic progress may be so rapid and extensive that the lids cannot be closed over the eyes, so that ulcerations of the cornea may result. These ulcerations may become infected and may even lead to loss of the eye. Rarely, the optic nerve may be involved by papilledema, papillitis, or retrobulbar neuritis, causing blindness. Patients with the above-described eye signs often have only mild hyperthyroidism, and some may be euthyroid or even have a mild hypothyroidism.

The causes of the manifestations in progressive exophthalmos are not well understood. It is quite likely that the milder eye signs, such as lid retraction,

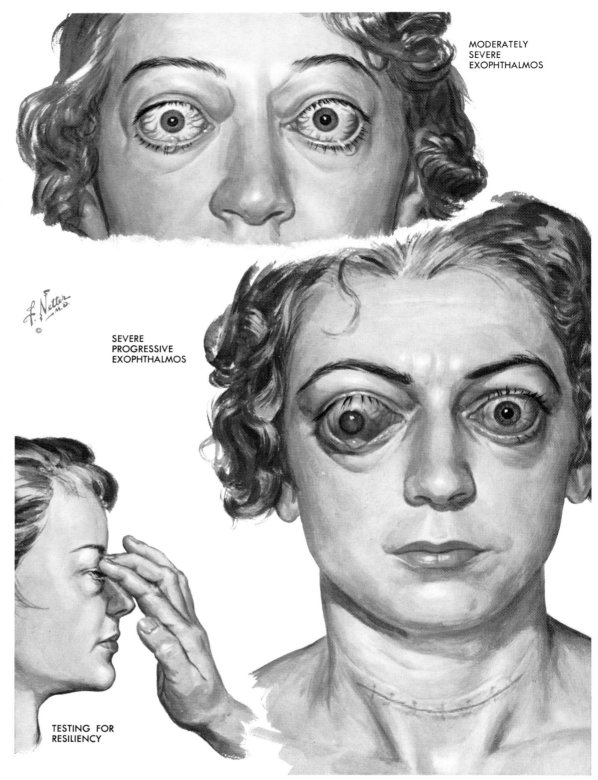

MODERATELY SEVERE EXOPHTHALMOS

SEVERE PROGRESSIVE EXOPHTHALMOS

TESTING FOR RESILIENCY

dilatation of the pupils, and even lid lag, may be related to an increased sympathetic activity. The proptosis, however, represents an increase in retrobulbar mass, and this probably can be attributed to an increased extra-ocular muscle mass due to fluid lymphoid infiltrate and increased retrobulbar fat.

The course of this type of ophthalmopathy is unpredictable. The onset may be chronic or acute. On occasion, exophthalmos involving only one eye may be seen, but, if the opposite eye is carefully examined, some abnormalities in that organ also are often found; although one eye may appear normal, while the other is so exophthalmic as to require decompression, eventually an involvement of the second eye will be observed.

It is extremely uncommon for the eyes to return to a perfectly normal state. However, if these patients sleep with their heads elevated, limit the intake of fluids, and are maintained on a slightly more than physiological dose of thyroid hormone (180 to 240 mg per day), frequently some (occasionally, a marked) decrease in the degree of exophthalmos will take place. Glucocorticoid therapy has improved the status of the eyes by reducing the inflammatory reaction around the eyeball and by lessening the retro-orbital lymphocytic infiltration. Orbital decompression and pituitary stalk section are ultimate measures rarely required. The general opinion is that it is undesirable to thyroidectomize patients with severe exophthalmos. In the presence of marked hyperthyroidism, treatment with radioactive iodine is more advisable. As far as the exophthalmos is concerned, better results are obtained if this form of treatment is administered in repeated small doses of radio-iodine than in one dose, large enough to produce rapid destruction of the thyroid.

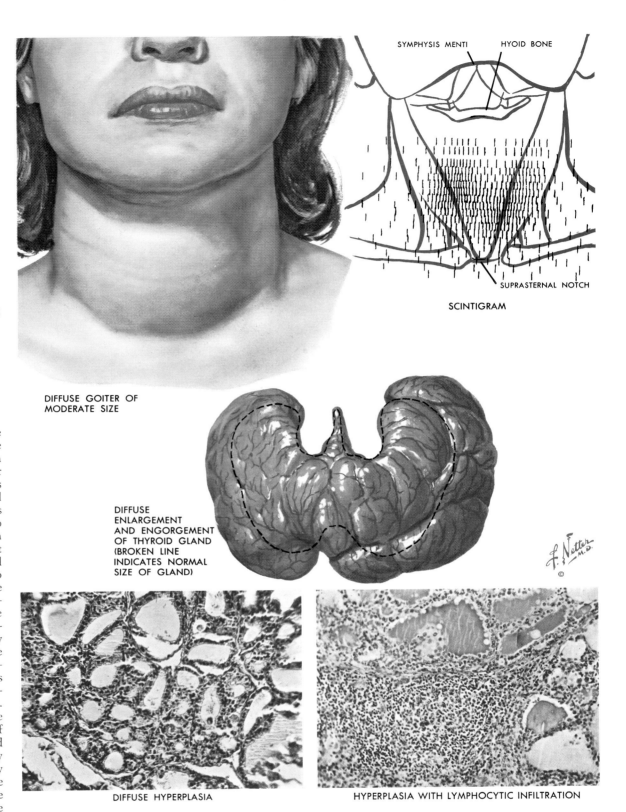

SCINTIGRAM

DIFFUSE GOITER OF
MODERATE SIZE

DIFFUSE
ENLARGEMENT
AND ENGORGEMENT
OF THYROID GLAND
(BROKEN LINE
INDICATES NORMAL
SIZE OF GLAND)

DIFFUSE HYPERPLASIA

HYPERPLASIA WITH LYMPHOCYTIC INFILTRATION

Thyroid Pathology in Diffuse Hyperthyroidism (Graves' Disease)

In patients with Graves' disease, the most dramatic anatomical changes are those found in the thyroid gland, though characteristic changes, in organs other than the thyroid, also are involved in this malady. The thyroid, which in normal adults living in nongoiter belts weighs between 15 and 20 gm, is usually two to four times its *normal size* in patients with Graves' disease. In extreme situations it may be as much as ten times the normal size. In contrast, a rare patient fails to show any significant enlargement of the thyroid. *Diffuse enlargement* and *engorgement* of the thyroid occur in a more or less symmetrical fashion. These features can very well be demonstrated by a *scintigram* of the thyroid after the administration of a test dose of radioactive iodine. As shown here, the thyroids of such patients concentrate the radioactive iodine very diffusely and evenly. Notwithstanding the diffuseness of the process and the apparent symmetry of the thyroid, some surgeons have called attention to the fact that one lobe may be somewhat larger, though minimally so, than the other. Characteristically, the *pyramidal lobe*, which extends above the isthmus on one or the other side of the trachea, is enlarged enough to be easily palpable. The enlarged thyroid gland is smooth to palpation. Typically, it is very vascular, as evidenced by an audible bruit (which may be heard usually over the superior poles of either lobe) and, in some instances, by a palpable thrill over the lateral lobes. The untreated thyroid gland, being vascular and friable in this disease, can be a source of serious bleeding during surgery.

Histological examination of the untreated thyroid reveals a very characteristic *microscopic picture* of *diffuse hyperplasia*. Ordinarily, the colloid is completely lost from within the follicle. Any colloid which remains is pale-staining and, presumably, is considerably less dense than normal colloid. The thyroid

cells are hypertrophied and hyperplastic. The acinar cells, which normally are low cuboidal, become high cuboidal or columnar and, by measurement, may be more than twice as high as those in the normal thyroid gland. In some instances the hyperplasia of the acinar cells is so great that an intra-acinar papillary infolding takes place.

Along with the marked hyperplasia, there is a pronounced increase in avidity for radioactive iodine. Whereas the normal iodine uptake is seldom greater than 45 per cent of a test dose in 24 hours, in patients with this malady it is nearly always more than 50 per cent and may be as great as 80 or 90 per cent.

In a small number of patients with long-standing Graves' disease, *hyperplasia* is accompanied by significant to extensive *lymphocytic infiltration* of the thyroid parenchyma, occasionally with large lymph follicles being present. Postoperative hyperthyroidism

is more likely to develop in patients whose thyroids show lymphocytic infiltration, especially when massive.

Other anatomical and functional changes include those in the eyes, skeletal muscles, heart, liver, thymus, and the lymphoid tissues. The eyes are frequently proptosed; associated with this condition are enlarged, edematous, extra-ocular muscles, with increased fluid and fat in the retro-orbital space. These muscles, and the skeletal muscles as well, show edema, round cell infiltration, hyalinization, fragmentation, and destruction. The heart may be somewhat enlarged, but it does not present any characteristic or classical pathological changes. The liver has been reported to show fatty infiltration, with focal and central necrosis. Characteristically, the thymus and lymphoid tissues are enlarged, displaying simple hypertrophy.

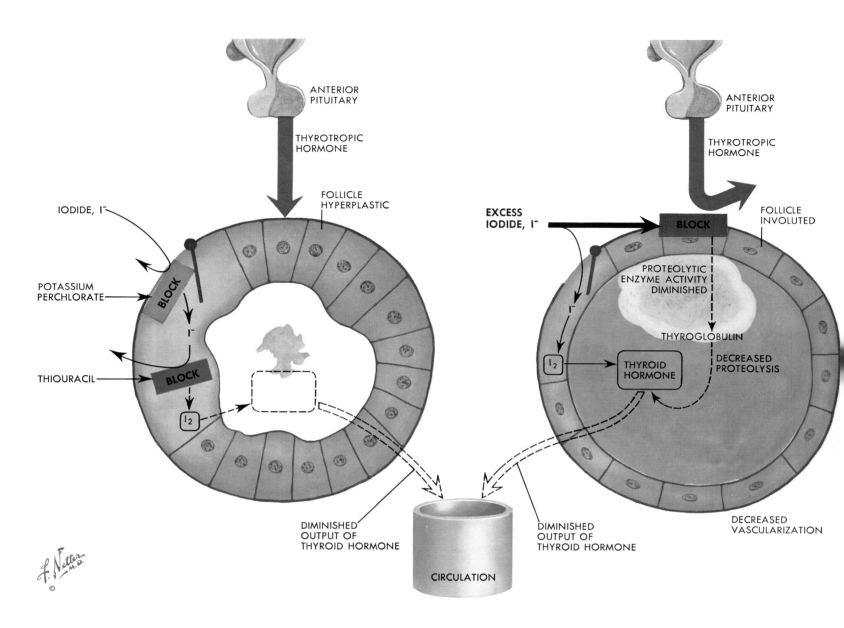

IODIDE, I⁻

POTASSIUM PERCHLORATE

THIOURACIL

ANTERIOR PITUITARY

THYROTROPIC HORMONE

FOLLICLE HYPERPLASTIC

BLOCK

BLOCK

I⁻

I₂

DIMINISHED OUTPUT OF THYROID HORMONE

CIRCULATION

EXCESS IODIDE, I⁻

ANTERIOR PITUITARY

THYROTROPIC HORMONE

BLOCK

FOLLICLE INVOLUTED

PROTEOLYTIC ENZYME ACTIVITY DIMINISHED

THYROGLOBULIN

I⁻

I₂

THYROID HORMONE

DECREASED PROTEOLYSIS

DIMINISHED OUTPUT OF THYROID HORMONE

DECREASED VASCULARIZATION

SECTION II—PLATE 14

EFFECTS OF THERAPY IN DIFFUSE HYPERTHYROIDISM (GRAVES' DISEASE)

It was first shown in mice that the classical TSH leads to a discharge of thyroxine rather quickly (in a matter of 2 to 4 hours), whereas the thyroid-stimulating factor found in the blood of patients with Graves' disease does so in 12 to 14 hours only, and has thus been termed "long-acting thyroid stimulator (LATS)". It belongs to the S_7 class of globulins and is thus an antibody which may combine with an intrathyroidal inhibitor of TSH activity, producing hyperthyroidism. Ordinary TSH is not usually found in excess in the plasma of such patients, although this may be demonstrated quite regularly in myxedema. It appears that either an excessive secretion of LATS, with, possibly, an increased sensitivity of the thyroid gland to TSH, accounts for the excessive thyroid hormone secretion. The possibility that, in certain cases, a spontaneous, diffuse overactivity of the thyroid gland (not caused by any overproduction of a thyrotropic hormone) may be the basis of hyperthyroidism must still be considered. However, there is pro-

gressively less evidence for this, and it seems more likely that diffuse hyperthyroidism is, in fact, a disease due to extrathyroidal overstimulation of the gland.

LATS has been derived from isolated lymphocytes from patients with hyperthyroidism. Its titer is particularly high in pretibial myxedema. Blood levels gradually fall with improvement of Graves' disease and may be markedly diminished with cortisone-type therapy. It is not elevated at all with toxic adenoma.

Characteristically, the *acinar cells* of the thyroid *follicle* are *hyperplastic* and *high columnar* in structure. The *follicles*, becoming overcrowded, may show papillary *infolding*. Because of excessive secretion of thyroid hormone, the *colloid*, which acts as a storage reservoir, is *lost* from the follicles. The hypertrophic gland is *highly vascular*.

Functionally, the gland is trapping iodide at a rapid rate, utilizing it quickly in the genesis of thyroid hormones, and releasing it promptly into the *circulation*. *Iodide* (I^-), used in the treatment of this disease for over 40 years, acts by inhibiting the enzymatic release of thyroxine and tri-iodothyronine from the thyroglobulin stored in the colloid, possibly by blocking the action of TSH. Unfortunately, this block is eventually broken through; however, increased doses of iodide may again be effective in patients whose hormonogenesis cannot be controlled by lesser amounts. *Potassium perchlorate*, an agent now used in treating certain patients who are

sensitive to some of the other antithyroid drugs, acts by blocking the iodide trap, thereby precluding adequate synthesis of the thyroid hormone. Potassium thiocyanate acts similarly. *Methyl-* and *propylthiouracil* and methimazole *reduce thyroid hormone production*. These antithyroid drugs act by blocking the oxidative enzyme system of the thyroid, thereby preventing the oxidation of iodide ($2I$) to *iodine* (I_2), which is necessary for the iodination of tyrosine, the precursor amino acid which leads to the thyroid hormones.

The aim of therapy, in the presence of *hyperplastic*, hyperfunctioning *thyroid glands* in Graves' disease, is to diminish the excessive secretion of thyroid hormones, thereby removing the systemic manifestations secondary to the hormonal excess. Formerly, the success of a subtotal thyroidectomy depended on the removal of an optimal amount of tissue to bring about a euthyroid state. On occasion, myxedema was produced, or subsequent recurrence of the hyperthyroid state followed an excessive regrowth from the remnant left behind. Hoarseness, due to damage to the recurrent laryngeal nerve, and tetany, due to removal of the parathyroid glands, were other complications. The advent of compounds designed to block the synthesis of thyroid hormone, and the use of radioactive iodine to destroy parts of the hormonogenic tissue (an improvement over external radiation, previously available) have made the therapeutic approach more satisfactory but also more complicated.

(*Continued on page 55*)

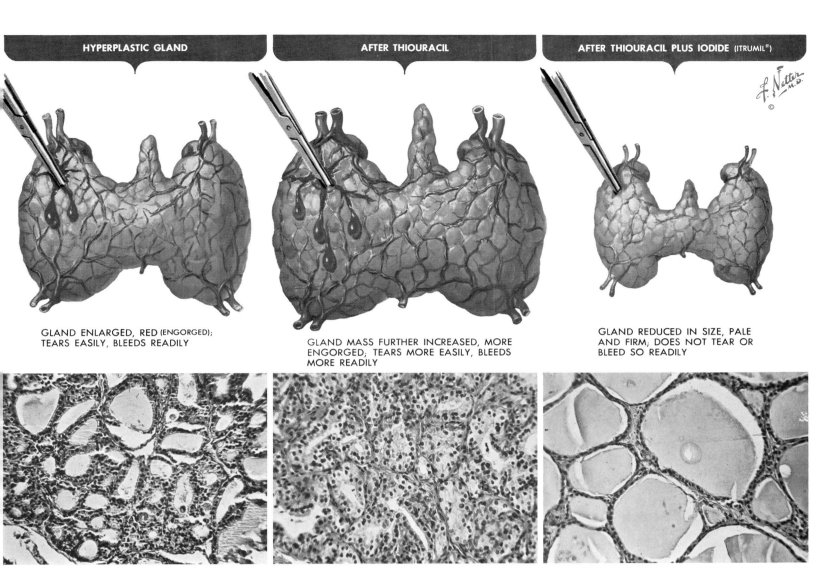

HYPERPLASTIC GLAND	AFTER THIOURACIL	AFTER THIOURACIL PLUS IODIDE (ITRUMIL®)

GLAND ENLARGED, RED (ENGORGED); TEARS EASILY, BLEEDS READILY

GLAND MASS FURTHER INCREASED, MORE ENGORGED; TEARS MORE EASILY, BLEEDS MORE READILY

GLAND REDUCED IN SIZE, PALE AND FIRM; DOES NOT TEAR OR BLEED SO READILY

ACINAR HYPERPLASIA AND LOSS OF COLLOID (MEAN ACINAR CELL HEIGHT 12 MICRA)

INCREASE IN ACINAR CELL HYPERPLASIA; COMPLETE LOSS OF COLLOID (MEAN CELL HEIGHT 17 MICRA)

INVOLUTION OF ACINAR EPITHELIUM; STORAGE OF IODINE—POOR COLLOID (MEAN CELL HEIGHT 9 MICRA)

SECTION II—PLATE 15

EFFECTS OF THERAPY IN DIFFUSE HYPERTHYROIDISM (GRAVES' DISEASE)

(Continued from page 54)

Chemical blockers eventually prevent the synthesis of thyroid hormones, resulting in lowered plasma levels. This leads secondarily to an *increased hyperplasia* of the thyroid gland, since a fall in circulating thyroxine will increase the release of thyrotropin. It should be noted that some goitrogenic antithyroid agents also augment the action of thyrotropin. In contrast, in patients treated with iodide, one finds *involution* of the thyroid, with *shrinkage of the* thyroid *acinar epithelium,* and *decreased vascularity,* but an increased storage of colloid within the thyroid follicles. Some experimental evidence supports the thesis that *excess iodide* blocks the utilization or the action of TSH on thyroid tissue. This would account for the reduction in acinar cell height and the *decrease in proteolytic enzyme activity* within the thyroid follicle, allowing more *thyroglobulin* to accumulate within the follicle while *less thyroid hormone is secreted*. With a reduction in the release of thyroid hormone *into the circulation*, a fall in the rate of oxygen consumption and other symptoms of hyperthyroid-

ism ensue. Whereas there is a marked hypertrophy of the thyroid gland with the organic blocking agents, there is a reduction in both size and vascularity, at least temporarily, with iodide treatment. Agents such as propylthiouracil, given over long periods of time, may actually result in the development of myxedema, whereas this is seen extremely rarely in patients receiving iodides.

In preparing patients for thyroid surgery, a rigorous attempt must be made to induce euthyroidism before undertaking the procedure. Nowadays, this is achieved by administering organic blocking agents. Since the gland becomes more vascular as well as hypertrophic after the administration of an agent such as *thiouracil,* tears more easily, and *bleeds* more readily, it is advantageous to administer iodide as well. In patients *treated with both thiouracil* (or imidazole derivatives) *and iodide, the cell height* in the follicles is markedly reduced, and, once again, *colloid* is stored in the acini. This will *reduce the size of the gland and make it firm* and far *less vascular*. A *ready-made combination of thiouracil and iodide* may be employed. If this is not used, it is advisable to start the chemical blocking agent at least a few days in advance of the iodide, since the former is far less effective initially when the gland contains large amounts of inorganic iodine.

The use of radio-iodine in the treatment of diffuse hyperthyroidism, except during pregnancy, has steadily increased in popularity. Doses ranging from 2 to 6 millicuries are administered

by mouth, and there follows a gradual reduction in the signs and symptoms of hyperthyroidism. It may take over 6 months to reach euthyroidism. Depending on the dosage of radio-iodine given, euthyroidism may be achieved after 3 months, or a degree of hyperthyroidism may still remain. In that case, an additional dose of radio-iodine is administered. In some instances, hypothyroidism and myxedema develop, requiring substitution therapy. It seems doubtful that the production of invasive neoplasia in the thyroid, following radio-iodine treatment, has ever been proved in man, although islets of highly abnormal cells have been well demonstrated in carefully studied cases. Since the production of neoplasia in the thyroid has, however, been established in animals following radio-iodine therapy, conservative management calls for administering radio-iodine only to patients over the age of 40 years, or below this age only in special instances. There are those who feel that overtreating, so as to produce a completely atrophic thyroid gland and myxedema, with thyroid substitution which will reduce TSH secretion to very low levels, provides additional security in terms of a possible development of neoplasia of the thyroid in later years.

It is apparent that each type of therapy carries its special indications and complications. These can be evaluated by pathophysiological considerations, so that the proper choice may be made, and any ensuing complications may be dealt with effectively.

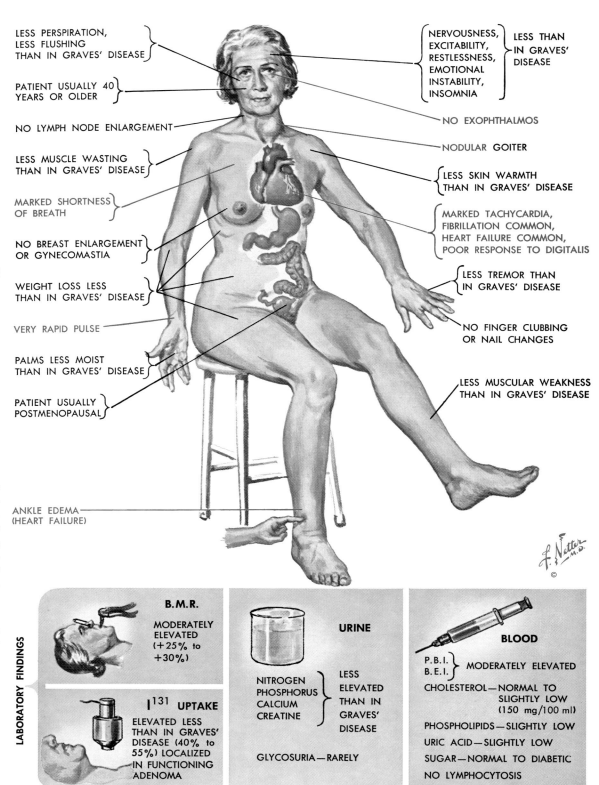

LESS PERSPIRATION, LESS FLUSHING THAN IN GRAVES' DISEASE

PATIENT USUALLY 40 YEARS OR OLDER

NO LYMPH NODE ENLARGEMENT

LESS MUSCLE WASTING THAN IN GRAVES' DISEASE

MARKED SHORTNESS OF BREATH

NO BREAST ENLARGEMENT OR GYNECOMASTIA

WEIGHT LOSS LESS THAN IN GRAVES' DISEASE

VERY RAPID PULSE

PALMS LESS MOIST THAN IN GRAVES' DISEASE

PATIENT USUALLY POSTMENOPAUSAL

ANKLE EDEMA (HEART FAILURE)

NERVOUSNESS, EXCITABILITY, RESTLESSNESS, EMOTIONAL INSTABILITY, INSOMNIA — LESS THAN IN GRAVES' DISEASE

NO EXOPHTHALMOS

NODULAR GOITER

LESS SKIN WARMTH THAN IN GRAVES' DISEASE

MARKED TACHYCARDIA, FIBRILLATION COMMON, HEART FAILURE COMMON, POOR RESPONSE TO DIGITALIS

LESS TREMOR THAN IN GRAVES' DISEASE

NO FINGER CLUBBING OR NAIL CHANGES

LESS MUSCULAR WEAKNESS THAN IN GRAVES' DISEASE

LABORATORY FINDINGS

B.M.R. MODERATELY ELEVATED (+25% to +30%)

I^{131} UPTAKE ELEVATED LESS THAN IN GRAVES' DISEASE (40% to 55%) LOCALIZED IN FUNCTIONING ADENOMA

URINE

NITROGEN PHOSPHORUS CALCIUM CREATINE — LESS ELEVATED THAN IN GRAVES' DISEASE

GLYCOSURIA—RARELY

BLOOD

P.B.I. B.E.I. — MODERATELY ELEVATED

CHOLESTEROL—NORMAL TO SLIGHTLY LOW (150 mg/100 ml)

PHOSPHOLIPIDS—SLIGHTLY LOW

URIC ACID—SLIGHTLY LOW

SUGAR—NORMAL TO DIABETIC

NO LYMPHOCYTOSIS

CLINICAL MANIFESTATIONS OF HYPERFUNCTIONING THYROID ADENOMA

A *nodular goiter,* due to a hyperfunctioning adenoma producing hyperthyroidism, may develop in a thyroid as a single adenoma or as a multinodular goiter containing a variety of adenomas manifesting varying degrees of functional capacity. The clinical picture of this type of hyperthyroidism differs very significantly from that observed in patients with Graves' disease.

Patients with adenomatous goiters with hyperthyroidism are *usually over the age of 40 years.* They generally come from a goiter belt and often give a history of having had either a multinodular thyroid or a single nodule in the thyroid for a long time. As a rule, they have cardiovascular symptoms, and frequently they have been referred to a cardiologist before being sent to a thyroidologist or endocrinologist. They complain of *marked shortness of breath* and have *tachycardia,* frequently with *fibrillation.* The *heart failure,* common in these patients, usually responds poorly, or not at all, to *digitalis.* When in heart failure they may manifest all the signs and symptoms of this disease, except that they usually do not have an increased circulation time, as in Graves' disease. Characteristically, these patients *do not have* exophthalmos. Rarely, one may observe a minimal lid retraction or even a minimal lid lag. However, in general, this is uncommon. There is no clubbing of the fingers. Patients with this type of hyperthyroidism have *less of the muscular weakness* so characteristic of Graves' disease. The *basal metabolic rate* is not as markedly elevated as it is in Graves'

disease, and these patients are *not especially nervous or excitable.* They do *not show signs of marked weight loss* or *of muscle wasting,* both of which are so striking in Graves' disease. Since a large percentage of women patients are *postmenopausal, gynecomastia* and the changes in the menstrual cycle, often seen in Graves' disease, are not present.

Patients with this malady have a *moderate elevation in protein-bound iodine* and *in butanol-extractable iodine.* The *serum cholesterol* is only *slightly lowered,* as are other *lipids.* These individuals *do not* characteristically *show a lymphocytosis* in the peripheral blood. They do not have the marked *creatinuria* or loss of nitrogen, phosphorus, and calcium observed characteristically in Graves' disease.

Studies with radioactive iodine are highly useful

in examining these patients, especially if the site of concentration of the radioactive iodine is localized. Although the uptake of radioactive iodine may not be as great as is observed in classic Graves' disease, in this malady the *radioactive iodine* is usually concentrated primarily in the *hyperfunctioning adenoma,* with practically none in the remainder of the thyroid gland. A scintigram may locate the adenoma.

Patients with hyperfunctioning adenomas and hyperthyroidism characteristically are unresponsive to treatment with iodides. They may require very large doses of the thiouracillike drugs to control hormonogenesis by the adenoma. It has also been observed that the deposited dose of radioactive iodine, per gram of diseased thyroid, is greater than that necessary to control the hyperthyroidism of Graves' disease.

PATHOPHYSIOLOGY OF HYPERFUNCTIONING THYROID ADENOMA

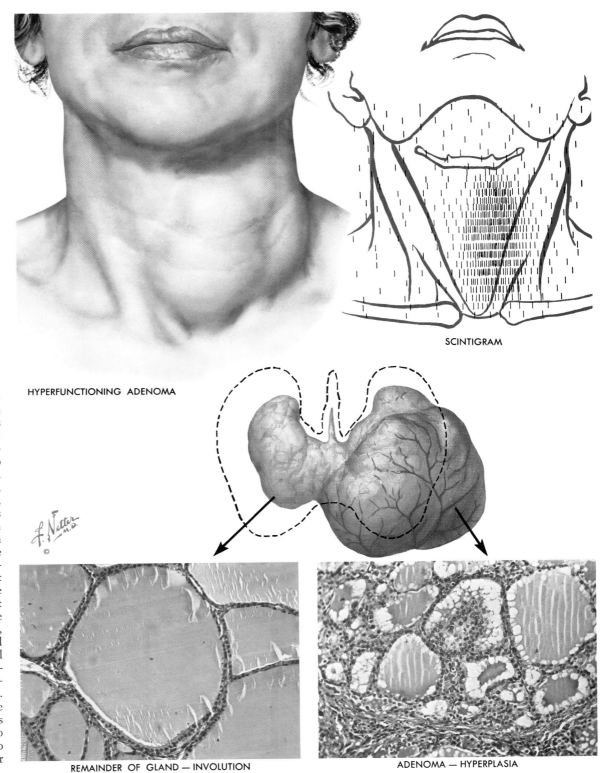

SCINTIGRAM

HYPERFUNCTIONING ADENOMA

REMAINDER OF GLAND — INVOLUTION

ADENOMA — HYPERPLASIA

Hyperthyroidism arising in a *hyperfunctioning adenoma* of the thyroid is probably much more common than was realized prior to the advent of modern studies with radioactive iodine. This syndrome usually occurs in patients who previously had nontoxic nodular goiters. In the most clear-cut and classic setting, the patient, usually a middle-aged female, presents with cardiovascular symptoms varying from complaints of palpitation and dyspnea to the picture of fibrillation and frank heart failure. The heart failure of hyperthyroidism exhibits a few characteristic features which should direct the physician to an investigation of the thyroid. Such patients have high-output failure, with a decreased circulation time in spite of an elevated venous pressure, and they do not respond well to the usual doses of digitalis. Other extrathyroidal pathology in patients with hyperthyroidism arising from hyperfunctioning adenomas of the thyroid is uncommon. Patients do not develop the typical eye signs of Graves' disease. These patients do not have the muscle weakness so characteristic of Graves' disease, nor do they show the hypertrophied thymic or lymphoid tissue.

Pathologically, the most classic feature of this disease is that found in the rare patient with "single" hyperfunctioning adenoma of the thyroid, which may be significantly enlarged, while the rest of the thyroid gland remains uninvolved. No palpable nodules are present in the remainder of the gland, which may actually be *smaller than normal*. In such unique situations, the examiner may be impressed by the small size or the impalpability of the unaffected lobe, as contrasted with the large, single nodule in the opposite lobe. It is extremely uncommon to hear a bruit or to detect a thrill over a hyperfunctioning adenoma of the thyroid. If a test dose of radioactive iodine is administered to the patient and a *scintigram* is made over the neck at the end of 24 or 48 hours, all the radio-

active iodine will be found to be in the nodule, the remainder of the gland having concentrated none.

Grossly, the nodule may be red, whereas the rest of the gland is pale in color.

Histological examination of the hyperfunctioning adenoma will demonstrate a uniform hypertrophy and *hyperplasia of the acinar cells*. Some papillary infolding may be present, though this is much less common than in the diffusely hyperplastic gland of Graves' disease. Lymphocytic infiltration is not found in this type of hyperplastic thyroid lesion. The *remainder of the gland* shows *involution*. If the acinar cells are measured, the cell height will be uniformly increased, averaging around 12 to 14 microns, whereas the cell height of the uninvolved tissue may be less than that of a normal thyroid, averaging around 5 to 6 microns.

The more common type of hyperfunctioning ade-

nomatous goiter, the "multinodular" type, occurs in the patient who, prior to developing hyperthyroidism, had a long-standing multinodular goiter, with a number of adenomas within the gland. Some of these nodules may be highly undifferentiated adenomas, and, rarely, even a cancerous lesion may be found within one of the nodules. If all multinodular thyroids could be examined, it is quite possible that in many of them the structure of undifferentiated adenomas would be present, others would show varying degrees of differentiation, and a few would exhibit the structure of a well-differentiated functional adenoma. With autoradiographic techniques it may be found that many of the latter would even have hyperfunction, as compared to the uninvolved nonadenomatous thyroid tissue. Some of these could later be the source of hyperthyroidism, which would develop insidiously.

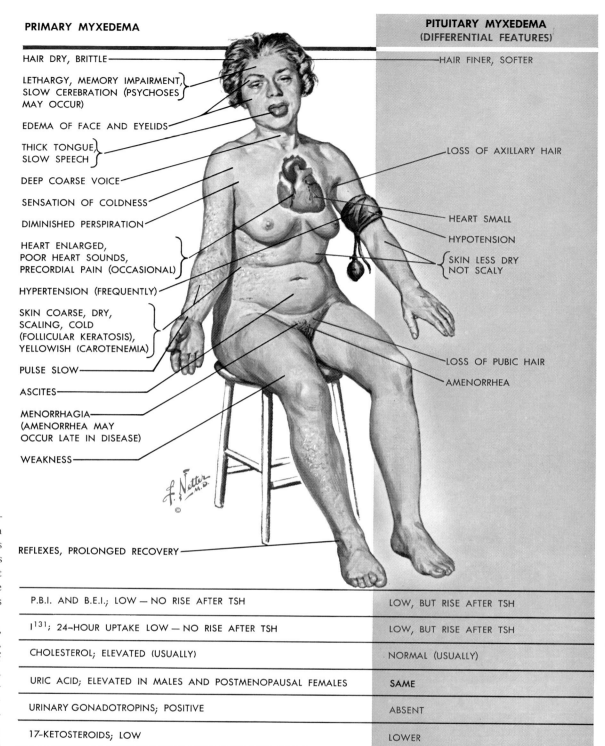

PRIMARY MYXEDEMA

HAIR DRY, BRITTLE

LETHARGY, MEMORY IMPAIRMENT, SLOW CEREBRATION (PSYCHOSES MAY OCCUR)

EDEMA OF FACE AND EYELIDS

THICK TONGUE, SLOW SPEECH

DEEP COARSE VOICE

SENSATION OF COLDNESS

DIMINISHED PERSPIRATION

HEART ENLARGED, POOR HEART SOUNDS, PRECORDIAL PAIN (OCCASIONAL)

HYPERTENSION (FREQUENTLY)

SKIN COARSE, DRY, SCALING, COLD (FOLLICULAR KERATOSIS), YELLOWISH (CAROTENEMIA)

PULSE SLOW

ASCITES

MENORRHAGIA (AMENORRHEA MAY OCCUR LATE IN DISEASE)

WEAKNESS

REFLEXES, PROLONGED RECOVERY

PITUITARY MYXEDEMA (DIFFERENTIAL FEATURES)

HAIR FINER, SOFTER

LOSS OF AXILLARY HAIR

HEART SMALL

HYPOTENSION

SKIN LESS DRY NOT SCALY

LOSS OF PUBIC HAIR

AMENORRHEA

ADULT MYXEDEMA

Clinical Manifestations and Etiology

Symptoms and Signs

Primary myxedema, although not described until 1874, is not an uncommon disease. In one general hospital it has been encountered about one tenth as frequently as is diabetes mellitus. It occurs about seven or eight times more often in females than in males, as does hyperthyroidism.

Myxedema is characterized by *dry, brittle hair* which, if previously curly, has lost its curl or may be incapable of taking a curl. Patients may be lethargic, their *cerebration* is *slow*, and their *memory* is often *impaired*. Individuals suffering from profound myxedema may actually manifest many *psychotic* features, which have been labeled "myxedema madness". Myxedema is associated with *edema of the face and of the eyelids*, or even with a round or moon facies (see Plate 19). The *tongue* is *thick*, the speech is *slow*, and the *voice* is *deep* and *coarse*, with a relative lack of inflection. The *skin* is *cool* and *dry*, because of *diminished perspiration*, and may be *coarse*. Often, a sandpapery *follicular keratosis* occurs over the extensor surfaces of the arms and elbows, frequently on the lateral thoracic wall and over the lateral thighs, and, occasionally, over the shoulders. The skin of the hand or of the face frequently acquires a *yellowish color*, suggesting *carotenemia*. The red cheeks on the light yellow background led early British clinicians to term this the "strawberry and cream" color of myxedema. These patients generally

	PRIMARY MYXEDEMA	PITUITARY MYXEDEMA
P.B.I. AND B.E.I.;	LOW — NO RISE AFTER TSH	LOW, BUT RISE AFTER TSH
I¹³¹;	24-HOUR UPTAKE LOW — NO RISE AFTER TSH	LOW, BUT RISE AFTER TSH
CHOLESTEROL;	ELEVATED (USUALLY)	NORMAL (USUALLY)
URIC ACID;	ELEVATED IN MALES AND POSTMENOPAUSAL FEMALES	SAME
URINARY GONADOTROPINS;	POSITIVE	ABSENT
17-KETOSTEROIDS;	LOW	LOWER
B.M.R.;	USUALLY LOW, BUT VERY VARIABLE	SAME

have a *slow pulse;* they may have *hypertension*, usually with an elevated diastolic pressure, which may improve following correction of the myxedema. *Precordial pain* (angina) is found *occasionally*. A typical feature is that the *heart* is *enlarged* in all directions, owing to myxedematous fluid in the myocardium and to pericardial effusions, which may also be associated with pleural effusions and even with *ascites*. *Heart sounds* are *poor*. Such effusions usually have an elevated protein content. Younger female patients may have *menorrhagia* severe enough to require surgical curettement. Later in the disease, reversible *amenorrhea* occurs. A *prolonged relaxation phase of the ankle jerk* may serve as a diagnostic sign. This may be quantitated with the aid of a modified electrocardiogram and can thus serve in the follow-

up therapy as well. There is generalized *weakness*.

Primary myxedema must be differentiated from *pituitary myxedema*. The history of patients with the latter disease often includes a severe postpartum hemorrhage, followed by absence of lactation and failure of the menstrual cycle to return after recovery from the postpartum period. Usually, the picture of myxedema does not develop until some time after the first sign of pituitary insufficiency; i.e., *amenorrhea* without hot flushes. These individuals usually complain of extreme weakness, somnolence, intolerance to the cold, impaired memory, and slow cerebration. On physical examination they differ from patients with primary myxedema by *finer, softer hair, loss of axillary* and *pubic hair, a small heart* (in contrast to the

(Continued on page 59)

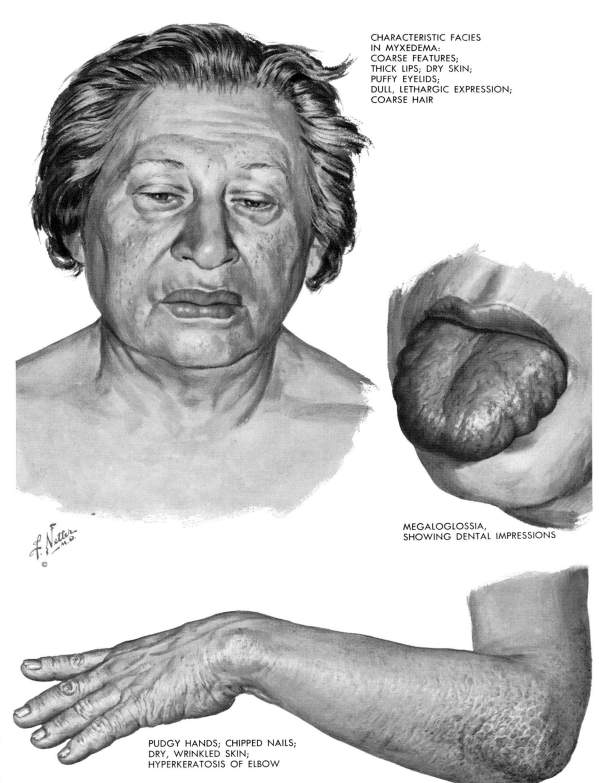

CHARACTERISTIC FACIES
IN MYXEDEMA:
COARSE FEATURES;
THICK LIPS; DRY SKIN;
PUFFY EYELIDS;
DULL, LETHARGIC EXPRESSION;
COARSE HAIR

MEGALOGLOSSIA,
SHOWING DENTAL IMPRESSIONS

PUDGY HANDS; CHIPPED NAILS;
DRY, WRINKLED SKIN;
HYPERKERATOSIS OF ELBOW

ADULT MYXEDEMA

Clinical Manifestations and Etiology

(*Continued from page 58*)

enlarged heart of patients with primary myxedema), some degree of *hypotension,* and a *skin less dry* and *not scaly*.

In primary myxedema the *protein-bound iodine* (P.B.I.) and the *butanol-extractable iodine* (B.E.I.) are low and do not rise after the administration of *thyrotropic,* or *thyroid-stimulating, hormone* (TSH). In pituitary myxedema they are also low but tend to increase after TSH. The *uptake of radioactive iodine* (I^{131}), in both types of myxedema, is low, but it rises in patients with pituitary myxedema after TSH. The *cholesterol* is usually high in primary myxedema but normal or low in patients with pituitary myxedema. In both types, the blood *uric acid* is elevated in males and in elderly postmenopausal women. In primary myxedema the *urinary gonadotropins* are positive, especially in postmenopausal women, whereas they are absent in patients with pituitary myxedema. The *17-ketosteroids* are low in primary and lower in pituitary myxedema, and the *basal metabolic rate* (B.M.R.) usually is low in both. A hypochromic anemia, if present, may be of any type—microcytic or normocytic; occasionally, a normochromic macrocytic anemia is found.

Etiology

The immediate cause of this malady is a deficiency in the secretion of thyroid hormone. This may result from destruction or removal of the thyroid, or from thyroid atrophy and subsequent replace-

ment by fibrous tissue. Myxedema may also develop with goiters which are incapable of synthesizing thyroid hormone, either owing to the administration of some agent which inhibits the organification of iodine or because of some defect in the enzymes necessary to the synthesis of thyroid hormone. It may also result from a chronic thyroiditis, such as Hashimoto's struma.

In considering the etiology of myxedema, it is necessary to separate the two types—primary myxedema of thyroid origin and secondary myxedema of pituitary origin with loss of the thyrotropic hormone, which is necessary for the normal function of the thyroid gland.

The causes of *primary myxedema,* due to a deficiency in the thyroid, may be classified as iatrogenic

or spontaneous (owing to changes within the thyroid gland itself). Probably the most common are the iatrogenic causes. A significant number of patients, who have undergone *thyroidectomy* in the treatment of nontoxic goiter or of Graves' disease, develop myxedema. A too-radical or a complete removal of the thyroid would certainly be followed by postoperative myxedema. Since the treatment of hyperthyroidism with *radioactive iodine* has become a widely used therapeutic modality, it has been noted that a significant percentage of the patients who have received this form of therapy developed post-treatment myxedema. This complication depends, to a great extent, on the dose of radioactive iodine deposited and held in the thyroid gland. It has also been reported, though not

(*Continued on page 60*)

ADULT MYXEDEMA

Clinical Manifestations
and Etiology

(Continued from page 59)

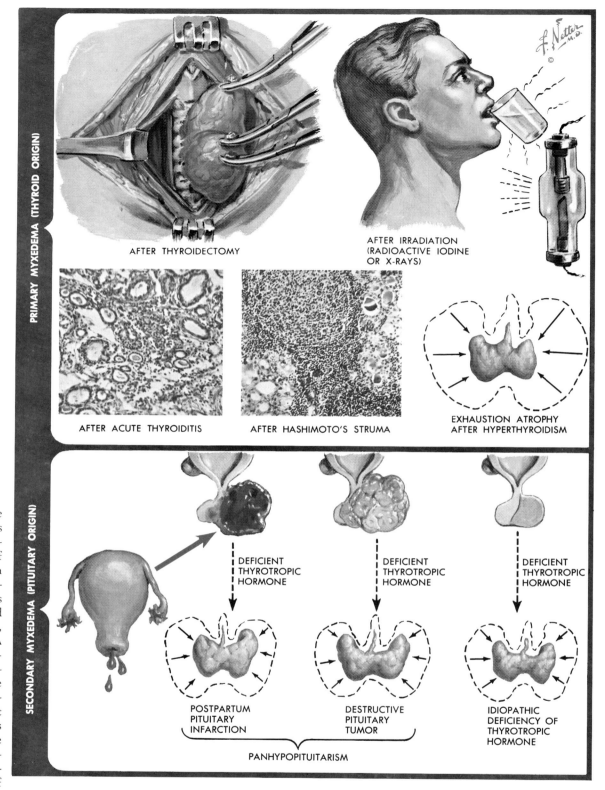

PRIMARY MYXEDEMA (THYROID ORIGIN)

AFTER THYROIDECTOMY

AFTER IRRADIATION
(RADIOACTIVE IODINE
OR X-RAYS)

AFTER ACUTE THYROIDITIS

AFTER HASHIMOTO'S STRUMA

EXHAUSTION ATROPHY
AFTER HYPERTHYROIDISM

SECONDARY MYXEDEMA (PITUITARY ORIGIN)

DEFICIENT
THYROTROPIC
HORMONE

DEFICIENT
THYROTROPIC
HORMONE

DEFICIENT
THYROTROPIC
HORMONE

POSTPARTUM
PITUITARY
INFARCTION

DESTRUCTIVE
PITUITARY
TUMOR

IDIOPATHIC
DEFICIENCY OF
THYROTROPIC
HORMONE

PANHYPOPITUITARISM

very commonly, that patients who have received *X-ray* treatment for neoplasms in the neck, near the thyroid, have developed myxedema. With the advent of thiouracil and related *drugs,* it has been possible to inhibit completely the production of thyroid hormone, and, in patients treated with such agents over a long period of time, without appropriate follow-up, myxedema has occurred occasionally. A number of instances of myxedema, following prolonged treatment of hypertension with potassium thiocyanate, have also been reported. Myxedema has developed as a complication of the treatment with cobalt of certain blood dyscrasias and of childhood tuberculosis with some of the sulfones. The various drug-induced myxedematous states are usually associated with the development of large, vascular, hyperplastic thyroids which developed as a compensatory reaction to the suppression of adequate secretion of thyroid hormone.

Spontaneous myxedema may follow *acute thyroiditis,* presumably owing to some viral agent involving the thyroid. Instances have been described in which the histological picture of *Hashimoto's struma* was found in the thyroids of patients presenting a classical picture of myxedema. Myxedema following long-standing Graves' disease has also been seen. In such instances, the change has been attributed to an *exhaustion atrophy of the thyroid.* Finally, a significant group of patients develop myxedema from un-

known causes and are classified as of the idiopathic type. Presumably, for some reason, in these people the thyroid has been exhausted and the glandular tissue has been replaced by fibrous tissue.

The *secondary myxedemas* can be attributed to some process in the pituitary, resulting in a *loss of the thyroid-stimulating hormone.* Such an isolated deficiency is present in rare instances. A number of patients have developed a *panhypopituitarism* following an *infarction* of the *pituitary* which developed after a *postpartum hemorrhage.* A loss of gonadotropic and thyrotropic hormones usually occurs in these patients, following recovery from the postpartum hemorrhage. The patients generally give a history of amenorrhea, without hot flushes; absence of milk, following delivery of the baby; a loss of libido; and

symptoms of hypothyroidism. Another group of patients presenting a picture of panhypopituitarism includes those whose pituitaries have been destroyed by a *pituitary tumor.* Some situations are suggestive of a pituitary insufficiency associated with a pituitary myxedema, in which we can find no overt cause to explain the panhypopituitarism. The myxedema of these patients is associated with a loss of axillary and pubic hair. Their hearts are not enlarged, as they are in patients with classical primary myxedema. Their thyroids are small and incapable of concentrating radioactive iodine or of producing thyroid hormone. Finally, these patients have a very poor tolerance for thyroid hormone, unless one of the adrenal cortical hormones is given concurrently; failure to do so has, on occasion, led to adrenal crises.

CRETINISM

Cretin is the term given to those unfortunate individuals who suffer from a congenital absence of the thyroid hormone. This may occur as a result of a congenital absence of the thyroid gland itself (*athyrotic cretinism*), or it may be associated with nonfunctioning goiters or with goiters incapable of synthesizing thyroid hormones, owing to an impairment in the "assembly line" at one level or another (*goitrous cretinism*). This malady occurs most frequently in endemic goiter regions, but goitrous cretins have been observed in areas where goiters are quite uncommon. Athyrotic cretins may have experienced some type of intra-uterine thyroiditis (accounting for the destruction of the thyroid gland), or the absence of thyroid tissue may be simply developmental.

In addition to the changes seen in adult myxedema, cretins present two other very obvious alterations, *viz.*, a failure of skeletal growth and maturation, and a marked retardation and deficiency in intellect. The development of centers of ossification is markedly delayed, and the epiphyses show a characteristic stippling. Delayed ossification of bone, of epiphysial union, and of dentition is observed. Body height may be reduced to as little as 55 inches, as in the 69-year-old *elderly cretin* shown. The base of the skull is usually short; there may be a persistence of the cartilaginous junctions between the pre- and postsphenoid bones, which normally ossify in the eighth month of fetal life. Furthermore, due to a delay in ossification of the membranous bones, the frontal suture is usually wide and the anterior fontanels are exceptionally large.

The *face* of a cretin, as a rule, is *round*, with a more or less *stupid expression* and a *yellowish color*. The *eyelids* are *puffy*, and the *palpebral fissures* are generally *narrowed* but horizontal, in contrast to the slant observed in Mongoloids. The *nose* is frequently *flat* and *thick;* the *lips* are *thick;* the *mouth* remains *open,* and a *large, thick tongue protrudes.* The voice is flat and harsh, and the hoarse cry of a cretin in the nursery is nearly diagnostic by itself. The *neck* is usually *short* and *thick.* The skin is dry and cool and presents a picture of nonpitting edema. In juvenile myxedema and in young cretins, there is usually a marked hyperkeratosis in the skin over the anterior abdominal wall. The hair is fine, lifeless, dry, and often quite sparse. In the juvenile myxedematous patient there may also be a marked growth of fine, short hair, of a lanugo type, over the shoulders, upper arms, and face.

Early, the cretin will have a *protuberant abdomen* and *umbilicus* and, nearly always, a sizable umbilical hernia. As

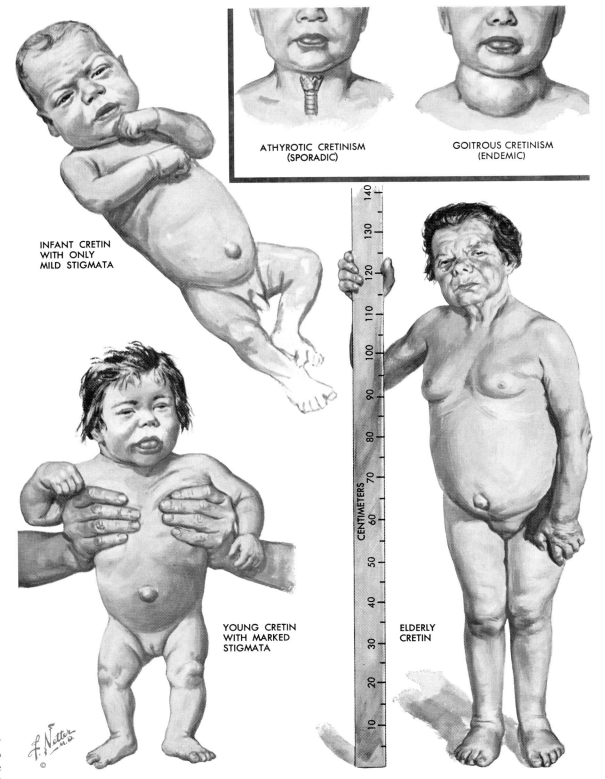

INFANT CRETIN WITH ONLY MILD STIGMATA

ATHYROTIC CRETINISM (SPORADIC)

GOITROUS CRETINISM (ENDEMIC)

YOUNG CRETIN WITH MARKED STIGMATA

ELDERLY CRETIN

the disease progresses, if it is untreated, these symptoms will be exacerbated, and feeblemindedness will be more apparent and totally irreversible.

The diagnosis of cretinism can be confirmed by demonstrating a low level of serum protein-bound iodine. The use of butanol-extractable iodine is far more reliable than the protein-bound iodine, which tends to be somewhat higher, as a rule. A low (or no) uptake of radioactive iodine is diagnostic. Finally, by X-ray examination the typical epiphysial dysgenesis, with its stippling effect, can be demonstrated.

Cretinism should be differentiated from Mongolism and from juvenile, or acquired, myxedema. Physical examination reveals that the Mongoloid has finer features and lacks the coarse skin of the cretin. The eyes are slanted, in contrast to the puffy, straight eyes of cretinism. The presence of a "simian line" in the palms and the excessive extensor flexibility of the

fingers are found in Mongoloids but not in cretins. Furthermore, the Mongoloid is considerably more active than the cretin and, naturally, would record normal thyroid functional studies. The importance of an early differentiation lies in the fact that the earlier high-dose thyroid replacement is started in a cretin, the better will be the ultimate I.Q. and bone development.

Hurler's disease, or gargoylism, is readily distinguishable from cretinism (see page 229).

Children with juvenile, or acquired, myxedema can be differentiated from the cretin by a history of normal growth and development, normal dentition, and the absence of feeblemindedness. Usually, their skeletal X-rays demonstrate perfectly normal growth of the epiphysial centers up to the time of the onset of developing myxedema; thus, the bone age may be only 2 or 3 years behind the chronological age.

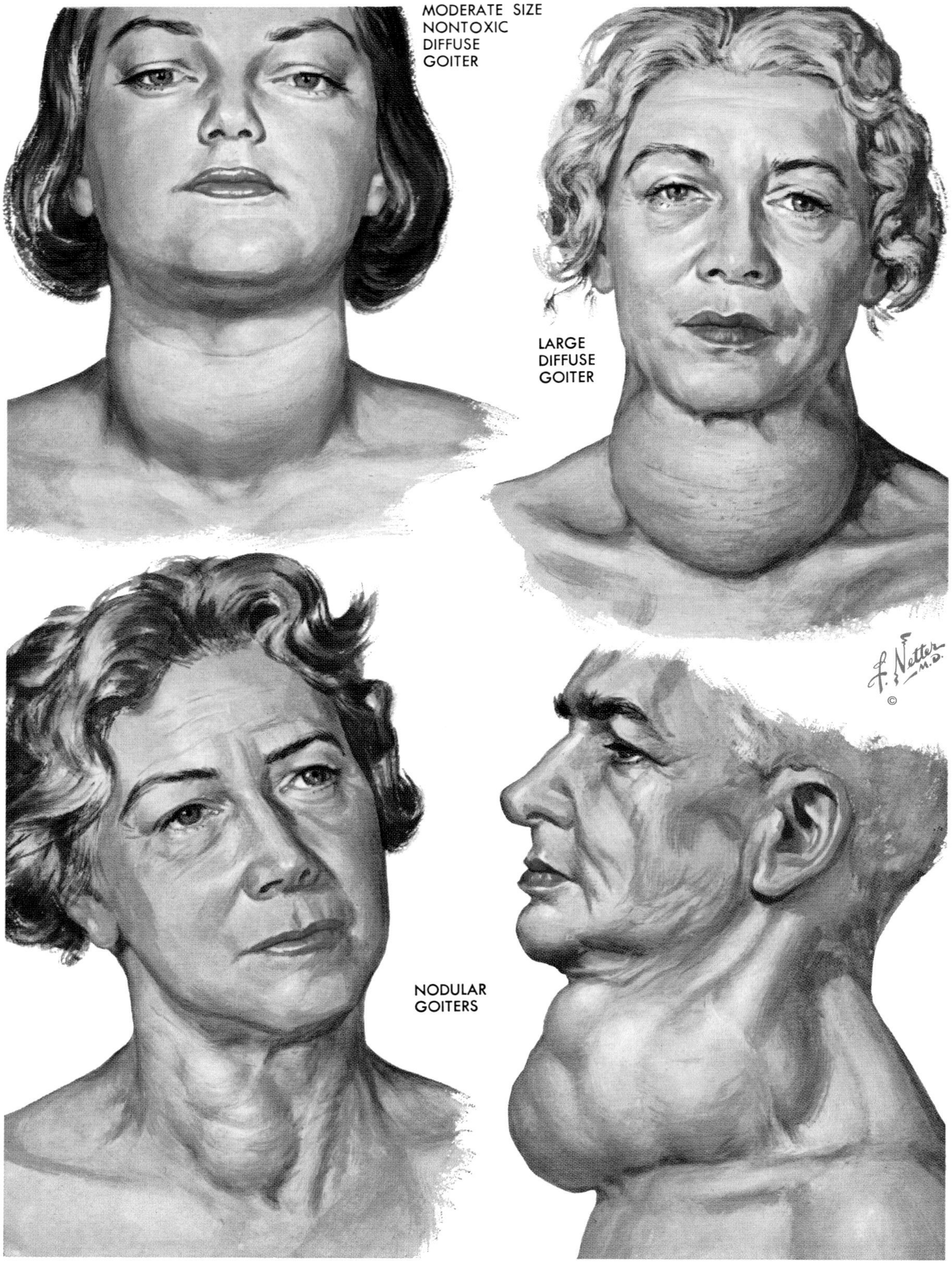

SIMPLE GOITER

MODERATE SIZE
NONTOXIC
DIFFUSE
GOITER

LARGE
DIFFUSE
GOITER

NODULAR
GOITERS

Nontoxic goiters occur throughout the world, in certain areas more frequently than in others. They seem to be more common in areas where the iodine content in the water and soil is low, as around the Great Lakes and also in mountainous areas. It has been suggested that these nontoxic goiters are more likely to be found in localities where the water contains large amounts of calcium carbonate and thus is quite hard. Characteristically, enlargement of the thyroid with a *moderate-sized nontoxic, diffuse goiter* occurs in both males and females at about the time of puberty. The enlargement may be progressive during the adolescent years, but may then level off or even appear to become smaller. In the female, however, it again increases in size with each pregnancy. In adolescent males, nontoxic goiters seem to be less persistent, unless there is a highly active goitrogen in the diet or some dietary deficiency contributing to the development of the goiter, in which case it may become quite prominent, but rarely as prominent as in females.

Such goiters are diffuse in the early stage; later, they may become *nodular*, feeling hard in one area or cystic in another. Nodular goiters may be more or less symmetrical or quite asymmetrical. Such a goiter, if allowed to continue, may

descend beneath the sternum and produce the picture of an intrathoracic goiter. With the increase in size of the goiter, especially if some of it is lodged beneath the sternum, obstructive symptoms may result from distortion of the trachea or of the esophagus. Occasionally, a nodular goiter may enlarge in one area very suddenly, producing pain which may be referred to the ear, neck structures, or shoulder. This is frequently explained on the basis of a hemorrhage into a follicle or into an adenoma or large cyst in the thyroid.

In such multinodular goiters, adenomas of various types may be observed, and these may present various kinds of histological structure. Some of them may be capable of function and may develop hyperfunction, resulting in a clinical picture of hyperthyroidism in

an adenomatous goiter, a so-called "hot nodule".

Cancer is much less common in these multinodular goiters than in those thyroids presenting a single nodule. However, the fact that the goiter is a multinodular one does not rule out the possibility of cancer developing or being found in it.

The indications for surgical removal of such thyroids may fall into several categories: One is for cosmetic reasons which may impel the patient to seek surgical removal of the gland. Another indication would be a sudden enlargement of the gland, especially if the site of rapid growth is hard, suggesting a neoplastic change. Finally, the most important reason is to correct any obstructive symptoms produced by the impingement of such a large mass on either the trachea or the esophagus.

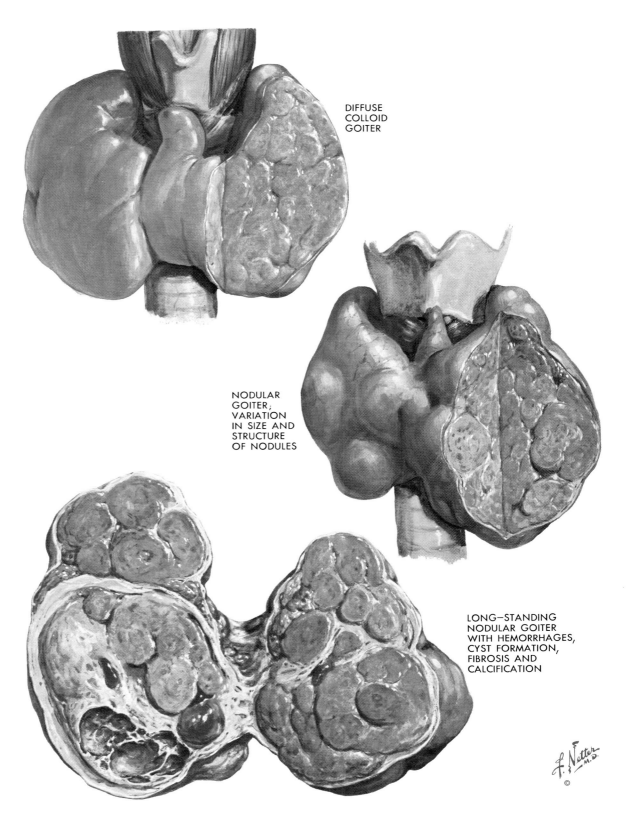

DIFFUSE
COLLOID
GOITER

NODULAR
GOITER;
VARIATION
IN SIZE AND
STRUCTURE
OF NODULES

LONG–STANDING
NODULAR GOITER
WITH HEMORRHAGES,
CYST FORMATION,
FIBROSIS AND
CALCIFICATION

GROSS PATHOLOGY OF
GOITER

Early in the history of a nontoxic goiter, the gland is usually diffusely and quite uniformly enlarged, with an increase in the size of the pyramidal lobe. This is known as a *diffuse* nontoxic, or *colloid, goiter.* Such glands may be two or three times the normal size, or they may be even larger. The patient may become aware of the condition because others have commented on the fullness of the neck, because the collar may feel too tight, or because it may become difficult to swallow.

The gland feels firm but not hard. In the early stage, microscopic examination discloses a diffuse, extreme hyperplasia of the thyroid. As the process progresses, with the advancing age of the patient, the thyroid may become *asymmetrical* and *multinodular,* which is evident on gross examination of the gland. Significant *variations in the size and structure of the nodules* become apparent. In the very *long-standing, nodular goiter, hemorrhages* into various sites in the gland, *cyst formation, fibrosis,* and even *calcification* are likely to be observed. On X-ray examination, any retrosternal extension of such a goiter may, if calci-

fied, initially simulate intrapulmonary calcifications.

Microscopic examination of such a nodular goiter may reveal every conceivable type of benign adenoma, including a highly undifferentiated trabecular pattern or the earliest stage of differentiation of tubular structure, the structure of microfollicles, or, finally, the picture of a hyperplastic adenoma.

Rarely, within these nodules may be seen various types of cancerous growths, such as adenocarcinoma or papillary carcinoma of the thyroid. However, the cancerous changes in such thyroids are much less common than they are in those of patients presenting a single nodule in the thyroid. Local pressure symptoms represent the most important indication for therapeutic interference, but the rare occurrence of a small malignancy must always be kept in mind.

ETIOLOGY OF GOITER

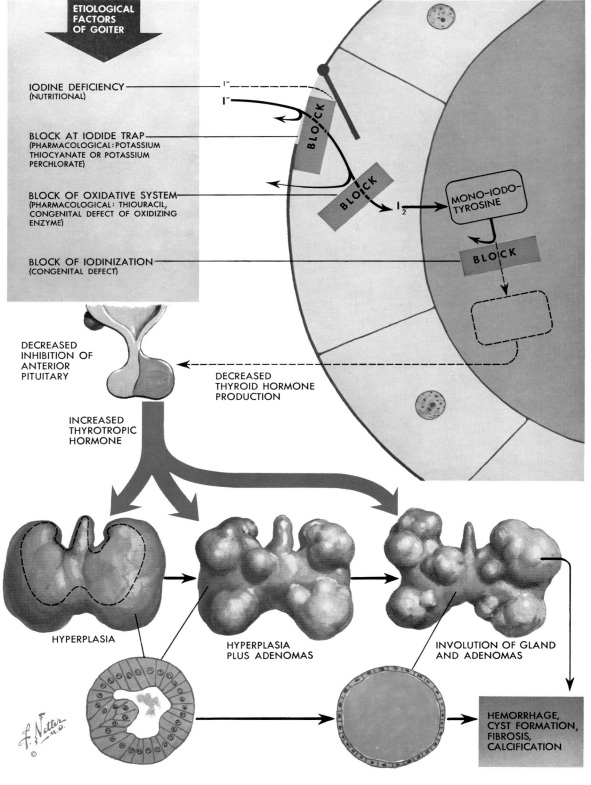

Nontoxic *goiter* is not traceable to any single cause. Basically, its development can be attributed to a deficiency in thyroid hormone secretion, to which the *pituitary* responds with an increased output of thyroid-stimulating hormone.

Lack of thyroid hormone, resulting in a hypothyroid state, may be predicted to result from nutritional deficiencies of elements or compounds necessary for the synthesis of thyroid hormones, yet the only known deficiency state that may be goitrogenic is the *dietary deficiency of iodine.* Such iodine deficiencies are related to geographic areas where the soil and water lack iodine, such as around the Great Lakes. The use of iodized table salt has markedly reduced the incidence of the iodine-deficiency goiter.

Impairment of, or interference with, the synthesis of thyroid hormone is today the most common cause of goiter. A growing number of clinical situations exist in which congenital deficiencies of enzyme systems, necessary to the intrathyroidal metabolism of iodine or to the synthesis of thyroid hormone, have explained the congenital hypothyroidism and the development of nontoxic goiters in goitrous cretins.

A decrease in thyroid hormone will be followed by a compensatory increase of the thyroid-stimulating hormone. This, in turn, produces a nonfunctioning growth of the thyroid, or goiter. The *iodide trap* may be impaired spontaneously in some patients. In others, the ingestion of *potassium thiocyanate* or *potassium perchlorate* results in a paralysis of the iodide trap and an impairment of hormone synthesis. The *oxidative*

system, which turns iodide ($2I^-$) to iodine (I_2), may be defective *congenitally* or may be blocked by natural goitrogens, which act like *thiouracil* and related agents to prevent the synthesis of thyroid hormone by paralyzing the thyroid peroxidase or other oxidative enzymes. It has been suggested that the sulfonamides and related agents prevent the utilization of iodine, even after it has been oxidized from iodide, by competing with tyrosine as a receptor of iodine.

Another group of goitrous cretins has been explained on the basis of a block of the enzyme systems necessary to the interconversion of *mono-iodotyrosine* to di-iodotyrosine and the *coupling* of these to form thyroid hormone. In this connection a very interesting congenital defect is the finding of an impaired dehalogenase which interferes with thyroid hormone synthesis. Here, administration of I[131]-labeled di-iodotyrosine does not, as normally, lead to excretion of

urinary I[131] iodide revealing a dehalogenase deficit.

The hypothyroid states, developing from lack of iodine in the diet, from the administration of goitrogenic drugs which block the synthesis of thyroid hormones, or from congenital defects of systems necessary for the synthesis of thyroid hormone, result in *increased thyrotropic hormone.* This leads to a maximum growth stimulus of the thyroid gland, with a manifold increase in thyroid size and extreme *hyperplasia* and hypertrophy of the thyroid. After a prolonged period of thyroid hyperplasia, *adenomas* of various types develop within the hyperplastic thyroid. Finally, after a period of extreme hyperplasia, exhaustion or *involution* occurs. The epithelium becomes flat, the follicles fill with a viscous colloid, and, eventually, *hemorrhagic cysts* may occur, some becoming *calcified* or *fibrosed.* Rarely, carcinoma may form within such a hyperplastic gland.

TRABECULAR
(EMBRYONAL)
ADENOMA

TUBULAR
(EMBRYONAL)
ADENOMA

MICROFOLLICULAR
(FETAL)
ADENOMA

MICRO- AND
MACROFOLLICULAR
ADENOMA

MACROFOLLICULAR
(COLLOID)
ADENOMA

HYPERPLASTIC
ADENOMA
(FUNCTIONAL OR
NONFUNCTIONAL)

HISTOLOGY OF THYROID ADENOMAS

HISTOLOGY OF THYROID ADENOMAS

Nodular goiters, on microscopic examination, usually are benign. Many of the nodular lesions prove to be well-encapsulated benign adenomas. Such adenomas present a variety of histological patterns, some of which are similar to the histological structures of the thyroids seen in various stages of embryonic development. Thus, some of these have been labeled embryonal or fetal adenomas, depending upon the degree of differentiation.

The least-differentiated tumors of the thyroid present a pattern of cords of solidly packed cells and resemble the least-differentiated embryonal thyroid. This type of adenoma has been labeled trabecular, or embryonal, or solid adenoma. Radio-iodine (I¹³¹) is not taken up by this kind of adenoma, which, like highly undifferentiated embryonic thyroid tissue, is nonfunctional.

Another class, which may be grouped with the trabecular adenomas as an embryonal adenoma, and which resembles the first stage of differentiation of the embryonic thyroid, is known as a tubular adenoma. Such tumors are characterized by loosely packed cords of cells surrounding a lumen like the walls of a tubule. Radio-iodine studies of these adenomas indicate that they also are incapable of function.

The next stage of differentiation is represented by the microfollicular, or fetal, adenoma. It can be compared to the thyroid of the 14- to 15-week-old human fetus or to that of the 12- to 14-day-old chick embryo. It is characterized by small, uniformly sized and uniformly shaped follicles, which are lined by cuboidal cells and contain faintly staining colloid. Such tumors are functional, being capable of concentrating signifi-

cant amounts of radio-iodine but less than that trapped by normal thyroid tissue.

Another group has been classified as the micro- and macrofollicular adenomas of the thyroid. Such tumors differ from the microfollicular (fetal) adenomas by virtue of a variation in the size and shape of the follicles and the somewhat flattened epithelium. Usually, these tumors are also capable of concentrating radioactive iodine but, again, less than that trapped by normal thyroid tissue.

Macrofollicular, or colloid, adenomas of the thyroid differ from the structure of a diffuse colloid goiter only by virtue of a capsule or pseudocapsule surrounding the nodule. These nodules are characterized by large colloid-filled follicles surrounded by flat epithelium. The functional capacity of the colloid adenomas, as measured with radio-iodine techniques, is variable. Some may have measurable function but

less than that possessed by normal thyroid tissue, and others may have minimal function to none at all.

Two types of hyperplastic adenomas are seen in the thyroid, each presenting a pattern of hypertrophied and hyperplastic follicular cells which may invaginate into the follicular lumen. These tumors can be differentiated by studies with radioactive iodine and by measuring the height of the acinar cells. In one group, the adenomas are functional, having an excellent iodine-concentrating capacity which is greater than that of the adjacent normal thyroid tissue, and their follicular cells are uniformly hyperplastic. Such tumors are capable of hyperfunction and even of producing hyperthyroidism. The other hyperplastic adenomas are nonfunctional, and their cells, though hyperplastic, are much less uniform in size, as can be shown by a frequency curve of the recorded acinar cell heights.

DIFFUSE INFILTRATION OF THYROID STROMA

ACUTE AND SUBACUTE THYROIDITIS

Acute Thyroiditis

Acute thyroiditis, which is also known as acute diffuse thyroiditis, acute non-suppurative thyroiditis, or pseudotubercular thyroiditis, is characterized by *fever,* extreme *malaise,* and a firm, very *tender enlargement* of the *thyroid gland.* This is usually asymmetrical, and the gland may be two to three times its normal size. In a majority of patients, the principal symptoms of this malady can be related to the thyroid and the structures near it. A swelling of the neck is definitely present, as is *pain* in the thyroid, which may be *referred* to the mandibular joints or to the ears. A marked *tenderness* in the thyroid, and even in *lymph nodes* near the gland, is evident, and the patient may complain of *dysphagia.* Characteristically, these patients have *spiking temperatures,* which may be dangerously high in the very acute stages of the disease. In some people the general malaise, even with muscle pains, is so marked that the nature of the disease in the thyroid is not at first recognized.

The cause of this disease is not known, although a viral etiology has been suspected. Several patients have manifested symptoms and signs of herpangina or other indications of the Coxsackie viral infections. Notwithstanding the strongly suggestive signs and symptoms, attempts to demonstrate the Coxsackie virus in the thyroid or in the body fluids of such patients have been fruitless. Thyroiditis is oftentimes associated with mumps. Recently, the mumps virus has been recovered from the thyroids of patients with thyroiditis. It is quite likely that several viruses may affect the thyroid as well as other types of glandular tissue.

Following a primary insult, the release of thyroglobulin or denatured thyroid tissue into the circulation may result in an immunological sensitization and the production of auto-immune antibodies. These, in turn, may damage the thyroid tissue as they combine with it and superimpose a local allergic reaction upon the

initial inflammatory one. The examination of biopsy specimens from such thyroids reveals an *inflammatory reaction* which is characterized by the *infiltration of thyroid stroma* with mononuclear cells, a proliferation of fibrous tissue, and giant cell formation within various parts of the specimen.

In patients with this malady, tracer studies with *radioactive iodine* have demonstrated that the thyroids do not concentrate significant amounts of iodine. Indeed, the uptake is usually in the neighborhood of 1 to 5 per cent. This very low avidity for radioactive iodine may be altered by the administration of thyrotropic hormone. In contrast, the *protein-bound iodine* (*P.B.I.*) of patients with acute thyroiditis is, characteristically, somewhat elevated above the normal level. Some evidence suggests that this elevation simply reflects a release of thyroglobulin into the circulation, and that this thyroglobulin does not repre-

sent an increased level of free thyroxine. The combination of a low I[131] uptake and a normal or high P.B.I. very strongly suggests the presence of thyroiditis.

Subacute Thyroiditis

Subacute thyroiditis presents a self-limited course. The milder cases can be controlled by agents such as aspirin, and the symptoms, in such instances, may last only a few weeks. In others, the disease may last for several months and may require more drastic forms of therapy. X-ray therapy has been helpful in such patients, as has the prolonged administration of goitrogenic agents such as propylthiouracil. It is in this group that the adrenal steroids seem to have their greatest usefulness. The administration of such agents not only produces marked relief of symptoms but may actually shorten the course of the disease.

CHRONIC THYROIDITIS

Hashimoto's Struma, Riedel's Struma

Hashimoto's Struma

Hashimoto's struma (struma lymphomatosa, or lymphadenoid goiter) is a progressive disease of the thyroid, which occurs much more commonly in females than in males. Though it may develop at any age, it is found most frequently in patients between 20 and 40 years of age.

The symptoms of Hashimoto's struma are insidious, beginning with a gradual enlargement of the thyroid. Tenderness of the gland is noted only rarely. Fever does not develop. Occasionally, a patient's history may include a previous period of nervousness and some weight loss. The sedimentation rate is normal, and leukocytosis does not occur. There may be a relative lymphocytosis. The basal metabolic rate is usually below normal.

On physical examination, it is impressive, if the borders of the thyroid can be clearly felt, that these are *scalloped* with pseudopodia, which are much *more definite on the lower than on the lateral borders.* Characteristically, such goiters are *lobulated* and gray on section.

Microscopically, there are macrofollicles and microfollicles showing hyperplasia and involution, with a marked infiltration of lymphocytes and plasma cells. Large hyperplastic lymph follicles, with germinal centers, are frequently present. Such lymphadenoid goiters exhibit varying degrees of interacinar fibrosis. There may be a number of atrophic acini with acidophilic cells.

In recent years, evidence has accumulated to support the thesis that Hashimoto's struma is an auto-immune disease caused by *"spillage" of thyroglobulin* into the circulation, against which *lymph nodes* and *plasma cells* produce *antithyroglobulin antibodies.* It has been demonstrated that the administration of rabbit thyroglobulin (in a Freund's adjuvant) to rabbits results in the development of antibodies directed against thyroglobulin. The thyroids of the animals in which the antibodies have been produced present a histological picture like that of Hashimoto's struma. Subsequent studies by various clinical investigators have demonstrated that a significant number of patients with Hashimoto's struma have *antibodies* against thyroglobulin in their *serum.* In a recent report it was stated that 98 per cent of the patients with Hashimoto's struma had antibodies to thyroglobulin; 83 per cent of the patients with myxedema, 67 per cent of those with Graves' disease, and 33 per cent of those with nontoxic nodular goiters also had thyroid antibodies. This test, though important in determining possible mechanisms as to the development of lymphadenoid goiter, is not specific enough to merit a precise pathological

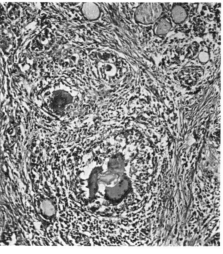

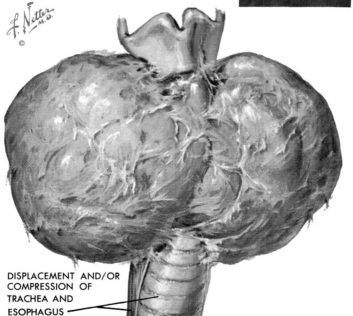

diagnosis of a nodular goiter in a given patient. The radio-iodine uptake tends to be low, whereas the protein-bound iodine may be elevated on account of the spillage of thyroglobulin from the gland.

Riedel's Struma

Riedel's struma, or ligneous thyroiditis, occurs very infrequently and then predominantly in males. It is a chronic, proliferative, fibrosing process involving the thyroid. It may extend to *displace and/or compress the trachea and esophagus,* and the overlying fascia and muscles. Riedel's struma is characterized by a stony-hard, enlarged thyroid, which is firmly adherent to adjacent structures but not to the skin. Oftentimes, the gland may be asymmetrical, with greater enlargement of one side than of the other. Subjectively, patients with Riedel's struma may complain of pres-

sure, which may be severe enough to require decompression of the trachea by subtotal thyroidectomy.

Microscopically, this disease is characterized by a marked diffuse sclerosis, with considerable invasion of the normal thyroid tissue. A woodlike, hard texture is characteristic. The unaffected portions of the gland reveal varying numbers of persistent acini, which appear to be compressed by the surrounding dense, fibrous stroma. The cells of the persistent follicles are not remarkable; unlike those in Hashimoto's struma, they do not show acidophilic degeneration or any other signs of atrophy.

The etiology of Riedel's struma is unknown. Some authors have suggested that this is an end stage of a previous Hashimoto's struma. Although some evidence exists to support this theory, much conflicts with it, and it is important to note that Riedel's struma is much less common than is Hashimoto's struma.

MAY HAVE MULTIPLE FOCI

PAPILLARY CARCINOMA

USUALLY PRESENTS AS SOLITARY NONFUNCTIONING NODULE

TWO DIFFERENT PARTS OF TUMOR

Papillary Carcinoma of the Thyroid

METASTASIZES: CHIEFLY TO REGIONAL LYMPH NODES (CERVICAL AND MEDIASTINAL)

SECONDARILY TO LUNGS (MILIARY SPREAD)

RARELY TO SKELETON

VERY RARELY TO BRAIN

Papillary carcinoma is the *most common malignant tumor of the thyroid gland.* Its *incidence, according to age,* is greatest in young adults, but it may be seen as late as the eighth decade or in the very young child. This disease occurs more frequently in females than it does in males and, in the female, is found about eight times more commonly during the childbearing years.

Papillary carcinomas may be very small, or they may be readily palpable. Often, however, such a tumor presents only as an enlarged lymph node in the neck, and it is found in the thyroid only after intensive search of the excised gland. Papillary carcinomas of the thyroid frequently show *multiple foci.* It is not uncommon to find two or more lesions in the thyroid of a patient who presented with a lymph node in the neck, which, on biopsy, proved to be a papillary lesion of thyroid origin.

Histologically, this cancer shows a picture of papillary cords, with a delicately vascularized connective tissue which is lined by one to many layers of cuboidal and columnar cells. Characteristically, colloid is absent from a pure papillary carcinoma of the thyroid gland. However, many do have areas of follicular carcinoma with well-differentiated colloid-filled follicles.

Papillary carcinoma *metastasizes* frequently to the *cervical and upper mediastinal lymph nodes.* If this type of cancer spreads beyond the confines of the neck, it is usually to the *lungs secondarily.* In this setting an *X-ray* of the *chest* reveals *miliary nodules* fanning out from the hilus. Such X-rays are often confused with those of miliary tuberculosis, of sarcoidosis, or of silicosis. This type of X-ray picture may also be seen in patients with metastases arising from primaries in the breast, stomach, lung, or pancreas. *Skeletal metastases* occur quite infrequently. When the bones are involved, the patient is usually in the older age group. Rarely, metastases may be

found in the *brain.*

This type of cancer is one of the least aggressive and *least malignant* of the cancers occurring in the human body. However, it is capable of causing death. It may be very aggressive in children under the age of 7 years or in adults beyond the fifth decade.

Studies reveal that this cancer has a very *low degree of function,* as measured by its capacity to concentrate radioactive iodine. However, in some patients with metastatic papillary carcinoma of the thyroid, it has been possible to induce function in the metastases by removing the normal thyroid gland and administering thiouracil, or related antithyroid drugs, over a long period of time. In such patients it may be possible to induce even maximum function in the tumors, so that cancericidal doses of radioactive iodine may be administered.

Studies in experimental animals have demonstrated

that prolonged administration of goitrogenic antithyroid agents not only may produce extreme hyperplasia of the thyroid but also, if the drugs are given long enough, may bring about lesions that are comparable to a variety of benign adenomas of the thyroid. In a high-cancer strain of mice or rats, the administration of such goitrogenic drugs will result in the development of thyroid cancers, many of which have a structure not unlike that of papillary carcinoma. It has been suggested that the pituitary is necessary for the development of cancer of the thyroid. On this basis, it has been advocated that patients with papillary carcinoma of the thyroid be treated with large doses of thyroid hormone. Unfortunately, such medication cannot effect a cure, but the ultimate growth of the tumor may be somewhat delayed. In general, this tumor has a reasonably good prognosis if treated early by radical neck dissection.

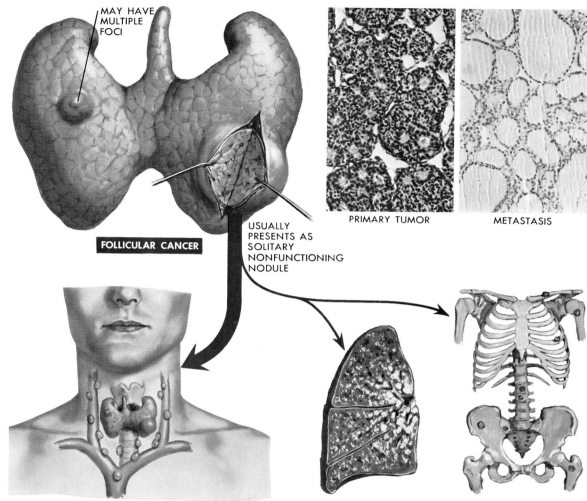

MAY HAVE MULTIPLE FOCI

FOLLICULAR CANCER

USUALLY PRESENTS AS SOLITARY NONFUNCTIONING NODULE

PRIMARY TUMOR   METASTASIS

FOLLICULAR CARCINOMA OF THE THYROID

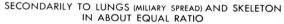

METASTASIZES: CHIEFLY TO REGIONAL LYMPH NODES (CERVICAL AND MEDIASTINAL)

SECONDARILY TO LUNGS (MILIARY SPREAD) AND SKELETON IN ABOUT EQUAL RATIO

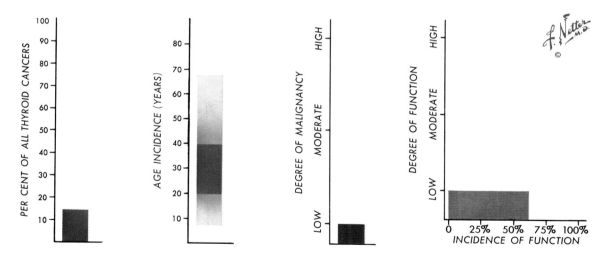

Follicular cancers of the thyroid are much less common than papillary cancers, accounting for about *12 to 15 per cent* of all cancers arising in this organ. They may occur at any age, but, most commonly, they are seen between the ages of *20 and 40 years,* and much more often in females than in males.

Follicular cancer may present as a small nodule or as a large mass within the thyroid. Like the papillary cancer, this lesion may have *multiple foci.*

Histologically, follicular cancer of the thyroid shows a fairly well-organized follicular pattern, with small but frequently irregular follicles lined by high cuboidal epithelium. The follicles often appear in clusters. The follicles with a more orderly arrangement commonly contain colloid. Such colloid-containing follicles have been demonstrated, by autoradiographic techniques, to concentrate radioactive iodine. Extensive examinations of these cancers will reveal that a large percentage of the follicular type contain sizable areas which present the histological pattern of a papillary cancer; a similar study

of many papillary cancers will reveal that a sizable fraction present follicular patterns. In some follicular cancers, not only may areas of papillary structure be found, but there also are regions with less differentiation, showing tubular and even trabecular structure.

These cancers, even though they are not highly malignant, frequently *metastasize* early to the cervical and *mediastinal lymph nodes.* Later, they metastasize to the *lungs,* with a diffuse *miliary type of spread* fanning out from the hilar areas. *Skeletal metastases* also occur, but usually late in the disease. However, occasionally, patients may be encountered who present themselves with symptoms of one or more skeletal metastases which, when biopsied, look like perfectly normal thyroid tissue. Such lesions have been mislabeled "benign metastasizing strumas".

Studies of *function* have demonstrated that a majority of follicular cancers are capable of concentrating radioactive iodine; however, practically none can concentrate more than a small fraction of the amount trapped by normal thyroid tissue. This natural avidity of the tumor for radioactive iodine can be greatly enhanced, in a majority of the patients studied, by removing the normal thyroid and by administering thiouracil, or related goitrogenic agents, for varying periods of time.

Regarding *malignancy,* although this type of cancer is likely to be nonaggressive, it is apt to be more so than papillary cancer of the thyroid. It has a very good prognosis, especially if it is diagnosed and treated, before the age of 40 years, by radical neck dissection.

SOLID ADENOCARCINOMA OF THE THYROID

SOLID ADENOCARCINOMA

CERVICAL LYMPH NODES NOT USUALLY INVOLVED

LUNG (DISCRETE NODULES)

SKELETON

LIVER

KIDNEY

MOST COMMON SITES OF METASTASIS

LESS COMMON SITES OF METASTASIS

PER CENT OF ALL THYROID CANCERS

AGE INCIDENCE (YEARS)

DEGREE OF MALIGNANCY — HIGH MODERATE LOW

DEGREE OF FUNCTION — HIGH MODERATE LOW

INCIDENCE OF FUNCTION — 0 25% 50% 75% 100%

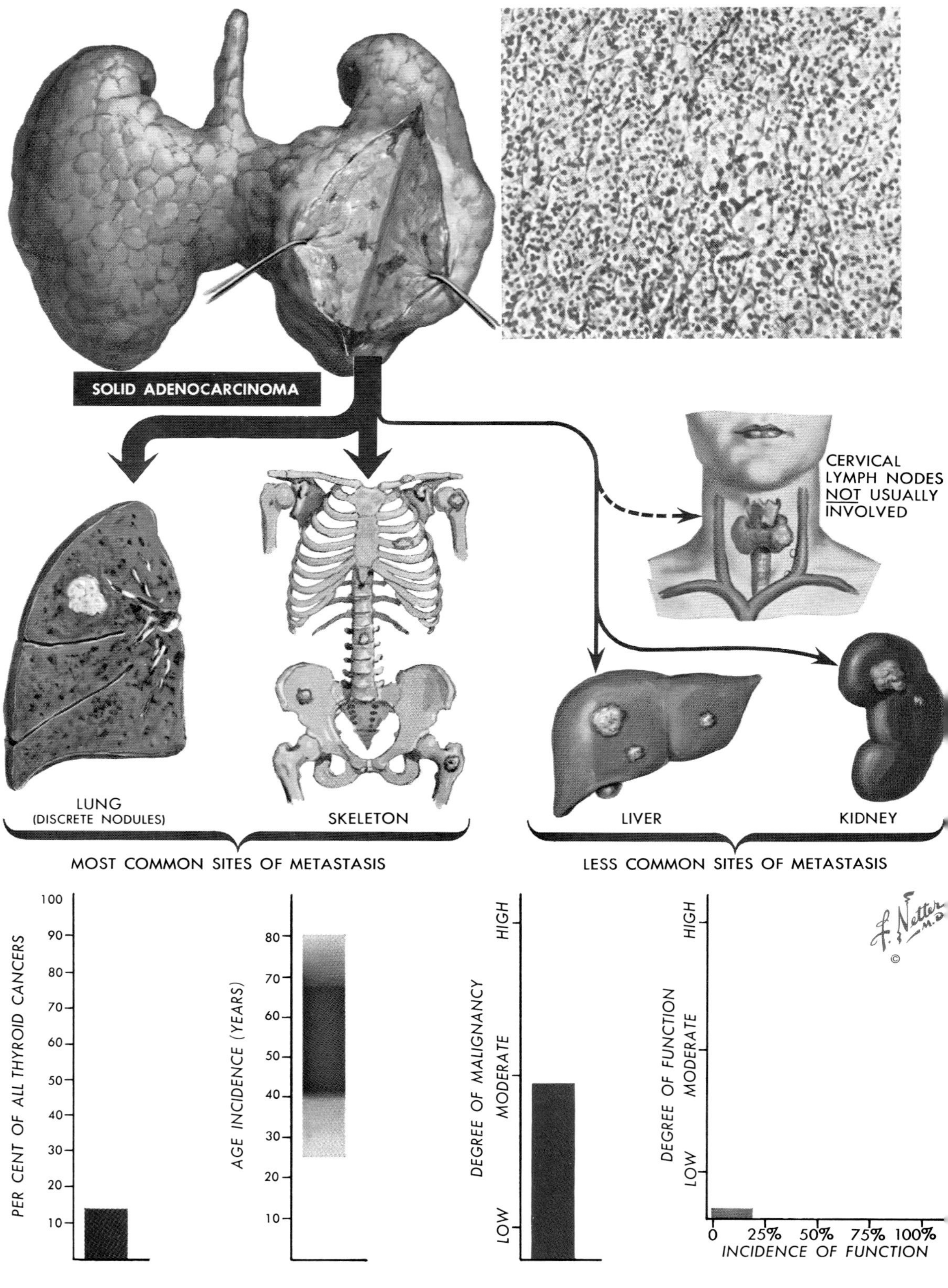

The *solid adenocarcinoma,* or trabecular carcinoma, of the thyroid constitutes about *15 per cent of the cancers of the thyroid* seen in one series. Although this cancer may appear in the early part of the third decade, it is observed most commonly *after the age of 40 years,* in what is known as middle life. It is found more often in females than in males.

These cancers may present as small, discrete nodules. More commonly, however, they are large, bulky, and hard. Usually, they are localized to one lobe, and, unlike the papillary and follicular cancers of the thyroid, it is uncommon to find multicentric lesions.

On *histological examination,* such tumors present a solid trabecular pattern of closely packed cells, with considerable variation in the size of the nuclei and with hyperchromatism; though most are of the solid, cellular type exclusively, there may be areas which present a follicular structure.

These cancers usually *metastasize* distantly by way of the blood stream. Although metastatic deposits may be found in the *cervical lymph nodes,* such metastases are *uncommon* with this particular histological type. *Pulmonary* and *skeletal metastases* are more characteristic. The pulmonary metastases usually occur as single, *discrete nodules.* The skeletal metastases may be multiple or single and are, usually, a mixture of osteolytic and osteoblastic types. This is one cancer of the thyroid which relatively frequently metastasizes to the *liver.* It occasionally leaves its metastatic deposits in the *kidneys,* which may cause confusion as to the primary tumor, *i.e.,* tumor of the thyroid with renal metastases or cancer of the kidney with thyroid deposits.

Studies with radioactive iodine have revealed that this type of thyroid cancer has little or no *function.*

Although this cancer would be listed as only moderately aggressive, it is a great deal more *malignant* and aggressive than the papillary, follicular, or Hürthle cell cancers of the thyroid, and thus it does not carry the same favorable prognosis. However, it does have a much better prognosis than has the giant and spindle cell cancer of the thyroid.

HÜRTHLE CELL CARCINOMA OF THE THYROID

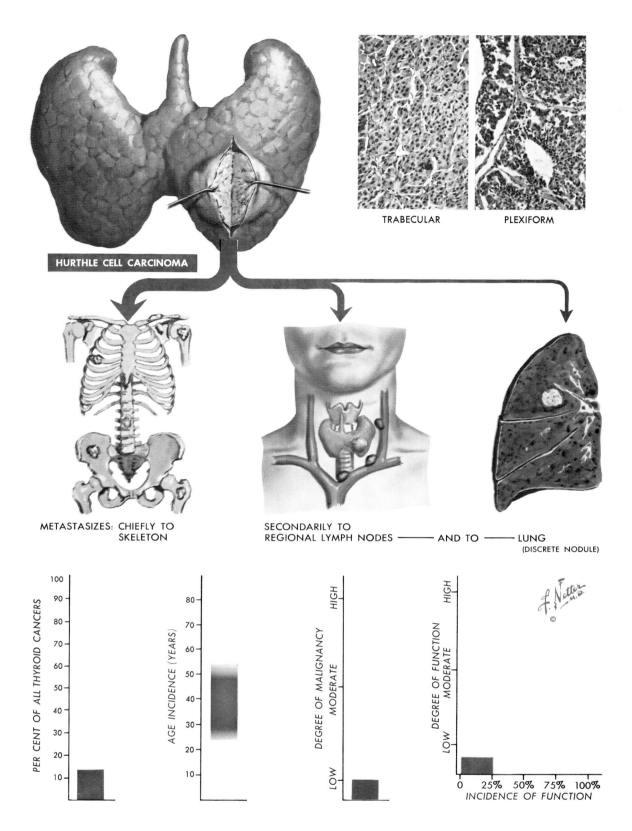

HURTHLE CELL CARCINOMA

TRABECULAR   PLEXIFORM

METASTASIZES: CHIEFLY TO SKELETON

SECONDARILY TO REGIONAL LYMPH NODES —— AND TO —— LUNG (DISCRETE NODULE)

PER CENT OF ALL THYROID CANCERS

AGE INCIDENCE (YEARS)

DEGREE OF MALIGNANCY — HIGH / MODERATE / LOW

DEGREE OF FUNCTION — HIGH / MODERATE / LOW
INCIDENCE OF FUNCTION — 0 25% 50% 75% 100%

Hürthle cell carcinoma of the thyroid is relatively uncommon, making up about *12 per cent* of any large series of thyroid cancer. It occurs most often between the ages of *20 and 50 years,* and anywhere from four to eight times more frequently in females than in males.

Anatomically, it usually presents as a single nodule and is only moderate in size; it may be barely palpable, or it may be large enough to involve one entire lobe of the thyroid.

Histologically, it is characterized by the appearance of bright, opaque, pink-staining cells, which are high cuboidal to low columnar and which may occur in an orderly *trabecular* arrangement, with each column being separated by a rich, thin-walled capillary blood supply, or may be stratified in *plexiform* groups, which also are separated by the capillaries of the rich blood supply.

Although this type of tumor is relatively benign, it may metastasize, even to vital structures, resulting in the death of the patient. As a rule, the *metastatic spread* is via the blood stream to the *lungs* and, chiefly, to the *skeleton.* Some metastases may be demonstrated in the *regional lymph nodes,* presumably reaching these nodes via the lymphatics.

The *function* of this particular type of cancer, as determined by measuring its avidity for radioactive iodine, is extremely low to absent. However, the metastases of a few such tumors have been observed to acquire maximum function following the removal of the normal thyroid gland and the administration of such agents as thiouracil or propylthiouracil. Actually, histological examination of at least one of these metastatic lesions presented the appearance of a follicular carcinoma of the thyroid rather than of the undifferentiated structure observed in the primary Hürthle cell carcinoma.

A growing opinion is that most thyroid cancers are closely related and that the histological patterns are only variants of one large pattern. This may explain the differences in the histological patterns of metastases from those of the primary tumors such as have been cited here.

With a low degree of malignancy, this tumor has a fair prognosis.

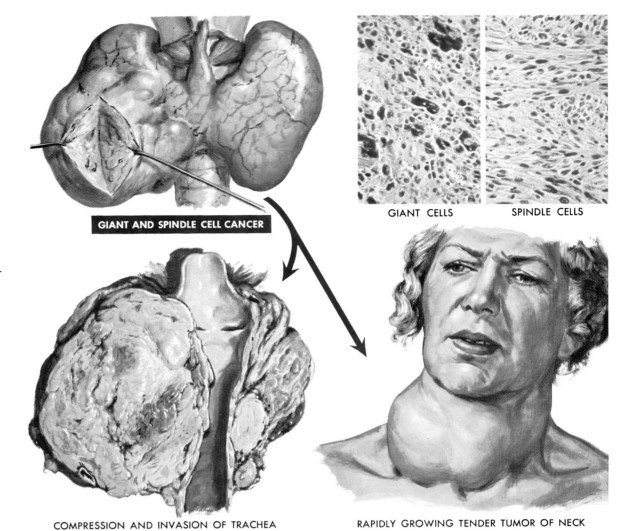

GIANT AND SPINDLE CELL CANCER

GIANT CELLS   SPINDLE CELLS

COMPRESSION AND INVASION OF TRACHEA   RAPIDLY GROWING TENDER TUMOR OF NECK

GIANT AND SPINDLE CELL CARCINOMA OF THE THYROID

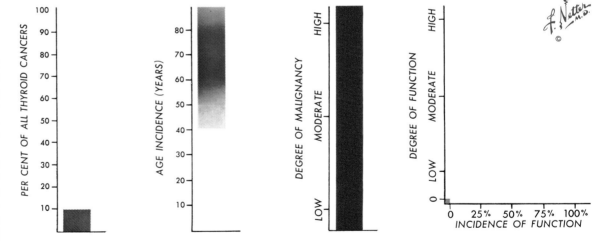

The *giant and spindle cell cancer* of the thyroid is one of the most *malignant* and deadly of all carcinomas occurring in man. It accounts for less than *10 per cent* of one large series of thyroid cancers. It usually occurs *after the age of 50,* without predilection for either sex.

The giant and spindle cell carcinoma develops as a *rapidly growing, tender tumor of the neck,* and it never shows any sign of hormonal *function*. Oftentimes, the patient can give the exact date of onset (usually a very recent one) and describes a rapid growth, causing pressure symptoms, dysphagia, and even tenderness or pain in the mass. Examination of the nodule reveals a large, hard mass, which may be fixed. It is usually tender; heat, and even redness in the skin over the nodule, may be present.

The findings of tenderness, local heat, and even redness may suggest to the uninitiated the diagnosis of an abscess of the thyroid. Such lesions often contain a great deal of yellowish necrotic tissue and, when opened after removal, do, in fact, look like an abscess. However, in considering an abscess in the differential diagnosis of such tumors, the clinician should keep in mind that abscesses

of the thyroid are extremely uncommon. A large hemorrhage into a thyroid adenoma or into a thyroid cyst may present a clinical picture which is similar to that of this type of neoplasm. Rarely, a unilateral subacute thyroiditis must be differentiated from such a cancer. This clinical picture, in a patient beyond the fifth decade, should be considered as a giant and spindle cell carcinoma until it can be ruled out.

Histologically, this tumor is a solid, highly anaplastic growth, with *spindle cells* predominating but with a great number of *large giant cells* occurring throughout the tumor.

This cancer, which is so highly malignant, seldom metastasizes widely. Its rapid growth is local and invasive, into the surrounding neck structures, usually causing death by direct *invasion of* the *trachea,* result-

ing in *compression* and asphyxiation. It also frequently invades the esophagus and the hypopharynx, and may extend into the lungs. Rarely, it may metastasize to the skin over the chest wall.

The lesion is almost never curable by surgery. It usually recurs within months after surgical removal, even though the lesion appeared, at operation, to have been completely eradicated. It is extremely resistant to radiotherapy. Studies with radioactive iodine have repeatedly demonstrated that such lesions are devoid of any radio-iodine-concentrating capacity. Thus, any attempt to treat these tumors with radioactive iodine would have no effect whatsoever.

It is extremely uncommon for a patient with this type of cancer to survive more than 12 months after the diagnosis has been made.

TUMORS METASTATIC TO THE THYROID

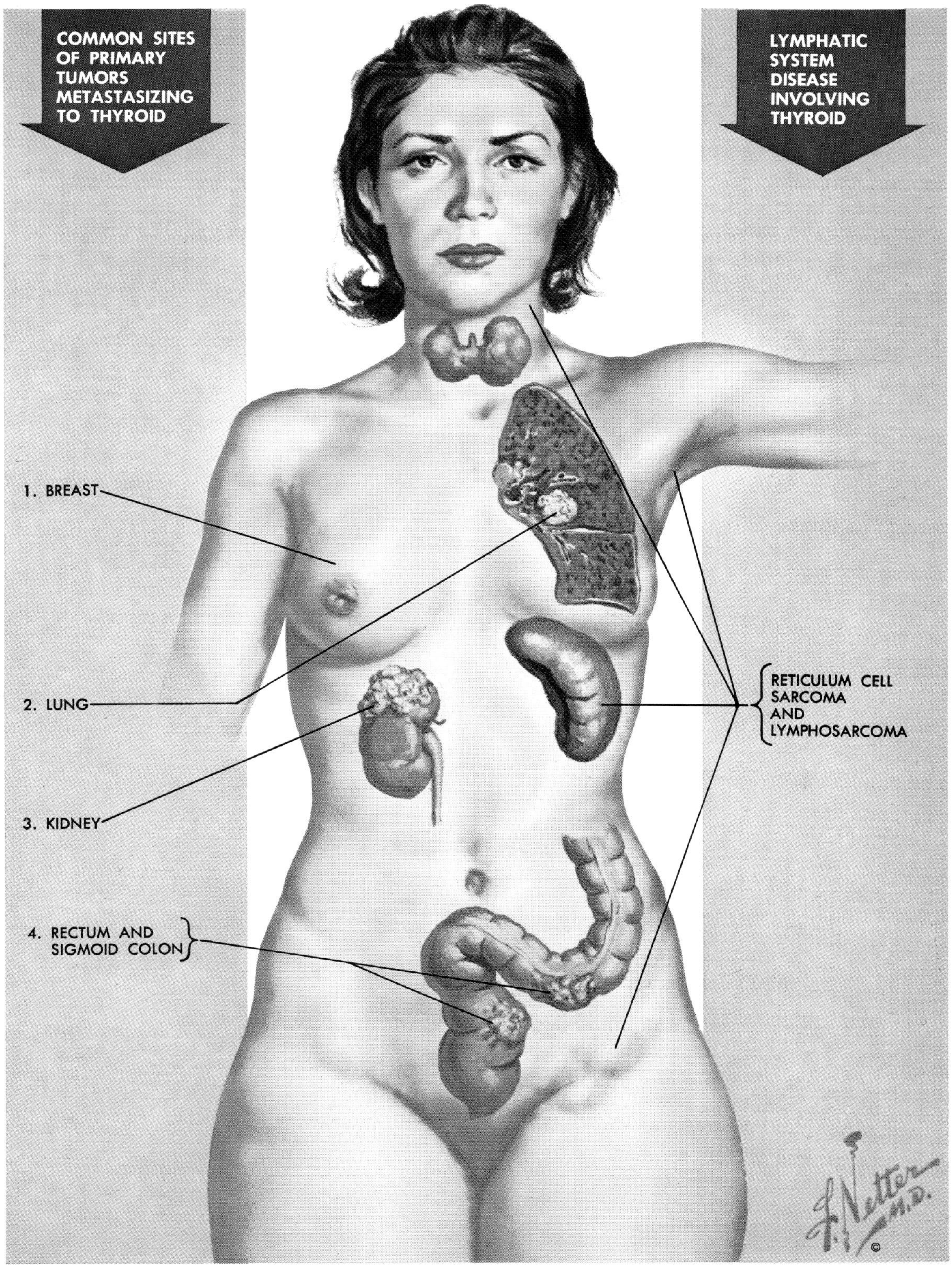

COMMON SITES OF PRIMARY TUMORS METASTASIZING TO THYROID

LYMPHATIC SYSTEM DISEASE INVOLVING THYROID

1. BREAST
2. LUNG
3. KIDNEY
4. RECTUM AND SIGMOID COLON

RETICULUM CELL SARCOMA AND LYMPHOSARCOMA

Until fairly recently, it was commonly thought that cancers arising in other organs did not metastasize to the thyroid gland. However, as a result of more careful examinations of the thyroid at necropsy and in life, it is now well established that cancers from various organs may, in fact, metastasize to the thyroid.

Cancer of the *breast* is the most common metastatic lesion in the thyroid; it has been found, at autopsy, in 30 per cent of patients who died of breast cancer.

Not infrequently, *cancer* of the *lung*, usually of the bronchogenic type, metastasizes to the thyroid.

A very interesting lesion, which also may be found in the thyroid, is metastatic hypernephroma, or the clear cell *cancer* of the *kidney*. This lesion may be confused with an intrinsic tumor of the thyroid, such as the solid adenocarcinoma or the Hürthle cell cancer. Any bulky, solid adenocarcinoma of the thyroid which is at all atypical should raise the

question of a primary renal cell cancer. This type of cancer apparently metastasizes to the thyroid via the vertebral veins, a route taken by lesions of other pelvic viscera.

One noteworthy case, seen by the author, who had an admitting diagnosis of Graves' disease and cancer of the thyroid, proved to have a carcinomatous pheochromocytoma, which accounted for the hypermetabolism and metastases in the thyroid and cervical lymph nodes, and this, in turn, accounted for the clinical diagnosis of thyroid cancer.

Cancers of the *rectum* and of the *large bowel* occasionally metastasize to the thyroid gland. Other metastatic lesions, found in the thyroid on rare occasions, have arisen in the mouth, the salivary glands, the stomach, and the prostate.

Reticulum cell sarcoma and *lymphosarcoma* may occur in the lymphoid tissue of the thyroid during the course of these systemic diseases. Rarely, both lesions may appear in the thyroid gland and, later, disseminate to other lymph-node-bearing areas of the body.

Clinically, metastatic tumors of the thyroid present as masses, on palpation during a physical examination, and patients who have this condition often are generally debilitated. A thyroid scan, after the administration of radioactive iodine (I^{131}), will reveal negative areas on the scintigram, suggesting that the masses do not take up iodine, unlike the surrounding normal thyroid tissue. If a primary source is not apparent, an open biopsy of the thyroid will usually reveal the true nature of the lesion.

Section III

THE SUPRARENAL GLANDS (ADRENAL GLANDS)

by

FRANK H. NETTER, M.D.

in collaboration with

EDWARD G. BIGLIERI, M.D.
Plates 16-18 and 20

E. S. CRELIN, Ph.D.
Plate 1

CALVIN EZRIN, M.D.
Plate 11

PETER H. FORSHAM, M.D., M.A. (Cantab)
Plates 6-10, 12-15, 21-28

MAURICE GALANTE, M.D.
Plates 2 and 3

ROY O. GREEP, Ph.D.
Plate 5

PROF. G. A. G. MITCHELL, O.B.E., T.D., M.B., Ch.M., D.Sc.
Plate 4

DAVID H. P. STREETEN, M.B., D. Phil.
Plate 19

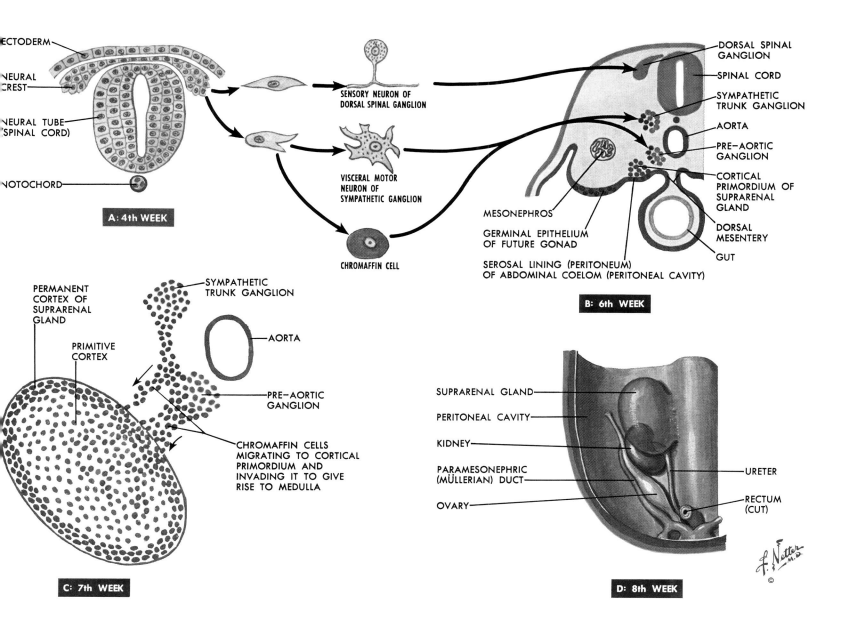

ECTODERM

NEURAL CREST

NEURAL TUBE (SPINAL CORD)

NOTOCHORD

A: 4th WEEK

SENSORY NEURON OF DORSAL SPINAL GANGLION

VISCERAL MOTOR NEURON OF SYMPATHETIC GANGLION

CHROMAFFIN CELL

DORSAL SPINAL GANGLION

SPINAL CORD

SYMPATHETIC TRUNK GANGLION

AORTA

PRE-AORTIC GANGLION

CORTICAL PRIMORDIUM OF SUPRARENAL GLAND

DORSAL MESENTERY

GUT

MESONEPHROS

GERMINAL EPITHELIUM OF FUTURE GONAD

SEROSAL LINING (PERITONEUM) OF ABDOMINAL COELOM (PERITONEAL CAVITY)

B: 6th WEEK

PERMANENT CORTEX OF SUPRARENAL GLAND

PRIMITIVE CORTEX

SYMPATHETIC TRUNK GANGLION

AORTA

PRE-AORTIC GANGLION

CHROMAFFIN CELLS MIGRATING TO CORTICAL PRIMORDIUM AND INVADING IT TO GIVE RISE TO MEDULLA

C: 7th WEEK

SUPRARENAL GLAND

PERITONEAL CAVITY

KIDNEY

PARAMESONEPHRIC (MÜLLERIAN) DUCT

OVARY

URETER

RECTUM (CUT)

D: 8th WEEK

SECTION III — PLATE I

DEVELOPMENT OF THE SUPRARENAL (ADRENAL) GLANDS

Each suprarenal (adrenal) gland actually consists of two parts, a *cortex* and a *medulla*, which, secondarily, become combined within a common capsule. The two parts have separate origins. The cortex is derived from mesodermal tissue and the medulla from *ectodermal* tissue (A and B). The cortex and medulla normally occur as separate glands in fish. There is an increasingly close relationship between the two parts in higher animals up to the mammals, in which the cortex encapsulates the medulla.

From the fifth to the sixth week of development, the cortical portion of each suprarenal gland begins as a proliferation of cells which originate from the developing peritoneal epithelium at the base of the *dorsal mesentery* near the cranial end of the *mesonephros* (B). The cells proliferate rapidly and penetrate the retroperitoneal mesenchyme to form the *primitive cortex*. The primitive cortex soon becomes enveloped by a thin layer of more compactly arranged cells that become the *permanent cortex* (C), the cells being derived from the same source as those of

the primitive cortex. By the eighth week the cortical tissue has an intimate relationship with the cranial pole of the kidney. Toward the end of the eighth week, the cortical mass attains a considerable size, separates from its peritoneal mesothelial cell layer of origin, and becomes invested in a capsule of connective tissue. At this time the *developing suprarenal gland* is much larger than the developing *kidney* (D).

The primitive, or fetal, cortex constitutes the chief bulk of the organ at birth. By the second week after birth, the suprarenals have lost a third of their weight. This is the result of the degeneration of the bulky primitive cortex, which disappears by the end of the first year. The outer permanent cortex, which is thin at birth, begins to differentiate as the inner primitive cortex undergoes involution; however, full differentiation of the permanent cortex into the three zones of the adult gland—*viz.*, glomerulosa, fasciculata, and reticularis — is not completed until about the third year after birth.

Certain *ectodermal cells* arise from the *neural crest* and migrate from their source of origin to differentiate into *sympathetic neurons* of the autonomic nervous system. However, not all of the cells of the primitive autonomic ganglia differentiate into neurons. Some become endocrine cells, which are designated as *chromaffin cells* because they stain brown with chromic acid salts (A). This staining reaction is presumed to be due to the presence within these cells of the hormone epinephrine. Certain chromaffin cells

migrate from the primitive *autonomic ganglia* adjacent to the developing cortex, to give rise eventually to the medulla of the suprarenal gland. When the cortex of the suprarenal has become a prominent structure (during the seventh week), masses of these *migrating chromaffin cells* come into contact with the cortex and begin to *invade* it on its medial side (C). By the middle of fetal life, some of the chromaffin cells have migrated to a central position within the cortex. Chromaffin cells are widely scattered throughout the embryo; however, the only chromaffin cells which usually persist in the adult are those constituting the medulla of the suprarenal gland.

True accessory suprarenal glands, consisting of both cortex and medulla, are rarely found in the adult. When they do occur, they may be within the celiac plexus or embedded in the cortex of the kidney. Accessory suprarenals, composed of only cortical substance, occur frequently. Accessory, separate cortical or medullary tissue may be present in the adult in the spleen, in the retroperitoneal area below the kidneys, along the aorta, or in the pelvis (see page 106). Since the suprarenals are situated close to the gonads during their early development, accessory tissue may also be present in the spermatic cord, attached to the testis in the scrotum, attached to the ovary, or in the broad ligament of the uterus. Although one suprarenal gland may be absent occasionally, complete absence of the suprarenals rarely occurs.

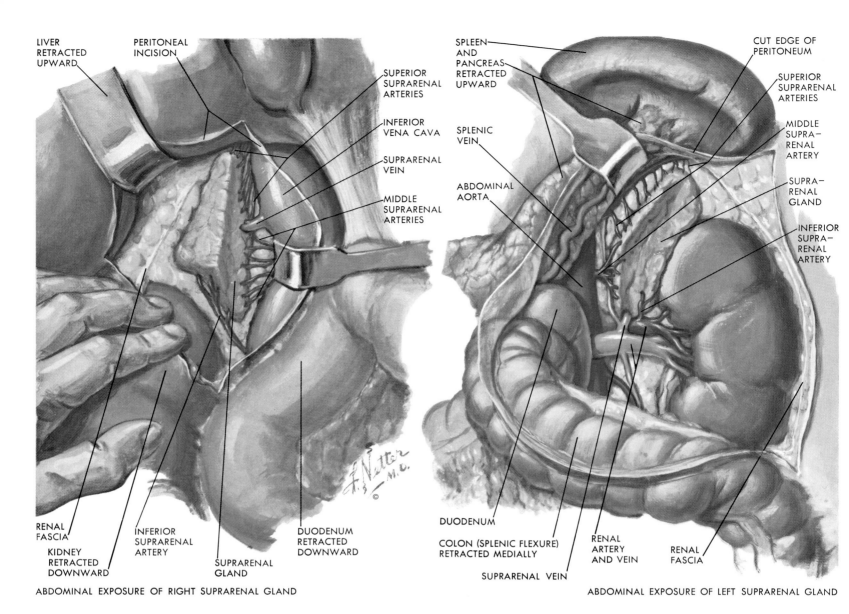

LIVER RETRACTED UPWARD

PERITONEAL INCISION

SUPERIOR SUPRARENAL ARTERIES

INFERIOR VENA CAVA

SUPRARENAL VEIN

MIDDLE SUPRARENAL ARTERIES

SPLEEN AND PANCREAS RETRACTED UPWARD

SPLENIC VEIN

ABDOMINAL AORTA

CUT EDGE OF PERITONEUM

SUPERIOR SUPRARENAL ARTERIES

MIDDLE SUPRARENAL ARTERY

SUPRARENAL GLAND

INFERIOR SUPRARENAL ARTERY

RENAL FASCIA

KIDNEY RETRACTED DOWNWARD

INFERIOR SUPRARENAL ARTERY

SUPRARENAL GLAND

DUODENUM RETRACTED DOWNWARD

DUODENUM

COLON (SPLENIC FLEXURE) RETRACTED MEDIALLY

SUPRARENAL VEIN

RENAL ARTERY AND VEIN

RENAL FASCIA

ABDOMINAL EXPOSURE OF RIGHT SUPRARENAL GLAND

ABDOMINAL EXPOSURE OF LEFT SUPRARENAL GLAND

SECTION III—PLATE 2

ANATOMY AND BLOOD SUPPLY OF THE SUPRARENAL (ADRENAL) GLANDS

The suprarenal glands are two small triangular structures, located extraperitoneally at the upper poles of the kidneys. They are found on the posterior parietal wall, on each side of the vertebral column, at the level of the eleventh thoracic rib and lateral to the first lumbar vertebra. Normally, the weight of each suprarenal gland may vary from 4 to 14 gm in the adult, the average being from 3.5 to 6.0 gm. The surface of the gland is corrugated or nodular, to a variable extent. Each gland measures from 20 to 30 mm in width, from 40 to 60 mm in length, and from 3 to 6 mm in thickness. Each is surrounded by areolar tissue, containing much fat and covered by a thin fibrous capsule attached to the gland by many fibrous bands. The suprarenal glands have their own fascial supports, so that they do not descend with the kidneys when these are displaced. The glands appear golden-yellow, distinct from the paler surrounding fat. The cut section presents, within the golden cortical layer,

a flattened mass of darker, reddish-brown medullary tissue.

The *right suprarenal gland* is pyramidal or triangular in shape. It occupies a somewhat higher and more lateral position than does the left one. Its posterior surface is in close apposition to the right diaphragmatic crus. The gland is located retroperitoneally in the recess, bounded superiorly by the postero-inferior border of the *right lobe* of the *liver* and medially by the right border of the *inferior vena cava*. The base of the pyramid is found in close apposition to the anteromedial aspect of the upper pole of the *right kidney*.

The *left suprarenal gland* is generally elongated or semilunar in shape, and a little larger than the right. It is more centrally located, its medial border frequently overlapping the lateral border of the *abdominal aorta*. Its posterior surface is in close relationship to the diaphragm and to the splanchnic nerves. The upper two thirds of the gland lie behind the posterior peritoneal wall of the lesser sac. The lower third is in close relationship to the posterior surface of the body of the *pancreas* and to the *splenic vessels*.

The suprarenal glands have a very rich vascular supply, characterized by the following features: (1) Unlike those in other organs, the arteries and veins do not usually run together. (2) The arterial supply is abundant, as many as fifty to sixty terminal small arterioles having been counted in some glands. (3) The venous blood is channeled almost completely through

a large, single venous trunk, easily identified.

Arterial blood reaches the suprarenal gland through a variable number of slender, short, twiglike *arterioles,* encompassing the gland in an arterial circle. Three types must be distinguished: short capsular arterioles, intermediate cortical ones, and long branches that go through the cortex to the medulla and its sinusoids. These arterioles are terminal branches of the *inferior phrenic artery* superiorly, of the *superior suprarenal artery* supramedially, of the *middle suprarenal artery* medially, and of the *inferior suprarenal artery* inferomedially on the right and left sides, respectively. This general pattern is occasionally supplemented by additional branches from vessels adjacent to the gland, such as the ovarian artery in the female or the internal spermatic artery in the male (on the left side).

Venous blood from the right suprarenal gland empties into the vena cava through the *right suprarenal vein*. This vein is short, generally measuring only 4 to 5 mm in length, and is located in an indentation on the anteromedial aspect of the right suprarenal gland at the junction of the upper and middle thirds. On the left side the *left suprarenal vein* is situated inferomedially and empties directly into the *left renal vein*. The left suprarenal vein is often joined by the *left inferior phrenic vein* before it empties into the left renal vein.

The nature of the pathological process and the degree of diagnostic accuracy determine,

(*Continued on page 79*)

ANATOMY AND BLOOD SUPPLY OF THE SUPRARENAL (ADRENAL) GLANDS

(Continued from page 78)

primarily, the surgical approach to the suprarenal glands, as does the build of the patient, with reference to how far downward his rib cage extends. No one particular approach can be considered suitable for all cases, and the removal of a diseased gland or an adrenal tumor may, at times, present formidable difficulties. The necessity for localizing the pathological process at the time of surgery, or for exploring the supposedly normal contralateral side, often makes the transabdominal approach the operation of choice.

EXTRAPERITONEAL LUMBAR APPROACH: This is generally considered to be the most direct and least difficult of all approaches to the suprarenal glands. It is particularly indicated in cases where the adrenal cortical pathology is well established and localized, as in cases of unilateral tumors well demonstrated preoperatively.

TRANSABDOMINAL APPROACH: Two incisions may be utilized: (1) an upper muscle-splitting, horizontal semicircular incision, crossing the midepigastrium at the midline and extending subcostally on each side; or (2) an upper, vertical midline incision, extending from the tip of the xiphoid to a point 1 to 2 inches inferior to the umbilicus.

The *right suprarenal gland* is exposed by *retracting* the *liver* and gallbladder superolaterally and the stomach and *duodenum* medially. The peritoneal reflection is divided vertically along the right border of the *vena cava*. The *peritoneal incision* should be extended in a lateral direction along the posterior aspect of the liver, in order to gain better access to the adrenal gland, which occupies a high position and two thirds of which lie behind the liver and the vena cava. Extension of the peritoneal incision inferiorly beyond the upper pole of the right *kidney* will facilitate caudal *retraction* of this organ.

To gain *access to the left suprarenal gland,* the lesser peritoneal sac is entered through an incision in the gastrohepatic or gastrocolic ligament, the posterior parietal *peritoneum is opened* just to the left of the midline, and the adrenal gland is localized, posterior to the pancreas, by retracting the latter inferiorly. The author's preference is a route whereby the *spleen* and *pancreas are mobilized supramedially,* after incising the lateral peritoneal reflection, and the *splenic flexure of the colon is retracted inferomedially,* thus exposing the adrenal gland. This approach requires more time but has the advantage of providing better exposure.

TRANSTHORACIC APPROACH: This approach has its optimal utility for the removal of the left suprarenal gland. It is a rather extensive procedure, inviting the hazards of additional postoperative

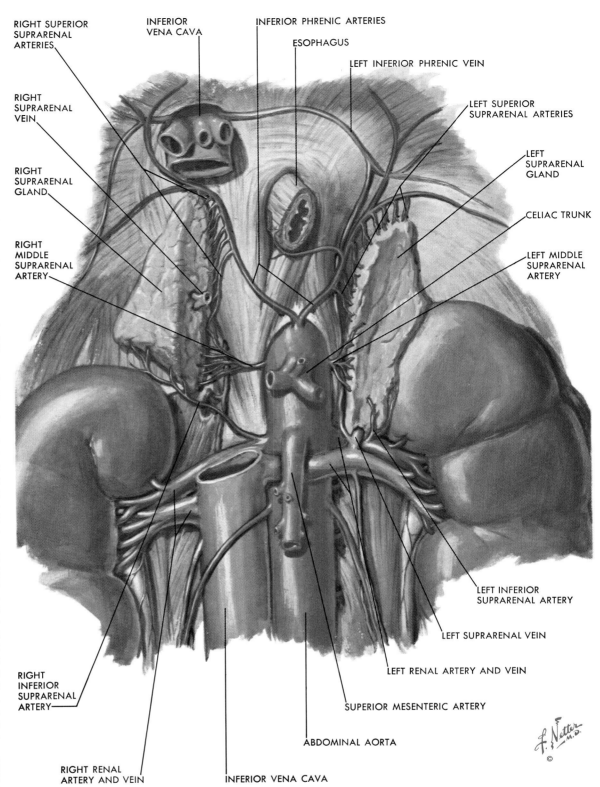

complications, but advantageous when used for the removal of very large tumors of the gland.

GENERAL CONSIDERATIONS: Successful surgery of the suprarenal glands presupposes several indispensable requirements. Division of the perirenal fascia (Gerota's capsule) is necessary in order to enter the proper retroperitoneal space and to gain easy access to the suprarenal glands. Familiarity with the gross pathology of the glands is necessary, because the marked variation in appearance, configuration, and consistency can be treacherous and makes more hazardous any premature conclusions or irreversible decisions. Unless the gland contains an easily identifiable tumor, it should be dissected free, so that both anterior and posterior surfaces can be inspected and palpated with ease throughout their entire extent. Occasionally, it is difficult to make a correct evaluation of the pathological process, even with the gland

freely dissected. Familiarity with the vascular anomalies of the *blood supply* of the suprarenal glands is also indispensable. The numerous *arterioles,* frequently arranged like the teeth of a comb around the superior, medial, and inferior borders of the gland, should be secured with ligatures or clips, because they have been known to be the source of troublesome hemorrhage both during and after operation. The *suprarenal vein* should preferably be divided after controlling the arterial blood supply, in order to minimize bleeding in the event that the suprarenal gland is opened. The vein should be secured with a transfixation ligature of fine material, since simple ligatures have been known to slip away, causing profuse hemorrhage, pre- or postoperatively, from the vena cava. Finally, the gland should be handled gently, as it fractures easily when traumatized, jeopardizing its complete removal.

RIGHT PHRENIC NERVE
ANTERIOR VAGAL TRUNK
RIGHT GREATER THORACIC SPLANCHNIC NERVE
RIGHT LESSER THORACIC SPLANCHNIC NERVE
RIGHT AORTICO-RENAL GANGLION
RIGHT LEAST THORACIC SPLANCHNIC NERVE
RIGHT (POSTERIOR) RENAL GANGLION

LEFT PHRENIC NERVE
POSTERIOR VAGAL TRUNK
LEFT GREATER THORACIC SPLANCHNIC NERVE
CELIAC GANGLIA
LEFT LESSER THORACIC SPLANCHNIC NERVE
LEFT AORTICO-RENAL GANGLION
LEFT LEAST THORACIC SPLANCHNIC NERVE
LEFT RENAL GANGLION

RIGHT SYMPATHETIC TRUNK
RIGHT 1st LUMBAR SPLANCHNIC NERVE
SUPERIOR MESENTERIC GANGLION
LEFT SYMPATHETIC TRUNK
LEFT 1st LUMBAR SPLANCHNIC NERVE

T10
T11
T12
L1
SPINAL CORD
SYMPATHETIC TRUNK
SPLANCHNIC NERVES
CELIAC GANGLION
POSTGANGLIONIC FIBERS SUPPLY BLOOD VESSELS
PREGANGLIONIC FIBERS RAMIFY ABOUT CELLS OF MEDULLA
SUPRARENAL GLAND
CORTEX
MEDULLA

INNERVATION OF THE SUPRARENAL (ADRENAL) GLANDS

The suprarenal (adrenal) glands show considerable species variation, and this is true also of their nerve supply, which is autonomic in origin. The information given here refers to the arrangement in man. Relative to their size, these glands have a richer innervation than other viscera.

The *sympathetic preganglionic fibers* for these glands are the axons of cells located in the intermediolateral columns of the lowest two or three thoracic and highest one or two lumbar segments of the *spinal cord.* They emerge in the anterior rootlets of the corresponding spinal nerves, pass in white rami communicantes to the homolateral *sympathetic trunks,* and leave them in the *greater, lesser,* and *least thoracic* and *first lumbar splanchnic nerves,* which run to the *celiac, aorticorenal,* and *renal ganglia.* Some fibers end in these ganglia, but the majority pass through them, without relaying, and enter numerous small nerves which run outward, on each side, from the celiac plexus to the suprarenal glands. These nerves are joined by direct contributions from the terminal parts of the greater and lesser thoracic splanchnic nerves, and they communicate with the homolateral *phrenic nerve* and renal plexus. Small ganglia exist on the suprarenal nerves and within the actual *suprarenal medulla;* a proportion of sympathetic fibers may relay in these ganglia, and the glandular nerves may contain a higher content of postganglionic fibers than is usually stated.

Parasympathetic fibers are conveyed to the celiac plexus in the celiac branch of the *posterior vagal trunk,* and some of these may be concerned with suprarenal innervation and may relay in ganglia in

or near the gland; some authors deny that the vagi supply the suprarenals. Kuré *et al* (1931) suggested that the suprarenal parasympathetic supply emerges via posterior spinal nerve root efferent fibers, which enter the thoracic splanchnic nerves and, thereafter, follow the same course as the sympathetic fibers, but the existence of such posterior root efferents is still unproved.

The possibility that some of the nerve fibers are afferent is also unproved, although Kiss (1951) claimed that afferents from the suprarenal cortex enter the cord through the ninth to the eleventh thoracic spinal nerves.

On each side, the suprarenal nerves form a suprarenal plexus along the medial border of the suprarenal gland. Filaments associated with occasional ganglion cells spread out over the gland to form a delicate subcapsular plexus, from which fascicles or solitary

fibers penetrate the cortex to reach the medulla, apparently without supplying cortical cells en route, although they do supply cortical vessels. The majority of the branches of the suprarenal plexus, however, enter the gland through or near its hilus as compact bundles, some of which accompany the suprarenal arteries. These bundles run through the cortex to the medulla, where they ramify profusely and mostly terminate in synaptic-type endings around the medullary chromaffin cells; some fibers invaginate, but do not penetrate, the plasma membranes of these cells. The preganglionic sympathetic fibers end directly around the medullary cells, as these cells are derived from the sympathetic anlage and are the homologues of sympathetic ganglion cells.

Other fibers innervate the suprarenal vessels, including the central vein, which has an unusually thick, and often eccentrically arranged, muscle coat.

HISTOLOGY OF THE SUPRARENAL (ADRENAL) GLANDS

The suprarenal glands are composed of two separate and distinct endocrine tissues, the *suprarenal cortex* and the *suprarenal medulla,* each being entirely different in embryological origin, structure, and function (see page 77). In the adult the cortex comprises about 90 per cent of the suprarenal gland and completely surrounds the thin layer of centrally located medulla. In histologic sections the cortex is seen to be composed mainly of radially oriented cords of cells. During embryogenesis, cells destined to form the medulla migrate through the cortex. *At birth* there is present, in addition to a thin outer layer of *permanent cortex,* a thick band of *fetal cortex,* which soon involutes.

The cells of the suprarenal cortex are typically epithelioid in appearance, with centrally placed nuclei having two or more prominent nucleoli. The cytoplasm features a variable abundance of lipid-containing vacuoles, in addition to mitochondria and the Golgi apparatus.

In the suprarenal cortex, three concentrically arranged cell layers, or zones, can be identified on the basis of the grouping of cells and the disposition of cell cords. In the thin outermost layer, the *zona glomerulosa,* the cells occur in arched loops or round balls. The middle layer, or *zona fasciculata,* is much the widest of the three zones and is composed of cells arranged in long straight cords, or *fascicles.* The innermost layer, or *zona reticularis,* is contiguous with the medulla. Here, the cell cords are entwined, forming a reticulum. The two inner zones are entirely dependent on hypophysial corticotropin (ACTH) for the maintenance of their structure and function. The zona glomerulosa, on the contrary, remains structurally and functionally normal in the absence of the hypophysis. Under normal conditions the cortical cells at the inner border of the cortex have few lipid vacuoles and are referred to as *compact cells,* in contrast to the lipid-laden light (*clear*) cells that occupy the midportion of the cortex. Under *ACTH stimulation* the layer of compact cells increases in width at the expense of the layer of light cells.

The zona glomerulosa is primarily responsible for the secretion of aldosterone, a mineralocorticoid having the prime function of regulating the metabolism of sodium and potassium. The function of the zona glomerulosa is essentially independent of that of the remainder of the cortex. The control of aldosterone secretion appears to involve the renal juxtaglomerular apparatus and the renin-

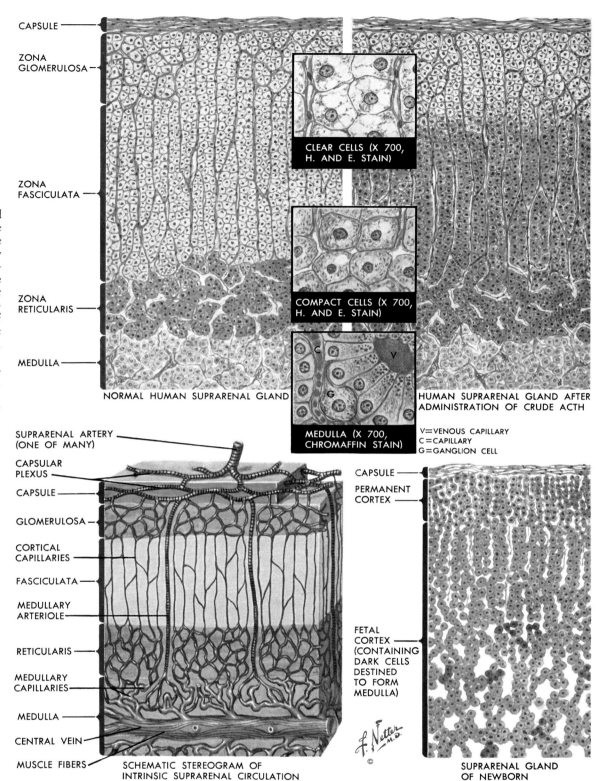

CAPSULE

ZONA GLOMERULOSA

ZONA FASCICULATA

ZONA RETICULARIS

MEDULLA

CLEAR CELLS (X 700, H. AND E. STAIN)

COMPACT CELLS (X 700, H. AND E. STAIN)

MEDULLA (X 700, CHROMAFFIN STAIN)

C
V
G

NORMAL HUMAN SUPRARENAL GLAND

HUMAN SUPRARENAL GLAND AFTER ADMINISTRATION OF CRUDE ACTH

V=VENOUS CAPILLARY
C=CAPILLARY
G=GANGLION CELL

SUPRARENAL ARTERY (ONE OF MANY)

CAPSULAR PLEXUS

CAPSULE

GLOMERULOSA

CORTICAL CAPILLARIES

FASCICULATA

MEDULLARY ARTERIOLE

RETICULARIS

MEDULLARY CAPILLARIES

MEDULLA

CENTRAL VEIN

MUSCLE FIBERS

SCHEMATIC STEREOGRAM OF INTRINSIC SUPRARENAL CIRCULATION

CAPSULE

PERMANENT CORTEX

FETAL CORTEX (CONTAINING DARK CELLS DESTINED TO FORM MEDULLA)

SUPRARENAL GLAND OF NEWBORN

angiotensin system (see page 95). The zonae fasciculata and reticularis can best be regarded as a functional unit, having, as its primary purpose, the secretion of the glucocorticoid cortisol and some adrenal androgens. Cortisol plays a prominent rôle in regulating the catabolism of protein, facilitating glucogenesis, and suppressing inflammation through its inhibitory action on connective tissue (see page 84).

The suprarenal gland receives blood from 30 to 50 small *arteries* which penetrate the *capsule* at different points and form the *capsular plexus* of arterioles. These supply the *capillaries* that extend radially through the *cortex* and separate the cords of cells. The suprarenal *medulla* has both a *venous* and an *arterial blood supply.* Capillaries from the cortex extend into the medulla as venous capillaries; a few *medullary arterioles* extend through the cortex to form arterial *capillaries in the medulla.* Both categories of vessels

join to form veins that drain through the single large *central suprarenal vein.* The venous tributaries enter the latter between thick bands of *smooth muscle,* longitudinally disposed in its wall.

The *suprarenal medulla* is comprised of *columnar cells* which secrete the catecholamines epinephrine and norepinephrine. Since the catecholamines are readily darkened by the oxidizing agent potassium dichromate, the medulla is often referred to as *chromaffin tissue.* It has been demonstrated, by histochemical means, that some islets of chromaffin cells secrete mainly epinephrine, whereas others secrete norepinephrine. Preganglionic sympathetic fibers enter the medulla and terminate directly on the parenchymal cells or scattered sympathetic ganglion cells. Fibers from the latter are believed to innervate only muscle cells in the walls of the vessels in the cortex and medulla.

BIOSYNTHESIS AND METABOLISM OF ADRENAL CORTICAL STEROID HORMONES

The hormones derived from the *adrenal cortex* are steroids, in common with those from the gonads. The steroids produced by the adrenal cortex may be grouped broadly into GLUCOCORTICOIDS, 17-KETOSTEROIDS or adrenal androgens, mineralocorticoids (notably ALDOSTERONE), ESTROGENS, and PROGESTEROIDS. Some of these are highly potent biologically; others are relatively inactive.

The structure, growth, and secretory activity of the adrenal cortex are regulated entirely by the anterior pituitary corticotropin, also known as adrenocorticotropic hormone (*ACTH*), except for *aldosterone*, which is regulated largely by *angiotensin II* and changes in *blood volume* and *sodium* and *potassium* levels. The ACTH is produced and released from certain basophils as well as large chromophobe cells of the anterior pituitary (*adenohypophysis*) (see page 11), the release being governed by two independent processes. Only cortisol or cortisone with a 17-hydroxyl group, among the glucocorticoids, inhibits ACTH release when present in higher than physiological levels in the blood stream. If there is a fall in cortisol level, ACTH secretion commences through a so-called "servomechanism" and, thereby, raises the cortisol level again, which turns off ACTH. This is accompanied by a diurnal variation in ACTH secretion. In man, maximal adrenal activation occurs between 2 a.m. and 8 a.m. In contrast, after 8 a.m. there is a gradual daytime fall in ACTH activity and cortisol secretion, under basal conditions, so that, by late evening, the adrenal cortex is far less active. The diurnal variation is revealed by blood 17-hydroxycorticoid levels which, normally, in the afternoon are only half the morning levels. Changes in urinary 17-hydroxycorticoid levels follow plasma levels with a brief lag. This diurnal rhythm is abolished in Cushing's syndrome, owing to bilateral adrenal hyperplasia or tumor, or to destruction of the pretectoral or temporal lobes as well as other central nervous system lesions (see page 85). This continuous feed-back inhibition of ACTH by cortisol may be interrupted at any time by an overriding mechanism, *viz.*, *stress*. Stressful stimuli reaching the *cerebral cortex* release the inhibition of the reticular formation or of the limbic system upon *hypothalamic centers* in and around the tubero-infundibular nucleus and the median eminence. Large *neurons* then *secrete* corticotropin-releasing factor (CRF), a polypeptide hormone mediator. Vasopressin, or antidiuretic hormone (ADH), as well as other synthetic short-chain peptides, also has a corticotropin-releasing effect. The CRF travels down the *portal circulation* of the pituitary stalk

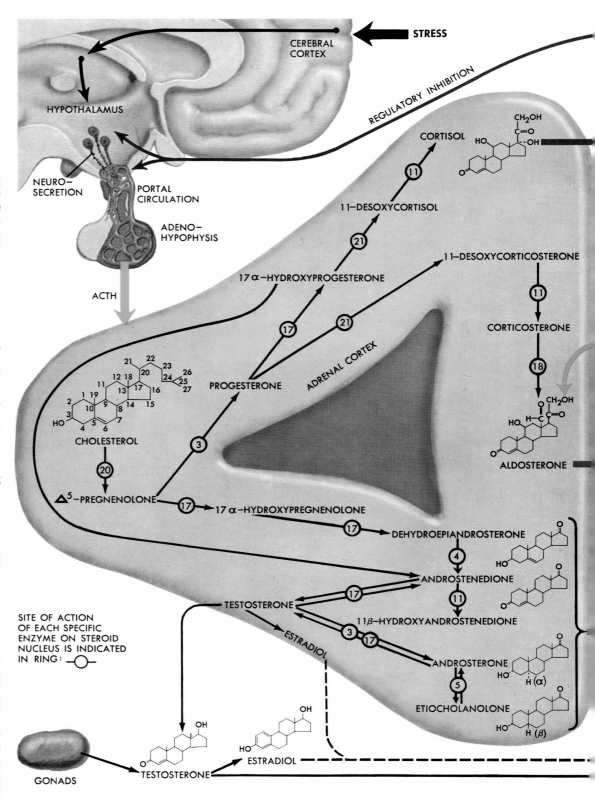

to the anterior pituitary, releasing ACTH, which activates the adrenal cortex. The greater the stress, the more ACTH is secreted. The upper secretory limit of human adrenals is around 250 mg a day of cortisol.

The biosynthesis of adrenal cortical steroids depends on ACTH, since, in its absence, only 10 per cent of the normal synthetic rate of steroid hormone formation takes place. *Cholesterol* arises from acetate and is stored in profusion in the adrenal cortex. Its basic cyclopentenophenanthrene ring, which is numbered as shown, is modified by enzymes which induce hydroxyl groups into the ring (hydroxylases), while other enzymes (dehydrogenases) may remove hydrogen from an OH group, and others (oxidases) remove hydrogen from a CH group, each at specific positions. Compounds isolated from the adrenal vein may be divided as follows: the glucocorticoids as distinguished by an α-ketol group and an 11-hydroxyl

group. These include the all-important *cortisol,* of which about 15 to 20 mg are secreted daily in adults under basal conditions, and *corticosterone,* of which 2 to 5 mg are secreted daily.

The 17-ketosteroids, or 17-oxosteroids, representing weak androgens, are characterized by an oxygen atom in the 17 position. *Testosterone,* which has sixty times the androgenic potency of even the most potent 17-ketosteroid, has also been isolated from the adrenal cortex but carries a 17-hydroxyl group. Of the 17-ketosteroids, about 75 per cent are in the form of *dehydroepiandrosterone* (DEA). It is secreted in about the same quantity (20 to 25 mg daily) as cortisol. Among mineralocorticoids, the most important is *aldosterone,* of which 75 to 125 μg are secreted daily on a normal salt intake (see page 99). Found usually in only very small amounts in body fluid is *11-desoxycorticosterone,* which, in its regulation

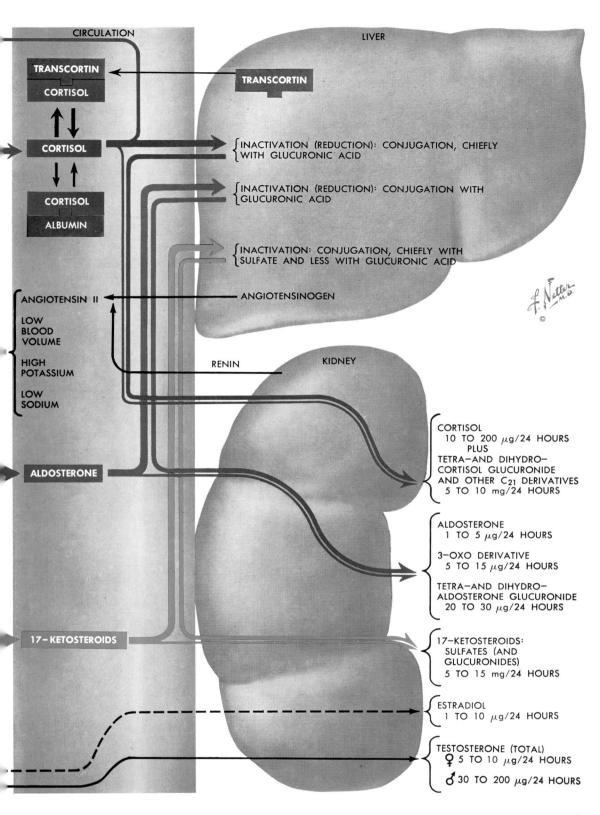

CIRCULATION

LIVER

TRANSCORTIN
CORTISOL

TRANSCORTIN

CORTISOL

CORTISOL
ALBUMIN

{ INACTIVATION (REDUCTION): CONJUGATION, CHIEFLY
WITH GLUCURONIC ACID

{ INACTIVATION (REDUCTION): CONJUGATION WITH
GLUCURONIC ACID

{ INACTIVATION: CONJUGATION, CHIEFLY WITH
SULFATE AND LESS WITH GLUCURONIC ACID

ANGIOTENSIN II

LOW
BLOOD
VOLUME

HIGH
POTASSIUM

LOW
SODIUM

ANGIOTENSINOGEN

RENIN

KIDNEY

ALDOSTERONE

17-KETOSTEROIDS

CORTISOL
10 TO 200 μg/24 HOURS
PLUS
TETRA–AND DIHYDRO–
CORTISOL GLUCURONIDE
AND OTHER C₂₁ DERIVATIVES
5 TO 10 mg/24 HOURS

ALDOSTERONE
1 TO 5 μg/24 HOURS

3-OXO DERIVATIVE
5 TO 15 μg/24 HOURS

TETRA–AND DIHYDRO–
ALDOSTERONE GLUCURONIDE
20 TO 30 μg/24 HOURS

17-KETOSTEROIDS:
SULFATES (AND
GLUCURONIDES)
5 TO 15 mg/24 HOURS

ESTRADIOL
1 TO 10 μg/24 HOURS

TESTOSTERONE (TOTAL)
♀ 5 TO 10 μg/24 HOURS
♂ 30 TO 200 μg/24 HOURS

behaves more like cortisol and is a less potent sodium container than aldosterone. The adrenal cortices secrete small amounts of *estradiol* (derived from testosterone) and estrone (derived from *androstenedione*), both of them becoming important after menopause when the adrenals are the only source of estrogens. Up to 1 mg a day of *progesterone* and closely related compounds arises from the adrenal cortices simply because progesterone is the major direct precursor of all corticosteroids.

Maximal suppression of pituitary ACTH secretion, by the administration of potent cortisol derivatives, reduces urinary 17-hydroxycorticoids, 17-ketosteroids, and estrogens, but affects aldosterone only slightly. Maximal stimulation with ACTH in an 8-hour period will increase urinary 17-hydroxycorticoids as well as estrogens three- to fivefold, but 17-ketosteroids and aldosterone only twofold in normal subjects, as a rule.

Cortisol represents over 80 per cent of the total 17-hydroxycorticoids, or Porter-Silber chromogens, found in the blood stream. About one half circulates in the form of the original molecule. The remainder circulates as the reduced, inactive *tetrahydro derivative, conjugated* at C-3 with *glucuronic acid* and, to a much smaller extent, with sulfate or phosphate. The biologically active, unconjugated cortisol in the plasma is bound, to some extent, by *albumin* and also to an α-globulin, derived mainly from the *liver*. This latter substance is called *transcortin*, or corticosterone-binding globulin (CBG). The CBG mechanism assures a ready source of available circulating hormone, since 20 to 30 per cent are always dissociated off the carrier which protects the remaining bound material from inactivation and conjugation in the liver. In addition, CBG solubilizes cortisol, which, of itself, has only limited solubility. The binding mechanism

affects the unconjugated metabolites very little, the conjugated material not at all. The production of CBG is increased markedly by estrogen therapy. In the later stages of pregnancy, the titer of CBG-bound cortisol is much increased, yet there are no manifestations of hyperadrenocorticism, since most of the active hormone is not available to the tissue. Conversely, a lowering of transcortin occurs in various conditions which are characterized by abnormalities of serum proteins, *e.g.*, cirrhosis, nephrosis, and multiple myeloma. The relative excess of unchanged cortisol rapidly suppresses ACTH secretion, so that hyperadrenocorticism does not usually develop.

The half-life of free cortisol in the plasma, determined with C-14-labeled cortisol in tracer amounts, is normally about 2½ hours. This period is markedly increased by liver dysfunction and decreased by thyrotoxicosis. This results from changes in the catabolism of cortisol in the liver.

The degradation of cortisone into inactive metabolites is quite similar to that of cortisol. Since cortisol and cortisone are freely interchangeable by enzymic action in the adrenal and the liver, a considerable amount of tetrahydrocortisone and cortisone may be found in the urine, particularly in the hyperthyroid state.

In the metabolism of 17-ketosteroids, dehydroepiandrosterone (known in the past as dehydro-isoandrosterone) is a precursor of a number of adrenal 17-ketosteroids, including *etiocholanolone* and *androsterone*. It has been shown to be present largely as the water-soluble sulfate in the adrenal cortex itself. It is apparently carried to enzyme sites in this form, and, in the presence of sulfatase at these enzyme sites, it is hydrolyzed and then transformed. In addition to the production of 17-ketosteroids, the adrenal, like the *testis* and (to a smaller extent) the *ovary*, produces *testosterone*. It is excreted as the *glucuronide*, with small amounts of free testosterone. *Total urinary testosterone* rarely exceeds 10 μg per day in normal women, but much larger amounts are found in males (especially younger ones), arising mostly from the testicles.

The 17-*ketosteroids*, such as dehydroepiandrosterone, are degraded in the liver and also directly *conjugated* at the C-3 position, mainly by *sulfate*, whereas *etiocholanolone* and *androsterone* are found mainly as *glucuronides*. Both are solubilized forms which are rapidly excreted in the urine. Daily *excretion* of 17-ketosteroids amounts, normally, to 10 mg ± 5 mg in females, 12 to 15 mg ± 5 mg in males.

Aldosterone follows the same metabolic pattern as cortisol, consisting of intrahepatic reduction and biologic *inactivation*, and *conjugation of the tetrahydro derivative* with glucuronate at the C-3 hydroxyl group. Twenty to thirty μg of this conjugate are excreted daily in the urine. In addition, 5 to 15 μg of the aldosterone 3-*oxoglucuronic acid conjugate* are found as pH1 hydrolyzable material. A much smaller fraction of aldosterone—between 1 and 5 μg—appears in the urine in the free form.

THE BIOLOGICAL ACTIONS OF CORTISOL

In man, the most abundant glucocorticoids are cortisol and cortisone. Their various physiological actions, when exaggerated by excessively high levels, will lead to Cushing's disease (see page 85).

Glucocorticoids are *catabolic* hormones leading to diversion of *amino acids* from *muscle* to the liver for deamination. *Muscle wasting,* with weakness, results. Decreased protein synthesis and *increased resorption of bone matrix* occur. These, together with the fact that glucocorticoids sharply suppress secretion of pituitary growth hormone in children given excess glucocorticoids therapeutically, lead to growth arrest.

Amino acids that are blocked from entry into muscle go to the *liver,* where they are deaminated, the carbon skeletons forming carbohydrate (notably *glycogen*) and fat. This increased *gluconeogenesis* raises *blood glucose,* which is immediately reduced by *increased excretion of insulin* from the β-cells. However, these will eventually become *exhausted* in patients with poor insulinogenic reserve having a family history of diabetes, and permanent diabetes may result. The increased *fat* is distributed characteristically, as in Cushing's disease (see page 85). Excess glucocorticoids lead to a rise in serum lipids and cholesterol. There is *increased gastric acidity,* with a greater secretion of hydrochloric acid and pepsin and a thinning of mucus in the stomach, *aggravating ulcers* already present or predisposing to *ulcer formation.* Changes in calcium metabolism lead to a marked *increase in renal excretion of calcium, decreased absorption* of it in the *intestines* by counteracting *vitamin D,* and bone effects as mentioned above. Together with a catabolic attack on bone matrix, a creeping osteoporosis is induced when excess cortisol is given. *Retention of sodium* at the *renal tubular level* occurs, but it is far less in magnitude than that exerted by aldosterone. Exchanging with the reabsorbed sodium at the tubular level, potassium and hydrogen are secreted, so that cortisol excess leads to *potassium depletion,* weakness, and alkalosis. There is a marked *increase in glomerular filtration,* and this, together with the direct antagonism of cortisol to antidiuretic hormone in the collecting tubule, leads to *diuresis.* Cortisol diverts amino acid from lymphoid tissue as well, leading to marked reduction in size and to actual *lysis of the nodes.* This is accompanied by an initial *release of antibodies* stored in lymph nodes but, eventually, by a marked *decrease* in over-all *antibody production,* which, together with breakdown of inter- and intracellular barriers to the diffusion of particles, raises susceptibility to viral and bacterial infections.

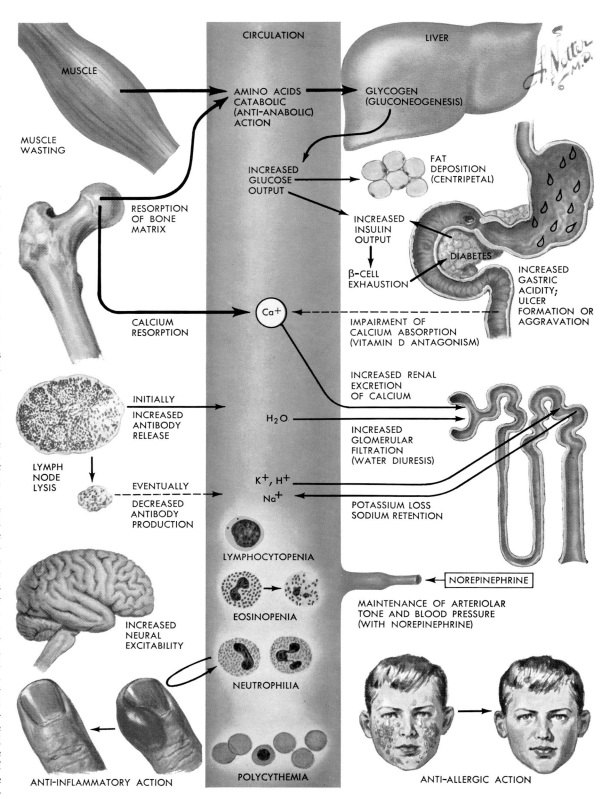

An over-all *increase in neural excitability,* with a lowered threshold for epileptic seizures, is found on the one hand; marked excitability and sleeplessness, with euphoria, on the other.

In a permissive fashion, cortisol is necessary for the *vasoconstrictive action* of *norepinephrine* and other vasoconstrictors. This leads to the use of large doses of cortisol, or its synthetic derivatives, in nonhemorrhagic shock.

The blood picture is markedly affected by cortisol, giving rise to *lymphocytopenia* and marked *eosinopenia* in the face of significant *neutrophilia.* There appears to be more rapid destruction of eosinophils in the circulation and, particularly, in lungs and spleen. *Polycythemia* with excess cortisol contrasts with the normocytic normochromic anemia in adrenal insufficiency.

Most important is the *anti-inflammatory action* shown by only those glucocorticoids with a 17-hydroxyl group, such as cortisol and cortisone. The cellular response to a noxious or infectious agent is reduced by decreasing the accumulation first of neutrophils and second of lymphocytes, and, finally, by inducing delayed fibroplasia. Thus, the exudative inflammatory response is abolished. By the same token, cortisol is markedly *anti-allergic,* and, here, both a decrease in the formation of histamine and histaminelike substances by the affected cells and some surface protection of cells that would normally react to an antigen-antibody complex are involved. These actions of glucocorticoids form the basis of their widespread clinical use. As inflammatory and allergic responses are decreased, eventual fibrosis is minimized and subsequent degeneration reduced. Thus, cortisol abolishes manifestations of disease without directly antagonizing the causative agent.

CUSHING'S SYNDROME

Clinical Findings

This syndrome (or disease) carries the name of the Boston neurosurgeon, Harvey Cushing, who first described its signs and symptoms and linked it to a basophilic adenoma of the anterior pituitary gland.

It is a relatively rare condition, found in about 1 of 1000 autopsies. It occurs far more frequently (4 to 1) in females than in males. The highest incidence is in the third and fourth decades, and it occurs somewhat more often following pregnancy, suggesting that pituitary over-activity during gestation may be predisposing to the development of a pituitary ACTH-producing tumor.

One may be dealing simply with an *overactive pituitary ACTH mechanism* unduly stimulated by some disturbance in the hypothalamus, which no longer responds to the normal regulatory mechanism. A *basophil adenoma* of the *pituitary* is a rare cause of Cushing's disease. It seldom leads to an enlargement of the gland sufficient to cause a deviation from the *normal sella turcica*. With certain *chromophobe adenomas* that produce large amounts of *ACTH*, especially those arising after bilateral adrenalectomy for Cushing's disease, an *enlarged sella turcica* may be found. The resulting *hyperplasia* of the *adrenal cortices* leads to a sharp increase over the normal weight of 4 to 6 gm per gland, running as high as 15 to 20 gm. In the presence of adrenal cortical hyperplasia, one may deal, very rarely, with an ACTH-producing tumor such as a bronchogenic carcinoma or a carcinoma of the gallbladder. In those cases the adrenal cortices are extremely large, and overproduction of cortisol is excessive (see page 231). In about 15 per cent of the cases, Cushing's disease may be produced by an independent *adenoma* of the *adrenal cortex* or by an *adenocarcinoma* which, by producing excess cortisol, inhibits pituitary ACTH, thereby leading to a characteristic *atrophy* of the *contralateral adrenal*.

The secretion of excess cortisol is predominant over that of other corticosteroids, except with carcinoma, where 17-ketosteroids are markedly elevated. In practice, most cases of Cushing's disease fall somewhere in the spectrum between two extremes: the adrenogenital syndrome, with an excess of 17-ketosteroids (see page 94), or Cushing's disease with, mainly, an excessive cortisol secretion.

Other pathological changes include atherosclerosis of the larger vessels, nephrosclerosis and, sometimes, calcinosis of the kidney, at times with parathyroid adenomas, gonadal atrophy, pancreatic islet cell hyperplasia, and, occasionally, fat necrosis of the pancreas. Thymic tumors have been described, and, here,

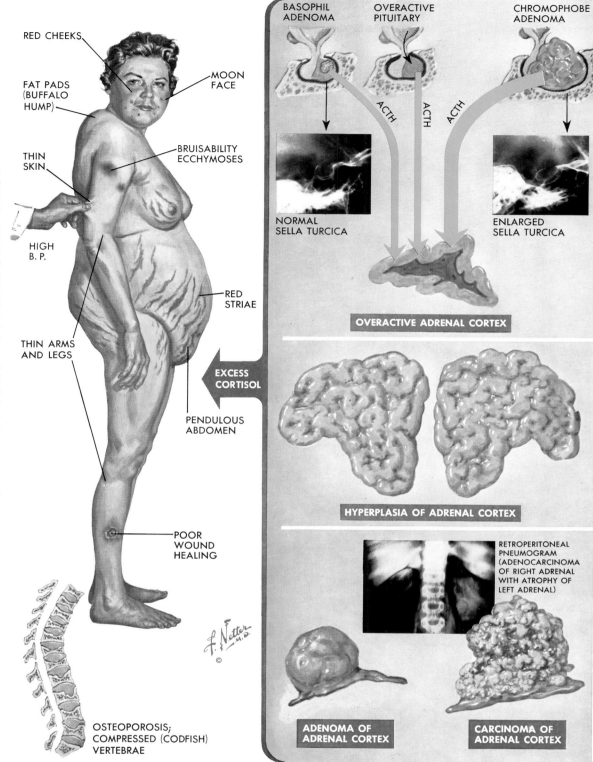

one suspects that ACTH-like substances may arise from the thymus.

Excess cortisol leads to excitability and, sometimes, psychoses, as well as to abnormal fat distribution without a marked gain in weight, characterized by the establishment of a *moon face*, a *pendulous abdomen*, and *fat pads supraclavicularly* and over the 7th vertebra (known as the *buffalo hump*). Characteristically, the *arms* and *legs* look *thin*.

The over-all catabolic effect of excess cortisol brings about marked muscle wasting, especially in the quadriceps femoris group, with early inability to mount stairs. The *skin* is *thin* and almost paperlike. Its transparency produces unnaturally *red cheeks*, revealing the underlying vasculature with a coexisting polycythemia. Disappearance of elastic fibers (owing to the catabolic effect of excess cortisol), coupled with stretching (owing to abnormal accumulation of fat),

produces depressed *red-to-purple striae* over the abdomen, buttocks, upper thighs, breasts, and even down the arms. There is marked *bruisability*, with numerous *ecchymoses*, and, following venipuncture, subcutaneous leakage is the rule. *Poor wound healing* and high susceptibility to infection are characteristic. Severe *osteoporosis*, owing to decreased deposition of bone matrix, and a continuous loss of calcium in the urine lead to frequent *vertebral compression* fractures and *dorsal kyphosis* as well as rib fractures. The skull is often involved also. (The latter is hardly ever found in postmenopausal senile osteoporosis.) Diabetic glucose tolerance tests are common (80 per cent incidence). Remissions and exacerbations occur until the patient gets weaker, has vertebral fractures and, eventually, becomes bedridden. If untreated, death ensues within 5 years, as a result of general debility, vascular accidents, and, more rarely, diabetic coma.

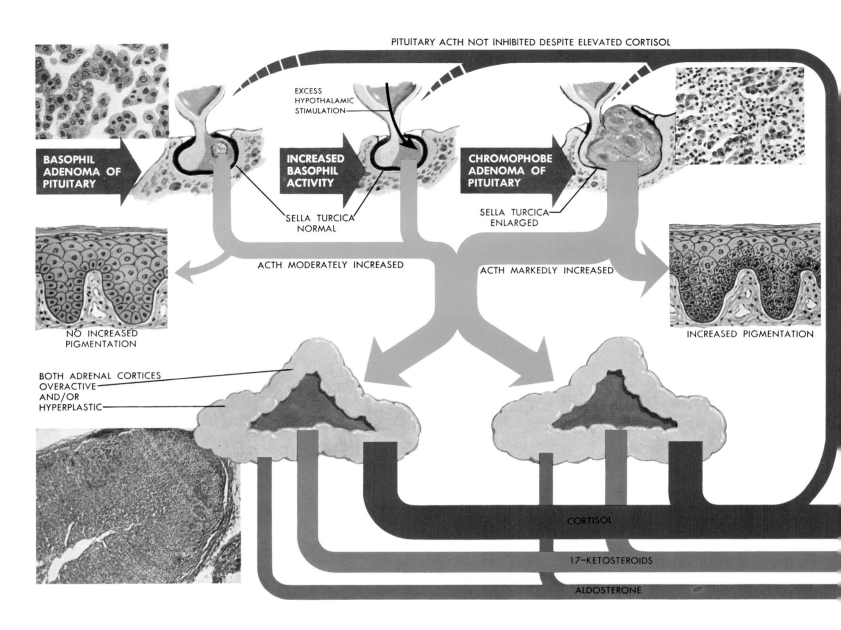

PITUITARY ACTH NOT INHIBITED DESPITE ELEVATED CORTISOL

EXCESS HYPOTHALAMIC STIMULATION

BASOPHIL ADENOMA OF PITUITARY

INCREASED BASOPHIL ACTIVITY

CHROMOPHOBE ADENOMA OF PITUITARY

SELLA TURCICA NORMAL

SELLA TURCICA ENLARGED

ACTH MODERATELY INCREASED

ACTH MARKEDLY INCREASED

NO INCREASED PIGMENTATION

INCREASED PIGMENTATION

BOTH ADRENAL CORTICES OVERACTIVE AND/OR HYPERPLASTIC

CORTISOL

17-KETOSTEROIDS

ALDOSTERONE

CUSHING'S SYNDROME

Pathophysiology

The signs and symptoms as well as the pathology of Cushing's syndrome, or Cushing's disease, are primarily referable to excess *cortisol,* but *17-ketosteroids* may be variably elevated. When a *basophil adenoma of the pituitary* is the source of *excess ACTH,* sections of the pituitary reveal a marked *increase in the basophilic element,* with areas of hyalinized basophils, known as Crooke's cells, present. The latter may also be seen in primary tumors of the adrenal cortex secreting too much cortisol, and they represent a form of irreversible atrophy of the ACTH-producing basophils. In the case of a basophil adenoma, there is only a *moderate increase in ACTH,* with *no increase in pigmentation,* and the *sella turcica* is usually *not enlarged.* The *adrenal cortices* are either *overactive* and/or frankly *hyperplastic* and, usually, weigh in excess of the average 4 to 6 gm per adrenal. The greatest weights found thus far have usually been in nonendocrine tumors secreting ACTH (see page 231), such as in an occasional bronchogenic adenoma or carcinoma. In the more frequently *increased basophilic activity* in general, due to *excess hypo-*

thalamic stimulation, the adrenal weights and cortisol secretion are both only moderately elevated. In the presence of anterior pituitary overactivity with bilateral hyperplasia of the adrenal cortices, *pituitary ACTH is not inhibited,* as it would be normally by elevated cortisol levels. An occasional *chromophobe adenoma of the pituitary gland* may secrete excess ACTH (see page 89). In such a case there may be frank *enlargement of the sella turcica,* produced by a rather large tumor, and the *marked increase in plasma ACTH* is associated with *increased pigmentation of the skin* owing to enhanced melanin formation. It is thought that there are instances of small chromophobe adenomas that do not lead to pigmentation yet are accompanied by large adrenal cortices secreting excess cortisol. It is usually after removal of both adrenals that such small tumors grow rapidly, and patients who previously were totally nonpigmented will then rapidly develop a brownish color.

In the presence of a benign *adenoma of the adrenal cortex,* there is a complete *inhibition of pituitary ACTH* production through the negative feed-back mechanism, whereby excess cortisol inhibits hypothalamic stimulation of the anterior pituitary ACTH-producing cells. This will lead to atrophy of both normal adrenals, but, usually, the tumor stands out, on X-ray, on the ipsilateral side. However, characteristically, there will be a void above the other kidney, with *atrophy of the contralateral adrenal cortex.* Typically, in a *benign adenoma of the adrenal cortex,*

the *cells* reveal *uniformity of size,* and the tumor usually responds excessively, and for a prolonged period of time, to administered ACTH.

A *carcinoma of the adrenal cortex* may be one in situ, in which case there is much *cellular pleomorphism* but no invasion of the veins. On the other hand, it may also be of a highly malignant type, with markedly invasive properties, and, when this occurs, metastases may go to the liver, spleen, and lungs. Here, too, inhibition of the contralateral gland takes place.

The secretion of *cortisol is markedly elevated* in all instances. That of *17-ketosteroids is less than normal,* usually, in adenoma of the adrenal cortex; only *moderately elevated* in *hyperplasia;* and *markedly elevated in adenocarcinoma.* *Aldosterone* is almost always *normal* with *hyperplasia* and *adenoma* but may, occasionally, be elevated with an *adenocarcinoma.* In spite of this, electrolyte changes are found, on occasion, which are those of aldosterone excess, *i.e.,* an *elevated serum sodium* and a *low potassium* with a *hypokalemic alkalosis.* In this case, high levels of cortisol are responsible.

The excess of the various hormones is clearly related to the symptomatology. Cortisol may be responsible for *moderate hypertension,* which is characteristically more of the systolic type at first, gradually becoming diastolic. Much of this is due to the rapidly advancing arteriosclerosis and nephrosclerosis. Excess cortisol leads to *muscular weakness,* as a consequence of the nitrogen loss and general catabolic action. *Obesity* is mostly

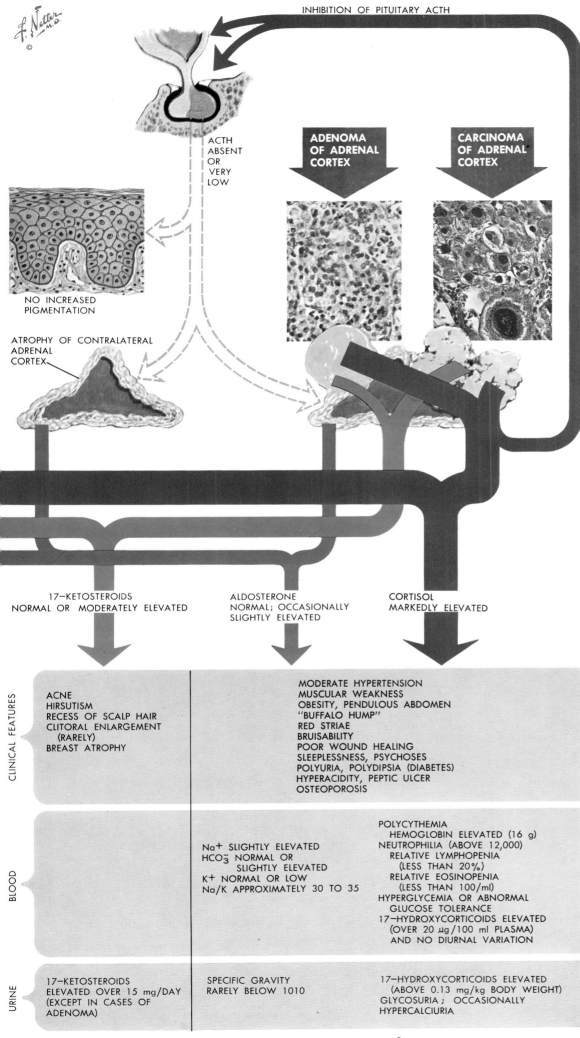

of a distributory nature, the body weight rarely exceeding 100 kg, or 220 lb, with a *pendulous abdomen, buffalo hump,* and supraclavicular fat pads. The subcutaneous *red striae* are due to a thinning in the dermis and dehiscence because of atrophy of the elastic fibers. *Bruisability* is a consequence of the decreased contractility of small blood vessels because of decrease in smooth muscle, and of their increased fragility because of excess catabolism of the connective tissue. *Poor wound healing* is a consequence of the inhibition of fibroblastic hyperplasia by cortisol, and of an excessive susceptibility to infection resulting from inadequacy of phagocytosis and antibody formation. *Sleeplessness,* as a precursor of *psychoses,* is related to the stimulatory effect of cortisol on the central nervous system. *Polyuria* and *polydipsia* are, usually, accompaniments of *diabetes.* Up to 80 per cent of the patients with Cushing's disease show an abnormal glucose tolerance test, but only 20 per cent have frank diabetes. The *hyperglycemia* of the *abnormal glucose tolerance* test is usually accompanied by excessive insulin levels, especially in the obese. There is growth arrest because of excess catabolism and because growth hormone secretion is completely suppressed by excess cortisol. Hypercalciuria, associated with osteoporosis, and increased urinary losses of calcium because of cortisol excess, are also responsible for polyuria. *Hyperacidity* is common, and *peptic ulcers,* though not necessarily more frequent than in the normal population, are far more severe and perforate more frequently, sometimes with gastric hemorrhages. Osteoporosis accounts for compression fractures of the vertebrae and kyphosis. *Osteoporosis* is irreversible in the adult, but in children cured of Cushing's disease there is excellent recalcification. In the blood, one characteristically finds *polycythemia* with *elevated hemoglobin, neutrophilia,* and *relative lymphopenia* and *eosinopenia.* The latter may disappear during the remissions, whereas lymphopenia usually persists for a while.

Plasma 17-hydroxycorticoids may be *elevated* above 20 µg per 100 ml but need not necessarily be that high. More characteristically, there is *no diurnal variation,* whereas, normally, the afternoon plasma samples show approximately one half the morning titers of 17-hydroxycorticoids. The *urinary 17-hydroxycorticoids* are elevated usually above 0.13 mg per kilogram of body weight, in contradistinction to the patient with obesity whose urinary 17-hydroxycorticoids will usually fall below this figure. More diagnostically, the urinary (unconjugated) cortisol will be elevated above the upper limit of 200 µg per day. Occasional *glycosuria* is found. This need not always reflect an excessively elevated blood sugar, since there is, occasionally, a renal loss of glucose in the presence of excess cortisol. *Hypercalciuria* is compatible with cortisol excess, in spite of reduced gastrointestinal absorption, because of antagonism of cortisol to vitamin D, resulting, at times, in reduced blood calcium levels. This may be the reason for the rare cases of coexisting secondary hyperparathyroidism and Cushing's disease.

Tests Used in the Diagnosis of Cushing's Syndrome

In Cushing's syndrome a hemogram will show a low relative lymphocyte count of less than 15 per cent of total leukocytes; a neutrophilia between 10,000 and 20,000, which may go up to 30,000 or 40,000 in the presence of infection; polycythemia with packed red cells of 50 per cent or more; and, especially during acute phases of the disease, a direct eosinophil count of 50 or less per cubic millimeter, as opposed to the normal of 100 to 300.

The diagnosis of Cushing's syndrome is strongly implied by total *urinary 17-hydroxycorticoids* (conjugated and unconjugated) higher than 10 mg per day, provided that simple obesity is corrected on the basis of 0.6 mg per pound of body weight. This figure may be falsely elevated in hyperthyroidism. The definite diagnosis must depend on an evaluation of the secretory dynamics of the adrenal cortices with regard to cortisol.

The *determination of plasma 17-hydroxycorticoids,* or Porter-Silber chromogens, will reveal the *absence* of the usual *diurnal variation,* which would normally show a 50 per cent decrease in titers between 8 a.m. and 6 p.m. A simpler test, however, is the one-dose 11-p.m. *dexamethasone suppression test.* This relies on the fact that 1 mg of dexamethasone, given orally at 11 p.m., will inhibit the outflow of ACTH from the pituitary at about 2 a.m., which is a normal prelude to the rise of cortisol levels to their maximum at 6 a.m. With a half-life of cortisol of less than 2 hours, plasma cortisol levels at 8 a.m. will be less than 5 μg per 100 ml in normal subjects. In Cushing's disease, however, the levels will remain above 10 μg per 100 ml, there having been no inhibition. In nearly all such patients an emotional upset may, occasionally, lead to a falsely elevated level, in spite of the administration of dexamethasone, but mild sedation with barbiturates will safeguard the normal suppression below 5 μg per 100 ml. This simple test will satisfactorily exclude Cushing's syndrome.

An *elevated urinary free cortisol* level represents the most specific demonstration of Cushing's disease.

The differentiation between *adrenal cortical hyperplasia* and *tumor* may be made in the least time-consuming fashion by the Metopirone® test (see page 14). This compound selectively blocks 11-β-hydroxylation in the steroid ring and therefore prevents the formation of cortisol. This effectively leads to an outpouring of ACTH, which will increase the

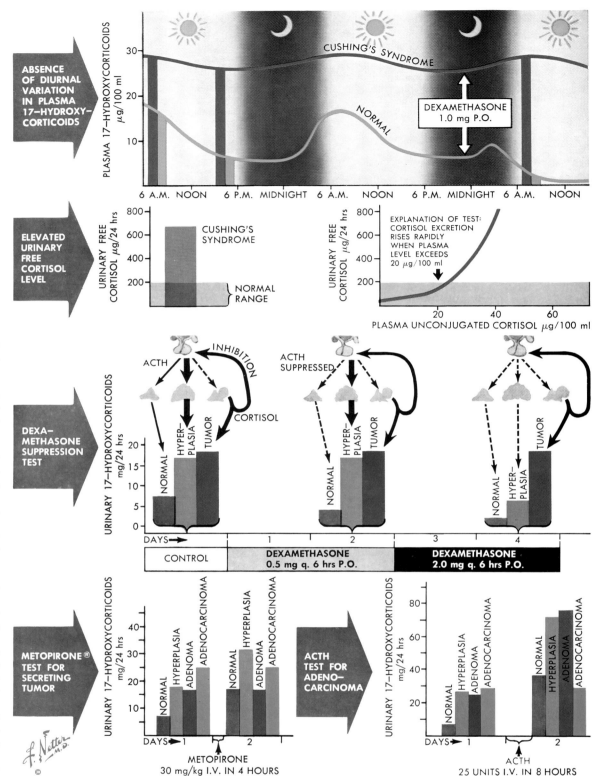

amount of cortisol precursors still measured as 17-hydroxycorticoids in the urine. In one type of test, a 24-hour control urine is obtained, and, on the following day, 30 to 60 mg of Metopirone® per kilogram of body weight is given as an intravenous infusion over a 4-hour period. During the test day a second 24-hour urine is obtained. Patients with normal adrenals and those with hyperplasia will about double their 17-hydroxycorticoid output. However, in patients with adrenal tumors, there will be no change, since the self-sufficient cortisol-producing tumor has long since suppressed pituitary ACTH production and secretion. The same differentiation between hyperplasia and tumor may be achieved by the more cumbersome *dexamethasone suppression test* of Liddle, the first part of which (2-mg-per-day dose) may serve to demonstrate the presence or absence of Cushing's syndrome. Whereas, on the 8-mg dose (per day) of

dexamethasone, patients with hyperplasia have a 50 per cent (or better) suppression of urinary 17-hydroxycorticoids, those with a *tumor* are totally unaffected.

The preoperative differentiation between the presence of a benign adenoma and a potentially malignant adenocarcinoma may often be made by an *8-hour intravenous ACTH test* or even by the injection of 80 units of ACTH gel, intramuscularly. Normally, there should be a three- to fivefold rise in 17-hydroxycorticoids, compared to a control day. This is often excessive with an *adenoma,* but most of the *adenocarcinomas* do not respond. They also usually produce excessive urinary levels of estrogen, dehydroepiandrosterone, and 11-desoxycortisol, to name a few.

Tumors may be located by careful tomograms of the adrenal region after good catharsis. Rarely, this requires a retroperitoneal pneumogram, using either oxygen or CO_2 as a contrast medium.

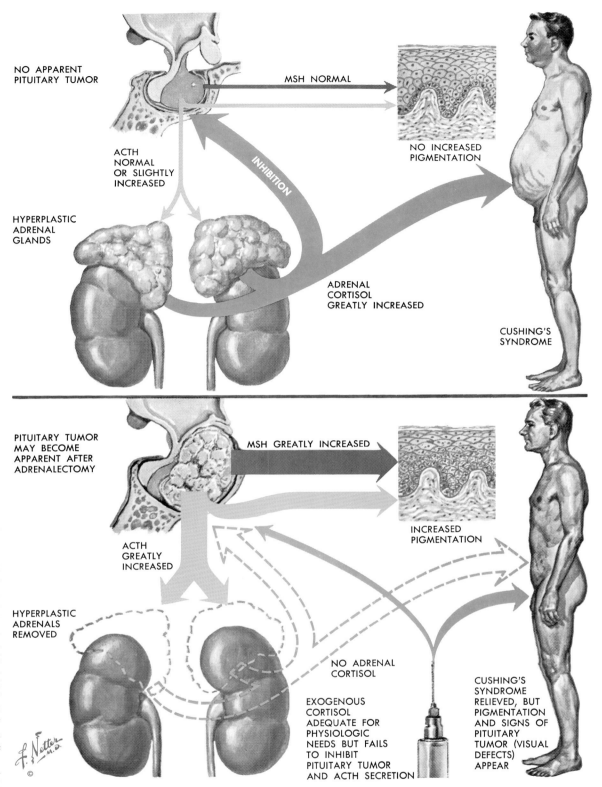

CORTICOTROPIN-PRODUCING CHROMOPHOBE TUMORS

Most of the clinical features of *Cushing's syndrome* are direct consequences of adrenal cortical hyperfunction, which produces a sustained excess of glucocorticoid hormones, chiefly *cortisol*. In the absence of an adrenal tumor and in the presence of *hyperplastic adrenal glands,* the syndrome is induced by increased amounts of some type of corticotropin of either pituitary or other origin (see page 231). Since Cushing's original description, the rôle of the pituitary in the pathogenesis of adrenal overactivity has been debated hotly. The hyaline change originally described by Crooke, which occurs in the β-1 subtype of basophils (see pages 10 and 11), is now generally considered to be a regressive phenomenon induced by prolonged high levels of circulating cortisol, since it can be found in patients who have been treated with ACTH and cortisone, as well as in all cases of spontaneous Cushing's syndrome. Pituitary tumors, of one kind or another, occur in about 15 per cent of the patients with bilateral adrenal hyperplasia producing this syndrome. Of these, only one third are predominantly basophil in staining reaction. Most of these are *too small to distort* the outlines of the *sella* or to press on the visual pathway. Only in 10 per cent is the *tumor* large enough to deform the sella and only some of these reduce the visual fields.

A derangement of the normal inhibitory mechanism, whereby a rising level of cortisol shuts off ACTH, is present in every case of Cushing's syndrome with bilateral adrenal hyperplasia, even when no ACTH-producing tumor is present. If this were not so, the disease would shut itself off. Excess ACTH has been demonstrated in plasma. By the administration of potent cortisol analogues, such as dexamethasone, Liddle has shown that *ACTH secretion* may be *inhibited* in many of these patients, but with higher doses than would be required in the normal patient (see page 88).

The rapid development of obvious *pituitary tumors after* bilateral *adrenalectomy,* in the treatment of Cushing's syndrome, is now a well-recognized clinical entity. These usually preexist but grow more rapidly after removal of the target glands. The patients generally show an *increased* deep, diffuse, brownish *pigmentation* of the skin, particularly prominent over the extensor surfaces of the limbs, since part of the ACTH molecule is identical with melanocyte-stimulating hormone (*MSH*). Skull X-rays, which were normal before operation, often show an intrinsically expanded sella turcica with destruction of the dorsum sellae and posterior clinoids. *Very high levels of ACTH* are found in the blood, and urinary assays for MSH may also be very high. In most of these tumors, the histology is that of an anaplastic or pleomorphic chromophobe adenoma or carcinoma. Rarely is there evidence of PAS-positive or basophilic granulation.

Some patients develop only part of the postadrenalectomy syndrome, in that only excessive pigmentation is noted without demonstrable tumor. The adrenalectomy seems to increase the growth potential of a previously slow-growing pituitary tumor. Even when doses of glucocorticoid, as high as were formerly secreted by the hyperplastic adrenals, are given to the postadrenalectomy tumor patient, inhibition of ACTH may not be obtained. X-ray treatment or surgery is helpful, but the melanin pigmentation of the patient usually persists. Pituitary tumors have been noted to develop mostly in patients who have undergone *adrenalectomy for adrenal hyperplasia;* therefore, in such patients, careful X-ray studies of the sella turcica, examination of the visual fields, and attention to the ease of suppressibility of ACTH by an agent such as dexamethasone (see page 88) should precede adrenalectomy if hyperplasia is thought to be present. These cases should have treatment directed primarily to the pituitary gland, with preference being given to surgical excision if the visual pathway is affected.

THE BIOLOGICAL ACTIONS OF 17-KETOSTEROIDS

The 17-ketosteroids (17-KS), produced by the adrenal cortex in both sexes, include dehydroepiandrosterone (by far the most abundant), *etiocholanolone,* and *androsterone,* together with many other compounds characterized by the presence of a ketone group in the 17 position of the steroid ring. The sum total of the 17-ketosteroids is modified in the *liver,* and they are excreted in the urine as sulfates, glucuronides, and very small amounts in the free form, the total being 10 mg ± 5 in females and 15 mg ± 5 in males, the difference being attributed to testicular contribution of 17-KS. The adrenal is also a significant source of testosterone, which has a 17-hydroxyl group in the molecule (see page 82).

The action of the 17-ketosteroids of adrenal cortical origin may be considered under various headings. In varying degrees, 17-ketosteroids have an *anabolic effect* and induce nitrogen retention, as has repeatedly been proved by nitrogen balance studies. In this *anabolic action,* amino acids are diverted from the liver to *muscle, bone matrix, sex organs, skin,* and *connective tissue,* where they undergo an intracellular transfer which is enhanced by the more active 17-ketosteroids. Once inside the cell, they are synthesized into protein. It is of interest that insulin and growth hormone exert the same type of anabolic action. Cortisol and its derivatives counteract this, being catabolic (see pages 84 and 225). Anabolic agents increase *muscle mass,* and this, in turn, is accompanied by an increased excretion of creatinine in the urine. Secondary *calcium deposition* follows the increased deposition of bone matrix with androgens. This is enhanced by increased tubular reabsorption of calcium under the action of anabolic agents. *Androsterone,* in very large doses which are not physiological, tends to lower *plasma cholesterol.* In addition, it has been found that a solvent, ethyl-*p*-chlorophenoxyisobutyrate, used in oral preparations of androsterone, also leads to the lowering of serum cholesterol.

A weak androgenic effect is exhibited by 17-ketosteroids, but (except for Δ[4]-androstenediol, more potent than testosterone, present in body fluids in quantities still unknown) the most potently androgenic 17-KS is still only one sixtieth as active as testosterone. Androgenic 17-ketosteroids stimulate male sex characteristics, consisting of an *increase in facial hair* and, at the same time, a *recession of the hair line* and *hypertrophy of sebaceous glands* (acne). There is *enlargement of the larynx,* which accounts for

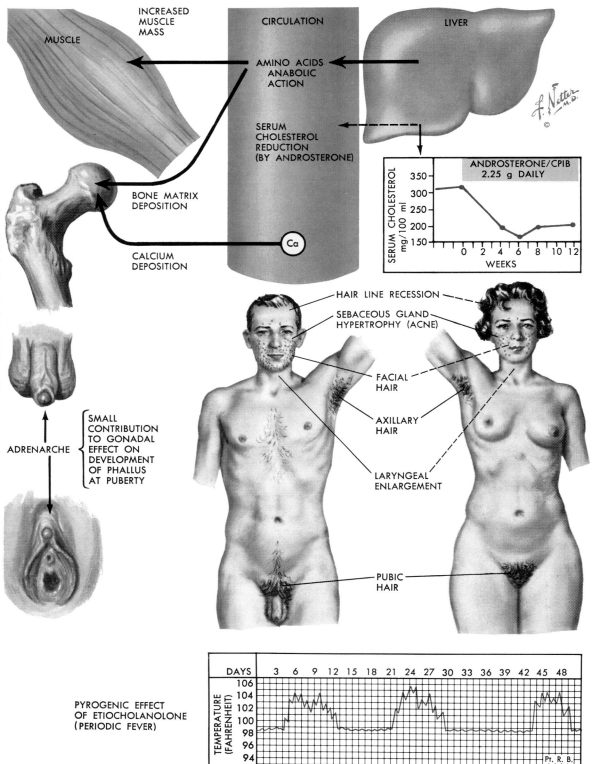

PYROGENIC EFFECT OF ETIOCHOLANOLONE (PERIODIC FEVER)

DAYS	3	6	9	12	15	18	21	24	27	30	33	36	39	42	45	48

TEMPERATURE (FAHRENHEIT) 106 104 102 100 98 96 94   Pt. R. B.

the deep male voice in contrast to that of females. It must be emphasized that the administration of androgens or weakly androgenic anabolic agents to women, in amounts to increase hair growth and deepen the voice, produces irreversible changes which must be guarded against by judicious dosage.

Sexual hair growth is enhanced by androgens. Growth of *axillary hair* is primarily related to an increase in 17-ketosteroids, of adrenal origin, at puberty, although testicular androgens, including testosterone, will also enhance this growth. *Pubic hair* growth is stimulated at puberty by 17-KS and by testosterone. In the male it is characterized by extension in the midline up to the umbilicus (known as the male escutcheon), whereas a triangular area only is covered in females. Hair growth over *chest* and *around the nipples* is also induced by androgens. On the other hand, it must be emphasized that the effect

of androgens on sexual hair growth is dependent not only on the presence of androgens but also on the genetic make-up of the hair follicles. Thus, the American Indian need not shave, yet shows all other signs of virility.

The development of the *phallus* accompanies a rise in 17-KS during the *adrenarche.* Although 17-KS contribute only a small part toward development of the phallus, they are nonetheless significant.

Etiocholanolone, an extremely weak anabolic agent and androgen, exerts a *pyrogenic* effect. Experimentally, it may be shown that, on infusion of either etiocholanolone or related compounds, a rather prompt hyperpyrexia occurs. This has clinical importance since, occasionally, patients with unexplained periodic fevers have been shown to have increased amounts of circulating etiocholanolone and definitely elevated urinary levels.

MAJOR BLOCKS IN ABNORMAL STEROIDOGENESIS

Starting with *cholesterol,* a great many chemical modifications are required of the adrenal cortex in order to produce a final biologically active steroid. Each of these steps in biosynthesis requires the action of one or more specific enzymes capable of modifying chemical groupings at specific locations within the cyclopentenophenanthrene ring. The specific enzymes are carried in the genes, and it is, therefore, not surprising to find that certain abnormalities in steroid biosynthesis are, in fact, familial and/or inherited. Each of the various types of the adrenogenital syndrome is produced by a variety of *blocks* to the addition or transformation of specific groups. The congenital androgenic states have a common deficiency of cortisol. This calls forth an excess of ACTH, which, in turn, stimulates the adrenal cortices to increased abnormal activity and enlargement.

I. The highest block in biochemical sequence is found in the syndrome of lipoid hyperplasia, first described by A. Prader and R. E. Seibenmann. In this rare disease the enzymes responsible for the breakdown of the side chain of cholesterol are absent. As a consequence, cholesterol does not serve as a precursor for all the active steroid hormones but accumulates in the adrenals, testes, and ovaries (see pages 92 and 93). During early fetal life, the intra-uterine Müllerian duct system of the female type is preserved. Genotypic males have female external genitalia. Sometimes, one finds true females; in other instances, male pseudohermaphrodites. Complete adrenal ovarian and testicular insufficiency leads to an early demise unless vigorously treated.

II. Next in line is a syndrome discovered by Bongiovanni and Eberlein, in which there is an absence of c-3-β-OL-DEHYDROGENASE and the linked ISOMERASE. Thereby the oxidation of the hydroxyl group in the 3 position of the ring and the shift of the double bond from C_5 to C_4 do not take place, so that *progesterone* cannot be formed from *pregnenolone.* There follows an accumulation of *dehydroepiandrosterone* and some of its derivatives. Characteristically, the Δ^5 unsaturation of pregnenolone is found in most of the urinary steroids. Since the abnormal derivatives have only a modest androgenic capacity, male patients, who form the majority of this group, show typical undermasculinization, with hypospadias but no cryptorchidism and are thus male pseudohermaphrodites. There is a marked deficit of cortisol as well as

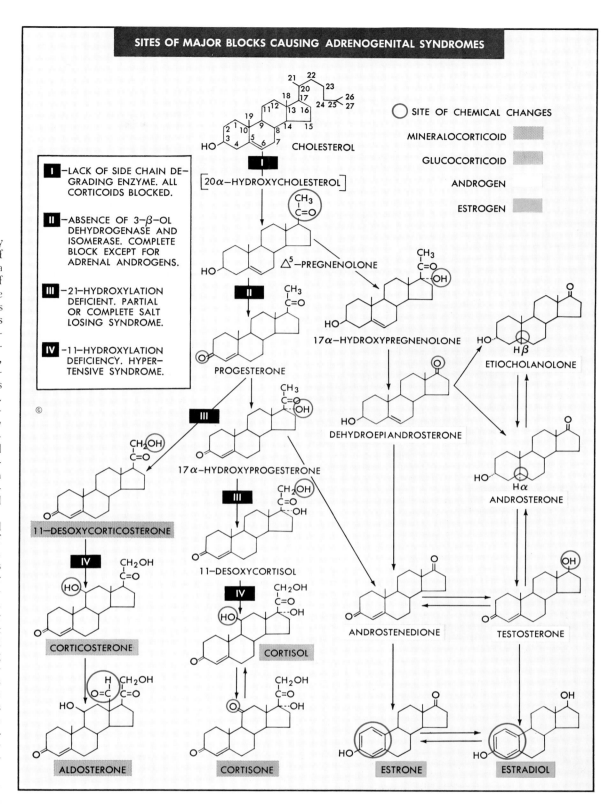

of aldosterone, leading to an early demise unless promptly treated. An excess of 17-ketosteroids is easily established, but there is no increase in pregnanetriol, derived normally from 17-α-hydroxyprogesterone, and so characteristic of most of the other adrenogenital syndromes of congenital origin.

III. By far the most common defect is the lack of 21-hydroxylation, which may be "partial" or, on rarer occasions, "complete". In patients with a very low level of cortisol, there is, more rarely, also a low level of aldosterone. Thus, with excessive androgenicity because of 17-ketosteroid overproduction, the *salt-losing type* is found in only one third of the cases associated with absent aldosterone (see page 92).

In another rare salt-losing type of defect, the oxidation of the 18-angular methyl group is impaired, and aldosterone is not formed.

IV. A much rarer syndrome is that of *11-hydroxy-*

lation deficiency, which leads to the *hypertensive syndrome* because of the accumulation of *desoxycorticosterone,* normally found in only very small amounts. With cortisol deficiency, an excess of ACTH leads to overproduction of 17-ketosteroids and adrenal hyperplasia with low serum potassium (see page 93).

Most of the adrenogenital syndromes are accompanied by a rise in testosterone as well as an increase of estrogens together with the 17-KS. Pregnanetriol is characteristically elevated, except in the Type II block. The ratio of 11-desoxy-17-ketosteroids to 11-oxygenated 17-ketosteroids (normal 0.25) may be as high as 2.3 in congenital adrenal hyperplasia and has been suggested as a useful measure. The anatomical abnormalities are best delineated by an intravenous urogram, by radiographic examination of the vagina and bladder with contrast media, and, on occasion, by culdoscopy or exploration of the pelvis.

HYPOTHALAMUS

LITTLE OR NO INHIBITION OF PITUITARY ACTH PRODUCTION BECAUSE OF DEFICIENT CORTISOL

ADENO-HYPOPHYSIS

PIGMENTATION DUE TO INCREASED ACTH

CORTISOL

11

BLOCK

ACTH GREATLY INCREASED

11-DESOXYCORTISOL

PREGNANETRIOL EXCRETED IN URINE

21

BLOCK

11-DESOXYCORTICOSTERONE

21

INFANTILE ADRENOGENITAL SYNDROMES

HYPERPLASIA OF ADRENAL CORTEX

17α-HYDROXYPROGESTERONE

17

BLOCK 11

PROGESTERONE

CHOLESTEROL

BLOCK 20

3 BLOCK

CORTICOSTERONE

Δ⁵-PREGNENOLONE

18

17

ALDOSTERONE

17α-HYDROXYPREGNENOLONE

17-KETOSTEROIDS (GREATLY INCREASED DUE TO LACK OF CORTISOL INHIBITION OF ACTH AND 21 BLOCK)

H. AND E. STAIN   FAT STAIN
LIPOID HYPERPLASIA OF ADRENAL CORTEX

In all instances of infantile adrenogenital syndromes, simple virilism is the consequence of faulty *biosynthesis* of *adrenal cortical steroids*. Because of the secondarily *excessive secretion of ACTH* consequent to the inadequate production of cortisol, such patients will have a variably deep melanin hyperpigmentation. Depending on the *locus of the block,* there may be either an abnormal loss of sodium in the *salt-losing* variety (21) of the congenital adrenogenital *syndrome* or else, far more rarely, an abnormal accumulation of *desoxycorticosterone* in the *hypertensive syndrome* (11). With enzymatic blocks high up in the biosynthetic chain (20), the syndromes of LIPOID HYPERPLASIA and, at position 3-ol, C-3-β-DEHYDROGENASE DEFICIENCY may rarely be produced.

One of the rarest of the adrenogenital syndromes is depicted as a *complete deficiency of steroid hormone production,* including *17-ketosteroids* and testicular as well as ovarian hormones, in lipoid hyperplasia. Here the enzyme *at C-20* that attacks the long side chain of *cholesterol* is deficient, and it accumulates as an unused precursor of hormones in the adrenals, ovaries, and testes. The *H. and E. stain* and the *fat stain* reveal the hypercellularity of the hyperplastic adrenal cortex, together with a marked accumulation of lipid (cholesterol). This defect can affect both males and females, but a *genotypic male* will develop *female external genitalia,* due to the absence of any androgenic influence in utero. This is the most severe defect known among these syndromes, leaving the patient essentially without steroid hormones. Almost as rare is the deficiency of the C-3-β-ol-dehydrogenase and mutase which normally transform *pregnenolone*

into *progesterone.* The resulting accumulation of the Δ⁵ unsaturated compounds, many of them androgens, leads to rather weak androgenicity, with hypospadias in the male (but not cryptorchidism), thus mild pseudohermaphroditism. Since *17α-hydroxyprogesterone* is not formed, there will be an increase in 17-ketosteroids without the usual elevation of pregnanetriol, as a rule so diagnostic of the congenital adrenogenital syndrome. The affected patients have been predominantly males to date, but, because of the rarity of the condition, this is not a significant observation.

The *block at C-21* is by far the most common. It will lead to *undersecretion of cortisol,* and this, in turn, will bring forth an *excess of ACTH, pigmentation,* and increased secretion of 17-ketosteroids derived from *17α-hydroxyprogesterone.* This syndrome occurs in two forms — *partial* and *severe.* In the partial C-21 defect, enough *cortisol* is produced to prevent

marked adrenal cortical insufficiency, and barely enough *aldosterone* is produced to prevent circulatory collapse. Two thirds of this group belong to the partial category. Under heavy stress, decompensation of the sodium-retaining mechanism occurs, however. It is generally agreed that under those circumstances a large number of incomplete steroid hormones are secreted, which will block the aldosterone at the tubular level, thereby acting as *salt-losing* hormones. Progesterone itself is diuretic, in normal subjects, for that reason. One third make up the severe salt-losing group. They have such a severe defect at C-21 that insufficiency of aldosterone exists continuously, and *dehydration* and *circulatory collapse* are a constant danger.

Both the partial and severe C-21-hydroxylase deficiencies are carried by an autosomal recessive gene. The disease is found in about 1 of 50,000 newborns, although the incidence reported has varied widely,

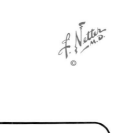

CORTISOL DEFICIENT OR ABSENT

PARTIAL BLOCK—ALDOSTERONE AND CORTISOL PRODUCTION ADEQUATE
TO PREVENT EXCESS SALT LOSS AND CIRCULATORY COLLAPSE
BUT VIRILISM OCCURS DUE TO EXCESSIVE 17-KETOSTEROIDS

SEVERE BLOCK
(SALT–LOSING
SYNDROME)

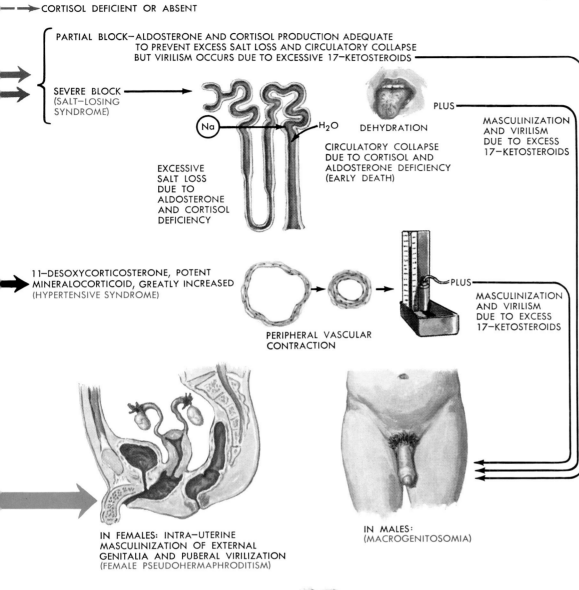

Na → H₂O

DEHYDRATION

PLUS

MASCULINIZATION
AND VIRILISM
DUE TO EXCESS
17–KETOSTEROIDS

CIRCULATORY COLLAPSE
DUE TO CORTISOL AND
ALDOSTERONE DEFICIENCY
(EARLY DEATH)

EXCESSIVE
SALT LOSS
DUE TO
ALDOSTERONE
AND CORTISOL
DEFICIENCY

11–DESOXYCORTICOSTERONE, POTENT
MINERALOCORTICOID, GREATLY INCREASED
(HYPERTENSIVE SYNDROME)

PLUS

MASCULINIZATION
AND VIRILISM
DUE TO EXCESS
17–KETOSTEROIDS

PERIPHERAL VASCULAR
CONTRACTION

IN FEMALES: INTRA–UTERINE
MASCULINIZATION OF EXTERNAL
GENITALIA AND PUBERAL VIRILIZATION
(FEMALE PSEUDOHERMAPHRODITISM)

IN MALES:
(MACROGENITOSOMIA)

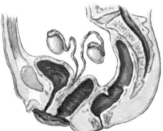

COMPLETE DEFICIENCY OF
STEROID HORMONES, INCLUDING
17–KETOSTEROIDS: TESTICULAR
ANDROGEN PRODUCTION ALSO
IMPAIRED (LIPOID HYPERPLASIA)

GENOTYPIC MALE
DEVELOPS FEMALE
EXTERNAL GENITALIA
DUE TO ABSENCE OF
MASCULINIZING INFLUENCE
OF ANDROGENS IN UTERO

depending on the country and the interest of the investigators. The condition is familial and appears in more than one sibling. Rarely, an acquired form of the partial defect is found in adults with high 17-ketosteroids together with an elevated pregnanetriol The always-present *virilization* leads to *macrogenitosomia* in the *male* and to *female pseudohermaphroditism* in the *female* with *puberal virilization*. In the male the *testicles* may be small or devoid of any palpable testicular tissue, raising the question of undescended testicles. Occasionally, however, one finds firm nodular testes that appear somewhat harder than normal. In these instances one is dealing with adrenal cortical rests that have been enlarged by the excessive ACTH present in the syndrome of congenital adrenal androgenic hyperplasia. In the female the changes in internal and external genitalia are governed by the time at which the excess 17-ketosteroids make

their presence felt during intra-uterine life (see page 122). If late, there is abnormality in the form of an *enlarged clitoris;* if early, the tissue dividing the urethra and the vagina is pushed back increasingly, leaving an ever-larger *urogenital sinus.* In the extreme, there may be a cloaca. Whereas bone growth is accelerated at first, with early maturation of the epiphyses, the end result is a reduction in height. Normal isosexual development does not take place, because of the suppression of gonadotropins by the elevated levels of androgen. The latter is responsible for frequent problems in interpersonal relationships and premature (often inappropriate) sexual behavior, which creates difficulties for teachers and family alike.

Another rare variant is the *block at C-11,* leading to the accumulation of not only 17-ketosteroids but *11-desoxycorticosterone* as well. This compound is a

potent *salt retainer.* Excess leads to *hypertension* and hypokalemia. Although only one thirtieth as potent as aldosterone, the relatively great quantity present gives rise to high levels of both diastolic and systolic blood pressure in the *hypertensive syndrome.* The sexual and somatic changes are the same as with the C-21 syndrome.

The diagnosis of the C-21- as well as the C-11-hydroxylase-deficiency syndrome, is made, first, on clinical grounds and, next, by demonstrating excessive urinary values for 17-ketosteroids and pregnanetriol. In children between 1 and 8 years of age, 17-ketosteroids do not normally exceed 2 mg per day. After that, there is a variable rise, reaching adult levels of 10- and 15-mg means for females and males, respectively, soon after puberty. In patients with the C-21 syndrome, values may rise to 100 mg of 17-ketosteroids daily at any age. Pregnanetriol, usually below 2 mg per day, may rise above 10 mg and is found elevated before 17-ketosteroids have risen. In making the diagnosis, it is imperative to show that administration of cortisol (or any other anti-inflammatory glucocorticoid) in divided doses, with a total not exceeding twice the normal secretion for the particular age, will lead to a significant (more than 50 per cent) fall in urinary 17-ketosteroids. In the salt-losing variety the serum Na/K ratio is below 30 because of the fall in serum Na and the rise in serum K, typical of Addison's disease (see page 103). In the partial defect these values are usually normal. In the hypertensive syndrome the reverse pertains, with serum sodium elevated and serum potassium depressed, so that the ratio lies above 30.

ADULT ADRENOGENITAL SYNDROMES

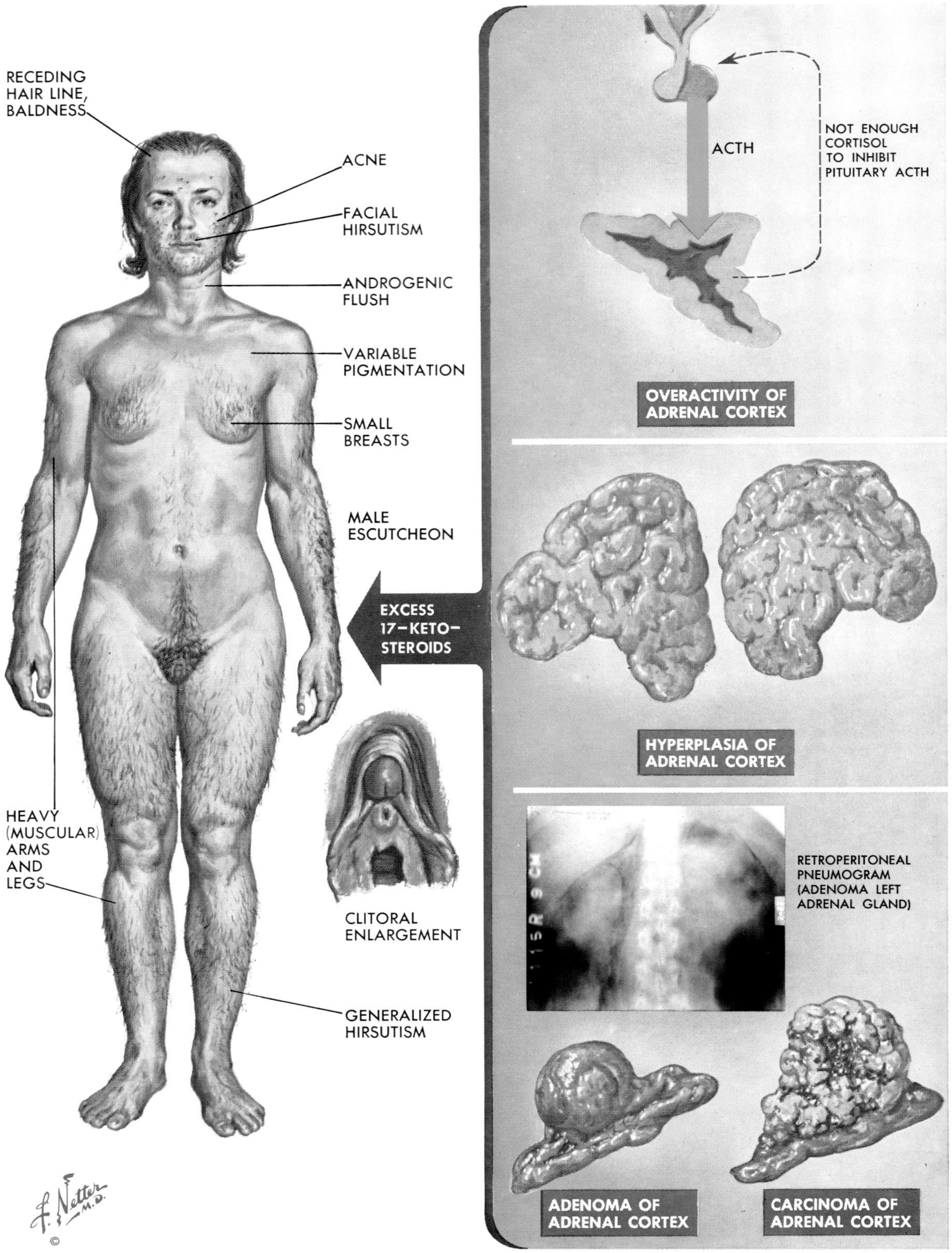

An excess of the various 17-ketosteroids will lead to masculinization that may go unrecognized in the male, adding to his natural prowess, but may prove devastating in the female. The adrenogenital syndromes vary in their clinical manifestations, depending on the sex affected, the age at onset of the abnormal production of 17-ketosteroids, and the precise nature of the biosynthetic abnormality present.

The adult female develops a *masculine habitus,* with *receding hairline, baldness, hirsutism of body and face, acne, small atrophic breasts* and uterus, a *male escutcheon,* and *enlargement of the clitoris.* The latter, together with an excess of androgen, is probably responsible for the frequent increase in heterosexual sex drive. Deepening of the voice, whether induced by the adrenogenital syndrome or by androgen therapy, is always irreversible. *Variable* degrees of melanin *pigmentation* are present, as is a red discoloration in the collar area, known as the *androgenic flush.* Menstruation usually ceases, as does ovulation. Feminine distribution of fat disappears, to be replaced by *heavier masculine musculature.* The skin, in contrast to that of Cushing's syndrome, which is thin and almost paperlike, becomes thick and resilient, reflecting the anabolic effect of the excess androgens. This condition may originate from *hyperplasia, adenoma,* or *adenocarcinoma* of the adrenal cortex.

This fully developed picture is relatively rare and must be differentiated from benign androgenic adrenal hyperactivity, which is seen far more frequently. In the latter condition, women are somewhat obese and have a quite feminine habitus, the only abnormality being increasing hirsutism and, sometimes, amenorrhea accompanied by a slight elevation of 17-ketosteroids.

Among patients with benign androgenic adrenal hyperplasia with, at most, a slight bilateral enlargement of the adrenal cortices, there are occasional cases which have the same biochemical blocks found in the prenatal varieties. This is characterized by a partial block of cortisol synthesis, an accumulation of pregnanetriol which is diagnostically elevated above the upper normal limit of 2 mg per day in the urine, and urinary 17-ketosteroids up to 30 mg per day.

In the adult the course, unless caused by a rapidly growing adenoma or adenocarcinoma, is usually benign, although it is psychologically and socially traumatizing.

The diagnosis depends on laboratory determination of urinary 17-ketosteroids, which are usually only moderately elevated in hyperplasia (15 to 20 mg per day). In the benign syndrome, 17-ketosteroids may be in the upper range of normal, remaining constant from day to day (even prior to ovulation) instead of rising as they do normally, implying an abnormal fixation of activity. In adenoma or adenocarcinoma, 17-ketosteroids are usually high (30 to 150 mg per day).

Any elevation in 17-ketosteroid excretion above 20 mg per day points to the adrenal as the source of excess androgen. In the absence of a 17-ketosteroid elevation, one is probably dealing with ovarian secretion of testosterone or androstenedione, and the 17-ketosteroids are not adequately suppressed by dexamethasone. Where abnormal amounts of androgen are being secreted by an ovarian or testicular tumor, 2000 units of chorionic gonadotropin, given intramuscularly on arising, may cause a three- to five-fold increase in testosterone excretion in the urine specimen obtained during the subsequent 24 hours. Where androgens are of adrenal origin, no such increase will be produced.

The differentiation between hyperplasia and tumor is made by the dexamethasone suppression test (see page 88). On 2 mg or 8 mg per day, there is no suppression of 17-ketosteroids with tumors; in hyperplasia, 17-ketosteroids are reduced 50 per cent or more. Unfortunately, differentiation between adenoma and adenocarcinoma, by the 8-hour intravenous ACTH test utilized in Cushing's syndrome, is not reliable in the adrenogenital syndrome. In searching for the site of a tumor in the adrenogenital syndrome, one must realize that the contralateral adrenal, as shown on the right in the *retroperitoneal pneumogram,* is not atrophic, since the tumor does not produce an excess of cortisol and thus does not inhibit ACTH.

RECEDING HAIR LINE, BALDNESS

ACNE

FACIAL HIRSUTISM

ANDROGENIC FLUSH

VARIABLE PIGMENTATION

SMALL BREASTS

MALE ESCUTCHEON

EXCESS 17-KETO-STEROIDS

HEAVY (MUSCULAR) ARMS AND LEGS

CLITORAL ENLARGEMENT

GENERALIZED HIRSUTISM

ACTH

NOT ENOUGH CORTISOL TO INHIBIT PITUITARY ACTH

OVERACTIVITY OF ADRENAL CORTEX

HYPERPLASIA OF ADRENAL CORTEX

RETROPERITONEAL PNEUMOGRAM (ADENOMA LEFT ADRENAL GLAND)

ADENOMA OF ADRENAL CORTEX

CARCINOMA OF ADRENAL CORTEX

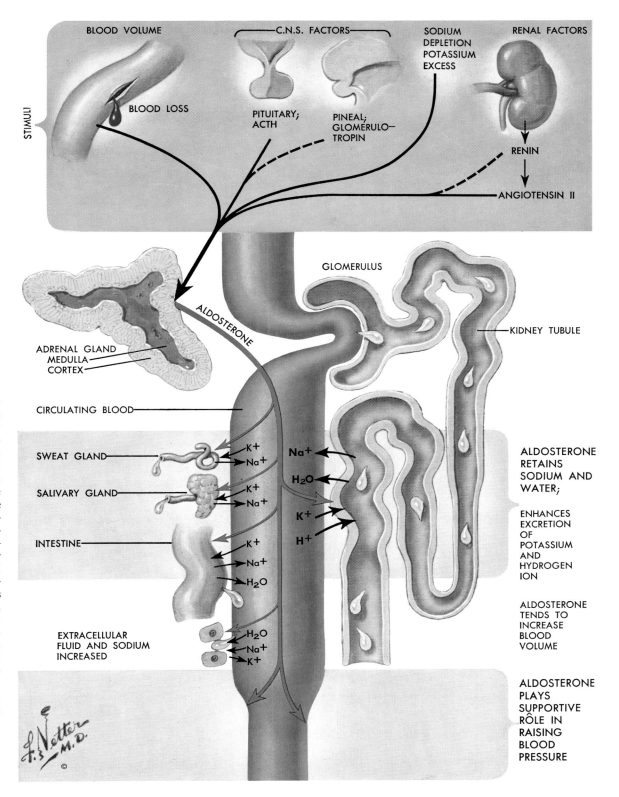

THE BIOLOGICAL ACTIONS OF ALDOSTERONE

The *pituitary* secretion of adrenocorticotropin (*ACTH*) regulates the secretion of cortisol by the adrenal gland. It may increase the secretion of *aldosterone,* produced in the zona glomerulosa, over a limited period of time only and to a small extent (two- to threefold). In contrast, a fall in blood volume may raise aldosterone secretion to thirtyfold. This suggests the existence of a separate aldosterone-stimulating substance. Ablation of the pituitary practically abolishes cortisol secretion but reduces aldosterone secretion by only 60 to 80 per cent. Although ACTH is not essential for the secretion of aldosterone, it does provide optimal conditions of the adrenal cortex for such production.

Recent evidence suggests that an aldosterone-stimulating substance may originate in the juxtaglomerular cells of the *kidney.* Alterations in *blood volume* provide potent stimuli to aldosterone secretion; a decrease stimulates and an increase depresses its secretion. These *stimuli* are, in part, transmitted to the *adrenal gland* by changes in the secretion of renin by the volume-sensitive juxtaglomerular cells. Thus, experimentally, the increase in aldosterone secretion, seen after *blood loss* in hypophysectomized animals, fails to occur in the absence of the kidney and of the pituitary. The enzyme *renin* changes angiotensinogen to angiotensin I, which, in turn, is rapidly converted to *angiotensin II* in the plasma. Angiotensin II acts as a potent stimulus to *aldosterone secretion* without significantly affecting the secretion of other adrenocortical hormones, provided the dose is not excessive. A substance, *glomerulotropin,* derived from the *pineal gland* or from the surrounding brain tissue, has been reported previously to increase aldosterone secretion. *Potassium* depletion decreases and potassium loading increases aldosterone secretion. The relative physiological importance of these latter stimuli is not clear, nor has their exact mode of action been elucidated.

Aldosterone is secreted in small amounts (100 to 150 μg per day) under conditions of normal sodium intake. The peripheral blood level is approximately 0.01 μg per 100 ml. Its half-disappearance time from plasma is rapid (20 to 30 minutes). Very little is bound to the corticosterone-binding globulin (transcortin), and most is bound loosely to albumin. No evidence suggests that aldosterone has significant glucocorticoid activity unless massive doses are administered.

The metabolism of aldosterone presents some differences from that of other adrenal steroids. A very small proportion of aldosterone is excreted unchanged; about 10 per cent is conjugated in such a way that acid hydrolysis at pH 1 releases the free hormone (3-oxo-conjugate); and 15 to 20 per cent of the secreted aldosterone appears as urinary tetrahydroglucuronide metabolites, devoid of biological activity.

Aldosterone is the electrolyte-regulating hormone of the *adrenal cortex.* Its major site of action is in the *distal tubule,* where it facilitates the exchange of sodium for *potassium* and *hydrogen ions.* Though its greatest quantitative effect is seen in the kidney, it acts in other organs as well. *Sweat, salivary secretions,* and the *stools* show decreased sodium and increased potassium content in the presence of aldosterone. The *retention* of *sodium* and *water increases extracellular fluid* and *blood volume.* In addition, aldosterone may play a rôle in regulating *blood pressure,* since its absence (as in Addison's disease) is associated with low blood pressure and its excess (as in primary hyperaldosteronism) leads to a high level.

Aldosterone is a potent hormone, the secretion of which is governed by a variety of stimuli which produce changes generally directed toward the maintenance of normal electrolyte composition, circulatory volume, and blood pressure.

PRIMARY HYPERALDOSTERONISM

In primary hyperaldosteronism the hormone is nearly always produced by a small *adrenal cortical adenoma* whose *cells* resemble the zona glomerulosa, the fasciculata, or both. The contiguous *adrenal gland* is usually of normal size and histology.

Hypertension is seen in nearly all patients with primary hyperaldosteronism, and, conversely, this condition may be a causative factor in up to 20 per cent of all hypertensives. *Potassium depletion* produces the clinical symptoms. A *low serum potassium level* is almost invariably found, but repeated determinations may be necessary to demonstrate this. Excessive *loss of potassium* and *hydrogen ions* occurs primarily from the kidneys. Excessive urinary excretion of potassium, in spite of a low serum potassium, suggests an abnormal hormone influence on normal kidneys. Other secretory products, such as sweat, saliva, and *stools,* also yield evidence of *increased potassium excretion.* The symptoms of potassium depletion usually appear as fatigue and loss of stamina. The resultant *hypokalemic alkalosis* may, at times, lead to *positive Chvostek's* and *Trousseau's signs.* Their presence, in an untreated hypertensive subject, is presumptive evidence of alkalosis and possibly of hyperaldosteronism. Potassium depletion also produces functional changes, and, at times, pathological vacuolization in the *renal tubule,* known as *hypokalemic nephropathy.* Alterations in renal tubular function are manifested by *polyuria, polydipsia,* and, often, marked nocturia. This abnormal function can be demonstrated by poor concentrating ability after dehydration or unresponsiveness to *antidiuretic hormone administration.*

Increased sodium and *water* reabsorption results in *hypernatremia* and, frequently, hypervolemia, without manifest edema. The *extracellular fluid* is *increased* and the blood volume enlarged, the latter being due primarily to an increase in plasma volume. These volume changes may be responsible for the almost complete suppression of peripheral renin concentration in primary hyperaldosteronism. A *low hematocrit* may reflect this dilutional phenomenon. It is the high and labile glomerular filtration of these patients which allows them to increase the filtered load of sodium to such an extent that marked edema does not occur, as a rule.

Headaches, weakness, nocturia, and paresthesias are the most prominent clinical symptoms. The benign hypertension frequently shows a postural fall. The pulse rate is usually slow and relatively fixed, regardless of changes in posture and activity, due to impairment of circulatory baroreceptor function often seen in this disorder.

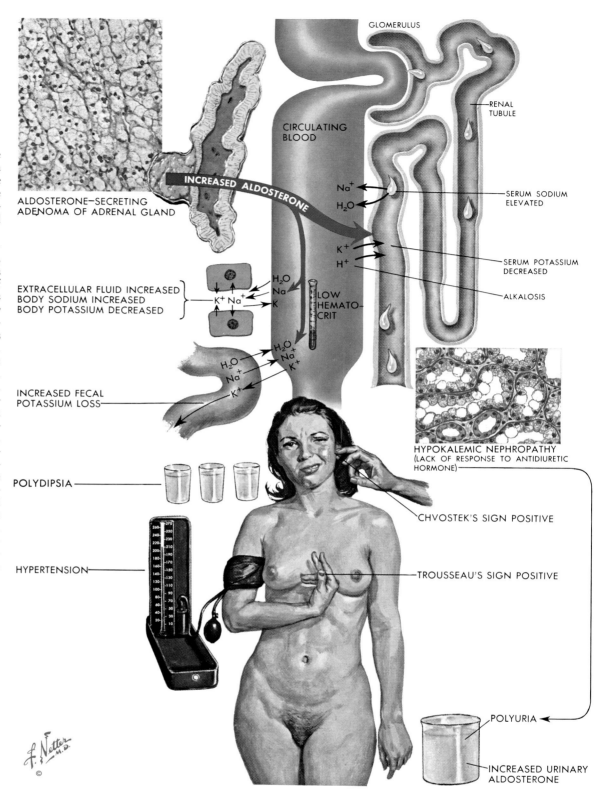

ALDOSTERONE–SECRETING ADENOMA OF ADRENAL GLAND

GLOMERULUS

CIRCULATING BLOOD

INCREASED ALDOSTERONE

RENAL TUBULE

Na⁺
H₂O

SERUM SODIUM ELEVATED

EXTRACELLULAR FLUID INCREASED
BODY SODIUM INCREASED
BODY POTASSIUM DECREASED

H₂O
Na
K⁺ Na⁺ K

LOW HEMATO-CRIT

K⁺
H⁺

SERUM POTASSIUM DECREASED

ALKALOSIS

H₂O
Na⁺
K⁺

H₂O
Na⁺
K⁺

INCREASED FECAL POTASSIUM LOSS

HYPOKALEMIC NEPHROPATHY (LACK OF RESPONSE TO ANTIDIURETIC HORMONE)

POLYDIPSIA

CHVOSTEK'S SIGN POSITIVE

HYPERTENSION

TROUSSEAU'S SIGN POSITIVE

POLYURIA

INCREASED URINARY ALDOSTERONE

Strong presumptive evidence of primary hyperaldosteronism can be obtained by routinely available laboratory determinations, such as the measurement of serum sodium and potassium, urinary potassium excretion, concentration tests and hematocrit and/or blood volume determinations. Hypernatremic, hypokalemic alkalosis, with increased plasma volume and excessive urinary potassium loss, are almost diagnostic. The single most useful determination is that of the *serum potassium.* At one time or another, most patients have demonstrated a low serum potassium, provided sodium intake was not restricted. Marked restriction of sodium intake limits the sodium available in the distal nephron for exchange with potassium and hydrogen, despite excessive aldosterone. Many of the metabolic abnormalities as well as the electrocardiographic changes caused by potassium depletion may be corrected during sodium restriction as potassium retention occurs. The electrolyte measurements should be performed during normal sodium intake.

Spironolactone, a peripheral antagonist of aldosterone, has proved useful in the diagnosis of primary hyperaldosteronism. If 1 gm of spironolactone is given by mouth daily for 3 days, it will bring serum potassium toward normal, temporarily, but, 5 to 7 days after cessation of the drug, the serum potassium will again fall to hypokalemic levels, since tumor secretion is not reduced but, frequently, is increased.

The definitive diagnosis of primary hyperaldosteronism is established by measuring the rate of secretion of *aldosterone* or the *daily excretion* of one of its metabolites (see page 95). Since volume depletion, achieved by salt restriction, may increase aldosterone secretion in normal subjects, the measurement of aldosterone should be performed during normal salt intake (5 to 8 gm NaCl) (see page 99).

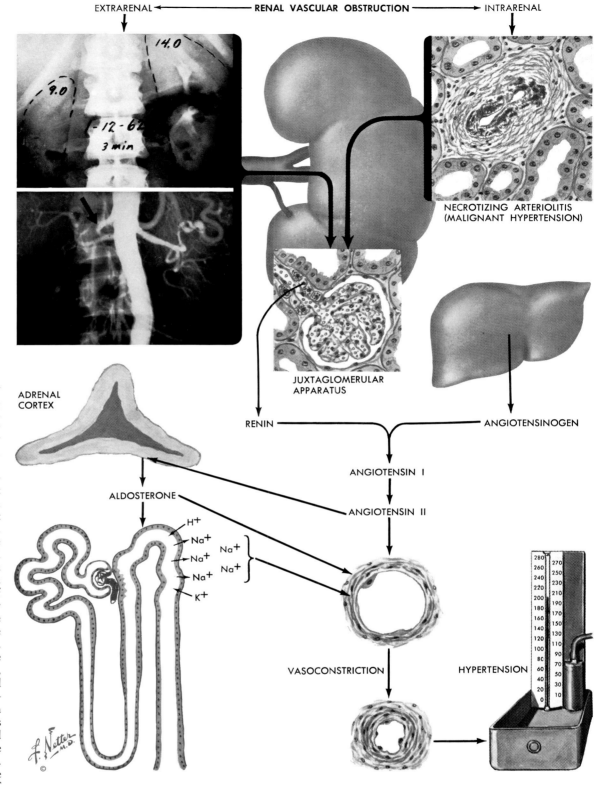

EXTRARENAL ← **RENAL VASCULAR OBSTRUCTION** → INTRARENAL

NECROTIZING ARTERIOLITIS
(MALIGNANT HYPERTENSION)

JUXTAGLOMERULAR
APPARATUS

ADRENAL
CORTEX

RENIN ——————————————— ANGIOTENSINOGEN

ALDOSTERONE

ANGIOTENSIN I

ANGIOTENSIN II

H⁺
Na⁺
Na⁺   Na⁺
Na⁺   Na⁺
Na⁺
K⁺

VASOCONSTRICTION   HYPERTENSION

RENAL HYPERTENSION

The existence of an endocrine relationship between the *adrenal gland* and the *kidney* has long been suspected and is now established by experimental evidence. *Renin,* an enzyme elaborated by the kidney, converts *angiotensinogen,* produced by the *liver,* into *angiotensin I.* In the plasma the latter is degraded further to *angiotensin II,* one of the most potent vasopressors. Besides its effect on the smooth muscles of the arterioles, it strongly stimulates *aldosterone* secretion. Aldosterone, too, has a hypertensive effect by a mechanism that is not well understood at this time. Its influence on sodium retention and potassium excretion in the kidney and on the distribution of these ions within the body is probably associated with this effect, whereby there is a rise in sodium concentration in the walls of arteries and other blood vessels.

Renin appears to be secreted by the *juxtaglomerular cells* located, usually, between the afferent renal arteriole and the proximal tubule. Increased granulation occurs in these cells when renin secretion is increased. Maneuvers such as reduction of renal pressure and blood flow through the kidney, as a consequence of salt deprivation, act as stimulants. The fact that blood volume changes are associated with increased secretion of aldosterone also suggests that the *juxtaglomerular apparatus* may well be the intrarenal volume receptor. Certainly, these cells are ideally located, in the wall of the afferent arteriole and near a tubule, to perform as a baroreceptor. Blood loss still raises aldosterone, even after removal of the pituitary. However, the failure of hemorrhage to stimulate aldosterone secretion in the hypophysectomized and nephrectomized dog is strong evidence that a regulatory volume-sensitive structure resides within the kidney.

In man, both *intrarenal* and *extrarenal* lesions are associated with increased secretion of aldosterone. A common factor in both disorders may be decrease in pressure and flow to the juxtaglomerular appara-

tus, the volume-sensitive region within the kidney. A thickening of the subendothelial layers, notably the smooth muscle in the renal arteries (fibromuscular disease, especially in women), and/or atheromatous deposits often lead to unilateral narrowing of a renal artery. This must be considered when the kidney size is found, by an intravenous urogram, to be less than 10 cm long on one side. A retrograde arteriogram may then reveal the site of vascular occlusion. The more frequent association of increased aldosterone secretion with *malignant hypertension* is not accompanied by overt vascular occlusions. The lesion may be more diffuse, involving smaller intrarenal vessels, thus making this a renovascular type of hypertension as well.

These consequences of increased renin secretion may, on occasion, lead to problems in the differential diagnosis of primary hyperaldosteronism. Hypertension, hypokalemia, and increased aldosterone secre-

tion are observed in primary hyperaldosteronism, frequently in malignant hypertension, and occasionally in renovascular hypertension. Useful distinguishing features in the latter two are (1) normal to low serum sodium concentrations and (2) normal or, more often, diminished rather than elevated total blood volume. The fact that there is almost complete suppression of peripheral renin concentrations in primary hyperaldosteronism will prove most useful in differential diagnosis. These observations are of greater importance as confirmatory findings in cases where differences in renal size and arteriographic evidence of occlusive disease are lacking.

The relative importance of the renin-angiotensin-aldosterone system, in maintaining normal pressure and volume relationships, is evident in the significant clinical disturbances produced by derangements in this mechanism.

PERIODIC PARALYSIS AND HYPOKALEMIA

Periodic paralysis is a disorder characterized by bouts of muscle paralysis, without impairment of sensation or loss of consciousness, in apparently robust, often very muscular, individuals. Attacks tend to occur during periods of relaxation and are decreased by muscular activity. The disease is more common in males. It is frequently *inherited* as an autosomal dominant trait (familial periodic paralysis) but may occur sporadically. In affected families there may be an increased incidence of migraine, epilepsy, and progressive muscular atrophy. Paralytic bouts, lasting from a few minutes to 2 or 3 days, usually start at or before puberty and tend to become less severe and less frequent with advancing years.

Attacks of paralysis commonly start *during* sleep or *relaxation*, or on *awakening*, especially after an *evening meal rich in carbohydrate*. The *paralysis* is flaccid in type, may be localized or generalized, but seldom involves the respiratory or facial muscles. Constipation, arrhythmias, or cardiomegaly suggest that smooth and cardiac muscle may be involved. Severe thirst, increased fluid retention, and weight gain frequently precede attacks, oliguria is present during paralysis, and diuresis and sweating often usher in the recovery phase. The *serum potassium*, usually normal between attacks, falls profoundly as paralysis develops, because of *movement of potassium ions* from the *extracellular fluid into the muscles*. This potassium shift is recognizable by arteriovenous differences in serum potassium, by appropriate changes in the electromyogram, and by direct measurement of potassium in biopsied specimens of paralyzed muscle. The *rise in intramuscular potassium concentrations* occurs without a detectable change in the chronically *elevated intracellular sodium concentration*. The consequent rise in the sum of intramuscular sodium and potassium concentration and rise in intracellular osmolality may be responsible for paralyzing the muscles.

Attacks of paralysis are readily induced by various "stresses" or by the administration of glucose, insulin, epinephrine, corticotropin, adrenal cortical extracts, or mineralocorticoids. In many patients with the disorder, though evidently not in all, spontaneous paralysis is preceded or accompanied by increased urinary excretion of *aldosterone* or aldosterone-like substances, often together with increased excretion of 17-ketosteroids and 17-hydroxycorticoids. The greater rate of carbohydrate metabolism, which normally follows a high-carbohydrate meal or the administration of glucose and insulin, has been shown to increase the sub-

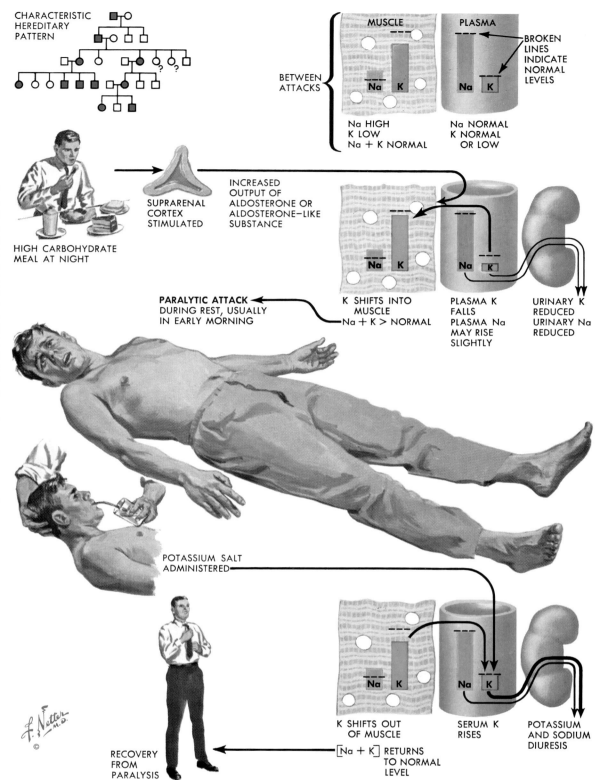

sequent urinary output of aldosterone-like material.

Death has occasionally occurred during a paralytic seizure, usually because of respiratory infections or paralysis. At autopsy, the only significant finding has been a vacuolar change within the muscle fibers. This change may be recognized in biopsies of paralyzed muscles and has been corrected by treatment with a low-sodium diet and diuretics.

Paralytic seizures are self-limiting but may be rapidly overcome by *administering larger doses of potassium salts* (by mouth or intravenously). The avoidance of attacks is most successfully accomplished by strict adherence to a diet low in sodium chloride (200 mg per day), together with the administration of a thiazide diuretic whenever the weight rises by more than 2 lb. Spironolactone, with its sodium diuretic effect, is also of value in preventing paralytic episodes.

Primary hyperaldosteronism (see page 96) may be differentiated from familial paralysis by the persistent hypokalemia between attacks and the associated hypertension. Periodic paralysis with low serum potassium levels is found, on occasion, with hyperthyroidism.

A rarer type of familial paralysis, called adynamia episodica hereditaria, usually starts in infancy, causes less severe paralysis, and commonly occurs during muscular activity during the day. In these patients, paralysis is associated with hyperkalemia and may be precipitated by the administration of potassium salts. No endocrine factors have been shown to be related to the paralytic attacks in this condition.

A condition of hysteria must always be ruled out presenting with a preponderance of females, the characteristic psychological features, the absence of chemical changes, and the retention of muscular responses to electrical stimulation.

SECONDARY HYPERALDOSTERONISM

Increased secretion of aldosterone is observed in certain edematous states, in malignant hypertension, and during salt deprivation. Though its secretion may be excessive, the phenomenon should be viewed as a physiologic consequence rather than a primary adrenal event.

In the primarily edematous states the consequences of excessive aldosterone secretion are not usually seen. Potassium depletion does not take place. Serum electrolytes are within physiological limits, unless diuretics have been used up to a week before the test. The normalcy of electrolytes relates to the fact that the intense proximal reabsorption of sodium diminishes its availability for competition with potassium and hydrogen ions in the distal tubule, thereby preventing the loss of potassium and hydrogen ions through the urine.

In *hepatic cirrhosis with ascites,* aldosterone secretion increases when ascitic fluid forms, as a continuous loss of plasma from the vascular compartment takes place. This event may be viewed as an "internal phlebotomy". It may well be the initiating stimulus for aldosterone secretion effected through the renin-angiotensin-aldosterone mechanism.

In right-sided *congestive heart failure,* the stimulus to aldosterone secretion may, again, be a decrease in pressure of "effective blood volume" affecting the juxtaglomerular cells in the kidneys, thereby leading to an increased secretion of aldosterone through the renin-angiotensin-aldosterone mechanism.

The combination of capillary leaks and massive proteinuria of *nephrosis* produces a persistent decrease in blood volume, which acts as a stimulus to increase aldosterone secretion. Frequently, patients with nephrosis have diminished or normal blood volume in the presence of markedly increased extracellular fluid.

The cause of increased aldosterone secretion in *cyclic idiopathic edema* is not clear. Often, an excessive secretion of pituitary antidiuretic hormone, under the influence of psychic stimuli, is the primary cause. The exact pathophysiologic mechanisms are complex, and aldosterone secretion is not always increased. When raised, it often is not responsive to the stimuli that would normally cause its decrease.

Aldosterone-blocking agents are usually effective in all those states in which aldosterone secretion is excessive.

In accelerated and *malignant forms of hypertension,* aldosterone secretion is invariably elevated, yet the metabolic abnormalities of aldosterone excess, such

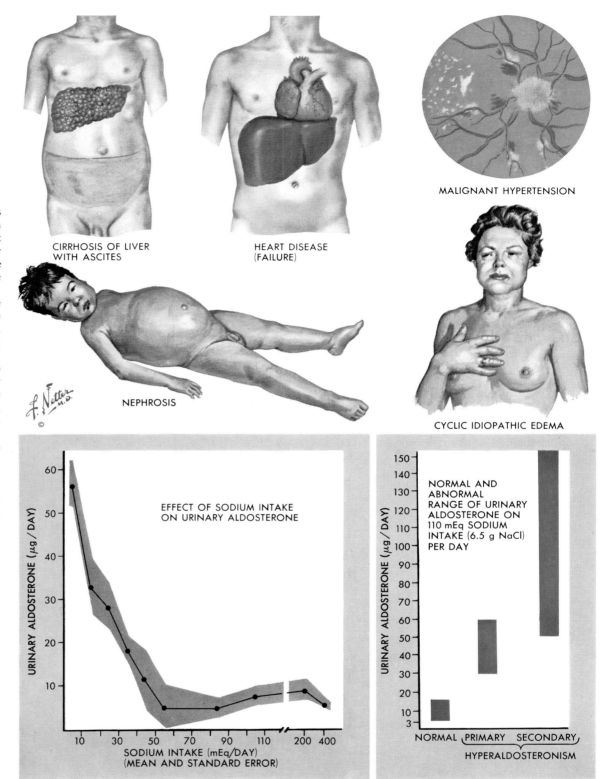

CIRRHOSIS OF LIVER WITH ASCITES

HEART DISEASE (FAILURE)

MALIGNANT HYPERTENSION

NEPHROSIS

CYCLIC IDIOPATHIC EDEMA

EFFECT OF SODIUM INTAKE ON URINARY ALDOSTERONE

URINARY ALDOSTERONE (µg / DAY)

SODIUM INTAKE (mEq/DAY) (MEAN AND STANDARD ERROR)

NORMAL AND ABNORMAL RANGE OF URINARY ALDOSTERONE ON 110 mEq SODIUM INTAKE (6.5 g NaCl) PER DAY

URINARY ALDOSTERONE (µg / DAY)

NORMAL   PRIMARY   SECONDARY

HYPERALDOSTERONISM

as hypernatremia, increased exchangeable sodium, expanded blood volume, and a very marked hypokalemia, are not observed. *Severe eyeground changes* (K-W grades 3 and 4) are seen, but they are practically absent in primary hyperaldosteronism, which is characterized by benign eyeground changes. These are useful differential diagnostic criteria. Though hypokalemia is occasionally present, it is not as severe as in primary hyperaldosteronism. The extrarenal unilateral stenosis of the renal artery may also give rise to secondary hyperaldosteronism, as do the intrarenal necrotizing vascular lesions of malignant hypertension. Both conditions lead to changes in the renin-angiotensin system and, thus, eventually to increased aldosterone secretion (see page 97). A definitive diagnostic separation between primary hyperaldosteronism and renovascular hypertension may be achieved by the measurement of plasma renin,

which is always low or absent in the former and high in the latter.

As previously described, the most potent stimulus to the secretion of aldosterone is a decrease in extracellular fluid volume and, in particular, in the intravascular compartment. *Sodium restriction* challenges the sodium-conserving mechanisms by producing decreases in the extracellular fluid and intravascular space. Progressive dietary sodium restriction leads to greater extracellular fluid loss and increased aldosterone secretion. Thus, it becomes apparent that, to establish unequivocally the presence of increased aldosterone secretion in primary hyperaldosteronism, the measurements must be performed while sodium intake is greater than 50 mEq per day. At an *intake level of 110 mEq (6.5 gm NaCl), primary* and *secondary hyperaldosteronism* are clearly distinguished from the *normal state.*

Acute Adrenal Cortical Insufficiency (Waterhouse-Friderichsen Syndrome)

Acute insufficiency is known as ADRENAL CRISIS. This may follow destruction of the adrenal cortex by infection, trauma, hemorrhage, or thrombosis, or it may follow stresses, such as surgery, anesthesia, or injury, in patients whose adrenal cortical reserve has already been diminished by disease, partial adrenalectomy, or previous treatment with glucocorticoids or ACTH. There is an insidious prodromal period of 8 to 12 hours before weakness, hyperpyrexia, and vascular insufficiency, with shock and loss of consciousness, develop. Pigmentation, which may have been unrecognized previously, may now become obvious, being accentuated by the inadequate circulation. However, it may not appear at all in acute adrenal crises, since the preceding cortical insufficiency may have been minimal or of too short a duration.

The diagnosis of acute adrenal cortical insufficiency must be made quickly, and, for this, a direct eosinophil count could well be helpful. In shock due to causes other than adrenal insufficiency, the count will be lower than 50 cu mm. In adrenal insufficiency, however, it is usually well above this level. Since one usually cannot wait for determination of plasma hydroxycorticoid levels or an analysis of serum electrolytes, it is well to start treatment empirically and prophylactically when in doubt.

In the WATERHOUSE-FRIDERICHSEN SYNDROME there is *hemorrhagic destruction* in both *adrenals,* together with a fulminating meningococcal septicemia, leading, at times, to acute adrenal insufficiency. This illness is found mostly in childhood, particularly under the age of 2 years, but it occurs well into early adulthood also. It is particularly prevalent in camps and wherever young people congregate. It is most common during months when there is a high incidence of meningococcal meningitis. The syndrome occurs in only approximately 3 per cent of patients with meningococcal infection, but, of those who die from the latter cause, close to 50 per cent have marked adrenal involvement.

The clinical picture is that of *extensive purpura, shock, prostration, cyanosis,* and *circulatory collapse,* with *marked hypotension.* In the presence of meningococcemia, there is a *characteristic biphasic fever chart,* which should arouse suspicion. The syndrome has been described, on occasion, with β-hemolytic streptococci and pneumococci, as well as other rare bacteria. Meningitis is frequently associated with the picture, and neutro-

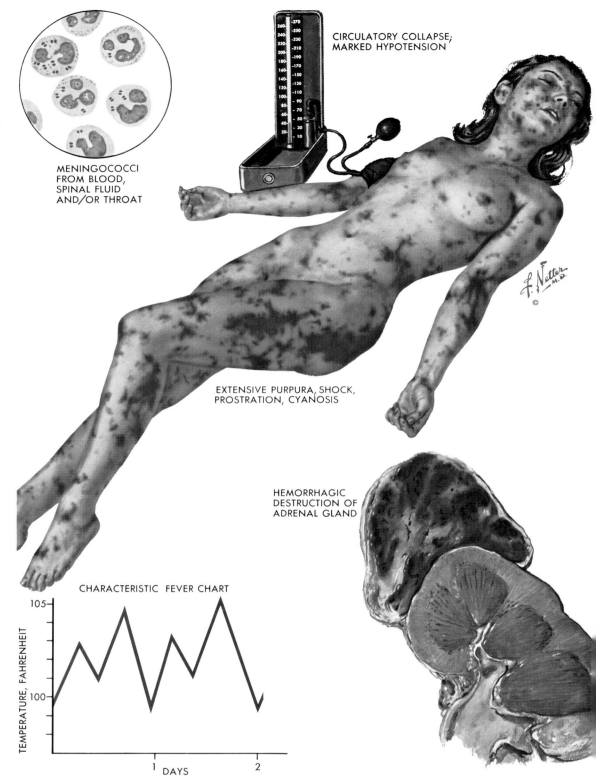

MENINGOCOCCI FROM BLOOD, SPINAL FLUID AND/OR THROAT

CIRCULATORY COLLAPSE; MARKED HYPOTENSION

EXTENSIVE PURPURA, SHOCK, PROSTRATION, CYANOSIS

HEMORRHAGIC DESTRUCTION OF ADRENAL GLAND

CHARACTERISTIC FEVER CHART

phils from both the *blood* and the *spinal fluid* characteristically show *meningococci* within the cytoplasm. The skin lesions are due to widespread destruction of the capillaries and arterioles, either because of bacterial embolization or as part of endothelial destruction through the Shwartzman phenomenon. This can be produced experimentally in rabbits by the intravenous injection of bacterial toxin. The first injection prepares and sensitizes the vascular bed. The second injection, given thereafter during a critical 6- to 32-hour interval, produces an accumulation of fibrinoid masses underneath the vascular endothelium, with hemorrhagic infarction in organs such as the adrenals. Exudation of blood through damaged vessels accounts for the purpura. The more extensive the purpura, the more likely will be involvement of the adrenals clinically. Direct invasion of the adrenals by meningococci is common. Apart from extensive bilat-

eral hemorrhage, a change also found in many stressful conditions is that of "tubular degeneration", whereby solid cores of cells of the zona fasciculata and, to a lesser extent, of the zona glomerulosa are transformed into hollow tubular structures. This change is due to depletion, in the involved cells, of adrenal cortical steroids and cholesterol and/or to the destruction of the vascular supply to the cells, leading to atrophy of whole columns of cells.

Treatment consists of the administration of sulfadiazine and soluble cortisol or other anti-inflammatory glucocorticoid preparations in very large doses, as well as pressor agents, notably angiotensin amide. Although survivals with Waterhouse-Friderichsen syndrome are now more common than 20 years ago, a minority of investigators presently feel that corticoids not only fail to contribute to therapy but actually lead to a more widespread septicemia.

CHRONIC PRIMARY ADRENAL CORTICAL INSUFFICIENCY (ADDISON'S DISEASE)

The normal adrenal cortex has an enormous functional reserve. Indeed, adrenal cortical deficiency does not become clinically manifest until nine tenths of the cortical tissue have been rendered unresponsive.

Obviously, therefore, with a secretory insufficiency often slowly progressive, the patient may live through a prolonged period of less apparent hormonal deficiency — a period during which secretion is adequate for everyday requirements, inadequate only when special stresses, such as operation, trauma, or infection, lead to crisis.

The most frequent cause of Addison's disease is *destructive atrophy,* which probably accounts for about 55 per cent of the cases in the United States. The exact reason for the atrophy is unknown, but toxic factors and, more recently, an auto-immune destructive process with demonstrable anti-adrenal antibodies have been considered responsible.

Today, in the United States, probably only about 40 per cent of the cases are due to *tuberculosis.* Whether of the bovine or the human strain, tubercular infection is almost always secondary to a focus elsewhere, usually in the lungs or genito-urinary tract.

The remaining 5 per cent of cases are accounted for by miscellaneous conditions such as hemorrhage due to *trauma, metastatic carcinoma, histoplasmosis,* amyloidosis, venous thrombosis, hemochromatosis, luetic gumma, etc.

Addison's disease is relatively rare in the United States, officially accounting for only 4 deaths per 1000. However, the actual number is undoubtedly far higher. Men and women are involved equally. Usually first noticed is *muscular weakness* and easy fatigability. The patient looks tired and acts weary; even speaking may be an effort. Mental weakness, along with physical weakness, increases as the day progresses, being least noticeable after a night's rest. The degree of muscle weakness depends not alone on the severity of the deficiency but also on the patient's muscular development prior to onset.

Acute prostration caused by a relatively minor infection, or an unexplained long convalescence, may be the first abnormality, suggesting that attention be given to the adrenal status. Since increased nervousness and irritability, with emotional instability and periods of depression often occur, one may be tempted to brand the patient a neurasthenic or psychoneurotic unless functional tests are carried out.

Pigmentation due to melanin is nearly always present in primary adrenal insufficiency. This pigmentation may serve to differentiate primary from secondary adrenal cortical deficiency due to pituitary corticotropin deficiency, since it is nearly always absent in the latter condi-

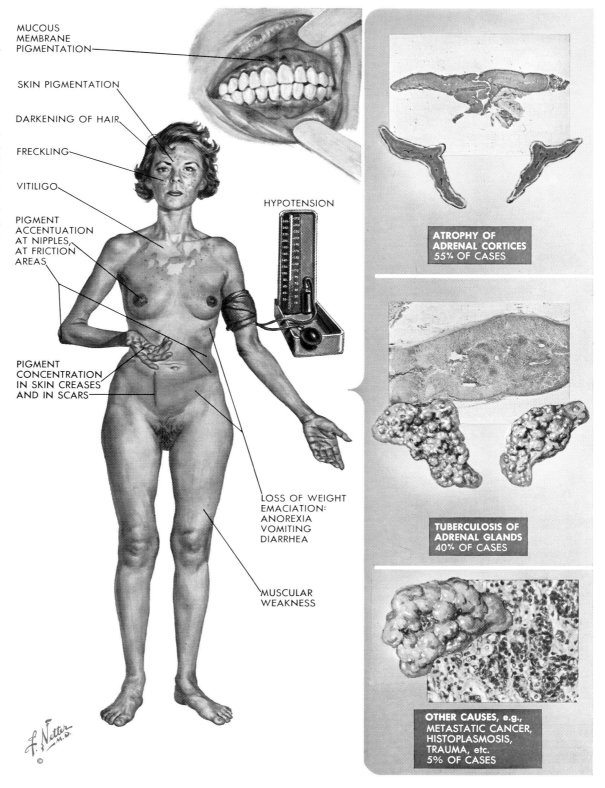

MUCOUS MEMBRANE PIGMENTATION

SKIN PIGMENTATION

DARKENING OF HAIR

FRECKLING

VITILIGO

PIGMENT ACCENTUATION AT NIPPLES, AT FRICTION AREAS

PIGMENT CONCENTRATION IN SKIN CREASES AND IN SCARS

HYPOTENSION

LOSS OF WEIGHT EMACIATION: ANOREXIA VOMITING DIARRHEA

MUSCULAR WEAKNESS

ATROPHY OF ADRENAL CORTICES 55% OF CASES

TUBERCULOSIS OF ADRENAL GLANDS 40% OF CASES

OTHER CAUSES, e.g., METASTATIC CANCER, HISTOPLASMOSIS, TRAUMA, etc. 5% OF CASES

tion. Assessment of pigmentation requires careful questioning as to the time of its development, previous exposure to sunlight, and racial characteristics of forebears as far back as three generations. *Skin pigmentation* may be generalized and is accentuated at the *nipples,* peri-anal and perigonadal areas, and wherever there are *areas of friction,* such as at the beltline and over the elbows and buttocks. The pigment shows concentration in the *palmar creases* and in *scars* contracted during the active phase of the disease. *Vitiligo* occurs in 15 per cent of the patients. *Mucous membrane pigmentation* is found quite rarely and is more common in patients of Indian, Negroid, or Mediterranean origin. *Darkening of the hair* occurs early. *Freckles* are common.

Loss of weight and dehydration are present. Not all patients are emaciated, but ALL will have suffered loss of weight in the recent past.

Hypotension and small heart size are found in all patients. However, those with previous hypertension may have blood pressure within the normal range, despite other signs of advanced adrenal disease.

Dizziness and syncopal attacks are caused by postural hypotension secondary to the dehydration, decreased plasma volume, hypotension, and muscle weakness. Hypoglycemic manifestations are found in less than half the patients; they may have suggestive symptoms, with relatively small reductions in blood sugar.

Growth of body hair is decreased in both sexes, but more strikingly in females, who may show complete absence of axillary hair. Otherwise, the secondary sex characteristics that are maintained by ovarian or testicular secretions are little affected, unless the patient is very emaciated, when amenorrhea and loss of potency are the rule.

LABORATORY FINDINGS IN PRIMARY ADRENAL CORTICAL INSUFFICIENCY (ADDISON'S DISEASE)

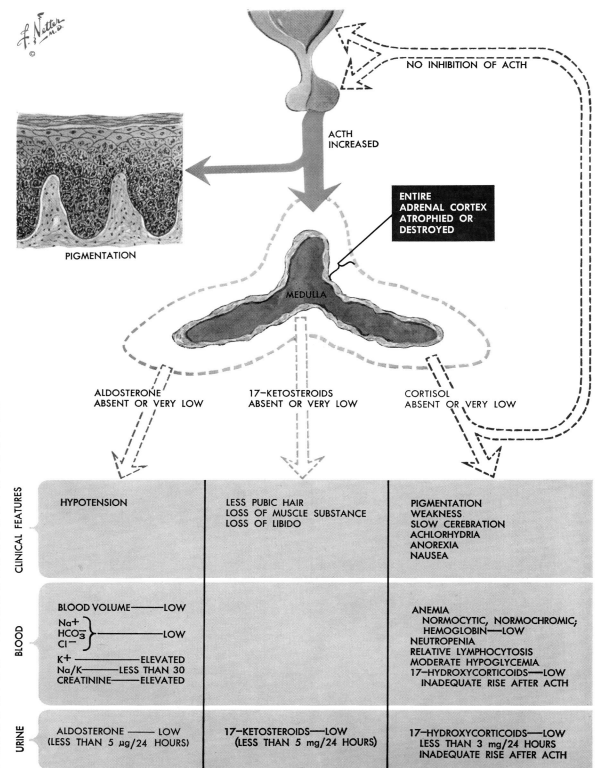

Primary adrenal cortical insufficiency may involve destruction of the adrenal cortices by granuloma, neoplasia, trauma, or atrophy, often on an auto-immune basis. The various signs and symptoms demonstrated by the patient with Addison's disease are related to deficiencies among the main adrenal cortical hormone groups and the increased secretion of pituitary ACTH and MSH. In the presence of *low levels of cortisol, the usual inhibition of ACTH production is absent,* so that *it rises above normal.* This and the concomitant rise in MSH will enhance melanin *pigmentation* of the skin and cutaneous appendages such as hair. The *adrenal cortices are atrophied* or *destroyed* to a varying extent, and there will be a variable deficiency of adrenal cortical secretions.

Aldosterone secretion may be absent or very low and is very low in the *urine* (less than 5 μg per 24 hours). *Hypotension* is the consequence. The *blood volume* is *reduced,* as is *serum Na* because of the increased loss of sodium in the urine, the intestinal glands, and the sweat glands. Corresponding anions, i.e., HCO_3^- and Cl^-, will also be *lowered.* In the absence of acidosis, one may calculate serum sodium quite adequately by adding these two in milliequivalents plus 10. Since the sodium exchanges, at the renal tubular level, for potassium and hydrogen, there will be marked *potassium retention* and a moderate acidosis. The *serum sodium/potassium ratio* will be *below 30,* and, because of some prerenal azotemia, serum *creatinine* and *BUN* will be elevated.

Secretion of 17-ketosteroids will be *reduced.* This results in *less pubic hair, loss of muscle mass,* weakness, and *loss of libido* in the female and, to a lesser extent, in the male. Urinary *17-ketosteroids* may be *extremely low* — less than 5 mg per 24 hours, as a rule.

Cortisol secretion will be reduced, and this will allow an increase in ACTH and

MSH secretion, which are responsible for *pigmentation.* The lack of cortisol will lead to *weakness* and *anorexia;* poor cerebration, with a slow rate of brain waves; a low voltage in the electrocardiogram; and *achlorhydria,* inducing alternating diarrhea and constipation, *nausea,* and vomiting. The blood picture will reveal a *normocytic, normochromic anemia* and *low hemoglobin.* There will be *neutropenia* with *relative lymphocytosis,* and tendency to eosinophilia.

Moderate hypoglycemia, especially reactive in type, is found in less than half the cases. Inadequate water diuresis is characteristic of adrenal cortical insufficiency, and it can be restored to normal only by the administration of cortisol or cortisone. *Plasma 17-hydroxycorticoids* tend to be lower than the usual mean of 9 μg per 100 ml, and, more importantly, they exhibit an *inadequate rise after ACTH* administration. *Urinary 17-hydroxycorticoids* are low — usually

less than 3 mg per 24 hours. Rarely, they may be normal but *will not reveal an adequate rise after ACTH* administration. There is, thus, a reduction in the adrenal cortical reserve of cortisol.

It is now possible to predict whether one is dealing with atrophy of the adrenal cortex or destruction by tuberculosis or similar diseases. In the former, the medulla is intact; in the latter, it is usually destroyed. The intravenous administration of 2-deoxyglucose (50 mg per kilogram of body weight for 30 minutes) will raise urinary epinephrine some five- to tenfold in a normal subject and in the patient with adrenal cortical atrophy; in the absence of the medulla, however, as in tuberculous destruction of the adrenal cortex, there will be no such rise in urinary epinephrine. In general, destruction of the zona glomerulosa reduces aldosterone secretion primarily; that of the zona fasciculata reduces mostly cortisol secretion.

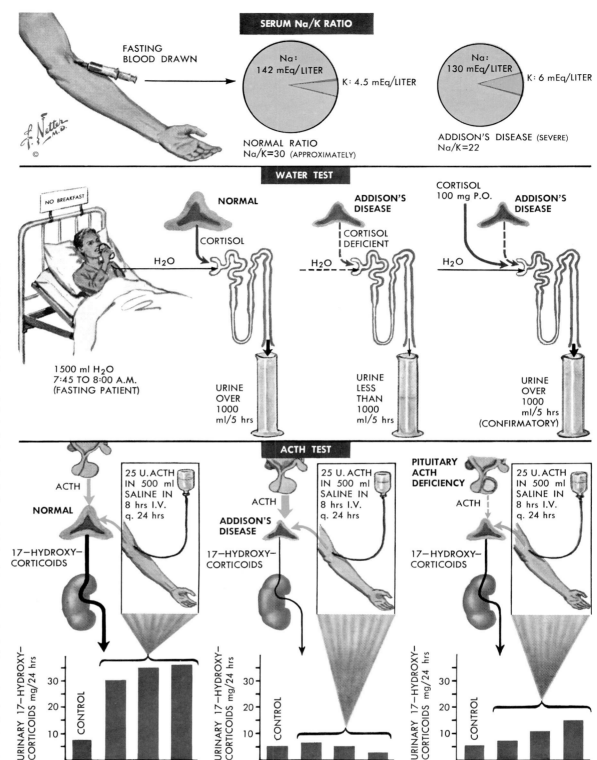

TESTS FOR PRIMARY ADRENAL CORTICAL INSUFFICIENCY (ADDISON'S DISEASE)

Because of the rather nonspecific symptoms, it is most important to establish the diagnosis of Addison's disease, beyond reasonable doubt, by specific laboratory measures. Moreover, the diagnosis should be established before treatment is commenced. Otherwise, it may be impossible, for many months, to rule out the possibility of a secondary deficiency caused by a lack of pituitary corticotropin.

Serum Na/K Ratio. In Addison's disease, deficiency of aldosterone causes a decrease in serum sodium with an increase in potassium. A determination of sodium alone might be misleading because of the concomitant dehydration. However, a calculation of the ratio between the two ions will, in effect, cancel out the hemoconcentration factor and is, thus, far more reliable. *Normally, the ratio is 30 to 1.* Anything significantly below this strongly suggests *Addison's disease,* such as 22 *in severe disease.* In practice, this is really all that is necessary for determining a deficiency in salt regulation and, by inference, aldosterone.

Effect of ACTH on Direct Eosinophil Count. This relatively simple office procedure, which is only an all-or-none test for adrenal cortical reserve, will exclude significant adrenal cortical insufficiency but will not prove the diagnosis. PROCEDURE: After a direct eosinophil count has been obtained from the patient, 25 units of lyophilized ACTH are injected intramuscularly, and, after 4 hours, blood is obtained for a second direct eosinophil count.

A fall of 50 per cent or more definitely excludes adrenal cortical insufficiency. Absence of such a fall is found in Addison's disease. However, it may be caused by an allergic eosinophilia or by inactivation of the ACTH in sensitized individuals.

Water Test. This test, which is based on the stimulating effect of cortisol on glomerular filtration, is probably the simplest and most widely used screening test for adrenal cortical insufficiency. PROCEDURE: The *fasting patient,* after urinating, drinks 1500 *ml of water* between 7:45 and 8 a.m. He remains *in bed* for 5 hours, collecting all urine passed. If the 5-hour specimen is *over 1000 ml* in volume, Addison's disease may be excluded; if much below, however, the diagnosis is likely. The procedure can then be repeated on the following day, 2 hours after a dose of 100 *mg of cortisol by*

mouth. If, this time, the 5-hour urine output is over *1000 ml,* the diagnosis is definite, and such conditions as heart failure and renal disease have been excluded.

ACTH Test. This is the most sensitive and specific test of all. It estimates, quantitatively, the actual functional cortisol reserve and, when repeated on successive days, measures the potential functional reserve as well. Thus, it may reveal potential Addison's disease in patients whose basal output is still normal. PROCEDURE: A total of 25 or 40 *units of ACTH in 500 ml saline is given intravenously* in *exactly 8 hours.* A 24-hour urine specimen is taken on the day before the test and, on each day, the test is repeated for *urinary 17-hydroxycorticoids. Normally,* there is a *three- to fivefold increase* in urinary 17-hydroxycorticoids on the first day of the test, with further small increases on successive days. In contrast, patients with *Addison's disease* show *no increase,* or even a slight fall, in

urinary 17-hydroxycorticoids. This test also serves to differentiate patients with Addison's disease from those having *pituitary ACTH deficiency.* Patients whose corticoid deficiency is secondary to a lack of corticotropin show a *gradual,* slight, but *sustained, increase* on successive days. As a rule, a definite diagnosis is possible after 2 days on ACTH.

Patients undergoing this test should be closely observed because, on occasion, an anaphylactic shock may occur.

In order to prevent these frightening, though rare, reactions, administration of 1 mg of dexamethasone just before starting the test, and again after 4 hours, has been recommended. This will not materially affect the results. Fortunately, ACTH with an amino acid chain length of 24 has now been synthesized. It works well intravenously and appears free of the risk of reactions due to foreign proteins.

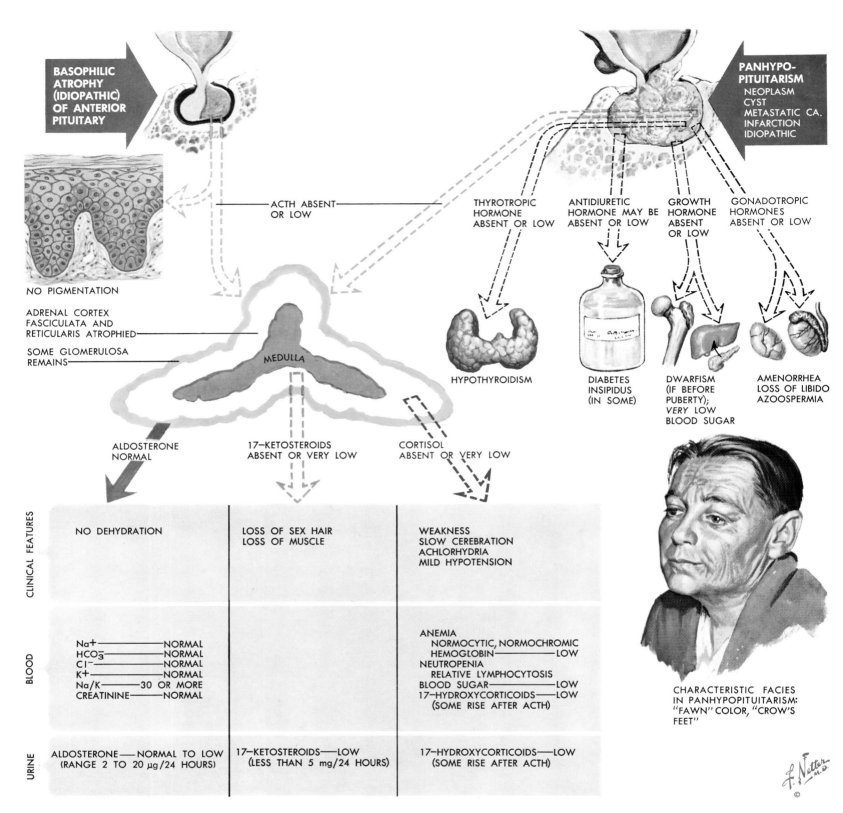

LABORATORY FINDINGS IN SECONDARY ADRENAL CORTICAL INSUFFICIENCY

This condition, often referred to as pituitary Addison's disease, differs from primary adrenal cortical insufficiency, or true Addison's disease. *ACTH* is either *absent* or very *low*. This may be due to *basophilic atrophy* of the *anterior pituitary* or to *panhypopituitarism* due to a *neoplasm*, a *cyst*, *metastatic carcinoma* (notably from the breast to the lung), septic *infarction* after delivery, and then pituitary insufficiency of an *idiopathic* nature, probably related to hypotha-lamic defects. In the isolated lack of ACTH, all the other target glands are intact. In panhypo-pituitarism there is *absence* or *lowering* of *thyrotropic hormone, growth hormone*, and *gon-adotropic hormones*. If much of the posterior pituitary is involved, *antidiuretic hormone may be absent or low*. As a consequence of such changes, there may be *hypothyroidism, dwarfism* (if the condition appears before puberty), *low blood sugar*, and insulin sensitivity, *amenorrhea, loss of libido, azoospermia*, and *diabetes insipidus* (in some). Diabetes insipidus may be of a very mild degree, since the loss of the anterior pituitary function markedly ameliorates polyuria caused by lack of antidiuretic hormone. In the absence of ACTH and MSH, there is *no increased pigmen-tation*; this is different from primary Addison's disease. In the *adrenal cortex* there is *atrophy* of the zonae *fasciculata* and *reticularis*, but most of the zona *glomerulosa* remains intact, since, to a large extent, this is independent of the trophic effect of ACTH. Thus, *aldosterone* levels are *normal*, whereas *17-KS are absent* or very *low*, and *cortisol* is markedly depressed. In panhypo-pituitarism there are *characteristic facies*, with *fawn-colored skin*, and *wrinkles* known as *crow's feet*. The *thinning of the lateral third of the eye-brows* is due to a lack of androgens and thyroid.

Because of the normal aldosterone levels, there is *no dehydration*. The *17-ketosteroids are low at less than 5 mg per 24 hours*. Unlike the response in primary adrenal cortical insufficiency, there will be some *rise of plasma 17-hydroxycorticoids after ACTH*. Urinary *17-hydroxycorticoids* also show some stepwise *rise after ACTH* has been given for 3 consecutive days (see page 102).

ADRENAL MEDULLARY HORMONES

The cells of the adrenal medulla are exodermal in origin, being derived from the neural crest. The adrenal medulla is essentially a sympathetic ganglion in which the postganglionic cells have lost their axons and have become specialized for secretion of their products directly into the blood stream. Incoming sensory stimuli descending through the *brain stem* or messages ascending through the *spinal cord* converge on the *hypothalamus,* whence they are relayed down the spinal cord. The *sympathetic outflow* from $T10$ *to* $L1$ forms the *splanchnic nerves* which, as preganglionic fibers, synapse in the *pre-aortic ganglia* and continue into the *adrenal medulla.* There, the polyhedral chromaffin cells are stimulated, by acetylcholine released at the nerve endings, to secrete *epinephrine* and *norepinephrine.* It appears that cells containing acid phosphatase secrete mostly epinephrine, whereas those showing fluorescence secrete norepinephrine. The fetal adrenal contains only norepinephrine, epinephrine appearing some time after birth. Chromaffin cells of the medulla respond to splanchnic nerve stimulation during emergency situations. Insulin hypoglycemia will deplete the epinephrine-secreting cells specifically, while reserpine, in low doses, causes the loss of norepinephrine exclusively.

Biosynthesis of catecholamines is accomplished by hydroxylation of phenylalanine to form *tyrosine.* This is turned into dihydroxyphenylalanine (DOPA) by the enzyme tyrosinase and is transformed into *dopamine* (hydroxytyramine) by decarboxylation which is then converted, by an α-hydroxylase, to norepinephrine and then, by N-methylation, to epinephrine. The methylating enzyme responsible for conversion of norepinephrine to epinephrine is found in high concentration only in the adrenal medulla. The average combined norepinephrine-epinephrine content of the normal human adrenal medulla ranges from 2 to 4 mg per gram of tissue in the adult. Of this, only up to 30 per cent is norepinephrine, whereas in all extramedullary catecholamine-secreting tissues most of the catecholamine is norepinephrine.

Both epinephrine and norepinephrine differ considerably in their *pharmacophysiology.* At one end of the scale, norepinephrine has far greater effect on *blood pressure* than does epinephrine. Norepinephrine acts by constricting most of the arteriolar supply in the body; epinephrine, while constricting the arterioles to the skin (which leads to blanching), causes dilatation of the blood vessels in liver and muscle.

Norepinephrine, while raising blood pressure through vasoconstriction, tends to decrease *cardiac output;* in contrast, epinephrine increases it. Epinephrine

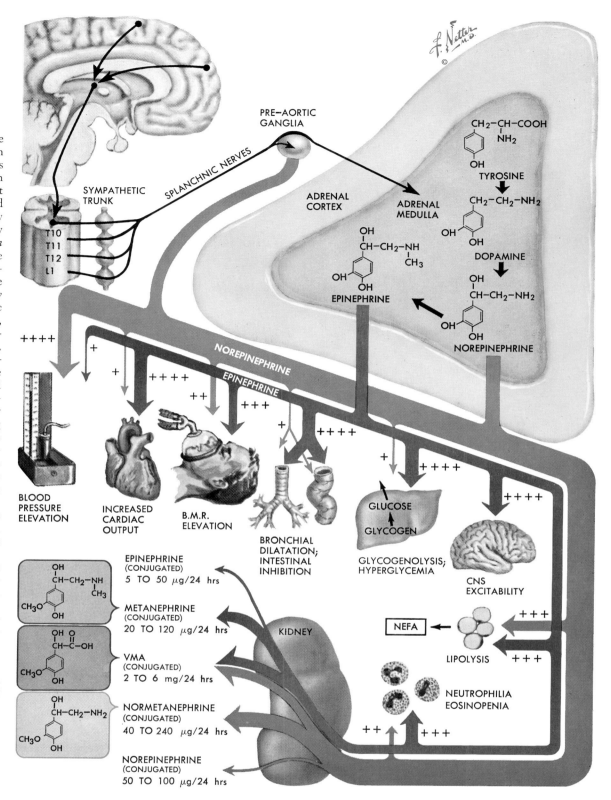

will also raise the *B.M.R.,* whereas norepinephrine hardly does so. Epinephrine will lead to marked *bronchial dilatation* and *inhibition of intestinal motility,* which are hardly shown at all by norepinephrine. Epinephrine, by activating the *glycogenolytic enzymes* and inhibiting insulin secretion, leads to marked *hyperglycemia,* not shared equally by norepinephrine, and increases *irritability* of the *central nervous system,* with a feeling of impending doom and anxiety, and marked dilatation of the pupils. The lipase of adipose tissue is activated by both catecholamines, leading to *lipolysis,* and an increased discharge of *NEFA* into the blood stream, with rises above the normal NEFA of 0.4 ± 0.2 mEq/l. It is of interest that patients with excess catecholamine-producing tumors are nearly never fat. Epinephrine, much more than norepinephrine, produces *neutrophilia* with *eosinopenia.* All these activities would favor the immediate survival of

an animal engaged in a fight, during flight, or while possessed by fright. This was first pointed out by Cannon in his theory of the "alarm reaction" and, subsequently, expanded to the "general adaptation syndrome" by Selye, including secondarily increased adrenal cortical activity.

The metabolism of catecholamines, mostly in the liver, consists of orthomethylation (80 per cent) and oxidative deamination (20 per cent) by specific catechol-O-methyl transferase (COMT) and a mono-amine oxidase (MAO). Less than 4 per cent of intravenously administered *epinephrine* or *norepinephrine* is found in the *urine,* whereas considerable quantities of *metanephrine, normetanephrine,* and the most extensively transformed vanyl mandelic acid (*VMA*) (3-methoxy-4-hydroxymandelic acid) are found normally and may all serve for quantitative estimation of adrenal medullary activity.

PHEOCHROMOCYTOMA

Pheochromocytomas are chromaffin tissue tumors, *90 per cent* of which occur in the *adrenal gland* itself. They are *flesh-colored* and often reveal a *hemorrhagic breakdown* in the substance of the tumor. Chromaffin tissue tumors may be found all along the course of the *aorta* along the sympathetic chain, in the *spleen*, in the *ovaries*, and, on occasion, in the *testes*. The *organ of Zuckerkandl*, at the *bifurcation of the aorta*, is a special site for tumor formation. Only the adrenal medullary tissue produces both *epinephrine* and *norepinephrine*. Rarely, ectopic tissue in the *bladder wall* may produce epinephrine, but, otherwise, extramedullary tumors secrete almost exclusively norepinephrine. Thus, removal of both adrenals will lead to a practical disappearance of epinephrine, but little change in norepinephrine, which is secreted mostly by the sympathetic nerve endings.

Adrenal pheochromocytomas are *bilateral in 10 per cent* of the cases (*more so in children*) and *multiple in 2 per cent*. They are, rarely, malignant, leading to functional liver metastases. The incidence is low, ranging from 1 in 1000 to 1 in 5000 at autopsy, but, as a rare cause of curable hypertension, they must be sought strenuously. Two major syndromes exist—that of *intermittent*, or paroxysmal, *hypertension* and that of *sustained*, or chronic, hypertension. The paroxysmal type is shown in less than 50 per cent of adults and in less than 10 per cent of children. Attacks of paroxysmal hypertension arise suddenly, lasting for minutes or hours. They are usually brought on by some emotional stress or other trigger mechanism, such as a sudden change in posture or, on occasion, by urination. In adults there is extreme *nervousness*, with anxiety, *sweating*, and *headache*. In older patients the increased heart rate may lead to angina. The attack usually ends with sweating, fatigue, and frustration. During menopause, generalized autonomic discharges, occasioned by some hypothalamic disturbance, may resemble such attacks. In children the visual complaints and sweating are more common. Constipation is frequently present, as is *abdominal pain*, and 10 per cent have puffy, red, cyanotic hands.

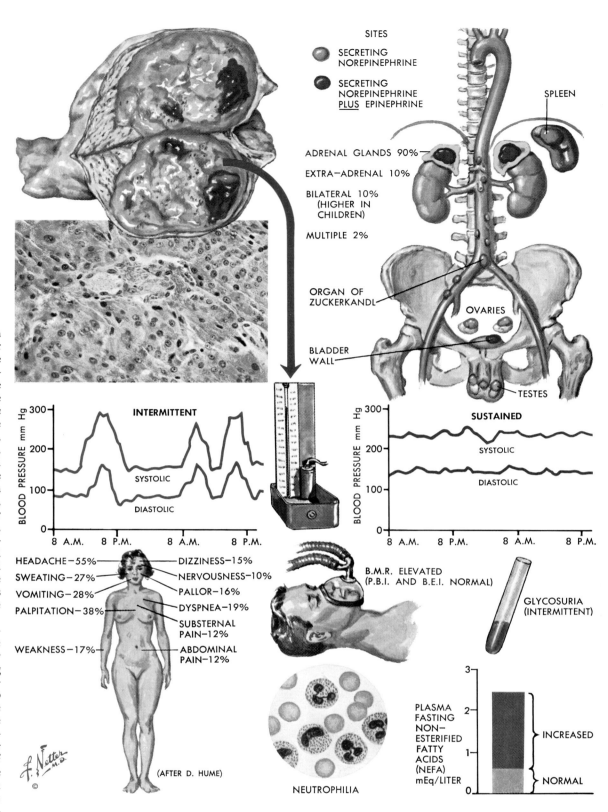

These symptoms are usually found infrequently in the adult. In children, hypertension and the demonstration of elevated catecholamines may, rarely, be related to the presence of a large spindle cell tumor in the retroperitoneal space, broadly classified as a neuroblastoma. An occasional one will be secretory, unlike the very rare ganglioneuroma found exclusively in adults, which is never secretory.

A pheochromocytoma should be suspected in patients with atypical paroxysmal attacks of hypertension or unexplained hypertensive reactions during induction of anesthesia, or shock during surgery under anesthesia, in the absence of hemorrhage. The sustained type of hypertension is nearly indistinguishable from essential or malignant hypertension, but it may, rarely, reveal its true nature by prodromal anxiety, with difficulty in focusing the eyes and with marked dilatation of the pupils. Suspicion should be raised in

continuous hypertension with signs of hyperthyroidism yet normal cholesterol levels and *normal protein-bound iodine values*, or with *intermittent glycosuria* and, occasionally, frank diabetes. Typically, there is marked *neutrophilia*, with a shift to the left, and *plasma fasting nonesterified fatty acids* are often well above the upper limit of 0.6 mEq/l. Characteristically, no patient with a pheochromocytoma is obese, and the vast majority have a history of a marked weight loss. Blood volume is usually below normal, in marked contradistinction to primary hyperaldosteronism, where it is elevated.

Any suspicion of the presence of a pheochromocytoma calls for the application of modern test procedures to eliminate this curable type of hypertension, and the question has been raised by some investigators whether screening tests should not be carried out on all hypertensives.

TESTS FOR PHEOCHROMOCYTOMA

Diagnostic work-ups for pheochromocytoma may be divided into bedside and laboratory tests.

The *phentolamine (Regitine®) test* is of value only during a hypertensive phase of the disease and is carried out as follows: After the patient has rested in bed for at least 10 minutes, an intravenous infusion of *5 per cent dextrose in water* is started. When the patient has reached the basal state, blood pressure readings are taken every minute and recorded for five consecutive readings. Then, so as not to disturb the patient, *5 mg of Regitine are given intravenously, through the tubing,* during a 1-minute period. Blood pressures are then taken every 30 seconds at first, then at 1-minute intervals. Blood pressure falls of 35 mm Hg *systolic* or 25 mm Hg *diastolic,* for 3 to 5 minutes, strongly suggest the presence of a catecholamine-secreting tumor. In normal subjects, hypotensive effects may be found, but, in the majority, there will be a slight rise of the blood pressure. To assure validity, patients should not receive any sedative, hypotensive, or narcotic agents for 3 days prior to the Regitine test. Reserpine should be discontinued for several weeks before the test is carried out. Any such medications may produce false positive reactions, generally found in uremic patients. However, if the patient is in so much need of hypotensive therapy that he cannot be taken off it, the test may still be performed, for, if there is no significant hypotensive response, pheochromocytoma is clearly ruled out. False negative tests may be found in hypertension whenever the pheochromocytoma has led to fixation of the hypertension as a result of secondary vascular changes.

The *provocative histamine test* is useful only during a lull in paroxysmal hypertension. It should be employed with the greatest of care, with 5 mg of Regitine being immediately available to cope with any excessive rise in blood pressure, usually observed within 1 or 2 minutes after giving the histamine. Histamine base is given intravenously during a 1- to 2-minute period (0.05 mg or less in 10 ml of saline). A significant rise in blood pressure (appearing within 2 minutes after the injection) of the order of 50 *mm Hg or more systolic* and *30 mm Hg or more diastolic,* after an *initial fall,* is suggestive of a catecholamine-producing tumor. Occasional false positive results occur. The marked flushing and histamine-type headaches are disadvantages.

Testing for a pressor response to tyramine has none of these side effects. It relies on the fact that tyramine releases an excess of catecholamines stored at

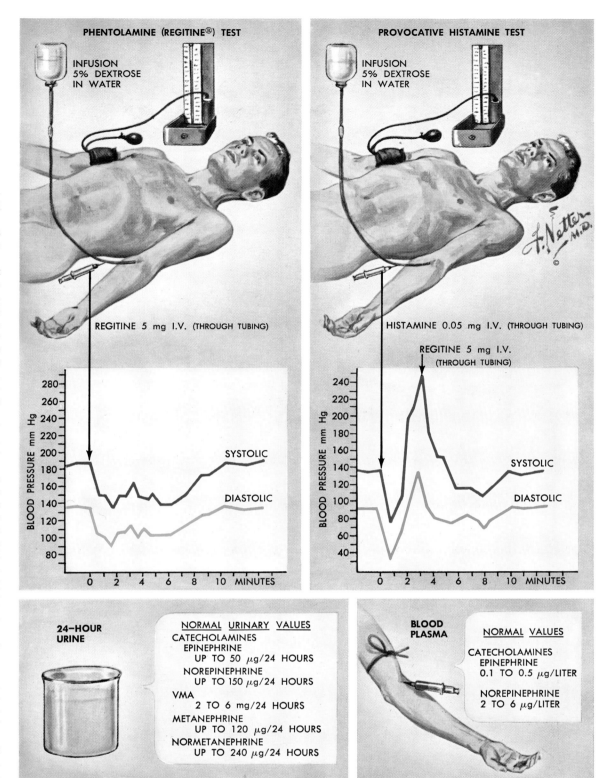

sympathetic nerve endings. Tyramine base is administered intravenously, during a 1-minute period, in doses from 250 to 1000 µg. If it provokes a pressor response greater than 30 mm Hg systolic, the test is positive. Antihypertensive medication, especially mono-amine oxidase, is an absolute contraindication, since it sensitizes the response more than tenfold.

Laboratory tests consist of the estimation of total *urinary catecholamines* and, usually, include techniques to separate epinephrine and norepinephrine. Values above *50 µg per 24 hours* of *epinephrine* and above *150 µg per 24 hours* of *norepinephrine* indicate the presence of a pheochromocytoma. Using *metanephrine* and *normetanephrine* is advantageous, because these stable metabolites occur in far greater quantity than the delicate catecholamines themselves. Vanyl mandelic acid (*VMA*) is the most stable and is present in milligram quantities. Values above 6 *mg*

per day are strongly suggestive of a pheochromocytoma. The patient should not use vanilla ice cream for 2 days prior to the test. The most sensitive procedure is to estimate *plasma epinephrine* and *norepinephrine,* and this may sometimes be combined with a provocative histamine test.

A pheochromocytoma may be localized by tomograms or retroperitoneal pneumography, since the majority are sufficiently large to be revealed by those means. If the blood pressure rises during induction of anesthesia, it may be controlled by administration of Regitine. Fatal postsurgical falls in blood pressure may be prevented by normalizing the typically low blood volume by means of presurgical transfusions and by administration of norepinephrine or angiotensin. An anterior abdominal approach, with thorough exploration of the entire length of the aorta, should be undertaken in all patients.

GENERAL THERAPEUTIC USES OF GLUCOCORTICOIDS

Potentiation of Vasopressors. On occasion, a *hypotensive state* unresponsive to pressor agents, such as norepinephrine, will yield promptly to a large dose (200 mg or more) of cortisol or an equivalent synthetic corticoid given intramuscularly. An immediate rise in blood pressure follows, in spite of a preceding normal level of 17-KS. Apparently, a sensitization of the vessel wall to the catecholamine is responsible.

Anti-inflammatory and Anti-allergic Action. These actions of the glucocorticoids form the basis of their widespread clinical use. *Inflammatory* or *allergic responses* are decreased, fibrosis is prevented, and subsequent degeneration is minimized, depending on how early in the particular disease their administration is begun. Thus, these hormones tend to abolish the manifestations of the disease without directly antagonizing the causative agent, yet, when given early, they help to prevent death during the acute phases of inflammatory or allergic disease. The best therapeutic use lies in the early, preventive administration of high doses or the late establishment of a maintenance regimen with a moderate, near physiologic dosage, allowing the disease to smolder.

Specific recommendations for therapy are beyond our present scope; however, a few words of a general nature may be desirable.

Whereas ACTH, or *adrenocorticotropic hormone*, will produce a mixture of the known adrenal cortical hormones, in which the 17-ketosteroids will counteract the catabolic activity of the glucocorticoids to some extent, *cortisol* and its derivatives will be relatively more catabolic. To date, none of the synthetic cortisol derivatives has revealed a dissociation of the anti-inflammatory and catabolic activities, which appear to be closely linked. Therein lies the ultimate limitation of corticoid therapy in allergic and inflammatory diseases. After reaching twice the normal adrenal cortical output of cortisol, *viz.*, 40 mg of cortisol per day, catabolic and other side effects mount rapidly, while the anti-inflammatory activity begins to lag behind. In attempts to eliminate or reduce the catabolic effect as well as the sodium-retaining activity of cortisol, numerous derivatives have been synthesized, some of which are shown below.

Compound	Relative Anti-inflammatory Potency Compared to Cortisol	Relative Sodium-Retaining Activity
Cortisol	1	+ +
Cortisone acetate	0.8	+ +
Prednisolone	4	+
Prednisone	3.5	+
Triamcinolone	5	o
6-Methylprednisolone	5	o
Haldranolone	10	o
Betamethasone	25	o
Dexamethasone	30	o
9-α-Fluorohydrocortisone	15	+ + + +

ACTH is used mostly in the form of long-acting repository preparations, such as gels. It has the disadvantage of being somewhat pigment-producing because of similarity to the MSH of part of the molecule. Many of the preparations show water retention because of contamination with posterior pituitary antidiuretic hormone.

The latter is not a factor in the synthetic 24-amino acid ACTH preparation now available for clinical use. The need for parenteral administration has led to a far more limited use than in the case of the corticoids.

In the THERAPEUTIC USE OF CORTICOIDS AND CORTICOTROPIN, clinical response is the ONLY CRITERION on which to base dosage, constantly weighing the improvement that may be produced against the side effects (discussed hereinafter).

HIGH DOSAGES of 60 to 1000 mg of cortisol or 2 to 30 mg of dexamethasone equivalent are required where MESENCHYMAL SUPPRESSION is desired. Doses of this magnitude may be administered, with benefit, for less than 1 week in the following conditions:
Aspiration pneumonitis
Lye and other burns of the esophagus
Acute serum disease, *e.g.*, penicillin reaction, beesting
Acute secondary glaucoma
Acute vascular collapse unresponsive to pressor agents

Dosages of the order mentioned above may be required for prolonged periods, in the following conditions, as lifesaving measures:
Pemphigus
Lupus erythematosus crises
Nephrosis unresponsive to intermittent therapy
Chronic pulmonary fibrosis no longer responding to moderate dosage
Acute phase of rheumatic fever, early in the course
Overwhelming polyarteritis, including trichinosis
Waterhouse-Friderichsen syndrome
Subacute lymphatic leukemia
Thrombotic thrombocytopenic purpura
Gram-negative bacterial shock

MODERATE DOSAGE, in the range of 30 to 60 mg of cortisol or 1 to 2 mg of dexamethasone equivalent, may be given for partial symptomatic control of the following diseases, while awaiting spontaneous remissions:
Allergic conditions: bronchial asthma, severe hay fever; allergic rhinitis; angioneurotic edema; atopic dermatitis; neurodermatitis
Blood dyscrasias: idiopathic thrombocytopenic purpura; allergic purpura; acquired hemolytic anemia
Eye diseases: acute uveitis; choroiditis; optic neuritis; sympathetic ophthalmia; macular degeneration
Collagen diseases: disseminated lupus erythematosus; dermatomyositis; only exceptionally, and in small dosage, in scleroderma and rheumatoid arthritis; erythema nodosum; nonsuppurative panniculitis
Gastro-intestinal diseases: ileitis; ulcerative colitis during the acute phase
Infectious diseases: in conjunction with specific antibiotics, but only for selected cases of pulmonary, urogenital, or bone tuberculosis, and in tuberculous meningitis
Miscellaneous conditions: Bell's palsy, at the very onset only, after which there are few successes; nasal polyps; sarcoidosis; nephrosis; pulmonary emphysema; acute gouty arthritis, only in patients sensitive to colchicine; adrenogenital syndrome; adrenal insufficiency; supportive therapy in terminal cases of leukemia, Hodgkin's disease, and carcinoma

One must constantly bear in mind that, when treating chronic disease, one should START WITH THE SMALLEST POSSIBLE DOSE, gradually increasing it, but never aspiring to more than 60 per cent clinical improvement. To expect more is to court the inevitable appearance of serious side effects. Of course, in life-threatening situations, one may be forced to start with a maximal dose, equivalent

to 200 mg of cortisol or 7 mg of dexamethasone. This should not be maintained for longer than 10 days and should then be reduced gradually. In general, the dose should be "from the bottom up" in long-range therapy and "from the top down" when handling acute, short-term, self-limited conditions.

Side Effects. 1. Weight gain (preceded by the characteristic distribution of fat) may be decreased by a high-protein, low-calorie diet. Retention of salt and water, leading to edema, is no longer important, because the newest synthetic corticoids are devoid of sodium-retaining effect.

2. Hypochloremic-hypokalemic alkalosis is rarely of disturbing magnitude. It may be prevented by giving supplemental potassium.

3. Negative nitrogen balance may be partly decreased by an anabolic agent such as methandrostenolone.

4. Thrombophlebitis and coronary occlusion tend to occur when the dose of corticosteroid is reduced or, especially, when treatment is stopped suddenly. These can be prevented by good hydration, exercise, and anticoagulation therapy, on the slightest suspicion.

5. Bleeding tendencies and ecchymoses, found increasingly with the use of more potent derivatives, are due to loss of vascular elastic tissue rather than blood dyscrasias, and, thus, superficial trauma should be avoided.

6. Gastric acidity and ulcer formation may be minimized by antacids and anticholinergics.

7. Glycosuria should be controlled by sulfonylureas or insulin when fasting blood sugar is above 130 mg per 100 ml, especially where there has been a family history of diabetes.

8. Sleeplessness can be minimized by giving the last dose of corticosteroid at 6 p.m. Sedatives or tranquilizers are helpful.

9. Psychosis, whose danger signals are inability to concentrate, weird dreams, and nightmares, is an indication that the dose should be decreased gradually. However, it must not be stopped suddenly, since this may be catastrophic in terms of the original disease.

10. Superinfection is a dreaded complication, to be minimized by extreme cleanliness, aseptic techniques, and appropriate — preferably bactericidal as opposed to bacteriostatic — agents.

11. With continuing ACTH or corticoid therapy, there is, unfortunately, early clouding of the lens and a tendency to posterior capsular cataract formation, which is often noticed by the patient as a blurring when looking into the light. This need have no connection with the accompanying disease and is a direct consequence of such therapy. There is no known way of prevention.

Termination of Therapy. After corticoids have been in use for more than 5 days, withdrawal should be slow in order to minimize the so-called corticoid withdrawal syndrome. In this, a cortisol type of adrenal insufficiency is associated, for a few days, with a flare-up of the initial disease. Since the suppressed pituitary ACTH returns before adrenal cortical responsiveness is back to normal, the adrenals may be sensitized by administering 80 units of ACTH gel every morning, for 1 week, at the end of corticoid therapy. Also, the corticoids should be withdrawn slowly, leaving a sentinel dose in the early morning for weeks, since this will not interfere with the nocturnal activation of the adrenals by pituitary ACTH. Finally, it is now apparent that intermittent administration of corticoids, such as every other day or once in the morning, will minimize side effects and withdrawal symptoms and is therapeutically nearly as effective as around-the-clock administration, except in the most severe forms of disease.

Section IV

SEX DIFFERENTIATION
THE GONADS

by

FRANK H. NETTER, M.D.

in collaboration with

PETER H. FORSHAM, M.D., M.A. (Cantab)
Plate 7

ARTHUR R. SOHVAL, M.D.
Plates 2 and 3, 24-27

SOMERS H. STURGIS, M.D.
Plates 20-23

JUDSON J. VAN WYK, M.D.
Plates 1, 4-6, 8-19

(The reader's attention is called to Volume 2, Reproductive System, THE NETTER COLLECTION OF MEDICAL ILLUSTRATIONS, in which many aspects of gonadal anatomy, physiology, and pathology are presented.)

Sex Chromatin and Chromosomal Sex

At the moment of fertilization, when the human zygote consists of a single undifferentiated cell, sufficient information is coded on the genes of the 23 chromosome pairs to direct the multiplication of cells into either a male or a female infant. In most individuals the differentiation of sex is an orderly process, and the child's sex will conform in every respect to the chromosomal sex determined at the moment of fertilization; however, when sexual development deviates from the expected normal pattern, we are led to probe into the multitude of intermediary stages to discover through what processes the genetic constitution directs the development of sexual characteristics.

Many of the spectacularly rapid advances in our knowledge of sex differentiation may be attributed to the recent acquisition of techniques which make it possible to visualize the chromosomal make-up of an individual. These skills, together with newly acquired information derived from steroid chemistry and experimental embryology, have made it possible to attribute many clinical abnormalities to some single specific error in sex differentiation.

Chromosomal Sex

Chromosomes which are actively engaged in directing cellular activities are not easily visualized by the light microscope. When cells are replicating, however, the genetic material condenses into discrete structures, which take stains specific for deoxyribonucleic acid (DNA). Chromosomes are most easily examined in metaphase. The study of large numbers of metaphase cells, usually from peripheral blood or bone marrow, has been made possible by tissue culture techniques. Cellular multiplication is arrested, in metaphase, by the introduction of colchicine or some other chemical agent, and a *"squash" preparation* is made of cells spread out under a cover slip. By applying such methods, Tjio and Levan demonstrated, in 1956, that the correct chromosomal number of man is 46, with 22 pairs of autosomes plus either an XX or an XY pair of sex chromosomes.

Mitotic chromosomes differ from one another primarily in size and in the position of the centromere (the point where the arms cross). In addition, certain autosomes have small satellites. An *arrangement of chromosomes from a single cell* is called an idiogram. The method of numbering follows the Denver system of nomenclature. The total number of chromosomes and the type of sex chromosomes present comprise the *karyotype*.

Precise identification of individual chromosomes is usually not possible. The X chromosomes resemble autosomes in

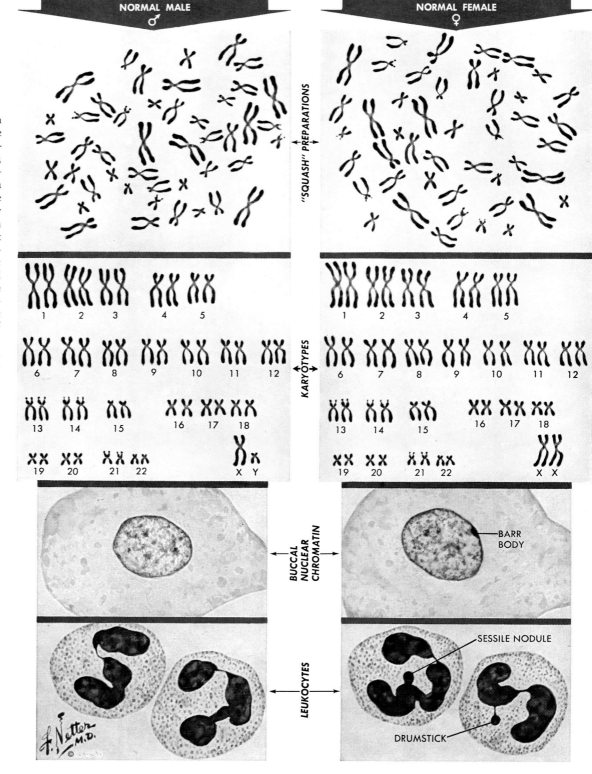

the group from 6 to 12 (particularly chromosome 6), and the Y chromosome is similar to 21 and 22.

Sex Chromatin and Nuclear Sex

It was Barr who first noted a spotlike condensation of *chromatin* in some somatic cells of females, but only infrequently in those of males. The chromosomal sex of an individual may be deduced from studies of *cells* scraped from the *buccal mucosa* (see page 111) or from white blood cells. After suitable stains have been applied to the former, a peripheral nuclear mass (*Barr body*) is readily discernible in over 40 per cent of cells from female subjects but in only a rare cell from males. The presence or absence of these chromatin masses in peripheral cells may thus be used to classify individuals as having either a positive or a negative nuclear sex or, more simply, as

being chromatin-positive or chromatin-negative. It is inaccurate to refer to this nuclear characteristic as the "chromosomal sex" or "genetic sex". The nuclei of *polymorphonuclear leukocytes* likewise exhibit sexual dimorphism, recognizable by *drumstick appendages* or *sessile nodules* in a small percentage of cells from female subjects.

The correlation between a positive nuclear sex and the presence of 2 X chromosomes, as determined by direct chromosomal counts, has, so far, been excellent. Cells from individuals with more than 2 X chromosomes usually contain more than 1 chromatin body. It is believed that the maximal number of chromatin bodies is always 1 less than the number of X chromosomes. Cogent evidence now supports Grumbach's hypothesis that the peripheral chromatin mass is derived from the heteropyknotic portion of a single X chromosome.

CORRELATION OF NUCLEAR CHROMATIN AND SEX CHROMOSOMES

The normal diploid resting nuclei of females (but not those of males) contain a specific chromatin blob known as the sex-chromatin mass, or the *Barr body*. These nuclei are designated as *chromatin-positive* (female nuclear sex), whereas those of males are called *chromatin-negative* (male nuclear sex).

The Barr body arises from part or all of one X chromosome which is positively heteropyknotic, relatively inert genetically, and a late replicator of deoxyribonucleic acid (DNA). It is best visualized in vesicular nuclei. *Buccal smears* and tiny skin biopsies provide readily accessible material for examination. The *technique* for obtaining an adequate buccal smear is important. The scraping of the mucosa must be sufficiently forceful to obtain cells of the deeper layers, and *fixation* in ether alcohol must be quick enough to preclude air drying of the film, so as to prevent artifacts.

The frequency of Barr bodies is quite variable, ranging from 40 to 60 per cent (Moore and Barr) in normal females. Though it may assume various shapes, the Barr body is most often planoconvex, with one side flattened against the nuclear membrane. Its nucleoprotein stains readily with basic dyes (hematoxylin, etc.). It persists throughout life, except for the *first 2 days after birth* when it may be reduced or absent. A similar phenomenon has been observed as a result of the *administration of ACTH* and *cortisone*. Cessation of treatment is followed by a return of the Barr bodies. The frequency of Barr bodies is unaffected by alterations in the sex hormonal status of the host.

Because of the variability in shape, the dimensions of the Barr body also vary, averaging about 1 micron in diameter. Unusually *small* and *large Barr bodies* are associated with X chromosomes of correspondingly abnormal size (see page 110). A reduction in size may also be noted temporarily when *antibiotics* are administered.

It is a peculiarity of one type of cell with a dense chromatin content, the neutrophilic leukocyte, that, with the attainment of mature segmentation, its Barr body gradually becomes extruded into the cytoplasm. When extrusion is partial, the chromatin mass is known as a *sessile nodule*. When extrusion has been completed, the sex-chromatin mass appears as a dense, ovoid nuclear appendage, about 1.5 microns in diameter, attached to the nuclear lobe by a slender

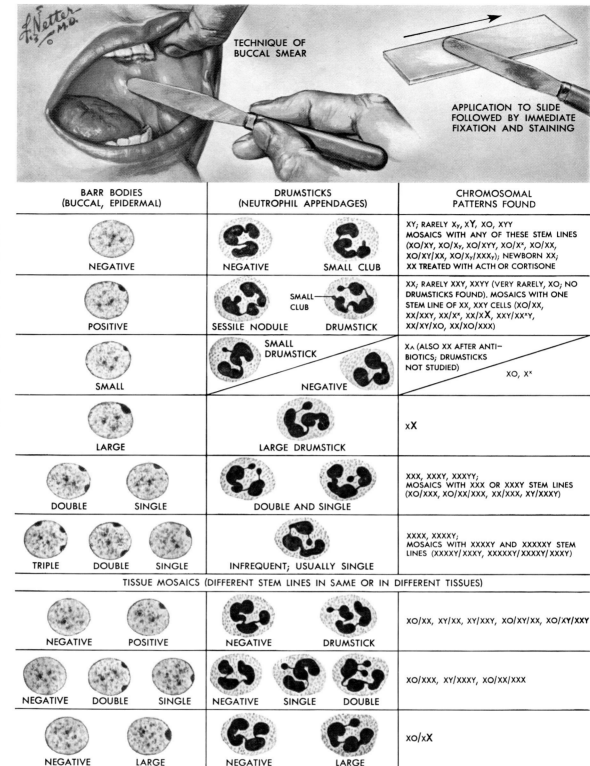

BARR BODIES (BUCCAL, EPIDERMAL)	DRUMSTICKS (NEUTROPHIL APPENDAGES)	CHROMOSOMAL PATTERNS FOUND
NEGATIVE	NEGATIVE — SMALL CLUB	XY; RARELY X$_Y$, XY, XO, XYY MOSAICS WITH ANY OF THESE STEM LINES (XO/XY, XO/X$_Y$, XO/XYY, XO/X^x, XO/XX, XO/XY/XX, XO/X$_Y$/XXX$_Y$); NEWBORN XX; XX TREATED WITH ACTH OR CORTISONE
POSITIVE	SESSILE NODULE — SMALL CLUB — DRUMSTICK	XX; RARELY XXY, XXYY (VERY RARELY, XO; NO DRUMSTICKS FOUND). MOSAICS WITH ONE STEM LINE OF XX, XXY CELLS (XO/XX, XX/XXY, XX/X^x, XX/X**X**, XXY/XX*$_Y$, XX/XY/XO, XX/XO/XXX)
SMALL	SMALL DRUMSTICK / NEGATIVE	X$_A$ (ALSO XX AFTER ANTI-BIOTICS; DRUMSTICKS NOT STUDIED) / XO, X^x
LARGE	LARGE DRUMSTICK	x**X**
DOUBLE — SINGLE	DOUBLE AND SINGLE	XXX, XXXY, XXXYY; MOSAICS WITH XXX OR XXXY STEM LINES (XO/XXX, XO/XX/XXX, XX/XXX, XY/XXXY)
TRIPLE — DOUBLE — SINGLE	INFREQUENT; USUALLY SINGLE	XXXX, XXXXY; MOSAICS WITH XXXXY AND XXXXXY STEM LINES (XXXXY/XXXY, XXXXXY/XXXXY/XXXY)

TISSUE MOSAICS (DIFFERENT STEM LINES IN SAME OR IN DIFFERENT TISSUES)

BARR BODIES (BUCCAL, EPIDERMAL)	DRUMSTICKS (NEUTROPHIL APPENDAGES)	CHROMOSOMAL PATTERNS FOUND
NEGATIVE — POSITIVE	NEGATIVE — DRUMSTICK	XO/XX, XY/XX, XY/XXY, XO/XY/XX, XO/XY/XXY
NEGATIVE — DOUBLE — SINGLE	NEGATIVE — SINGLE — DOUBLE	XO/XXX, XY/XXXY, XO/XX/XXX
NEGATIVE — LARGE	NEGATIVE — LARGE	XO/x**X**

thread. In this form it is known as a *drumstick*.

The frequency of drumsticks is quite variable from one female to another, the normal range being from 1 to 17 per cent, with an average of 2 to 3 per cent (Maclean). However, the number in any one individual tends to be quite constant. The examination is performed on a conventionally stained blood film, the usual procedure being to count the number of drumsticks found among 500 neutrophilic leukocytes.

Drumsticks must be distinguished from other nuclear appendages, especially those known as *small clubs*. The latter are found on the leukocytes of both males and females. These nonspecific appendages are considerably smaller than drumsticks but may have a similar configuration. As is the case with Barr bodies, *large* and *small drumsticks* reflect proportional changes in the size of X chromosomes.

In individuals with normal X chromosomes and in most persons with sex-chromosome abnormalities, there is a close correlation between the Barr body and the drumstick methods of determining nuclear sex. Discrepancies between the two usually signify the presence of *sex-chromosome mosaicism*. This is due to the fact that one *stem line* of cells may exist or predominate in one tissue, and a line with a different X complex may be present in another. Hence, both methods should be employed simultaneously.

Since Barr bodies and drumsticks are morphologically equivalent and are derived respectively from a single X chromosome, a general rule can be applied in most cases: The maximum number of either (for diploid cells) is 1 less than the maximum number of X chromosomes. However, the frequency of drumsticks in patients with 4 X chromosomes is apparently sharply reduced and not multiple, as might be expected.

PATHOGENESIS OF CHROMOSOMAL ABNORMALITIES

Aberrations of chromosome numbers result from abnormal chromosomal behavior and movement during nuclear *division*. They may appear during meiosis (maturation divisions of germ cells) or during mitosis (ordinary cell division after fertilization). *Numerical errors* may arise by one of four different mechanisms:

1. *Nondisjunction* is characterized by the failure of the longitudinally doubled chromosomes (sister chromatids) or of the members of a pair of homologous chromosomes to separate during anaphase. As a result, one daughter cell receives both chromosomes, while the other acquires none. Thus, the former has an extra chromosome, while the other lacks one (see page 126).

2. *Anaphase lag with simple loss* of a chromosome is usually due to failure of a metaphase chromosome to become oriented on the equatorial plate. Apparently, the centromere of one (but not of the other) member of a pair of chromatids is effective in drawing its daughter chromosome toward one pole of the nucleus. The chromosome with the inactive centromere fails to migrate to either pole, remaining in the cytoplasm, where it eventually disintegrates and is *lost*. Thus, one daughter cell lacks a chromosome while the other retains the normal number.

3. *Mosaicism* refers to the presence of chromosomally dissimilar cells in the same individual. The presence of two or more lines of cells with unlike karyotypes means that the chromosomal abnormalities originated after fertilization, usually at or soon after the first mitosis of the zygote (fertilized egg).

4. *Centric fusion,* a type of reciprocal translocation (see below), is a special variety which results in the loss of one chromosome. It involves two nonhomologous acrocentric (centromere near one end) chromosomes. *Breakage* close to the centromere occurs in the short arm of one chromosome and in the long arm of the other. Of the two newly produced chromosomes, one is necessarily a minute fragment, which is usually lost in a subsequent cell division.

Structural errors are due to breakage 'followed by improper reunion of the fragments. Abnormally short or long chromosomes are practically the only structural abnormalities presently recognizable. They are produced by one of four mechanisms, as follows:

1. *Reciprocal translocation.* If a translocation-produced chromosome lacks a centromere, or if it should have two centromeres, it will be eliminated.

2. *Isochromosome formation* occurs when a metaphase chromosome divides transversely instead of longitudinally. In terms of a normal X, the isochromosome of its long arms is expressed as

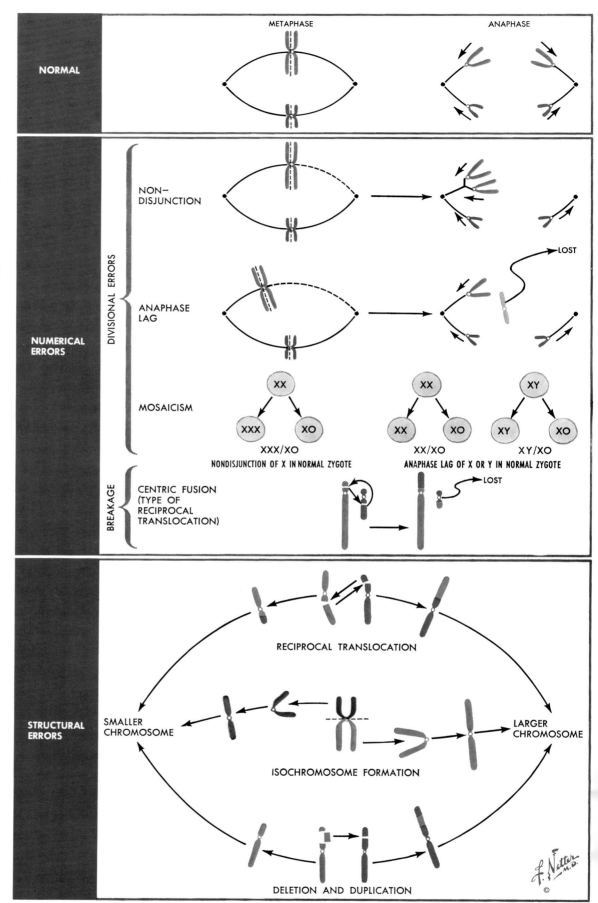

XX (see page 111); that of the short arms as XX.

3. *Deletion* is characterized by detachment and loss of a portion of a chromosome. The end result is a *smaller chromosome.* In comparison with a normal X, deletion of the short or long arms is expressed, respectively, as Xʌ or Xˣ (see page 111).

4. *Duplication* occurs when a segment deleted from a homologous chromosome is acquired in juxta-position to the genetically corresponding region. However, insertion of a deleted fragment from a nonhomologous chromosome also lengthens the recipient, though, in a strict genetic sense, this is not duplication.

Chromosomal abnormalities accounting for clinical disorders occur in about 0.5 per cent of the general population (Polani). Approximately three fourths of these involve the sex chromosomes.

DIFFERENTIATION OF GONADS

Factors Influencing Normal and Abnormal Gonadal Differentiation

Whether the primordial gonad differentiates as a testis or as an ovary is determined by genetic information coded on the X and Y chromosomes. Apparently, it is only at this initial step that the sex-determining genes exercise any influence on the sexual make-up of an individual. The differentiation of all the other anatomical and functional features which distinguish male from female are thought to stem secondarily from the effect of testicular or ovarian secretions on their respective primordial structures.

The Y chromosome possesses powerful male-determining genes which direct the primitive gonad to develop as a testis, even in the presence of more than one X chromosome. Two X chromosomes appear to be essential for the formation of normal ovaries, for individuals with a single X sex chromosome develop gonads which usually display only the most rudimentary form of differentiation.

Although many patients with congenitally defective gonads have been found to have an abnormal karyotype due to meiotic nondisjunction during meiosis (see page 126), similar patients may have normal-appearing sex chromosomes or chromosomal abnormalities not explainable on this basis.

In individuals with chromosomal mosaicism, the various tissues may have multiple cell lines of differing chromosomal make-up. Mosaicism arises from mitotic nondisjunction or chromosomal loss occurring after fertilization. In other patients, deletions or translocations of small chromosomal fragments may be recognized by experienced observers (see page 112). If these, perchance, involve a fragment bearing the sex-determining genes, the effect on gonadal structure may be as devastating as in instances where a total chromosome is lost.

In still other individuals, mutant sex-determining genes may cause a specific enzymatic error, leading to defective gonadal structure or hormonal secretion. Such conditions are usually hereditable, and no technique is yet available to visualize abnormalities at the level of the gene.

Stages in Gonadal Differentiation

UNDIFFERENTIATED STAGE. At the sixth week of gestation, the primitive gonad is represented by a well-demarcated *genital ridge* running along the dorsal root of the mesentery. The *cortical portion of the ridge* consists of a cloak of *coelomic epithelial cells*. The mature ovary is derived principally from these cortical cells. In these superficial layers are also found large *primordial germ*

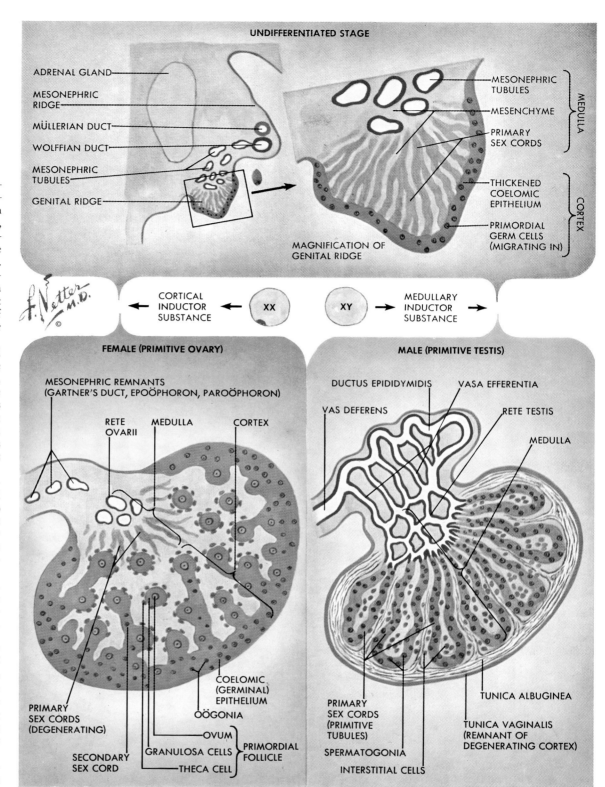

cells, capable of differentiating as either *oögonia* or *spermatogonia*.

The *medullary*, or interior, portion of the primitive gonad is composed of a *mesenchyme*, in which sheets of epithelial cells of uncertain origin are condensed to form the *primary sex cords*. This medullary portion has the potentiality for further differentiation as a testis.

TESTICULAR DIFFERENTIATION. If the primitive gonad is to become a testis, the inner portion of the *primary sex cords* becomes a collecting system connecting the seminiferous *tubules* with the mesonephric, or Wolffian, duct. The peripheral portions of the sex cords join with ingrowths of coelomic epithelium (containing primordial germ cells) to form seminiferous tubules. Most of the cortex, however, becomes isolated by the *tunica albuginea* and the *tunica vaginalis*, which are the only cortical vestiges in the mature testis. *Interstitial cells* of Leydig

become abundant at about 8 weeks and secrete the androgenic hormone necessary for the development of male external genitalia. Leydig cells disappear shortly after birth and are not seen again until the onset of adolescence.

OVARIAN DIFFERENTIATION. Ovarian development occurs several weeks later than does testicular differentiation. At this time the *cortex* undergoes intense proliferation, and strands of epithelial cells (called *secondary sex cords*) push into the interior of the gonad. Primordial germ cells are carried along in this inward migration. Clumps from the secondary sex cords fragment off to form *primordial follicles*. While the ovary is thus forming, the *primary sex cords recede* to the hilum, leaving stromal and connective tissue cells behind. Leydig cells and the *rete ovarii* persist as medullary *remnants* in the ovary. Proliferation of the cortex ceases at about 6 months.

DIFFERENTIATION OF GENITAL DUCTS

On page 113 it was pointed out that the early embryo of either sex is equipped with identical primitive gonads which have the capacity for developing into either testes or ovaries. In the case of the internal genital ducts, however, the early embryo has both a male and a female set of primordial structures. The *Müllerian ducts* have the potentiality of developing into *Fallopian tubes, uterus,* and the *upper portion* of the vagina. The *mesonephric,* or *Wolffian, ducts* have the capacity for developing into the *vas deferens* and the *seminal vesicles.* The large *Wolffian body,* containing the proximal *mesonephric ducts,* becomes the *epididymis.*

During the third fetal month, either the Müllerian or the Wolffian structures normally complete their development, while involution occurs simultaneously in the other set. Vestigial remnants of the other duct system, however, persist into adult life. In females the mesonephric structures are represented by the *epoöphoron, paroöphoron,* and the *ducts of Gartner.* In the male the only Müllerian remnant normally present is the *appendix testis.*

The direction in which these genital ducts develop is a direct consequence of the gonadal differentiation that occurred somewhat earlier. It is now clear, from the work of Alfred Jost and other experimental embryologists, that secretions from the fetal testis play a decisive rôle in bringing about regression of the Müllerian system and causing the derivatives of the mesonephric system to complete their normal male development. In the absence of these testicular secretions, the Müllerian structures proceed to become the uterus and Fallopian tubes, while the mesonephric structures become vestigial. It should be emphasized that female development is not dependent on any ovarian secretion, since, in the absence of any gonads at all, the uterus and Fallopian tubes develop normally.

The nature of the fetal testicular secretion which is responsible for male duct development is incompletely understood. It probably is not an ordinary androgenic hormone, since female babies who are subjected to high concentrations of androgen in utero, though externally virilized, fail to exhibit any masculinization of their internal ducts. Likewise, it has been shown experimentally that local applications of androgen fail to cause any regression of the Müllerian system, although, under conditions of extremely high dosage, there may be some abnormal retention of Wolffian remnants. Lastly, occasional male infants are born with morphologically normal testes but with an apparent inability to

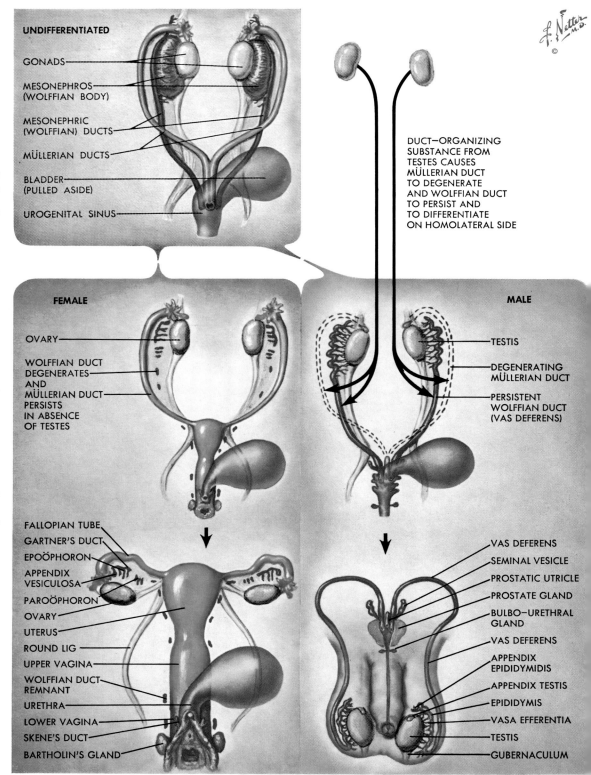

synthesize androgenic steroids. In such infants the internal duct system is always masculine (see page 123). For these reasons it is believed that the "duct-organizing substance" of the testis is not testosterone or a related steroid hormone. It appears to exert its action locally rather than through the systemic circulation. Experimentally, this was demonstrated by unilateral castration of a male fetus in the rat and in the rabbit. The duct on that side developed along female lines, whereas the contralateral duct developed along male lines. Similarly, the implantation of a testis on one side of a female fetus led to male development on that side, whereas it did not influence the female development on the other side.

The clinical counterpart of these studies is often encountered in babies with asymmetric gonadal differentiation, usually the result of chromosomal mosaicism. Such infants often are found to have an

undifferentiated gonad on one side and rudimentary testicular development on the other (see page 130). In such instances the side lacking in any gonadal differentiation will have a unicornuate uterus and vestigial vas deferens, whereas on the other side the testis will be attached to an epididymis and vas deferens. Similarly, in true hermaphrodites with ovotestes or with a testis on one side and an ovary on the other, the genital duct development again correlates well with the degree of testicular differentiation.

Although the nature of the testicular "duct-organizing substance" has not yet been determined, it is unassailable that the presence or absence of a fetal testis plays a decisive rôle in determining the fate of the primitive Müllerian and Wolffian ducts. This concept has proved to be of considerable value in predicting the anatomical findings in many disorders of sexual development.

DIFFERENTIATION OF EXTERNAL GENITALIA

Prior to the ninth week of gestation, both sexes have a urogenital sinus and an identical external appearance. At this *undifferentiated stage,* the external genitalia consist of a *genital tubercle* beneath which is a *urethral groove,* bounded laterally by *urethral folds* and *labioscrotal swellings.* The male and female *derivatives* of these structures are shown in the table and in the plate.

The *urogenital slit* is formed at an even earlier stage when the perineal membrane partitions it from a single cloacal opening. Thereafter, the bladder and both genital ducts find a common outlet in this sinus.

The *vagina* develops as a diverticulum of the urogenital sinus in the region of the Müllerian tubercle and becomes contiguous with the distal end of the Müllerian ducts. About two thirds of the vagina originates in the urogenital sinus and about one third is of Müllerian origin.

In normal male development the vaginal remnant is very tiny, since the Müllerian structures atrophy before this diverticulum develops very far. In male pseudohermaphroditism, however, a sizable remnant of this vaginal diverticulum may persist as a blind vaginal pouch.

In normal female development the vagina is pushed posteriorly by a downgrowth of connective tissue, so that, by the twelfth fetal week, it has acquired a separate external opening. In female pseudohermaphroditism the growth of this septum is inhibited, thus leading to persistence of the urogenital sinus.

The principal distinctions between male and female external genitalia, at this stage of development, are the location and size of the vaginal diverticulum, the size of the phallus, and the degree of fusion of the urethral folds and labioscrotal swellings.

Factors Determining Differentiation of External Genitalia. As in the case of the genital ducts, there is an inherent tendency for the external genitalia to develop along feminine lines. Masculinization of the external genitalia is brought about by exposure to androgenic hormones during the process of differentiation. Normally, the *androgenic hormone* is *testosterone,* derived from the Leydig cells of the *fetal testis.* The critical factor in determining whether masculinization will occur, however, is not the source of the androgen but rather its timing and its amount. In female pseudohermaphroditism due to congenital *adrenal hyperplasia,* the fetal adrenals secrete sufficient androgen to bring about some masculinization of the external genitalia. In other instances androgenic hormone may be derived from the *maternal circulation* (see page 122).

By the twelfth fetal week the vagina has migrated posteriorly, and androgens will no longer cause fusion of the urethral and labioscrotal folds. Clitoral hypertrophy, however, may occur at any time in fetal life or even after birth.

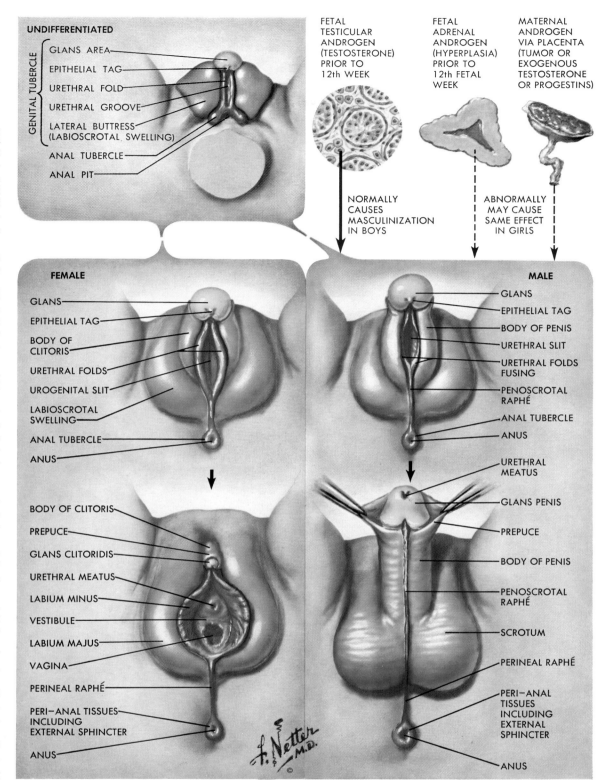

MALE AND FEMALE DERIVATIVES OF UROGENITAL SINUS AND EXTERNAL GENITALIA

MALE DERIVATIVE	PRIMORDIAL STRUCTURE	FEMALE DERIVATIVE
Prostatic utricle (vagina masculina)	**UROGENITAL SINUS**	Vagina (lower two thirds)
Prostate		Para-urethral glands (of Skene)
Bulbo-urethral glands (of Cowper)		Bartholin's glands
	EXTERNAL GENITALIA	
Penis	**Genital tubercle**	Clitoris
Corpora cavernosa		Corpora cavernosa
Glans penis		Glans clitoridis
Corpus spongiosum (enclosing penile urethra)	**Urethral folds**	Labia minora
Scrotum	**Labioscrotal swellings**	Labia majora

TESTOSTERONE AND ESTROGEN SYNTHESIS

Three glands having their origin in the coelomic cavity — the *adrenal cortex,* the *ovary,* and the *testis* — produce steroids under the influence of tropic hormones of the anterior pituitary, the *adrenocorticotropic hormone (ACTH),* and *gonadotropins.* Their secretions, in turn, are under the control of the hypothalamus, which is markedly inhibited by *estrogens* but only slightly by *androgens.*

For the majority of sex hormones, *cholesterol* is the precursor. In all of these steroid-secreting glands, the side chain of cholesterol is degraded to form *pregnenolone* and *dehydroepiandrosterone.* Pregnenolone is then transformed to *progesterone,* which, by degradation of the side chain, becomes *androstenedione* and is easily transformed to *testosterone.* Both of these are secretory products of the *Leydig cells,* which are found in abundance in the testis but are present in only small numbers in the hilar region of the ovary.

Testosterone is some sixty times more potent than most of the other naturally occurring androgens, except for Δ^4-androstenediol, which is the most potent substance occurring naturally in small amounts. Testosterone is transported in the *blood* adsorbed *on plasma proteins.* *Conjugation* with glucuronic acid takes place in the *liver.* Much of the conjugated testosterone is *excreted* in its water-soluble form by the *kidney* with a little free, unconjugated testosterone. The younger the *male,* the higher are the values found, the *normal* range for males varying from 30 to 200 µg per 24 hours of *total testosterone, i.e.,* glucuronide and free testosterone. In the *normal female* this age difference is not marked, and the total testosterone range is only from 5 to a maximum of 10 µg per day.

Dehydroepiandrosterone, a precursor of androstenedione and testosterone, is found mostly in the 17-ketosteroid fraction and is derived largely from the adrenal cortex. It is a weak androgen that makes up in excess of 60 per cent of the 17-ketosteroids. The *normal excretion* value for 17-ketosteroids is higher by 5 mg in the male than it is in the female, presumably because of the contribution by the testis of some dehydroepiandrosterone and a variety of other 17-ketosteroids.

The ovary contains at least three differential secretory zones: the *granulosa cells* of the follicle, engaged in estrogen formation; the *theca cells,* having a tend-

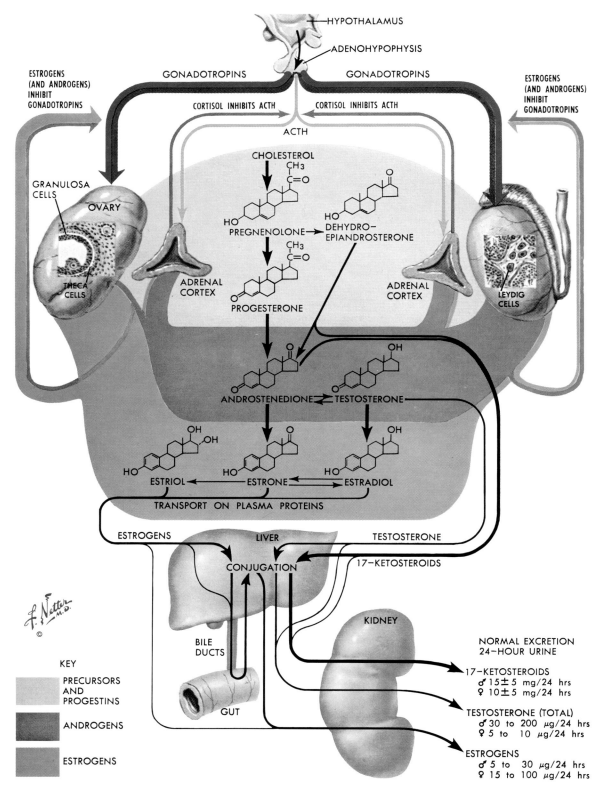

ency to produce somewhat more androgens; and the hilar cells, predominantly involved in androgen formation. The balance of these cellular elements assures a normal degree of femininity; conversely, an imbalance will lead to androgenicity. Within the ovary there are also the cells of the corpus luteum, which produce the bulk of progesterone.

Testosterone and *androstenedione,* respectively, appear to be the precursors of *estradiol* and *estrone.* Hydroxylation of the 19-carbon initiates a series of reactions that aromatize the A ring of the steroid nucleus, and this aromatization is, in fact, characteristic of estrogens. Estradiol is the most potent of some ten metabolites that have been isolated in human urine. In the presence of significant androgenicity (notably in the syndrome of polycystic ovaries), it is known that the enzymatic transformation of testosterone to estradiol is impaired. Estrone is second in

potency to estradiol, and *estriol* is purely an excretory product which is extremely weak biologically.

The *estrogens are carried on plasma proteins,* notably on albumin. Inactivation of estrogen occurs in the *liver* through conversion to less active estrogens (*i.e.,* estradiol to estrone to estriol), or by oxidation to totally inert compounds, or by conjugation to glucuronic acid. There is considerable enterohepatic circulation as estrogens are excreted in the *bile.* In the *normal male* 5 to 30 µg per day of total *estrogens* are *excreted in the urine,* whereas in the *female* 100 µg can be found, depending on the day of the menstrual cycle. There are two peaks in urinary excretion: one occurs just before ovulation, continuing for 4 to 5 days; the other, 3 to 4 days preceding the onset of the menstrual flow. It is, thus, of great clinical importance to know the exact date of the cycle when evaluating urinary estrogen levels.

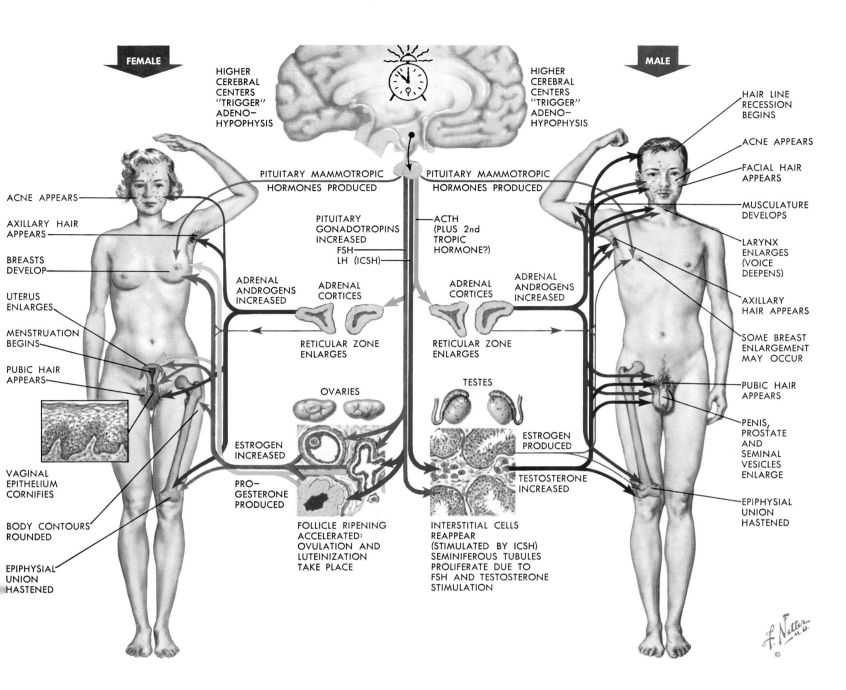

FEMALE

HIGHER CEREBRAL CENTERS "TRIGGER" ADENO-HYPOPHYSIS

HIGHER CEREBRAL CENTERS "TRIGGER" ADENO-HYPOPHYSIS

MALE

HAIR LINE RECESSION BEGINS

ACNE APPEARS

FACIAL HAIR APPEARS

MUSCULATURE DEVELOPS

LARYNX ENLARGES (VOICE DEEPENS)

AXILLARY HAIR APPEARS

SOME BREAST ENLARGEMENT MAY OCCUR

PUBIC HAIR APPEARS

PENIS, PROSTATE AND SEMINAL VESICLES ENLARGE

EPIPHYSIAL UNION HASTENED

ACNE APPEARS

AXILLARY HAIR APPEARS

BREASTS DEVELOP

UTERUS ENLARGES

MENSTRUATION BEGINS

PUBIC HAIR APPEARS

VAGINAL EPITHELIUM CORNIFIES

BODY CONTOURS ROUNDED

EPIPHYSIAL UNION HASTENED

PITUITARY MAMMOTROPIC HORMONES PRODUCED

PITUITARY MAMMOTROPIC HORMONES PRODUCED

PITUITARY GONADOTROPINS INCREASED FSH— LH (ICSH)—

ACTH (PLUS 2nd TROPIC HORMONE?)

ADRENAL ANDROGENS INCREASED

ADRENAL CORTICES

ADRENAL CORTICES

ADRENAL ANDROGENS INCREASED

RETICULAR ZONE ENLARGES

RETICULAR ZONE ENLARGES

OVARIES

TESTES

ESTROGEN INCREASED

ESTROGEN PRODUCED

PRO-GESTERONE PRODUCED

TESTOSTERONE INCREASED

FOLLICLE RIPENING ACCELERATED: OVULATION AND LUTEINIZATION TAKE PLACE

INTERSTITIAL CELLS REAPPEAR (STIMULATED BY ICSH) SEMINIFEROUS TUBULES PROLIFERATE DUE TO FSH AND TESTOSTERONE STIMULATION

f. Netter M.D.

NORMAL PUBESCENCE AND SEXUAL PRECOCITY

The Timing of Pubescence

Prior to the onset of pubescence, conspicuous physical differences between boys and girls are largely confined to the anatomy of their genital organs. Even then, however, in normal children the gonads are probably not totally without function, since the ovaries exhibit irregular ripening and involution of Graafian follicles, and the seminiferous tubules undergo some slight increase in size and convolutions.

Most of the physical changes which begin at puberty are attributable to a rise in androgens and estrogens from the gonads and reticular zone of the adrenal cortex. These glands are activated by *pituitary gonadotropic hormones,* which, until this time, are not secreted in measurable amounts in normal children. The secretion of pituitary gonadotropins appears to be initiated ultimately by the *hypothalamus* or by some adjacent area

of the brain which is sensitive to the general level of somatic maturation and which transmits this information to the *pituitary gland* by way of the *pituitary stalk.* The pituitary of a newborn rat, when grafted under the tuber cinereum of an adult hypophysectomized rat, secretes gonadotropins long before the donor rat would normally have reached puberty. Studies of children with sexual precocity likewise indicate that the hormonal events of pubescence are initiated in the central nervous system (CNS). It is not clear, however, whether, during childhood, the hypothalamus has not yet begun its secretion of gonadotropin-releasing factors or whether, during this period, there is active secretion of a gonadotropin inhibitor.

There is excellent correlation between the onset of pubescence and the maturation of the skeleton, and both may be hastened by exposure to sex steroids. Young children have been observed to secrete gonadotropic hormones and enter true adolescence following the removal of either virilizing or feminizing tumors. Similar observations have been recorded following the administration of exogenous androgens and estrogens. The development of adolescent sexual changes, under these circumstances, correlates well with the degree of skeletal advancement.

The female skeleton is normally, at all ages,

somewhat advanced beyond that of the male, and pubescence likewise occurs earlier in girls than in boys. These physiologic differences in timing are frequently exaggerated, since true sexual precocity occurs more commonly in females, whereas a physiologic delay in the onset of adolescence is predominantly a disorder of the male. Although ordinary methods of hormone assay fail to reveal significant sexual differences until the onset of pubescence, ovaries exhibit far more histologic activity during childhood than do testes. The autonomous secretion of small amounts of ovarian estrogen, during the prepubescent years, could readily explain the more rapid maturation of the female.

Hormonal Events in Female Pubescence (Plate 8)

With routine techniques, urinary gonadotropins first become measurable toward the end of the first decade of life, and a measurable rise in urinary estrogens is observed concomitantly. At this time the *ripening* and involution of *ovarian follicles* is intensified, the fibrous stroma becomes more abundant, and there is an exaggerated tendency toward the development of ovarian cysts and hyperthecosis.

(Continued on page 118)

117

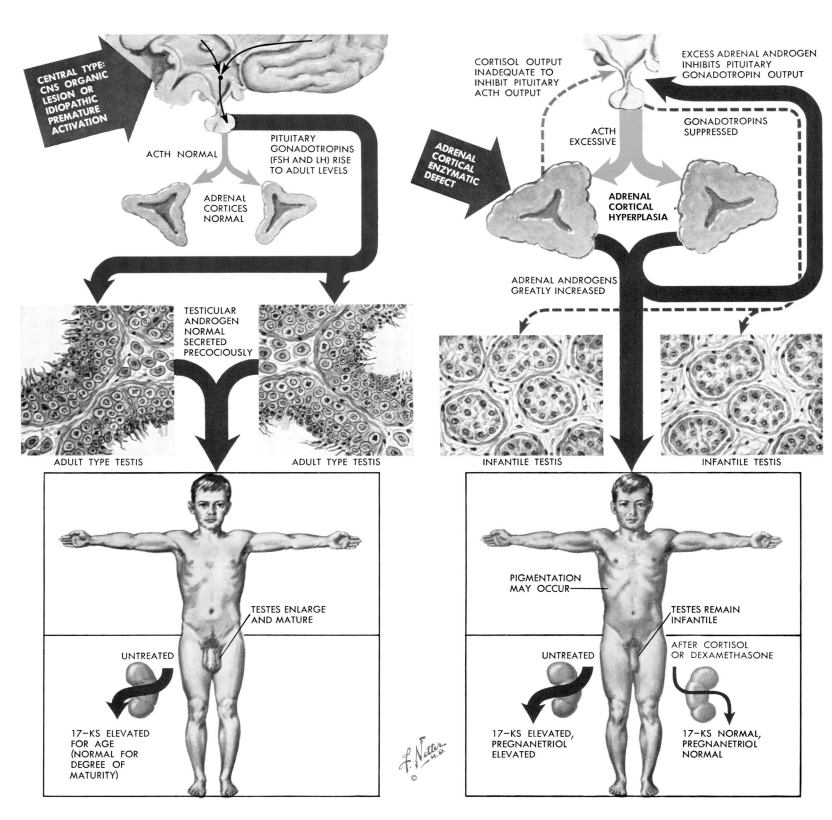

CENTRAL TYPE: CNS ORGANIC LESION OR IDIOPATHIC PREMATURE ACTIVATION

ACTH NORMAL

PITUITARY GONADOTROPINS (FSH AND LH) RISE TO ADULT LEVELS

ADRENAL CORTICES NORMAL

TESTICULAR ANDROGEN NORMAL SECRETED PRECOCIOUSLY

ADULT TYPE TESTIS

ADULT TYPE TESTIS

TESTES ENLARGE AND MATURE

UNTREATED

17-KS ELEVATED FOR AGE (NORMAL FOR DEGREE OF MATURITY)

CORTISOL OUTPUT INADEQUATE TO INHIBIT PITUITARY ACTH OUTPUT

EXCESS ADRENAL ANDROGEN INHIBITS PITUITARY GONADOTROPIN OUTPUT

ACTH EXCESSIVE

GONADOTROPINS SUPPRESSED

ADRENAL CORTICAL ENZYMATIC DEFECT

ADRENAL CORTICAL HYPERPLASIA

ADRENAL ANDROGENS GREATLY INCREASED

INFANTILE TESTIS

INFANTILE TESTIS

PIGMENTATION MAY OCCUR

TESTES REMAIN INFANTILE

AFTER CORTISOL OR DEXAMETHASONE

UNTREATED

17-KS ELEVATED, PREGNANETRIOL ELEVATED

17-KS NORMAL, PREGNANETRIOL NORMAL

F. Netter M.D.

NORMAL PUBESCENCE AND SEXUAL PRECOCITY

(Continued from page 117)

Rising estrogen levels produce *pubic hair growth* first, with *rounding of the body contours,* and *enlargement of the breasts,* owing to proliferation of duct tissue. There is thickening and *cornification of the vaginal epithelium.* The *uterus enlarges,* and the endometrium begins to proliferate.

In Caucasian females the average age of *onset of menstruation* (menarche) is 13.5 years, but *ovulation* does not occur until some additional months have elapsed. Until then, the menses are often highly erratic. *Progesterone* is secreted only as corpora lutea are formed following ovulation. When this occurs, the proliferative endometrium is transformed into a secretory type, and the breasts become further rounded as alveoli are stimulated to develop.

The capacity to secrete both androgens and estrogens is inherent in the adrenal glands as well as in the gonads of both sexes. *Enlargement of the reticular zone* of the *adrenal cortex* and increased excretion of 17-ketosteroids occur at about the same time that the ovaries exhibit heightened activity. Androgenic hormones from both the adrenals and ovaries increase the growth rate and the development of *pubic hair,* later *axillary hair,* and seborrhea and *acne.* Both androgens and estrogens have a stimulatory effect on *epiphysial maturation,* and, as fusion takes place, there is a rapid deceleration in the rate of linear growth (see pages 226 to 230).

The adrenal enlargement which occurs at adolescence cannot be accounted for by increased secretion of ACTH, since there is no proportional increase in the secretion of 17-hydroxycorticoids at that time. The administration of estrogen to a prepubescent child stimulates both enlargement of the reticular zone and an increase in urinary 17-ketosteroids. This effect is probably mediated through the pituitary, since it does not occur in hypopituitarism. Albright suggested that the "adrenarche" might be due to the secretion of luteinizing hormone (LH), but as yet this has not been confirmed.

"PREMATURE THELARCHE" AND "PREMATURE PUBARCHE". Two benign variants of female

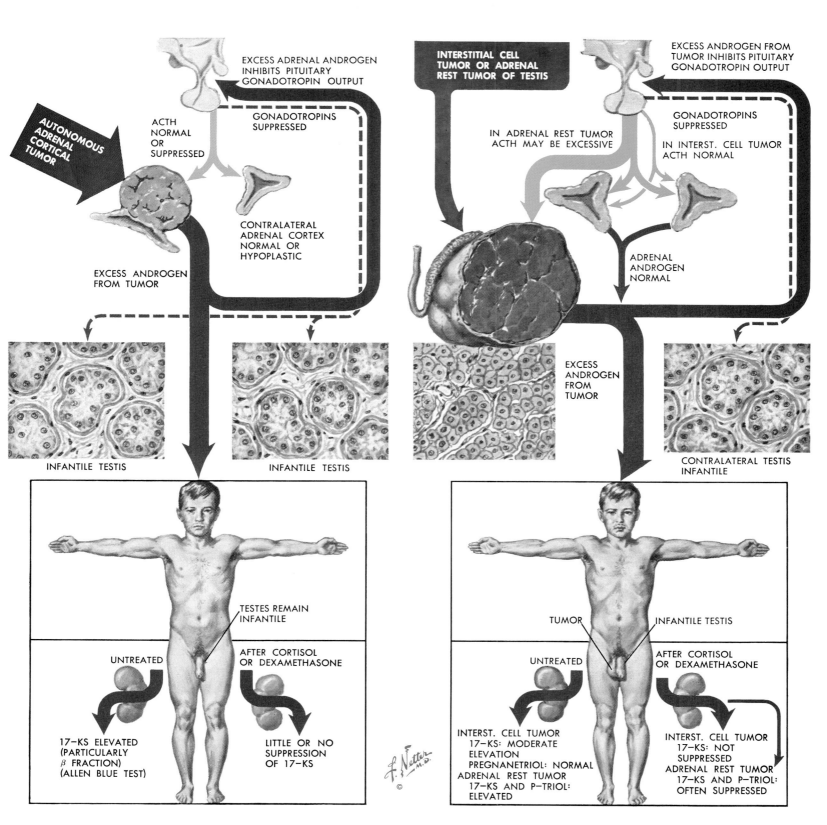

EXCESS ADRENAL ANDROGEN INHIBITS PITUITARY GONADOTROPIN OUTPUT

AUTONOMOUS ADRENAL CORTICAL TUMOR

ACTH NORMAL OR SUPPRESSED

GONADOTROPINS SUPPRESSED

CONTRALATERAL ADRENAL CORTEX NORMAL OR HYPOPLASTIC

EXCESS ANDROGEN FROM TUMOR

INFANTILE TESTIS

INFANTILE TESTIS

TESTES REMAIN INFANTILE

UNTREATED

AFTER CORTISOL OR DEXAMETHASONE

17-KS ELEVATED (PARTICULARLY β FRACTION) (ALLEN BLUE TEST)

LITTLE OR NO SUPPRESSION OF 17-KS

INTERSTITIAL CELL TUMOR OR ADRENAL REST TUMOR OF TESTIS

EXCESS ANDROGEN FROM TUMOR INHIBITS PITUITARY GONADOTROPIN OUTPUT

IN ADRENAL REST TUMOR ACTH MAY BE EXCESSIVE

GONADOTROPINS SUPPRESSED

IN INTERST. CELL TUMOR ACTH NORMAL

ADRENAL ANDROGEN NORMAL

EXCESS ANDROGEN FROM TUMOR

CONTRALATERAL TESTIS INFANTILE

TUMOR

INFANTILE TESTIS

UNTREATED

AFTER CORTISOL OR DEXAMETHASONE

INTERST. CELL TUMOR 17-KS: MODERATE ELEVATION PREGNANETRIOL: NORMAL ADRENAL REST TUMOR 17-KS AND P-TRIOL: ELEVATED

INTERST. CELL TUMOR 17-KS: NOT SUPPRESSED ADRENAL REST TUMOR 17-KS AND P-TRIOL: OFTEN SUPPRESSED

sexual development, which must always be differentiated from true sexual precocity, are premature development of breast tissue and of pubic hair. These conditions are often encountered as isolated findings.

In "premature thelarche" (benign infantile mammoplasia) the glandular tissue of the breast is moderately enlarged, but no pubic hair and no cornification of the vagina are observed. Hormonal assays are within normal limits. This condition may persist throughout childhood or may wax and wane. Rarely, there may be slight advancement of the bone age; in these cases there may be an early onset of true adolescence.

In "premature pubarche" the only abnormal finding is a growth of pubic hair. The 17-ketosteroids are normal or minimally elevated, and the bone age is only slightly advanced. The condition may persist throughout childhood, with normal adolescence occurring at a slightly early age.

Hormonal Events in Male Pubescence (Plate 8, page 117)

The male is physiologically less mature than the female throughout childhood, and pubescence occurs several years later. An increase in testicular size is usually the first manifestation of gonadotropic activity, occurring before there is any clinical evidence of increased androgen secretion. Testicular enlargement is due mostly to the increasing size and convolutions of the *seminiferous tubules*. Urinary gonadotropins usually become detectable at about the eleventh year, and at this time *interstitial*, or Leydig, *cells* can be identified in the interstitium. Formation of mature sperm normally occurs at about 14 to 15 years of age.

Androgens in the male are derived from both the *adrenals* and the *testes* (see page 116). The effects of androgen secretion on the development of *pubic hair, axillary hair,* and *facial acne* are similar to those in the female, but usually more intense. In addition, there are considerable *enlargement of the phallus, prostate, seminal vesicles,* and larynx; a *deepening of the voice;* a marked *increase in muscle mass;* an intensive growth spurt; and the appearance of *facial hair.* Androgenic hormones also cause gradual *recession of the temporal hairline,* with male-pattern baldness in individuals who are genetically predisposed.

(Continued on page 120)

NORMAL PUBESCENCE AND SEXUAL PRECOCITY

(Continued from page 119)

The urinary 17-ketosteroid levels reach their peak values between the ages of 14 and 18 years; even then, the levels found in males are only about one third higher than those in females. The 17-ketosteroids inadequately reflect the difference in androgenic status, since testosterone, the principal testicular androgen, is far more potent than the adrenal androgens while contributing very little to urinary metabolites.

Since *testosterone* serves as a precursor for the synthesis of *estrogenic hormones* (see page 116), male adolescence is accompanied by a rise in urinary estrogens. Adolescent *gynecomastia* occurs in about 80 per cent of normal boys and is probably due to estrogenic stimulation, although a direct effect of pituitary *mammotropic hormones* cannot be excluded.

Sexual Precocity in the Male
(Plate 9, pages 118 and 119)

Sexual Precocity of Central Origin. IDIOPATHIC SEXUAL PRECOCITY. No primary organic lesion can be discovered in approximately 50 per cent of boys exhibiting precocious sexual maturation. Pubescence proceeds in a normal pattern, with the sole exception that it begins earlier and is compressed into a shorter time. The *testes* undergo progressive bilateral *enlargement,* and biopsy reveals *interstitial cells* and *spermatogenesis* in accordance with the stage of physical maturity. Erections and ejaculations occur at an early age, and there is an increase in libido. The *adrenal glands* undergo normal adolescent enlargement. Gonadotropic hormones are usually easily detectable in the urine, but their levels are not excessive.

In sexual precocity of any type, the bone age almost always exceeds the height age. Thus, these children, who in childhood are exceptional for their tall stature, ultimately are somewhat dwarfed because of premature epiphysial fusion.

SEXUAL PRECOCITY DUE TO ORGANIC BRAIN LESIONS. Rarely, if ever, is sexual precocity of the central type the consequence of a primary tumor of the pituitary gland itself. Grumbach has demonstrated an abnormal electroencephalogram in a high percentage of children with "idiopathic" sexual precocity, but in only a small percentage of cases can specific neurologic lesions be diagnosed. The most common organic lesion is a tumor arising somewhere along the course of the third ventricle. This may be an astrocytoma, a meningioma, or a pinealoma.

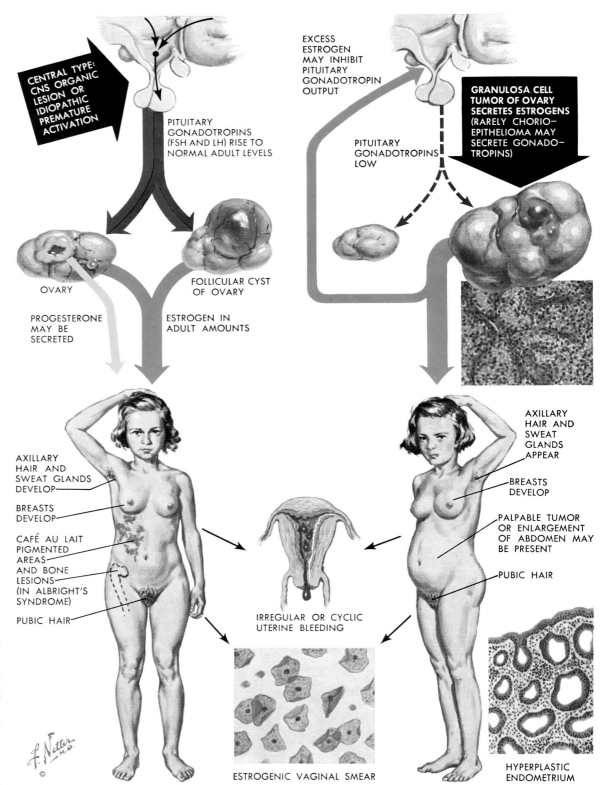

CENTRAL TYPE: CNS ORGANIC LESION OR IDIOPATHIC PREMATURE ACTIVATION

PITUITARY GONADOTROPINS (FSH AND LH) RISE TO NORMAL ADULT LEVELS

OVARY

PROGESTERONE MAY BE SECRETED

FOLLICULAR CYST OF OVARY

ESTROGEN IN ADULT AMOUNTS

AXILLARY HAIR AND SWEAT GLANDS DEVELOP

BREASTS DEVELOP

CAFÉ AU LAIT PIGMENTED AREAS AND BONE LESIONS (IN ALBRIGHT'S SYNDROME)

PUBIC HAIR

IRREGULAR OR CYCLIC UTERINE BLEEDING

ESTROGENIC VAGINAL SMEAR

EXCESS ESTROGEN MAY INHIBIT PITUITARY GONADOTROPIN OUTPUT

PITUITARY GONADOTROPINS LOW

GRANULOSA CELL TUMOR OF OVARY SECRETES ESTROGENS (RARELY CHORIO-EPITHELIOMA MAY SECRETE GONADOTROPINS)

AXILLARY HAIR AND SWEAT GLANDS APPEAR

BREASTS DEVELOP

PALPABLE TUMOR OR ENLARGEMENT OF ABDOMEN MAY BE PRESENT

PUBIC HAIR

HYPERPLASTIC ENDOMETRIUM

These patients usually have diabetes insipidus and defects in their visual fields. In other patients, sexual precocity may be associated with neurofibromatosis or a congenital malformation of the brain, often with severe mental retardation. Small hamartomas in the diencephalon have been found in several children with sexual precocity.

Sexual Precocity of Adrenal Origin. CONGENITAL ADRENAL HYPERPLASIA. In congenital adrenal hyperplasia the adrenals have been enlarged in utero, because excessive androgen was secreted early in pregnancy. Although this produces pseudohermaphroditism in the female, no gross anatomical abnormalities occur in the male. The adrenogenital syndrome can often be suspected at birth, however, because of *excessive phallic size* (macrogenitosomia), acne, and *Addisonianlike pigmentation* of the scrotum and peri-anal region. Most commonly, however, the simple viriliz-

ing form of adrenal hyperplasia in males is not recognized until many months later when there are further penile enlargement, appearance of *pubic hair,* and deepening of the voice. By this time there is great advancement of the height and an even greater advancement of the bone age.

As discussed in Section III, the fundamental abnormality in the adrenogenital syndrome is an inherited deficiency of one of the hydroxylase enzymes which are required for the synthesis of cortisol from 17-hydroxyprogesterone. The *impairment in cortisol production* thereupon activates the *pituitary* to secrete *excessive amounts of ACTH.* The *adrenal gland* undergoes compensatory *hypertrophy* and produces large quantities of cortisol precursors from which androgens are derived. These substances are detected in the urine as *pregnanetriol* and 17-ketosteroids

(Continued on page 121)

(17-KS). The *androgens*, in turn, *inhibit the pituitary gonadotropic mechanism,* so that the *testes* remain small and *infantile*.

The diagnosis is established by the *dexamethasone* or *cortisol suppression test* (see page 88). In this test the administration of exogenous glucocorticoids brings about a dramatic reduction in the excretion of urinary 17-ketosteroids and pregnanetriol. If substitution therapy with cortisol or other glucocorticoids is provided consistently, normal gonadal maturation will occur when the physiological maturation reaches the appropriate level. Wilkins and Cara have shown that, in those boys whose bone age is advanced to 12 to 14 years before treatment is begun, the institution of cortisol therapy will be promptly followed by the appearance of gonadotropins and normal adult maturation of the testes.

Several variants of the adrenogenital syndrome bring about different somatic defects (see pages 92 and 93). In the salt-losing variety, acute adrenal insufficiency develops within the early weeks of life and results in death unless adequate treatment is instituted. In the hypertensive variant, a deficiency of the 11-β-hydroxylase enzyme causes an accumulation of salt-retaining precursors of cortisol. The recently recognized C-3-β-ol-dehydrogenase defect produces a severe block in the synthesis of both adrenal and testicular steroids. Affected males may thus exhibit male pseudohermaphroditism along with severe adrenal insufficiency (see pages 92 and 93). No affected infants with this defect have yet survived infancy.

VIRILIZATION DUE TO ADRENAL CORTICAL TUMOR. The possibility of a virilizing *adrenal adenoma* or *carcinoma* must be considered in any child exhibiting premature masculinization. The clinical signs do not differ from those of the adrenogenital syndrome, although the *17-ketosteroids* are usually *higher* and, on fractionation, are found to be of a more primitive type. Since virilizing adrenal tumors function autonomously, the *urinary steroids* usually cannot be *suppressed* by the administration of exogenous *glucocorticoids*. The *gonads* and the *contralateral adrenal gland* may, on occasion, be *atrophic* due to *suppression* by the tumor of *pituitary gonadotropins* and *ACTH*. Usually, however, ACTH is suppressed in only those tumors which secrete excessive amounts of glucocorticoids.

Sexual Precocity Due to Testicular Tumors. INTERSTITIAL CELL TUMORS. Primary testicular neoplasms are a more rare cause of sexual precocity than are those previously described. These are usually detected, on physical examination, by *nodular enlargement of one testis*. The *contralateral testis* is often *infantile* due to *suppression of gonadotropins*. In true Leydig cell tumors the urinary 17-ketosteroids are elevated to a variable degree and are not suppressible by exogenous corticoids. The adrenals are normal.

HYPERPLASIA AND TUMORS OF ADRENAL RESTS. When the primitive gonads separate from the genital ridge (see page 113), clumps of adrenal cells are occasionally carried along and persist as adrenal rests in the hilum of the ovary or testis. This is particularly prone to occur in adrenal hyperplasia, where the fetal adrenal is excessively large. Males with the adrenogenital syndrome often have enlargement of one or both testes, owing to hyperplasia of these adrenal rests.

A number of patients, formerly thought to have Leydig cell tumors of the testes, have now been shown to have enzymatic abnormalities similar to those in adrenal hyperplasia. In such individuals, surgical excision of the tumor causes a temporary fall in the 17-ketosteroid excretion and some decrease in virilization, although, after a time, the adrenal glands may bring about a recurrence in the clinical picture. Before surgery is carried out in any such patient, it is important to study carefully the urinary 17-ketosteroid and pregnanetriol levels, as well as the possibility of a suppressive response to glucocorticoids.

TERATOMATOUS RESTS OF THE TESTIS. An exceedingly rare cause of sexual precocity is the presence of teratomatous rests which secrete large quantities of chorionic gonadotropin. These tumors are highly malignant, and usually metastasize before surgery can be carried out. The contralateral testis may undergo some true maturation under stimulation of this pituitarylike hormone.

Sexual Precocity in the Female
(Plate 10, page 120)

As in males, sexual precocity in the female may arise from a disturbance in the central nervous system or from an autonomous steroid-secreting tumor of the ovary. Adrenal tumors or adrenal hyperplasia in the female usually cause virilization rather than true sexual precocity.

Sexual Precocity of Central Origin. IDIOPATHIC PRECOCITY. The greater incidence of sexual precocity in females over that in males is largely accounted for by cases of idiopathic origin. A sexually precocious girl is less likely to have a demonstrable organic central nervous system lesion than is a boy, but it is not clear whether neurologic lesions producing sexual precocity are actually less common in females.

Girls with sexual precocity are advanced in stature and usually have a disproportionately advanced bone age. The *breasts* are enlarged, the *vaginal membranes* are thickened and *cornified,* and *pubic hair* and acne may be present. Although *axillary hair* is a late manifestation, observant mothers often first note the presence of adult perspiration odors in the axillae, where sweat glands develop, before any other signs have appeared. Rectal examination reveals the *uterus* to be enlarged, and irregular *menstrual bleeding* may occur for some months before a regular cyclic pattern is established. Spontaneous remissions of variable duration are not uncommon.

The urinary *estrogen values* are usually in the *adult female range*. The urinary gonadotropins may be undetectable or in the range of normal adults. The 17-ketosteroid excretion is elevated for age, consistent with the degree of maturity. In true sexual precocity the adrenal gland undergoes enlargement, just as it does in normal adolescence.

Stimulation of the gonads by *pituitary gonadotropins* may result in large *follicular cysts,* which are often difficult to distinguish from primary ovarian tumors. Such cysts are rich in estrogen content; if resected, there may be a temporary remission in the progress of the sexual precocity. Occasionally, after the removal of a unilateral cyst, the signs of sexual precocity may regress almost completely, and further sexual maturation may not recur for a number of years. Such observations suggest that some cysts develop autonomously, or at least that central stimulation does not always continue relentlessly.

ALBRIGHT'S SYNDROME. A special form of sexual precocity of central origin is that associated with Albright's syndrome of polyostotic fibrous dysplasia (see page 195). In this case true sexual precocity is associated with *lesions of the long bones* and hyperostosis of the basilar portion of the skull. *Café au lait* spots may be present, either unilaterally or bilaterally, often stopping at the midline. Thyroid enlargement is common, and, frequently, there may be a mild degree of thyrotoxicosis. These girls often have a prominent frontal bone or zygomatic arch and other features suggestive of acromegaly. Occasionally, they may have polycystic ovaries and marked hirsutism.

PSEUDOSEXUAL PRECOCITY IN PRIMARY HYPOTHYROIDISM. In untreated juvenile hypothyroidism the sexual maturation is usually retarded in proportion to the lag in bone age. Van Wyk and Grumbach have described several young hypothyroid girls, however, who, paradoxically, exhibited breast enlargement, precocious menstruation, and galactorrhea. Their bone ages were retarded, and no pubic hair was evident. All had an enlarged sella turcica and signs pointing to a pituitary tumor. After adequate replacement therapy with thyroid hormone, the signs of sexual precocity disappeared, and the pituitary fossa became smaller. It was postulated that the mechanism, in these patients, was an overlapping excessive secretion of gonadotropic and mammotropic hormones along with the high levels of TSH, the latter being appropriate in long-standing hypothyroidism.

Sexual Precocity Due to Ovarian Tumors. Feminizing tumors of the ovary account for about 15 per cent of all cases of sexual precocity in the female. The true frequency is undoubtedly less than this, owing to preferential reporting.

GRANULOSA–THECA CELL TUMORS. In most instances the histology is fairly characteristic (see CIBA COLLECTION, Vol. 2, page 202). These *tumors* can usually be easily *palpated,* on abdominal or rectal examination, when the child first comes to medical attention. Such tumors may secrete huge amounts of *estrogen,* causing the child to become intensely feminized in a very brief time.

Paradoxically, gonadotropic hormones are sometimes found in the urine of these girls, and the excretion of 17-ketosteroids may be as high as in true sexual precocity. There are, usually, definite growth of *pubic and axillary hair* and increased *axillary sweat secretion*. Such findings cannot be directly attributed to the secretion of estrogen but may be an indirect effect mediated through the pituitary (see Plate 8). The prognosis for a child with a granulosa cell tumor is good if the tumor can be completely removed without breaking the capsule. Occasionally, there is a recurrence in the contralateral ovary, but the frequency is sufficiently low that the normal ovary need not be removed.

LUTEOMAS AND CHORIO-EPITHELIOMAS. Other types of ovarian tumors are very rare, but two should be noted: Luteomas produce the same signs and symptoms as granulosa cell tumors, but they may be smaller and not easily palpable. Chorio-epitheliomas produce sexual precocity along with high urinary levels of chorionic gonadotropin. These tumors are exceedingly malignant.

Sexual Precocity Due to Exogenous Estrogens. In any young girl with sexual precocity, it is of utmost importance to rule out the possibility of exposure to exogenous estrogens. Such cases have been reported from the ingestion of stilbestrol tablets and of vitamin preparations which have been contaminated with estrogens, as well as from the use of cosmetics containing estrogens. Feminization has also occurred from eating certain portions of chickens which have been caponized by the implantation of stilbestrol tablets.

DISORDERS OF SEX DIFFERENTIATION

Classification

A hermaphrodite is an individual who possesses one or more physical features characteristic of the sex opposite to that in which he is being reared. In classical terminology a true hermaphrodite is a person who possesses both ovarian and testicular tissue. A *male pseudohermaphrodite* is one whose gonads are exclusively testes but whose genital ducts and/or external genitalia exhibit, to some degree, the phenotype characteristic of a female. A *female pseudohermaphrodite* is a person with exclusively ovarian gonadal structures but whose genital development exhibits some masculine traits.

As yet, no standard terminology or etiologic classification system has met with wide acceptance. A consideration of the various factors which control differentiation at each developmental level, as presented in pages 113 to 115, makes it possible, in most clinically encountered abnormalities, to localize, at least presumptively, the initial error and to predict the range of secondary consequences which may be expected.

CLASSIFICATION OF ERRORS IN SEX DIFFERENTIATION

I. Female Pseudohermaphroditism   Plate 11
  (a) Due to Adrenal Hyperplasia
  (b) Due to Androgenic Hormones of Maternal Origin
  (c) In Association with Malformations of the Intestine and Urinary Tract
II. Male Pseudohermaphroditism
  (a) Failure to Synthesize or Respond to Testicular Androgen (Duct-Organizing Substance Normal)   Plate 12
  (b) Specific Failure of Müllerian Ducts to Involute (Normal Androgen Secretion)   Plate 13
  (c) Mixed Types in Patients with Rudimentary Testes   Plates 13 and 19
III. Errors in Gonadal Differentiation
  (a) True Hermaphroditism   Plate 14
  (b) Syndrome of Seminiferous Tubular Dysgenesis (Klinefelter's Syndrome)   Plate 16
  (c) Syndrome of Gonadal Dysgenesis (Turner's Syndrome) (Gonadal Aplasia)   Plate 17
  (d) Gonadal Dysgenesis with Cortical Elements (Rudimentary Ovaries)   Plate 18
  (e) Gonadal Dysgenesis with Medullary Elements (Rudimentary Testes)   Plate 19

Female Pseudohermaphroditism (Plate 11)

Among the various sexual anomalies, female pseudohermaphroditism, in which

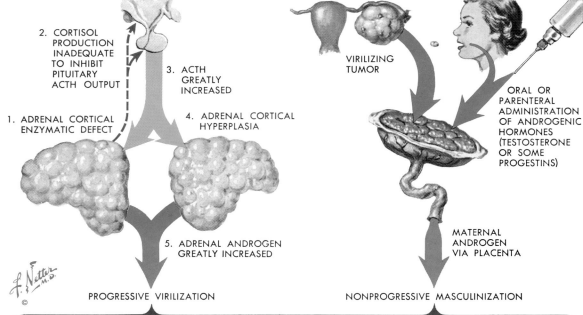

2. CORTISOL PRODUCTION INADEQUATE TO INHIBIT PITUITARY ACTH OUTPUT

3. ACTH GREATLY INCREASED

1. ADRENAL CORTICAL ENZYMATIC DEFECT

4. ADRENAL CORTICAL HYPERPLASIA

5. ADRENAL ANDROGEN GREATLY INCREASED

VIRILIZING TUMOR

ORAL OR PARENTERAL ADMINISTRATION OF ANDROGENIC HORMONES (TESTOSTERONE OR SOME PROGESTINS)

MATERNAL ANDROGEN VIA PLACENTA

PROGRESSIVE VIRILIZATION

NONPROGRESSIVE MASCULINIZATION

DEGREE OF GENITAL MASCULINIZATION DEPENDENT ON FETAL STAGE WHEN ANDROGEN EXPOSURE OCCURRED

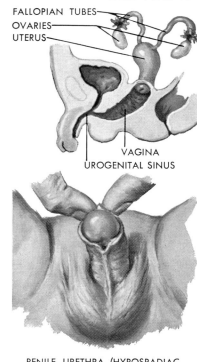

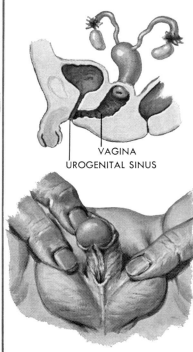

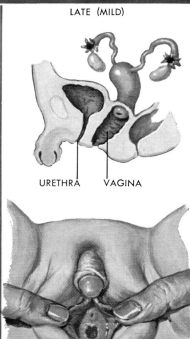

EARLY (PRIOR TO 12th WEEK: SEVERE)

LATE (MILD)

FALLOPIAN TUBES — OVARIES — UTERUS —

VAGINA — UROGENITAL SINUS

VAGINA — UROGENITAL SINUS

URETHRA   VAGINA

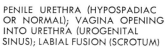

PENILE URETHRA (HYPOSPADIAC OR NORMAL); VAGINA OPENING INTO URETHRA (UROGENITAL SINUS); LABIAL FUSION (SCROTUM)

ENLARGED CLITORIS: VAGINA OPENING INTO UROGENITAL SINUS WITH ORIFICE AT BASE OF CLITORIS; PARTLY FUSED LABIA (BIFID SCROTUM)

SIMPLE ENLARGEMENT OF CLITORIS; GENITALIA OTHERWISE NORMAL

the gonadal structures are entirely ovarian, is the simplest to comprehend. Since, in the absence of testes, there is an inherent tendency for the genital ducts and external genitalia to feminize, a female fetus will exhibit masculinization only if it is subjected to an environment of androgen from an extragonadal source. Since androgens per se do not inhibit the development of Müllerian ducts, female fetuses exposed to androgen have normal internal duct structures, and the masculinization involves only the urogenital sinus and external genitalia.

Androgenic stimulation received *before the twelfth fetal week* inhibits the descent of the vagina and brings about a variable degree of *labioscrotal fusion*. The *urogenital sinus* is thus preserved, and a *single slitlike opening* will be situated anywhere from the normal urethral location to the tip of the *enlarged phallus*. An important point which differentiates

female pseudohermaphroditism from other types of hermaphroditism is that, since the *internal ducts are normal,* the *gonads* are rarely felt within the labioscrotal folds or in the vicinity of the inguinal rings. *Late androgenic stimulation,* after the twelfth fetal week or even in postnatal life, will lead to *clitoral enlargement,* but, by this time, the vagina will have descended normally, precluding a urogenital sinus, so no labial fusion can occur.

Congenital Adrenal Hyperplasia. The most common cause of female pseudohermaphroditism is congenital adrenal hyperplasia, which accounts for almost half of all infants born with ambiguous external genitalia.

Adrenal hyperplasia is caused by an autosomal recessive mutant gene; it involves male and female infants in equal numbers. The pathologic physiology in this disorder is discussed on pages 92 to 94, 118,

(Continued on page 123)

DISORDERS OF SEX DIFFERENTIATION

(*Continued from page 122*)

120, and 121. As virilization begins well before the twelfth fetal week, the external genitalia usually exhibit both labial fusion and clitoral hypertrophy. In more mildly affected infants, there may be only clitoral enlargement at birth.

With adequate glucocorticoid therapy, these girls grow normally and feminize at adolescence. A number of successful pregnancies have been reported in women with minor abnormalities who have been adequately treated.

Exposure to Androgens from Maternal Circulation. The early fetus is exquisitely sensitive to small amounts of androgen; hence, the treatment of pregnant women with low dosages of *androgen*, insufficient to produce masculinization in them, will often produce *masculinization of the fetal genitalia*. In recent years many female infants have been virilized by the administration of synthetic *progestational compounds* to mothers with habitual or threatened abortion. With the exception of esters of progesterone itself, most of the synthetic progestins are intrinsically androgenic to some degree, producing virilization of female fetuses when administered to gravid experimental animals.

A rarer cause of female pseudohermaphroditism is the presence of a *virilizing disorder in the mother,* usually due to an ovarian arrhenoblastoma.

Female Pseudohermaphroditism Associated with Malformations of the Intestine and Urinary Tract. Malformations of the female genitalia are sometimes found in association with imperforate anus, persistent cloaca, and other gross malformations of the lower intestine and upper urinary tract. In some cases bilateral renal agenesis has been present. The mechanism of these changes is certainly different from that of other forms of female pseudohermaphroditism, and they should properly be considered in the context of teratology rather than as specific abnormalities of sexual differentiation.

Male Pseudohermaphroditism (Plates 12 and 13)

Male pseudohermaphroditism (in which the only recognizable gonadal tissue is testicular) results if the fetal testis fails to produce either sufficient duct-organizing substance to cause involution of the Müllerian duct system or sufficient androgen to masculinize fully the external genitalia. This may be caused by a specific secretory error in a testis which has completed its anatomical differentiation, or it may be a secondary functional consequence when testicular development remains rudimentary. There is a growing tendency to restrict the term "male pseudohermaphroditism" to those individuals with relatively normal-appearing testes. Those patients whose testes exhibit only rudimentary development

should properly be considered as part of the spectrum of gonadal dysgenesis.

Failure to Synthesize or Respond to Testicular Androgen. SYNDROME OF FEMINIZING TESTES (Plate 12). Such patients appear to be females with normal external genitalia and secondary sexual characteristics, but they have *inguinal hernias* containing *well-developed testes* and *male genital ducts internally*. Affected individuals are genetic males, with a *normal XY karyotype.*

This disorder may be considered to be the consequence of an inherited inborn error of metabolism. Within a given sibship all the females will be normal, but half of the males will be affected and will be reared as females. Since affected individuals are infertile, it is not yet clear whether the mode in inheritance is by means of a sex-linked recessive or a sex-limited dominant mutant gene.

At birth, affected individuals may be indistinguishable from normal girls, except for somewhat prominent labia majora. The testes are located either in the labia majora, in the *inguinal canals,* or intra-abdominally. In less severely affected individuals there may be slight clitoral hypertrophy and labio-scrotal fusion. At adolescence, female secondary sexual characteristics appear, with *well-developed breasts* and cornification of the vagina. Menstruation, of course, does not occur, and examination reveals the *absence of a uterus* and cervix. The vagina is usually situated in its normal position but ends blindly. Because of their location and immobility, the testes are subject to injury. Biopsies of testes reveal them to be relatively normal in appearance except for *changes which might be associated with cryptorchidism.* There may be secondary spermatocytes or spermatids,

(Continued on page 124)

NORMAL FEMALE EXTERNAL GENITALIA (OR SLIGHTLY MASCULINIZED) VAGINA ENDS BLINDLY

RELATIVELY NORMAL FEMALE HABITUS (INGUINAL HERNIAE)

TESTES OPERATIVELY EXPOSED IN GROINS; LAPAROTOMY REVEALS COMPLETE ABSENCE OF UTERUS, FALLOPIAN TUBES AND OVARIES

SECTION OF TESTIS TYPICAL OF CRYPTORCHIDISM (ADENOMA IN UPPER LEFT CORNER)

NEGATIVE (MALE) NUCLEAR CHROMATIN, XY (MALE) CHROMOSOMAL PATTERN

URINARY GONADOTROPINS NORMAL

17-KS NORMAL OR SLIGHTLY ELEVATED

ESTROGEN (NORMAL LEVELS FOR FEMALE)

DISORDERS OF SEX DIFFERENTIATION

(Continued from page 123)

but spermatogenesis has not been reported. The testes are subject to malignant change, and it is usually considered advisable to remove them after they have brought about full feminization.

All the findings in this syndrome are compatible with an error in the peripheral responses to androgen. Incubation studies, carried out on testes removed from these patients, have revealed the production of estrogens, and there has been no apparent defect in the ability to synthesize testosterone. The testes are the ultimate source of estrogen in these women, since castration leads to a fall in the excretion of estrogens, as well as to the appearance of menopausal symptoms. The *urinary 17-ketosteroids* are slightly elevated, whereas the *excretion of estrogenic substances* is in the low-normal range for adult females. It is notable that some of these women are singularly devoid of sexual hair and acne, and, usually, the administration of testosterone has failed to produce these effects.

In some families the defect seems to be less complete, and the external genitalia exhibit some degree of masculinization at birth. In these girls the hormonal pattern, at adolescence, is likewise mixed, with inadequate breast development and some hirsutism. Instances have been reported in which the complete and the less complete forms have occurred within the same sibship.

MALE PSEUDOHERMAPHRODITISM DUE TO CONGENITAL STEROID HORMONE DYSGENESIS. Prader has described a group of male infants with severe adrenal insufficiency, enormous accumulations of lipid in the cells of the adrenal cortex and testes, and female or hermaphroditic external genitalia with male genital ducts (adrenal lipid hyperplasia).

Bongiovanni has studied similarly affected infants, and has ascribed his findings to a deficiency of C-3-β-ol-dehydrogenase in the patients' adrenal glands and testes. No synthetic step beyond cholesterol occurs, with consequent lack of adrenal and gonadal hormones (see page 116). This primitive defect severely limits the adrenal production of 17-hydroxycorticoids and androgens, thus leading to hyperplasia because of ACTH excess. Similarly, failure to synthesize testicular androgen fully explains the anomalous external genitalia.

The normalcy of the male genital ducts, in this syndrome and that of

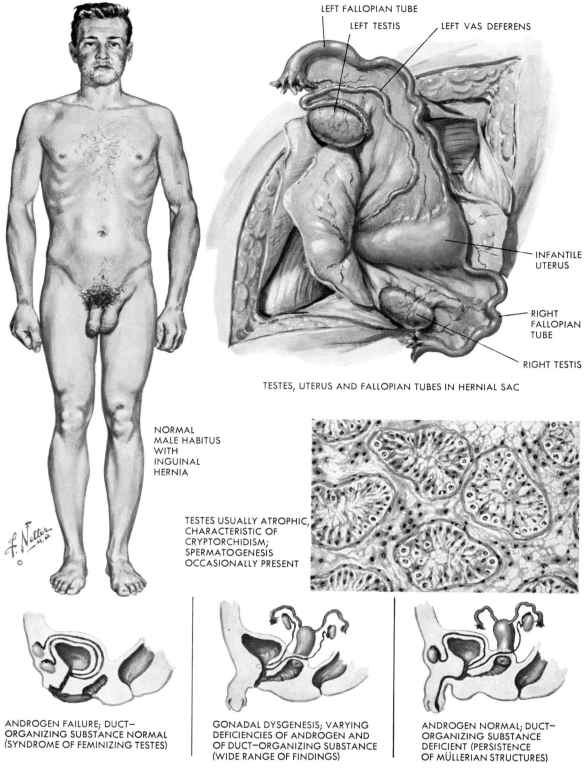

LEFT FALLOPIAN TUBE
LEFT TESTIS — LEFT VAS DEFERENS

INFANTILE UTERUS

RIGHT FALLOPIAN TUBE

RIGHT TESTIS

TESTES, UTERUS AND FALLOPIAN TUBES IN HERNIAL SAC

NORMAL MALE HABITUS WITH INGUINAL HERNIA

TESTES USUALLY ATROPHIC, CHARACTERISTIC OF CRYPTORCHIDISM; SPERMATOGENESIS OCCASIONALLY PRESENT

ANDROGEN FAILURE; DUCT—ORGANIZING SUBSTANCE NORMAL (SYNDROME OF FEMINIZING TESTES)

GONADAL DYSGENESIS; VARYING DEFICIENCIES OF ANDROGEN AND OF DUCT—ORGANIZING SUBSTANCE (WIDE RANGE OF FINDINGS)

ANDROGEN NORMAL; DUCT—ORGANIZING SUBSTANCE DEFICIENT (PERSISTENCE OF MÜLLERIAN STRUCTURES)

SOME VARIATIONS IN MALE PSEUDOHERMAPHRODITISM

feminizing testes, substantiates Jost's hypothesis that the duct-organizing substance is nonsteroidal in character. This evidence is particularly convincing in those cases of adrenal lipid hyperplasia, in which the normal synthesis of all biologically important steroid hormones fails.

Male Pseudohermaphroditism with Retention of Müllerian Ducts (Plate 13). In this illustration are represented the findings in a rare type of male pseudohermaphroditism, in which a *normal-appearing virile male* is found to have *retention of Müllerian elements.* Such individuals are considered, at birth, to be normal males. They grow normally throughout childhood and, at adolescence, virilize adequately.

In the few recorded patients with this syndrome (the frequency of which is unknown), the *testicular architecture* has been *normal,* rarely including full *spermatogenesis.* Some of these men have been known

to be fertile and to have sired normal children.

Beyond the presumption that the fetal testis somehow failed to secrete an adequate amount of *duct-organizing substance,* the etiology of this condition is unknown. Studies with modern chromosomal counting techniques have not yet been reported.

Male Pseudohermaphroditism with Rudimentary Testes. Although it is uncommon to encounter normal-appearing, well-virilized males with internal Müllerian structures, female internal duct structures are often found in males with hypospadias and more severe forms of hermaphroditic external genitalia. In such individuals, rudimentary testes are found either in the broad ligament or somewhere in the path of migration toward the scrotum. Development is frequently asymmetric. This type of male pseudohermaphroditism is more properly considered a form of gonadal dysgenesis (see page 130).

DISORDERS OF SEX DIFFERENTIATION

Errors in Gonadal Differentiation

True Hermaphroditism. In classic terms, true hermaphroditism exists only when both testicular and ovarian tissue are present in the same patient. In this group there may be an *ovary* on one side and a *testis* on the other, an *ovotestis* on each side, or any combination of these structures. These patients are rare, less than 100 authentic examples having been reported in the literature.

The ratio of patients with positive nuclear sex to those with negative nuclear sex is approximately 3 to 1. On a priori grounds it would be anticipated that chromosomal mosaicism would be encountered with the greatest frequency within this group; as of the present, however, this has not been borne out in the few available studies. In those individuals in whom the chromosomal sex has been studied, the karyotype has, for the most part, been euploid, with either an XX or an XY complement of sex chromosomes. It should be recalled, however, that exhaustive studies may be required to demonstrate chromosomal mosaicism, and chromosomal mosaicism limited to the gonads would be missed by studies limited to peripheral cells. In a similar fashion it is possible that further studies will reveal morphologically abnormal chromosomes due to translocations or deletions of small chromosomal fragments.

Clayton has reported a family in which bilateral ovotestes occurred in three siblings. The testicular structure in these individuals was indistinguishable from that in individuals with seminiferous tubular dysgenesis (Klinefelter's syndrome). Other instances of true hermaphroditism occurring within families have been reported, thus opening the possibility that, although the chromosomal morphology is normal, these individuals have inherited mutant sex-determining genes.

Regardless of the chromosomal or genetic make-up, true hermaphroditism may be regarded as arising from an extreme imbalance between the medullary and cortical primordia in one or both gonads, in which either the medullary or the cortical inductor substances have failed to inhibit differentiation of the heterologous component. It is of interest that Bradbury and Bunge have reported structures bearing a strong resemblance to *ova within the lumen of seminiferous tubules* in patients with ovotestes. These inclusions are encountered in tubules immediately adjacent to the ovotesticular junction.

The make-up of the internal genital ducts and external genitalia, in true hermaphroditism, may be predicted from the nature of the gonadal structures. In those individuals with an ovary on one

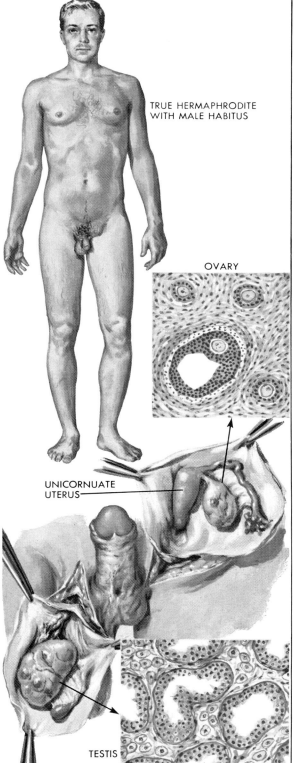

TRUE HERMAPHRODITE WITH MALE HABITUS

OVARY

UNICORNUATE UTERUS

TESTIS

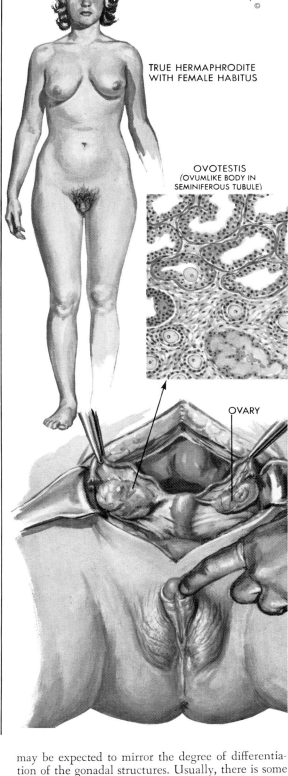

TRUE HERMAPHRODITE WITH FEMALE HABITUS

OVOTESTIS (OVUMLIKE BODY IN SEMINIFEROUS TUBULE)

OVARY

side and a testis on the other, *Müllerian structures* persist on the *side of the ovary,* whereas *atrophy of the Fallopian tube* and *well-developed Wolffian derivatives* are found *on the side of the testis.* The development of Wolffian structures is, in general, proportional to the degree of testicular maturation in those cases where both ovarian and testicular tissue occur on the same side. Where the testis has developed well, the gonadal structures are usually found in the scrotum, and there is a proportional decrease in Müllerian remnants. If the testis is rudimentary, on the other hand, the gonad is usually located in a broad ligament adjacent to a normal uterus. Usually, there is some degree of masculinization of the external genitalia, and the full spectrum of development, through and including a normal phallic urethra, may be encountered.

Adolescence and secondary sexual characteristics

may be expected to mirror the degree of differentiation of the gonadal structures. Usually, there is some amount of masculinization, and this may predominate. There are generally, however, some coincidental signs of active estrogen secretion. The breasts may enlarge, and menstruation may occur.

There is no absolute reason why the gonads in such individuals may not proceed to full spermatogenesis and oögenesis. Spermatogenesis is unlikely, however, if estrogens are secreted in any significant quantity, since they would tend to inhibit pituitary follicle-stimulating hormone, causing atrophy of the germinal epithelium. Regardless of the anatomical findings, it is no longer tenable to regard any form of hermaphroditism as a form of "sex reversal". The "true sex" of these individuals, as in normal males and females, is that one in which they can best adapt to society.

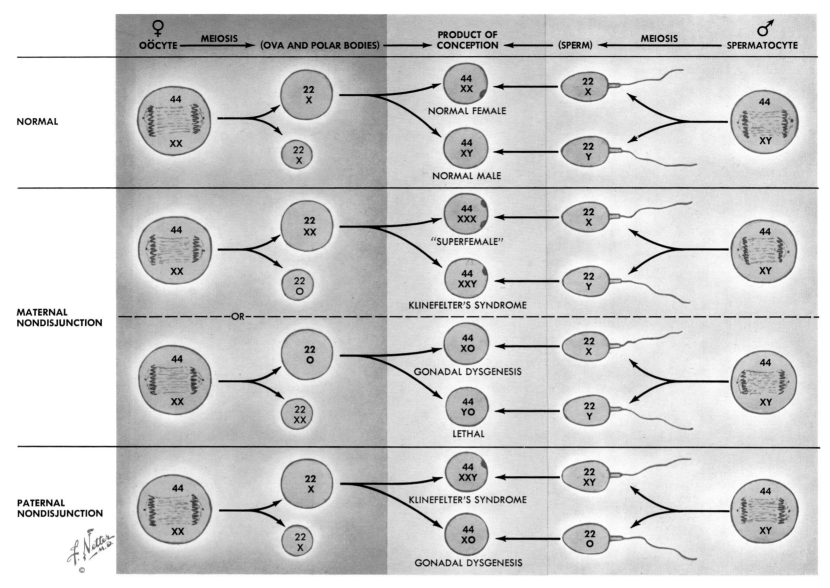

	OÖCYTE	MEIOSIS	(OVA AND POLAR BODIES)	PRODUCT OF CONCEPTION	(SPERM)	MEIOSIS	SPERMATOCYTE

NORMAL

44 XX → 22 X / 22 X

44 XX NORMAL FEMALE ← 22 X
44 XY NORMAL MALE ← 22 Y
← 44 XY

MATERNAL NONDISJUNCTION

44 XX → 22 XX / 22 O

44 XXX "SUPERFEMALE" ← 22 X
44 XXY KLINEFELTER'S SYNDROME ← 22 Y
← 44 XY

—OR—

44 XX → 22 O / 22 XX

44 XO GONADAL DYSGENESIS ← 22 X
44 YO LETHAL ← 22 Y
← 44 XY

PATERNAL NONDISJUNCTION

44 XX → 22 X / 22 X

44 XXY KLINEFELTER'S SYNDROME ← 22 XY
44 XO GONADAL DYSGENESIS ← 22 O
← 44 XY

F. Netter M.D. ©

SECTION IV—PLATE 15

ERRORS IN CHROMOSOMAL SEX

After the technique of determining sex chromatin became available, it was quickly ascertained that about 80 per cent of patients with Turner's syndrome were chromatin-negative and that many individuals with Klinefelter's syndrome were chromatin-positive. For a short time it was erroneously believed that the former group of phenotypic females were "chromosomal males" with an XY constitution, and that the latter group of phenotypic males were, in reality, "chromosomal females" with an XX constitution.

The cell culture technique of actually determining the karyotype soon disclosed, however, that individuals with chromatin-negative Turner's syndrome possessed only 45 chromosomes and that a solitary X chromosome was the only sex chromosome present. Similarly, patients with chromatin-positive Klinefelter's syndrome proved to have an XXY chromosomal constitution. Other sexual anomalies have been associated with XXX and other more bizarre chromosomal patterns. Many of the abnormalities in sex differentiation may now be attributed to errors in chromosomal number or to morphologic abnormalities in the sex chromosomes. A clue to the presence of such abnormalities is often provided by simple observation of the sex chromatin in buccal smears.

Errors in chromosomal number may be caused by faulty cell division of the parental gametocytes in *meiosis* or by faulty mitotic cell division in the zygote after fertilization (mitosis) (see page 112). It should be recalled that, in a normal individual, one of each pair of chromosomes is of paternal origin and the other is of maternal origin. During mitosis, each of the 46 chromosomes replicates itself exactly, so that each daughter cell again has the diploid number. A different process occurs in the production of germ cells, where each *primary spermatocyte* or *primary oöcyte* undergoes two meiotic divisions, to form, respectively, either 4 *sperm cells* or 2 *ova* and 2 *polar bodies*. Each of these cells contains the haploid number of 23 chromosomes. Although one of each chromosomal pair is represented in each ovum or sperm, it is entirely by chance that any given chromosome is of maternal or paternal origin. This process, in a single meiotic division, is illustrated in the upper section of the plate.

Although, ideally, exact halving of the chromosome number during meiosis and exact replication of the 46 chromosomes during mitosis take place, occasionally a chromosome becomes misplaced on the spindle and migrates to the wrong pole. In such instances one daughter cell will contain an extra chromosome, while the other daughter cell will be deficient. This accident, known as nondisjunction, may occur during either meiosis or mitosis. The *Xo individual with Turner's syndrome* or the *XXY individual with Klinefelter's syndrome* can, theoretically, result from either *maternal* or *paternal nondisjunction* during meiosis, but the *XXX "superfemale"* can arise only from maternal nondisjunction.

Studies of aneuploid individuals and their families for various X-linked characteristics, such as color blindness, provide evidence that Klinefelter's syndrome is most often caused by maternal nondisjunction, whereas Turner's syndrome is more frequently due to paternal nondisjunction. This conclusion correlates well with the observation that Klinefelter's syndrome is often associated with advanced maternal age, whereas Turner's syndrome is not.

SEMINIFEROUS TUBULAR DYSGENESIS (KLINEFELTER'S SYNDROME)

Klinefelter's syndrome is one form of faulty gonadal differentiation in which an abnormal make-up of sex chromosomes produces little or no abnormality until the age of adolescence, when *small testes with hyalinized seminiferous tubules* and *clumped Leydig cells, azoospermia, gynecomastia,* mild to moderate degrees of *eunuchoidism,* and, frequently, *elevation of the urinary gonadotropins* develop.

Although nearly always infertile, these patients may show a spectrum of inadequate masculinization ranging from moderately severe eunuchoidism to an almost normal male phenotype. Similarly, although the urinary gonadotropins are usually elevated after adolescence, this is not an essential feature. The degree of gynecomastia is highly variable, its etiology unknown. It is usually most marked in individuals with a tall eunuchoidal habitus and a high titer of urinary gonadotropins. It correlates very poorly with the quantity of estrogenic material excreted in the urine. Thus, it has been suggested that the gynecomastia is a response to the hypersecretion of various mammotropic pituitary hormones.

Characteristically, the *gonads* exhibit an irregular distribution of tubules and tubular scars, separated by loose connective tissue and clumps of Leydig cells. The number of Leydig cells is often increased, and nests of them may assume the configuration of adenomas. Urinary estrogens are somewhat elevated. There is considerable variation in the size of nonhyalinized tubules; some contain only *Sertoli cells,* and others reveal germ cells in early stages of maturation. The basement membrane of the *seminiferous tubules* is thickened and *sclerosed,* and many tubules contain large depositions of hyalin. The elastic membrane is frequently absent or poorly developed. Prior to adolescence, the testes are relatively normal, although subtle changes may be apparent to a pathologist skilled in testicular histopathology.

Since 1956 it has been found that the majority of these patients have 47 chromosomes, including an *XXY pattern* of sex chromosomes; in others seminiferous tubular dysgenesis may be associated with more than one chromatin body in the peripheral cells, and the karyotype may be XXXY or a more bizarre combination (see page 111). These individuals

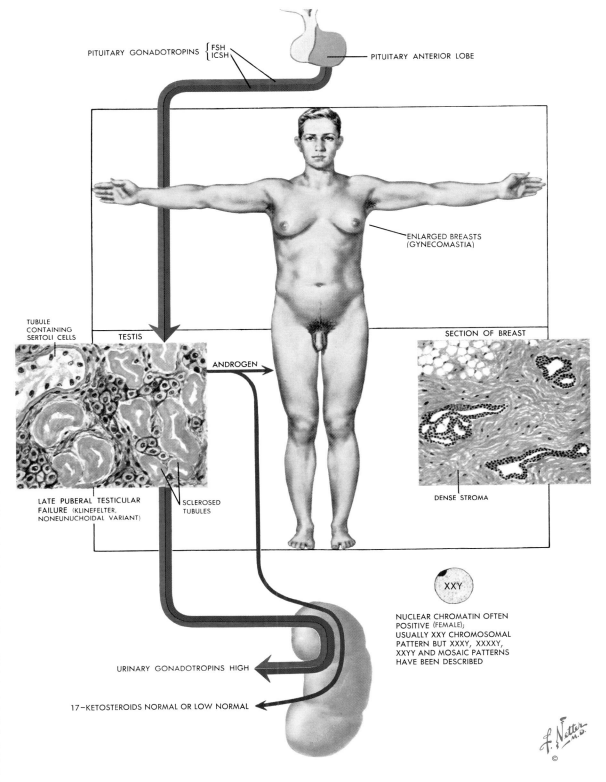

PITUITARY GONADOTROPINS {FSH / ICSH}

PITUITARY ANTERIOR LOBE

ENLARGED BREASTS (GYNECOMASTIA)

TUBULE CONTAINING SERTOLI CELLS

TESTIS

SECTION OF BREAST

ANDROGEN

DENSE STROMA

LATE PUBERAL TESTICULAR FAILURE (KLINEFELTER, NONEUNUCHOIDAL VARIANT)

SCLEROSED TUBULES

XXY

NUCLEAR CHROMATIN OFTEN POSITIVE (FEMALE); USUALLY XXY CHROMOSOMAL PATTERN BUT XXXY, XXXXY, XXYY AND MOSAIC PATTERNS HAVE BEEN DESCRIBED

URINARY GONADOTROPINS HIGH

17-KETOSTEROIDS NORMAL OR LOW NORMAL

usually are more seriously affected, with more severe mental deficiency and other congenital deformities.

The complete clinical syndrome usually associated with chromatin-positive seminiferous tubular dysgenesis may be encountered in the presence of a negative sex chromatin pattern. Testicular abnormalities similar to those in Klinefelter's syndrome can be brought about by irradiation damage, mumps orchitis, or other testicular injury. Such a history cannot usually be elicited, however, from the majority of infertile chromatin-negative men, and chromosomal analysis, likewise, is usually unremarkable. In general, those individuals with a negative chromatin pattern are less severely affected than those with chromosomal abnormalities.

Patients with Klinefelter's syndrome usually do not have multiple somatic abnormalities (as in Turner's syndrome), but they often have mild mental impair-

ment, with, characteristically, an I.Q. between 80 and 105. A high frequency of bizarre ideation bordering on frank schizophrenia is found along with a predilection toward various types of sexual perversion. Inmates of mental institutions have a positive nuclear sex in 1.2 to 2.4 per cent of phenotypic males.

Klinefelter's syndrome is probably the most common abnormality in sex differentiation, with a positive buccal smear in approximately 1 out of every 400 apparently normal newborn males.

Studies with associated sex-linked characteristics, such as color blindness and the Xg sex-linked blood group, indicate that Klinefelter's syndrome can arise by either maternal or paternal nondisjunction, but that maternal nondisjunction is more frequently the cause. This is corroborated by the observation that the mothers of such boys often were elderly when the patients were born.

Gonadal Dysgenesis

Syndrome of Gonadal Dysgenesis (Turner's Syndrome)

As classically described by Turner in 1938, patients with this syndrome are *dwarfed,* sexually *infantile girls* who display a variety of *congenital abnormalities,* such as *webbed neck, cubitus valgus,* and a broad, *shieldlike chest.* The physical similarities are so common that the diagnosis can often be made on sight. Although, initially, it was believed that the dwarfism and sexual infantilism were due to hypopituitarism, this has proved not to be the case, since the *urinary excretion of pituitary gonadotropins* is increased significantly above normal after the first decade of life. Pelvic exploration usually reveals a normal but *infantile uterus* and *Fallopian tubes,* with only *rudimentary gonadal development.* The gonads are usually represented by *fibrous streaks* in the *broad ligament* (see Plate 18). The sexual infantilism in this syndrome is thus secondary to failure in normal gonadal differentiation.

There is an inherent tendency for the genital ducts and *external genitalia* to *feminize,* and this propensity is not dependent on the presence of fetal ovarian tissue. Thus, prior to the advent of techniques to determine the sex-chromatin pattern or chromosomal sex, it was impossible to infer, from their feminine appearance, either the genetic or the gonadal sex of these patients. It has subsequently been the experience of many clinics that approximately *80 per cent* of individuals with classical Turner's syndrome have a *negative nuclear sex (chromatin-negative)* and *20 per cent* have a *positive nuclear sex (chromatin-positive).* Those who are chromatin-positive are indistinguishable, on physical grounds, from those who are chromatin-negative.

Chromatin-negative patients have proved, almost invariably, to lack one of the sex chromosomes. Thus, they have a karyotype of 45 chromosomes with a solitary X sex chromosome. Although such an individual could arise by either maternal or paternal nondisjunction (see page 126), studies with other sex-linked traits indicate that chromatin-negative Turner's syndrome most frequently results from paternal nondisjunction. This correlates well with the observation that advanced maternal age is not usually a factor, as it is so frequently in Mongolism and Klinefelter's syndrome.

Patients with a positive chromatin pattern are less easily understood. Although early reports indicated that these individuals had a karyotype of 46 chromosomes with a normal XX pattern, more detailed studies have shown that at least some patients have chromosomal *mosaicism,* or malformation of an X chromosome. Grumbach and Barr observed Xo/

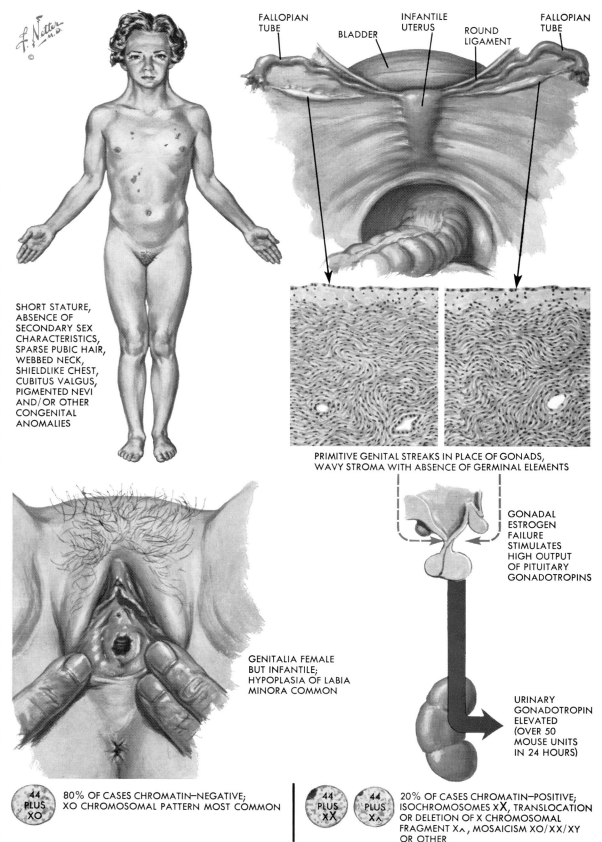

FALLOPIAN TUBE · BLADDER · INFANTILE UTERUS · ROUND LIGAMENT · FALLOPIAN TUBE

SHORT STATURE, ABSENCE OF SECONDARY SEX CHARACTERISTICS, SPARSE PUBIC HAIR, WEBBED NECK, SHIELDLIKE CHEST, CUBITUS VALGUS, PIGMENTED NEVI AND/OR OTHER CONGENITAL ANOMALIES

PRIMITIVE GENITAL STREAKS IN PLACE OF GONADS, WAVY STROMA WITH ABSENCE OF GERMINAL ELEMENTS

GENITALIA FEMALE BUT INFANTILE; HYPOPLASIA OF LABIA MINORA COMMON

GONADAL ESTROGEN FAILURE STIMULATES HIGH OUTPUT OF PITUITARY GONADOTROPINS

URINARY GONADOTROPIN ELEVATED (OVER 50 MOUSE UNITS IN 24 HOURS)

44 PLUS XO — 80% OF CASES CHROMATIN–NEGATIVE; XO CHROMOSOMAL PATTERN MOST COMMON

44 PLUS XX · 44 PLUS XΛ — 20% OF CASES CHROMATIN–POSITIVE; ISOCHROMOSOMES XX, TRANSLOCATION OR DELETION OF X CHROMOSOMAL FRAGMENT XΛ, MOSAICISM XO/XX/XY OR OTHER

XX/XXY mosaicism in one individual. Malformations have taken the form of deletions of parts of the X chromosomes, leaving only a *chromosomal fragment;* inversions of the long and short arms (*isochromosomes*); or *translocations* of chromosomal material to an autosome. Thus, it may be inferred that the failure of gonadal differentiation in this syndrome is usually, if not always, secondary to a deficit of sex-determining genes. The multiple congenital abnormalities usually associated with Turner's syndrome likewise may be attributed to the loss of other types of genetic information normally coded on the sex chromosomes.

ASSOCIATED SOMATIC DEFECTS. Patients with clas-

sical Turner's syndrome rarely reach 5 feet in stature and are usually abnormally short at birth and throughout childhood. The fact that they may display intrauterine growth retardation provides further evidence that the dwarfism is not of pituitary origin. Attempts to induce a more rapid growth rate in these children (by the administration of human growth hormone) have not, so far, been as effective as in control subjects. The bone age is usually normal or only slightly retarded.

In addition to dwarfism, the characteristic physical appearance includes an underdeveloped mandible;

(Continued on page 129)

GONADAL DYSGENESIS

(Continued from page 128)

high, arched palate; broad, shieldlike chest; and widely spaced, hypoplastic nipples. A shortened fourth metacarpal bone is found frequently, as are cubitus valgus and a short neck (often webbed). The hair line in back extends downward to the shoulders. *Pigmented nevi* and telangiectases are common. Abnormalities of the eyes and ears have been described. Coarctation of the aorta and other congenital cardiac malformations, osteoporosis, unexplained hypertension, renal anomalies, and a variety of other defects have been reported. Diabetes mellitus is said to occur with greater frequency than in the general population. The intelligence is usually normal or else only slightly less than that of other members of the family.

Babies with this syndrome often present with edema of the extremities and cutis laxa. The eponymic designation of the Bonnevie-Ulrich syndrome is applied to those patients in whom lymphedema is associated with other stigmata of gonadal dysgenesis.

Gonadal Dysgenesis with Cortical Elements (Plate 18)

Whereas individuals with an Xo sex-chromosomal make-up may be expected to have similar phenotypic characteristics, greater variability could be anticipated among those individuals with mosaicism and less severe morphologic abnormalities of an X chromosome. This has, indeed, proved to be the case, although complete correlations between the phenotype and chromosomal abnormality are not yet possible. In some individuals with other features suggestive of Turner's syndrome, the gonad differentiates beyond its primitive state and may be recognized as a primitive testis or ovary, depending on the preponderance of medullary or cortical elements. The cortex may differentiate to the extent of forming *primordial follicles* which are normal in appearance but *diminished* in number. Patients with a predominance of cortical elements are *more frequently chromatin-positive* than chromatin-negative.

Girls with primordial follicles eventually may experience *some breast enlargement* and scanty menstrual periods. These estrogenic manifestations usually develop late, however, and, at the usual age of adolescence, the classical picture is that of *sexual infantilism,* with elevated *urinary gonadotropins.* Such girls *may or may not exhibit* characteristic *stigmata of Turner's syndrome,* and often they are tall and *eunuchoid* rather than dwarfed. In the least severely affected individuals, there may be only infertility and subnormal development of the estrogen-dependent sexual characteristics. The reproductive difficulties of such women ordinarily would not be recognized as the result of a congenital abnormality in

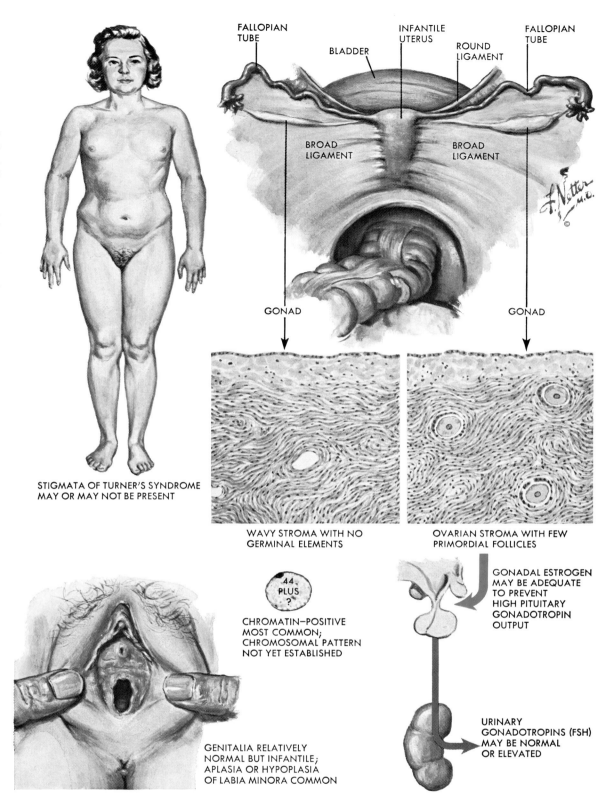

STIGMATA OF TURNER'S SYNDROME MAY OR MAY NOT BE PRESENT

FALLOPIAN TUBE

BLADDER

INFANTILE UTERUS

ROUND LIGAMENT

FALLOPIAN TUBE

BROAD LIGAMENT

BROAD LIGAMENT

GONAD

GONAD

WAVY STROMA WITH NO GERMINAL ELEMENTS

OVARIAN STROMA WITH FEW PRIMORDIAL FOLLICLES

44 PLUS ?

CHROMATIN–POSITIVE MOST COMMON; CHROMOSOMAL PATTERN NOT YET ESTABLISHED

GONADAL ESTROGEN MAY BE ADEQUATE TO PREVENT HIGH PITUITARY GONADOTROPIN OUTPUT

URINARY GONADOTROPINS (FSH) MAY BE NORMAL OR ELEVATED

GENITALIA RELATIVELY NORMAL BUT INFANTILE; APLASIA OR HYPOPLASIA OF LABIA MINORA COMMON

gonadal differentiation; for this reason, the frequency of such mild embryonic defects is not known.

Gonadal Dysgenesis with Medullary Elements (Plate 19)

If the medullary component of the primitive gonad develops beyond its rudimentary stage, it may be expected that the secretion of duct-organizing substances and androgen will parallel the morphologic development of the testis. If the testis remains rudimentary, the genital ducts and external genitalia likewise are ambiguous or hermaphroditic in appearance. Since the duct-organizing substance secreted from a testis exerts its action unilaterally, it is to be expected that asymmetric duct development will occur if the two testes do not mature equally.

In the most primitive of such *rudimentary testes,*

only *rete tubules* and nests of *Leydig cells* can be identified. In other instances, solid cords of cells, resembling the primary sex cords, are enmeshed within an *abundant mesenchymal matrix.* The spectra of testicular development in these cases find their counterparts in all the stages through which a normal testis passes in its embryonic differentiation.

When the genital ducts and external genitalia are unequivocally masculinized, the individual is usually classified as a male pseudohermaphrodite (see Plate 19 and page 124) rather than as an individual with Turner's syndrome. Regardless of the nomenclature, however, it should be recognized that, beginning with the Xo individual with classical Turner's syndrome and totally undifferentiated gonads, there is a steady progression of cases which represent every developmental level in male and female differentiation. In

(Continued on page 130)

GONADAL DYSGENESIS

(Continued from page 129)

this sense, the infertile female with rudimentary ovaries may be regarded as the counterpart of the hypogonadal male pseudohermaphrodite.

The further the phenotype deviates from the classical picture of Turner's syndrome, the more apt one is to encounter karyotypes which deviate from the typical Xo pattern. Thus, those individuals with asymmetric testicular development very frequently are found to be Xo/XY *mosaics*. Presumably, the less-well-developed gonad is derived from a preponderance of primordial cells with an Xo chromosomal constitution, whereas, among the primordial cells entering into the formation of the better testis, there is a higher frequency of *XY cells*.

The hormonal pattern which emerges at adolescence is frequently a recapitulation of the performance of the Leydig cells in utero. Thus, if these cells were sufficiently abundant to produce virilization of the external genitalia in utero, at adolescence they may be expected to produce androgenic hormones and bring about male secondary sexual characteristics. Likewise, gonads in which the cortical elements have differentiated beyond the primitive stage may be expected to bring about some degree of feminization at adolescence.

Considerations in Diagnosis and Management of Patients with Anomalous Sexual Development

In any infant suspected of abnormal sex differentiation, it is vitally important to make sufficient diagnostic studies, during the newborn period, to assign irrevocably the sex in which the child will be reared. Since, normally, the percentage of chromatin-positive cells is reduced for variable periods after birth, prompt establishment of the nuclear characteristic pattern is necessary. For such a differential diagnosis, determination of the nuclear sex chromatin and of the presence or absence of male genital ducts, as judged from the position of the gonads, is of utmost value to the clinician. In addition, chromosomal analyses, determination of the urinary 17-ketosteroids and pregnanetriol (for the exclusion of the adrenogenital syndrome), and, often, urethroscopy and exploratory laparotomy may be necessary before a final assignment of sex can be made. Unless the phallus is of adequate size, it is usually preferable to rear the child as a female. The surgical reconstruction of cosmetically acceptable and functionally adequate female genitalia is more simply accomplished than is the reconstruction of male genitalia.

In the case of true hermaphroditism, gonadal tissue heterologous to the sex of rearing should be removed at an early age, to preclude the emergence of a discordant

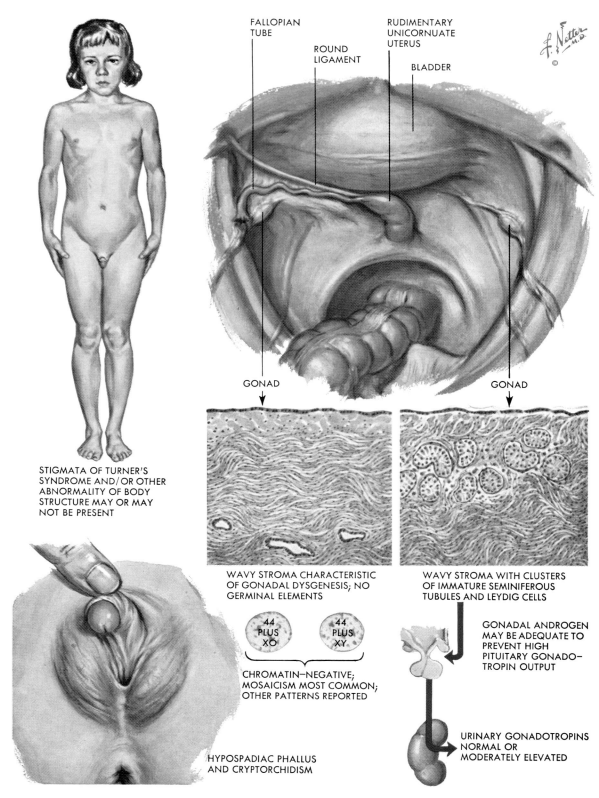

STIGMATA OF TURNER'S SYNDROME AND/OR OTHER ABNORMALITY OF BODY STRUCTURE MAY OR MAY NOT BE PRESENT

FALLOPIAN TUBE

ROUND LIGAMENT

RUDIMENTARY UNICORNUATE UTERUS

BLADDER

GONAD

GONAD

WAVY STROMA CHARACTERISTIC OF GONADAL DYSGENESIS; NO GERMINAL ELEMENTS

WAVY STROMA WITH CLUSTERS OF IMMATURE SEMINIFEROUS TUBULES AND LEYDIG CELLS

44 PLUS XO

44 PLUS XY

CHROMATIN-NEGATIVE; MOSAICISM MOST COMMON; OTHER PATTERNS REPORTED

GONADAL ANDROGEN MAY BE ADEQUATE TO PREVENT HIGH PITUITARY GONADOTROPIN OUTPUT

URINARY GONADOTROPINS NORMAL OR MODERATELY ELEVATED

HYPOSPADIAC PHALLUS AND CRYPTORCHIDISM

hormonal pattern during adolescence. Likewise, dysgenetic gonads, located within the abdomen, are often best removed in childhood to forestall the possibility of future malignancy. In such individuals, lifelong hormonal substitution therapy should be started at adolescence.

With modern techniques of surgical reconstruction, hormonal replacement, and psychologic management, it should now be possible to rear any child with anomalous sexual development in such a way that there will be no sense of ambiguity on the part of the parents or of the child himself. In most instances a satisfactory marital adjustment, in accordance with the sex of rearing, is a reasonable and attainable goal.

One of the most important lessons resulting from studies of individuals who were reared in the sex which was discordant with their chromosomal pattern, nuclear sex, gonadal sex, and genital duct sex

is that sexual orientation and drive are related to none of these things; rather, the gender rôle is an acquired characteristic derived from the early life experiences and environment in which a child is reared. Under normal circumstances the gender rôle is firmly established by the second year of life. Since ambiguous external genitalia, during infancy, form the greatest handicap in adopting a firm conviction of a sexual rôle, if possible, such genitalia should be surgically corrected before that time, in accordance with the assigned sex of rearing. If adequately managed in infancy, even the emergence of a paradoxical hormonal pattern at adolescence will not shake a conviction of gender rôle which has been firmly established. With proper diagnosis and management, anomalous sex differentiation should not, in itself, serve as a bar in the attainment of normal social and sexual relationships.

HIRSUTISM AND VIRILIZATION

The causes of *hirsutism* are many and diverse, from a racial or hereditary disposition toward superfluous hair growth to the advent of hyperplasias or tumors of elements of the adrenal (suprarenal) gland or of the ovary that may be a threat to health. Even minor degrees of hypertrichosis deserve careful consideration; the differential diagnosis necessarily depends on the validity of certain basic physiologic facts. First, each individual has an intrinsic sensitivity to androgenic and other stimuli with regard to hair growth. Widely used drugs may contain enough androgen to induce this response in sensitive individuals but not in the population at large. Second, the adrenal gland produces, in men and women, 17-ketosteroids that are weak androgens, and both ovaries and testes yield some of these, notably dehydroepiandrosterone. Yet the sixtyfold more potent testosterone is not a 17-ketosteroid. In the ovary much of the testosterone is normally transformed into estrogen. When the enzyme systems in either of these endocrine glands are disturbed, an abnormal growth of hair on the face or trunk of the female may be the first sign of the disorder.

Congenital causes of virilization of the newborn female infant include an *enzymatic defect in cortisol metabolism,* so that *ACTH* from the *pituitary* is not inhibited by the normal feedback mechanism, yet the adrenal continues to produce dehydroepiandrosterone and other androgenic precursors signalized by an *increase in the 17-ketosteroid metabolites* in the urine. As a result, *clitoral hypertrophy* and hypertrichosis may be apparent in the newborn. An excess of androgenic steroids from a *secretory ovarian* or *adrenal tumor* in the *pregnant mother,* as with *exogenous androgenic hormones provided in pill form or by injection* in early pregnancy, may cause the same changes, since these steroids can transgress the *placental* barrier into the fetal circulation. In some cases, refined studies of the *chromosomal karyotype* may indicate a condition of pseudohermaphroditism, where the external and internal genitalia may show phenotypic incongruity resulting from a *mosaic* pattern that has occurred early in embryonic life.

Secondary hirsutism and virilization may result from *androgenic prescriptions* or hormone preparations that may be metabolized into potent androgens by some individuals. In *old age,* facial hair is

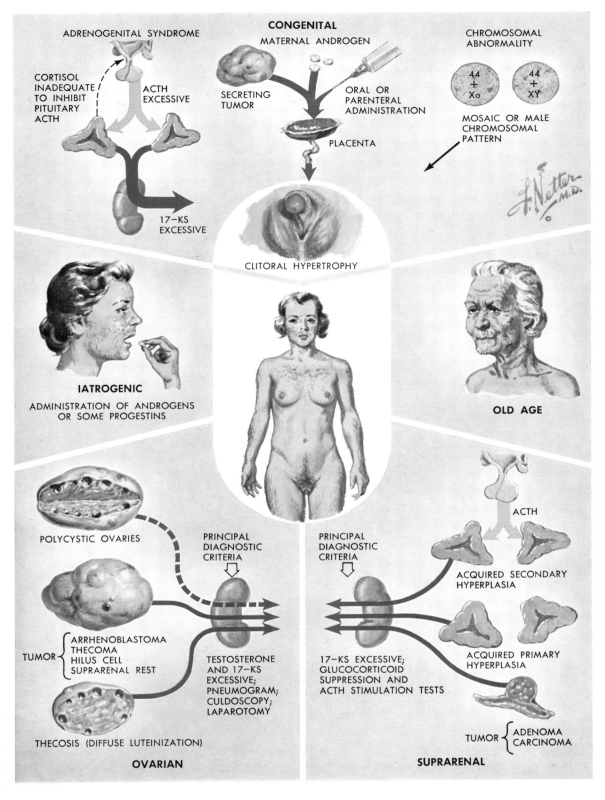

considered the result of adrenal androgenic corticoids that are not balanced by any of the estrogenic hormones after the time of ovarian failure at the menopause.

The more common causes of secondary hirsutism are seen in ovarian or adrenal disorders. With *ovarian disorders,* hirsutism is usually a concomitant to complaints of obesity, amenorrhea, and infertility. In most such cases, only a slight elevation of *17-ketosteroids* is found in the urine, but *testosterone* is significantly elevated. The diagnosis of *polycystic* (Stein-Leventhal) *ovaries* can be confirmed by *culdoscopy, pneumograms,* or *laparotomy.* Wedge resection and puncture of the multiple cysts often reduce excess androgen in these cases. *Masculinizing tumors of the ovary* can usually be totally excised, but a diffuse pattern of *stromal luteinization (thecosis)* cannot be corrected without complete gonadectomy.

Secondary adrenal causes of hirsutism and virilization may be due to a disturbance, primarily in cortisol metabolism, similar to that seen in congenital adrenal hyperplasia. Another group of cases derives from a *primary hyperplasia* of the adrenal cortex, a condition that can usually be differentiated from an adrenal adenoma or carcinoma by using either stimulation or suppression tests (see pages 88 and 94). A tumor, whether benign (*adenoma*) or malignant (*carcinoma*) tends to be autonomous; secretion of excessive 17-ketosteroids is not often increased, in such cases, by giving ACTH or suppressed by adequate doses of a glucocorticoid, in contrast to the response in functional adrenal hyperplasia.

From the psychological as well as the functional points of view, these complaints cannot be disregarded, and our diagnostic criteria for the causes of hirsutism and virilization are improving.

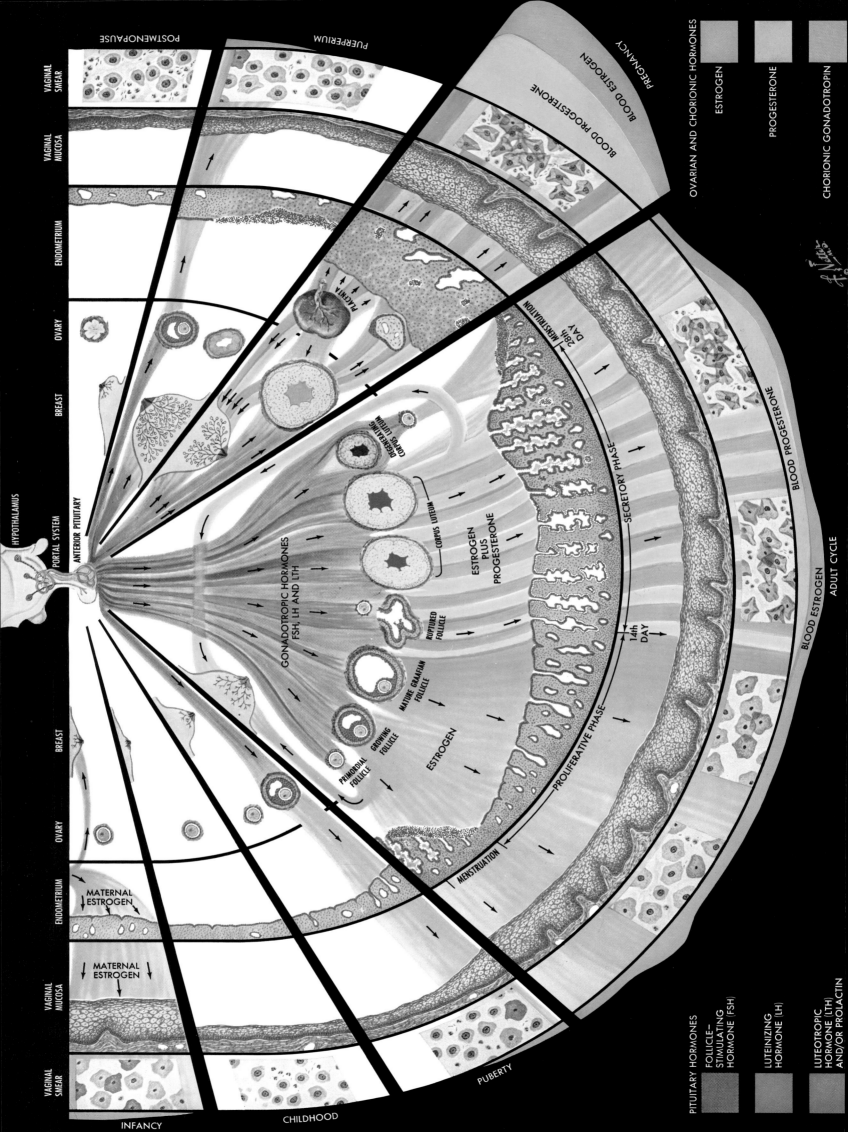

INFLUENCE OF GONADAL HORMONES ON THE FEMALE REPRODUCTIVE CYCLE FROM BIRTH TO OLD AGE

From birth to old age, all female mammals exhibit a succession of biologic events characterized by the phases of infancy, childhood, puberty (sexual maturation), the adult reproductive years, and, finally, postmenopause and senility. The physiologic indices that differentiate one phase from another are induced primarily by the secretion of ovarian estrogens.

Although ovulation may be considered the chief function of the ovaries, their production of estrogens and gestagens is no less essential to maintain and nourish all parts of the procreative apparatus and to play a part also in the function and maintenance of skin, hair growth, and the skeletal, vascular, and electrolyte systems. Finally, the effects of these hormones, in achieving emotional stability during adolescence, have their counterpart in psychological changes associated with estrogen deficiency after the menopause or following ovariectomy.

In the newborn infant there is abundant evidence that the placenta has provided no barrier to the high concentration of maternal estrogens prior to parturition. The female infant's breasts may show some enlargement, and witch's milk can occasionally be expressed from the nipples. The external genitalia are precociously developed, and the endometrium has been stimulated to proliferate. The vaginal mucosa is a manycelled layer of stratified epithelium. Vaginal smears are relatively free from pus cells and show the large, flat, polygonal cells characterized as estrogen-stimulated by their small pyknotic nuclei and extensive cornification.

Within a week or so after birth, all the above stigmata of estrogen stimulation recede. The newborn ovaries are small structures made up entirely of primordial follicles, disclosing no elements capable of producing estrogens.

In the decade of childhood, from the postnatal recessional changes to the time of puberty, the ovaries gradually show a buildup of interstitial tissue from an accumulation of fibrous stroma, as a constant succession of primordial follicles degenerate in atresia. The vaginal smear shows predominantly basal and parabasal cells mixed with bacteria and amorphous debris. The breasts remain infantile.

In the initiation of puberty, it is probable that pituitary maturation and consequent secretion of gonadotropins may well depend on higher centers in the hypothalamus, releasing some humoral factor into the hypophysial portal circulation at the time of puberty. The infant hypophysis has been found to contain gonadotropins. The infant ovary, in rodents, when grafted into a mature individual, is shown to be capable of response. A child's secondary sex organs will develop at any time, if they are subjected to estrogenic stimulation, yet such evidence is not usually seen until the young girl is at least 8 years old.

The uterus is first to respond to estrogenic hormones. The endometrium proliferates with the development of straight, tubular glands. Next, the vagina thickens and becomes stratified, with cornified superficial estrogenic cells appearing in the vaginal smear. In the ovary, primordial follicles progress beyond the stage of a one- or two-layer granulosa with a tiny antrum, and exhibit identifiable several-thickness granulosa and theca interna layers. In the breast, the areolae show pigmentation along with a domelike change, becoming elevated as a conical protuberance. Fat is deposited about the shoulder girdle, hips, and buttocks, and the adult pelvic and, later, the axillary hair patterns typical of the female begin to develop.

An intricate balance of stimulation and response between pituitary gonadotropins and ovarian steroids is essential for the proper sequence of events that result in normal ovulatory cycles. In adolescence as well as at menopause, minor disturbances are responsible for irregular, anovulatory uterine bleeding.

In the mature cycle, the upper two thirds of the endometrium are sloughed away in the first 48 to 72 hours of menstruation; the bleeding surface is rapidly repaired in the following 2 or 3 days from a spreading proliferation of epithelium from broken glands and arterioles, under the stimulus of estrogen secreted by numbers of ovarian follicles in response to follicle-stimulating hormone (FSH) from the anterior pituitary. By day 12 in a typical 28-day cycle, one follicle attains ascendancy and exhibits a rapid growth toward maturity, associated with thickening of the proliferative endometrium and increased desquamation of precornified and cornified cells from the vagina. The release of luteinizing hormone (LH) at midcycle on day 14 is responsible for ovulation of the mature follicle and for initiation of progesterone excretion from the rapidly forming corpus luteum, which is continued by luteotropic hormone (LTH), or prolactin. Endometrial glands become sawtoothed and secretory; the vaginal smear shows a regression toward intermediate cell types that are clumped together, with folded and wrinkled cytoplasm. If fertilization and implantation do not occur, the corpus luteum degenerates on about day 26, and, in consequence, with the rapid withdrawal of its estrogen and progesterone secretion, the endometrium shrinks, becomes ischemic, and breaks away with bleeding on day 28.

Through the changes described above, the juvenile breast has become mature, with branching and extension of both ducts (estrogens) and alveoli (progesterone). Toward the latter half of the cycle, there is often congestion of the lobules, with an increased sensitivity of the areolae and nipples.

Both estrogen and, to a lesser extent, progesterone are associated with not only the transient accumulation of edema fluid in the endometrium (most marked in the secretory phase) but, at times, a diffuse premenstrual edema in peripheral tissues, clinically recognized by subjective complaints of bloating, increased girth, and weight gain.

In the decade of adolescence, the skeletal system reacts to estrogen, first, by an accelerated growth rate of the long bones, and, second, by a hastening of epiphysial closure, the balance affecting final height.

When conception occurs, the early excretion of chorionic gonadotropin from the chorionic elements of a securely implanted embryo maintains the corpus luteum, preventing it from degenerating in 2 weeks. Thus, gonadotropin must become effective at least by day 25 or 26 of a standard cycle, although the titer is not high enough to be detected by any present tests until a few days after the typical menstrual flow was due. In pregnancy the peak production of chorionic hormone is seen by about day 90 after the last menstrual period, declining thereafter to a plateau. The corpus luteum is responsible for increasing progesterone and estrogens throughout the first 3 months, after which the placenta takes over until the end of the pregnancy. The augmentation of both estrogen and progesterone is approximately linear throughout the 9 months of gestation, accounting for the cessation of any demonstrable ovarian activity through the suppression of effective pituitary FSH and LH. The breasts react to the increasing steroid stimulation with an extension of both ductile and alveolar growth, and there is congestion without actual lactation. The vaginal smear shows the marked effect of the increased progesterone level, with massive clumping of the cells and the appearance of a particular form from the intermediate layer, called the navicular cell of pregnancy.

The puerperium is an inconstant phase of endocrine readjustment. The massive withdrawal of estrogen after placental delivery and the psychoneural mechanisms initiated by the suckling reflex bring about the release of prolactin, or lactogenic, hormone. Breast tissues, already conditioned by growth, respond with milk production. Ovarian activity is held in abeyance, during lactation and nursing, for several months in many cases, and even for a year or more, at times. However, reestablishment of the pituitary-ovarian cycle can, and often does, take place before weaning, so that another conception can occur before the advent of a menstrual flow. The raw and bleeding endometrial bed of the placental attachment takes from days to weeks to reepithelialize. The vaginal mucosa is thin, and the smear is relatively atrophic until ovarian estrogen is again produced.

In the United States menopause occurs late in the fourth or early in the fifth decade (mean age 49 ± 2). The ovaries no longer contain any follicles capable of responding to pituitary stimulation. Increasing amounts of FSH are built up, in the absence of any estrogen response. This estrogen deficiency is reflected by senile changes in the breasts, uterus, and vagina, also in the skin, bony skeleton, and vascular system.

The dominant factor in controlling endocrine relationships in the female reproductive tract is thus seen to be estrogen. Childhood and senility represent phases of tranquillity in gonadal activity. Proper hormonal interaction through the menstrual cycle, pregnancy, and the puerperium are determined fundamentally by appropriate modulations of estrogenic secretions.

133

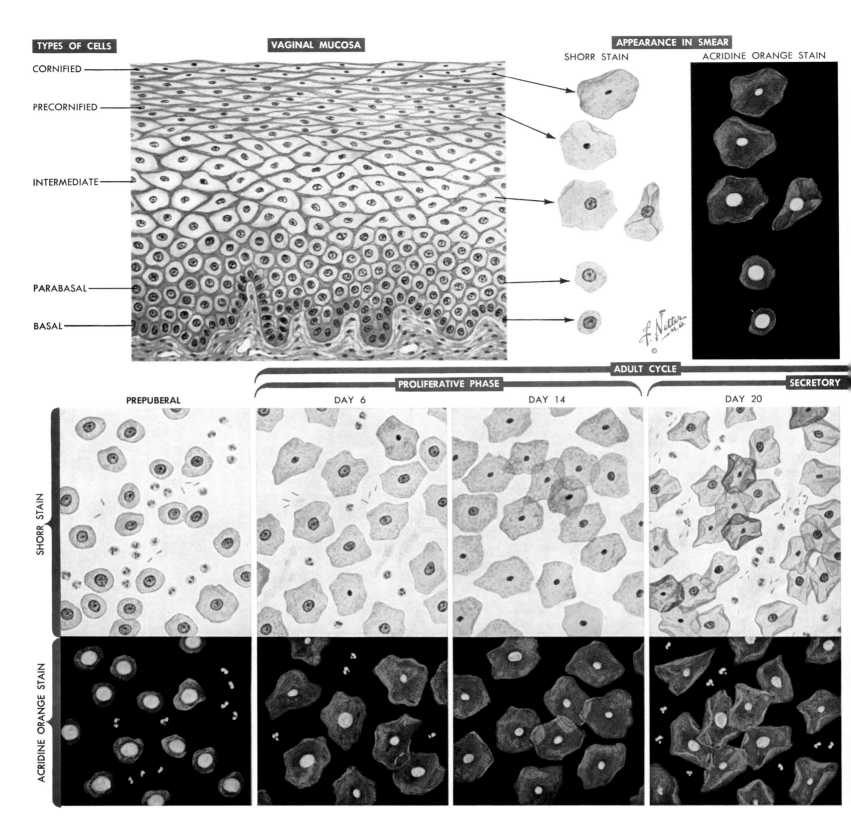

VAGINAL CYTOLOGY

As long ago as 1847, it was noted that cytological changes occur in the vaginal epithelium throughout the reproductive cycle in the human being. For many years, the only available test for estrogen from body fluids was an appropriate extraction technique; then came injection of the extract into immature or castrated rodents; and, finally, an evaluation of the vaginal smear from these animals, for specific estrogenic effects. At the present time the *vaginal smear* from the patient herself provides one of the easiest, most direct, and most economical tests for any steroid hormone. Recently, the *sediment from a voided urine specimen* has been shown to contain epithelial cells washed from the lower urethra, a structure with an embryologic derivation similar to that of the vagina, and, in the same way, these cells mirror ovarian steroid production.

In the fully *mature vaginal mucosa, five types of cells* are easily identifiable, from the lowest *basal layer* upward to the fully *cornified layer.* The *Shorr Trichrome staining technique* is widely used for its simplicity; the 10-second *acridine orange stain,* as modified by H. L. Riva and T. R. Turner, although involving *fluorescent microscopy,* provides startlingly clear cellular details.

Vaginal smears are best taken from the *middle third of the mucosa* after introduction of a Graves *speculum.* A *cotton-tipped applicator,* moistened with saline, is rubbed on the epithelial surface. It is then rotated on an albumin-coated *slide,* to release the cells. In preparing *urinary smears,* 50 ml from a freshly *voided specimen* are *centrifuged* for 10 minutes at 2000 rpm; the *supernatant* is *decanted, sediment* is *picked up* on the swab, and the *cells* are *spread* on the *slide.* Rapid fixation in alcohol ether is critical.

Cytological smears reveal not only the quantitative changes in estrogen but also the effect of progesterone.

In the *prepuberal* state, and also *postmenopausally,* the mucosa of the vagina and lower urethra is a thin layer made up almost entirely of *basal* and *parabasal cells.* The nuclei are large and round or oval; with acridine orange, using a critical acid pH, the DNA of the nucleus takes a yellow stain against the green of the cytoplasm,

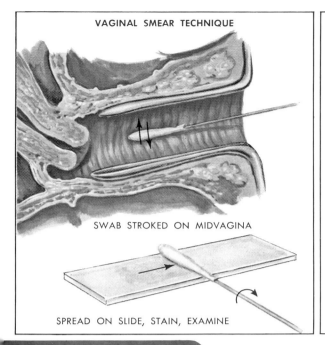

VAGINAL SMEAR TECHNIQUE

SWAB STROKED ON MIDVAGINA

SPREAD ON SLIDE, STAIN, EXAMINE

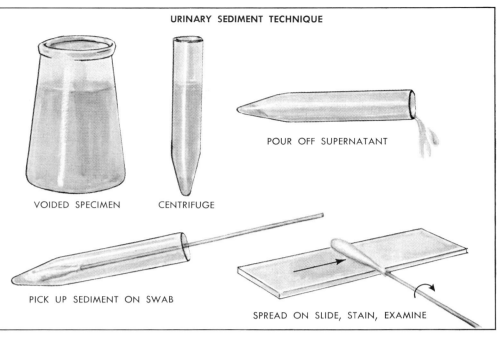

URINARY SEDIMENT TECHNIQUE

VOIDED SPECIMEN   CENTRIFUGE

POUR OFF SUPERNATANT

PICK UP SEDIMENT ON SWAB

SPREAD ON SLIDE, STAIN, EXAMINE

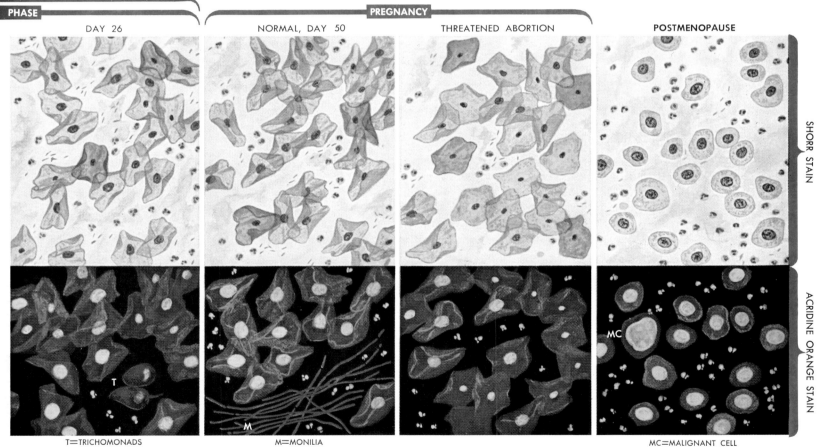

PHASE

PREGNANCY

| DAY 26 | NORMAL, DAY 50 | THREATENED ABORTION | POSTMENOPAUSE |

SHORR STAIN

ACRIDINE ORANGE STAIN

T=TRICHOMONADS   M=MONILIA   MC=MALIGNANT CELL

set against a black background. Bacteria are abundant, and these stain a bright red or red-orange.

In the normal menstrual cycle, by *day 6* most of the cells are from the *intermediate layer*, with *vesicular nuclei* and *polygonal, basophilic cytoplasm* (using Shorr's stain). At the time of ovulation, about *day 14,* these cells have progressed, under the peak stimulus of estrogen, to show a majority of *precornified cells* with *small pyknotic nuclei* and at least 20 per cent or more of fully cornified cells that take an acidophilic stain and may or may not have lost their nuclei. In the acridine orange preparation it is the *reduced size of the nuclei* that differentiates this increase in estrogenic stimulation from that found earlier in the cycle. *Bacteria are minimal or absent.*

By *day 20* in the normal cycle, ovulation has occurred, and the addition of progesterone to estrogen can clearly be noted. There is an increased number of *desquamated cells,* which are predominantly and progressively intermediate in type as the *secretory phase* develops. In contrast to the flat, *separated,* clearly outlined *cells of the proliferative phase,* in the latter half of the cycle, during the secretory phase, a *clumping together,* loss of cellular outline, and *wrinkling* and *folding* of the cell margins can be seen. Bacteria reappear. All these features, by *day 26,* give a "dirty" appearance to the slide; with Shorr stain, the cells are almost all *basophilic* again. Using acridine orange, amorphous clusters of cells are distinguished only by their relatively *large yellow nuclei. Trichomonads,* when present, take a brilliant red stain, shared by all other

microorganisms.

The above characteristics of a progesterone effect are continued and enhanced in the first trimester of *pregnancy.* In a *threatened abortion* due to progesterone deficiency, one of the earliest prognostic signs is a return of precornified or acidophilic cornified cells, with their dense, small nuclei. When these average 30 per cent or more of all the cells, the prognosis for the pregnancy is poor.

With acridine orange, the filaments of *monilia* stand out in bright red. In a *postmenopausal smear,* the large, eccentric nucleus of a *malignant cell* is easily observed.

The interpretation, by a trained cytologist, of the above changes, as seen in a series of vaginal or urinary smears, adds an important dimension to female endocrinology.

FUNCTIONAL AND PATHOLOGICAL CAUSES OF UTERINE BLEEDING

The *uterine mucosa* is the only tissue in the body in which the regular, periodic occurrence of necrosis and desquamation with bleeding is usually a sign of health rather than of disease. This periodic blood loss is controlled through a delicate balance of pituitary and ovarian hormones and results from the specific response of the target tissue, the *endometrium*. The normal ebb and flow of *estrogen* and *progesterone*, through a monthly cycle, first builds up and then takes away, in regular sequence, the support of the endometrium; therefore, a menstrual flow, characterized by repeated regularity in timing, amount, and duration of bleeding, bears witness to a normal and ordered chain of endocrine events for that individual. Irregularity in any of these characteristics suggests a functional disturbance or organic pathology. The major categories of pathologic states that can cause or be accompanied by either menorrhagia (heavy or prolonged flow) or metrorrhagia (spotting or bleeding between menstrual flows) are discussed below.

The concept of bleeding due to a *decrease* or *withdrawal of ovarian steroids* explains the unpredictable flow associated with persistent estrogen phases and anovulatory cycles. In the *normal cycle* a progressive *increase in estrogen production*, with a sharp rise from the maturing follicle toward the fourteenth day, causes a parallel development of all elements in the endometrium — stroma, glands, and coiled superficial arteries. At or soon after *ovulation,* the advent of progesterone from the *corpus luteum* slows up growth and proliferation and modifies the tissue into a secretory pattern. If conception and pregnancy do not occur, then the corpus luteum regresses in 14 days; its production of both estrogen and progesterone wanes; there are shrinkage of the endometrium, congestion of the nutrient arteries, anoxemia, necrosis, and desquamation. Occasionally, irregular shedding from an *imbalance* of the *estrogen-progesterone ratio,* producing a mixed *endometrium* with both proliferative and *secretory* glands in an *abnormal* luteal phase pattern, may cause menorrhagia. *Persistent estrogen production* from a series of follicles that fail to ovulate tends to build up a *hyperplastic endometrium* in which nests of *anaplastic glands* may develop. The circulating level of estrogen fluctuates in accordance with haphazard spurts of follicle growth. Sporadic reduction in circulating estrogen, spontaneously or through medication, undermines the vascular support of the uterine mucosa and initiates the changes inevitably followed by necrosis and bleeding. In *old age the hypoplastic, estrogen-deficient endometrium* some-

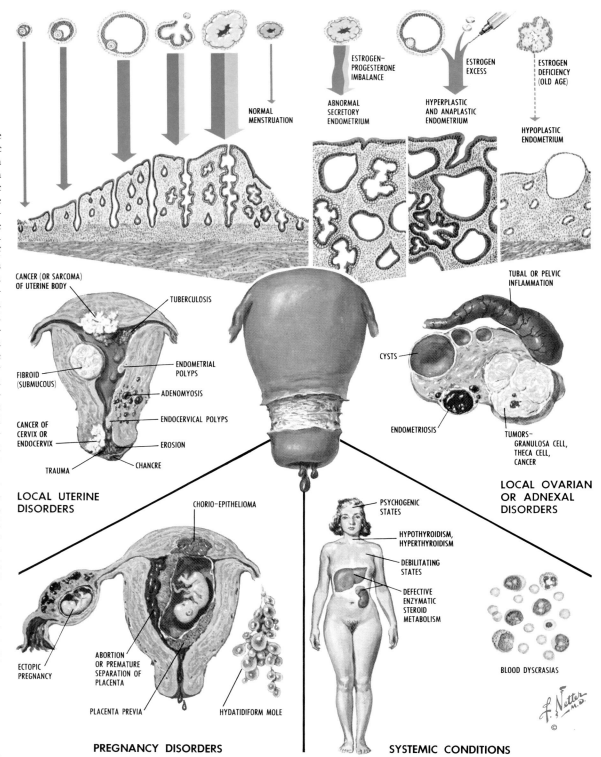

STEROID WITHDRAWAL BLEEDING

NORMAL MENSTRUATION

ESTROGEN-PROGESTERONE IMBALANCE — ABNORMAL SECRETORY ENDOMETRIUM

ESTROGEN EXCESS — HYPERPLASTIC AND ANAPLASTIC ENDOMETRIUM

ESTROGEN DEFICIENCY (OLD AGE) — HYPOPLASTIC ENDOMETRIUM

LOCAL UTERINE DISORDERS

CANCER (OR SARCOMA) OF UTERINE BODY
TUBERCULOSIS
FIBROID (SUBMUCOUS)
ENDOMETRIAL POLYPS
ADENOMYOSIS
CANCER OF CERVIX OR ENDOCERVIX
ENDOCERVICAL POLYPS
EROSION
TRAUMA
CHANCRE

LOCAL OVARIAN OR ADNEXAL DISORDERS

TUBAL OR PELVIC INFLAMMATION
CYSTS
ENDOMETRIOSIS
TUMORS— GRANULOSA CELL, THECA CELL, CANCER

PREGNANCY DISORDERS

CHORIO-EPITHELIOMA
ECTOPIC PREGNANCY
ABORTION OR PREMATURE SEPARATION OF PLACENTA
PLACENTA PREVIA
HYDATIDIFORM MOLE

SYSTEMIC CONDITIONS

PSYCHOGENIC STATES
HYPOTHYROIDISM, HYPERTHYROIDISM
DEBILITATING STATES
DEFECTIVE ENZYMATIC STEROID METABOLISM
BLOOD DYSCRASIAS

times breaks down and bleeds from a vulnerability to mild trauma or infection.

Local uterine disorders causing abnormal bleeding include *malignancy* of the *corpus* or *cervix,* benign *submucous fibroids* and *polyps, adenomyosis,* external *trauma* from force or noxious chemicals, and infections such as *tuberculosis* or a syphilitic *chancre.* Childbirth lacerations or *erosions* are, only rarely, the sole cause for undue bleeding.

Local ovarian or adnexal disorders may involve primary malignancies, including those *cystic* or *solid ovarian tumors* that secrete steroid compounds. *Pelvic inflammatory disease* and *endometriosis* may also cause irregular bleeding.

Pregnancy disorders, due not only to *placental dislocations* or to deficiencies as illustrated under systemic conditions, but also to *ectopic gestation* or degenerative conditions such as *hydatidiform mole*

or *chorio-epithelioma,* constitute the most frequent causes of uterine hemorrhage.

A variety of *systemic conditions* may be responsible for abnormal bleeding. Conditions such as *blood dyscrasias,* leukemia, purpura, scurvy, etc., usually show signs of bleeding elsewhere. Chronic and *debilitating disease states,* including iron-deficiency anemia and either *hypo-* or *hyperthyroidism,* can produce abnormal flow as well as undermine placental function. *Defects in steroid metabolism* or excretion, by the *liver* or *kidneys,* may produce a buildup in circulating estrogen, with consequent endometrial effects. Sometimes, *psychogenic states* appear to be the only causative factor for menstrual hemorrhage.

The confusing diversity of endocrine, neoplastic, gestational, and systemic conditions responsible for abnormal uterine bleeding presents a challenge to the diagnostic ability of the clinician.

DIAGNOSTIC STUDIES IN INFERTILITY

The Female Partner

The history (preferably obtained, at least in part, in the presence of the husband) must be complete, since it may provide important diagnostic clues. A detailed summary of the menstrual, obstetrical, and medicosurgical history yields information pertaining to ovulation and to incidents that may have adversely affected ovarian, tubal, uterine, and cervical factors in the fertility potential. Adequacy of coital practices should be investigated, and psychiatric screening is often helpful.

The physical examination must be general. In addition to evidence of gynecological infections and congenital anomalies, stigmata of endocrine disturbance should be sought. Routine laboratory tests include blood count, sedimentation rate, urinalysis, serology, blood typing, Rh factor, and chest X-ray. If an endocrine abnormality is suspected, especially if there is amenorrhea, determinations of the urinary 17-ketosteroids (and, in the future, urinary testosterone), 17-hydroxycorticoids, gonadotropins, basal metabolism rate, and serum protein-bound iodine, as well as a lateral film of the sella turcica, are indicated.

Methods for detecting ovulation, based essentially on various means of evaluating progestational activity, are of prime importance. The most useful and practical procedures are the following:

The *basal body temperature* (BBT) *curve,* a continuous graph of waking temperatures, is taken under basal conditions, just before the patient arises in the morning. Relatively lower levels are present during the preovulatory phase than in the postovulatory phase. The presence of a biphasic curve is suggestive, but not definite, evidence of ovulation. Even when ovulation occurs, it may take place a few days before or after the low point of the thermal shift.

Endometrial biopsy (see CIBA COLLECTION, Vol. 2, page 122) reveals the effects of progesterone (*viz.,* the secretory changes in the glands and in their glycogen-filled cells) and associated modifications of the stroma appearing after ovulation has occurred (see CIBA COLLECTION, Vol. 2, pages 118 and 119). It is a simple office procedure, preferably performed on the first menstrual day so as not to interfere with a fertilized ovum if one is present. The test furnishes presumptive, but not conclusive, evidence of ovulation.

Serial vaginal smears (see CIBA COLLECTION, Vol. 2, page 122) reveal a maximum number of cornified cells (reflecting a corresponding peak level of estrogen) at or just prior to ovulation (see page 134 and CIBA COLLECTION, Vol. 2, pages 108 and 109). Since it is necessary to observe a constantly changing cytology, single smears are of no value. Also, vaginal infections, as with

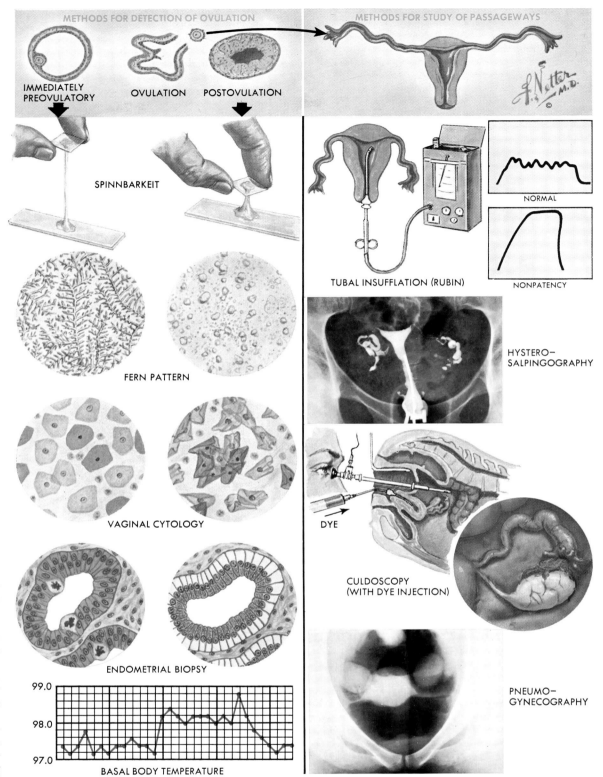

Trichomonas, may induce pseudocornification.

The *cervical mucus* is suitably studied in conjunction with the postcoital test. The latter provides a means of evaluating both the male and female under physiological conditions. It determines the adequacy of coital techniques, the receptiveness of the cervical mucus, and the quality of sperm migration. The mucus is withdrawn from the cervix, by aspiration or nasal polyp forceps, 12 to 18 hours after coitus at or near the estimated ovulation date. First, its *Spinnbarkeit* is tested. Immediately before ovulation, cervical mucus (under the influence of estrogen) is thin, clear, and stretchable up to 15 to 20 cm; at other times it is thick and viscid, and stretches only a few centimeters. Second, a drop is examined microscopically for leukocytes and live active sperm. Third, a heat-dried preparation is examined for *fern pattern.* This crystallization occurs under estrogen stimulation

but is inhibited by progesterone; *i.e.,* the arborization phenomenon is present before, but not after, ovulation.

Methods for studying passageways are necessary, in selected cases, after a study of possible physiological causes has been completed. *Tubal* status may be determined, before ovulation, by *insufflation* (employing CO_2), *hysterosalpingography* (which affords a good picture of the endometrial cavity), and *culdoscopy with dye injection,* to observe the tubes directly as well as the emission, through the fimbria, of dye instilled through the cervix (see CIBA COLLECTION, Vol. 2, page 123). Culdoscopy also provides for gross inspection of the ovaries. Additional data on the size of the ovaries and uterus are afforded by *pneumogynecography,* which consists of a flat film of the pelvis after introduction of CO_2 into the peritoneal cavity, with the patient's legs elevated.

DIAGNOSTIC STUDIES IN INFERTILITY

The Male Partner

It is estimated that somewhat under 50 per cent of barren marriages are attributable to the male. Certain items in the history are particularly important. These include mumps orchitis followed by fibrosis of the testes; diabetes mellitus; sexual habits such as those associated with inadequate erections, impotence, failure of ejaculation or intromission, and infrequent coitus; and noxious habits (excessive alcohol or tobacco, overeating). Some occupations and dress customs may result in deleterious increases in scrotal temperatures, with a marked fall in sperm count. Physical examination should be complete, with particular reference to congenital abnormalities (cryptorchidism, hypospadias), genital conditions (testicular atrophy, marked varicocele, prostatovesiculitis), and over- or undernutrition. Routine laboratory tests include serology, blood count, sedimentation rate, urinalysis, prostatic fluid examination, and chest X-ray. If an endocrine basis is suspected, determinations of urinary 17-ketosteroids, testosterone, gonadotropins, basal metabolic rate, and serum protein-bound iodine may be helpful.

The single most important diagnostic study is the *semen analysis*. The specimen, obtained after 4 days of sexual abstinence and produced by masturbation or coitus interruptus, is collected in a clean glass container and submitted for analysis within 2 hours. Care must be exercised to ensure completeness of the collection. Its fertility potential is evaluated in the light of several independent factors for which accurate criteria of normalcy are not yet fully delineated.

The freshly ejaculated specimen is a whitish coagulum which usually *liquefies* in about 15 minutes. Prolonged high viscosity suggests the possibility of interference with sperm migration. The normal *volume* is between 2.5 and 5 ml. Semen is almost always slightly alkaline, with a pH of about 7.7, so that a pH determination is rarely helpful in the over-all interpretation. In normal adult males the *sperm count* (performed in a hemacytometer) is quite variable and usually higher than 60 million per cubic millimeter. However, levels as low as 20 million per cubic millimeter are found in fertile men, provided the *motility* is good. Initially, the *percentage* of motile forms is 80 to 85. Another factor of importance is the *quality of motility* (progress forward), which is graded entirely subjectively. *Duration of motility* is another criterion. Two hours after liquefaction 60 to 70 per cent of the sperm should be actively motile. Estimations of motility are usually made again after 4, 6, and 24 hours. During the first 6 hours

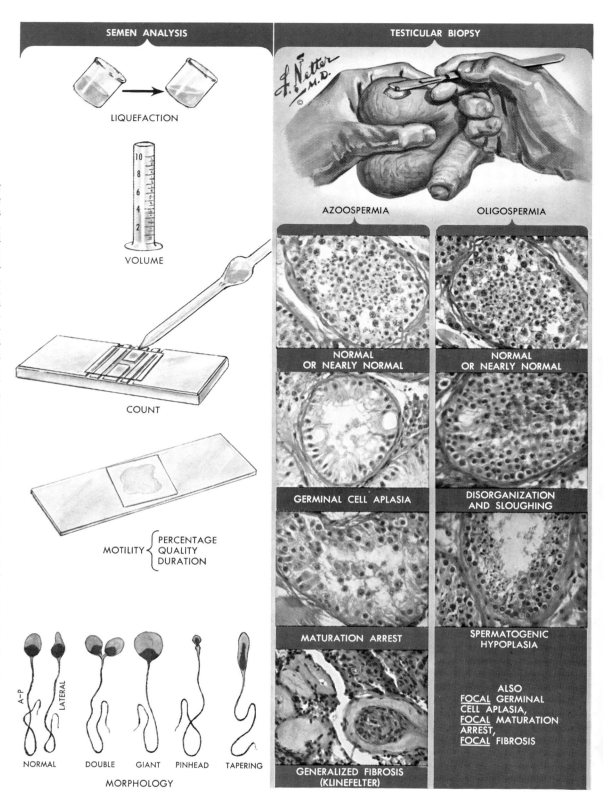

there is usually a decline in motile forms of about 10 per cent per hour. At the end of 24 hours an occasional, moderately active, sperm is found in a normal specimen.

The proportion of sperm with abnormal *morphology* is ascertained by oil immersion examination of a stained smear. Abnormal forms (which do not exceed 15 to 20 per cent in normal semen) include *double, giant, pinhead,* amorphous, and *tapering,* the last being particularly significant in male infertility. Determinations of seminal fructose levels may be helpful in the evaluation of androgenically normal azoospermic men. The absence of fructose, in such an instance, points to a bilateral congenital abnormality of the efferent duct system, presumably associated with seminal vesicle aplasia. In general, it should be emphasized that the semen quality of an individual is subject to considerable variation. Accordingly, it is

advisable to have at least two examinations before regarding the findings as truly indicative of the fertility potential.

In the presence of *azoospermia* and *oligospermia*, additional information for prognosis and therapeutic possibilities may be provided by *testicular biopsy* (see also CIBA COLLECTION, Vol. 2, page 86). About one fourth of all men with azoospermia have *normal* testicular histology (indicating duct obstruction, which may be surgically remediable). Among the remainder, the findings include *germinal cell aplasia, maturation arrest,* and *generalized fibrosis*. Normal histology is also found in occasional oligospermic men. About one half of the latter show *disorganization of the seminal epithelium, with excessive sloughing of cells*. *Spermatogenic hypoplasia* and *focal germinal cell aplasia, arrest,* or tubular *fibrosis* compose the remainder (see CIBA COLLECTION, Vol. 2, pages 77 and 79).

GYNECOMASTIA

Enlargement of the male breast, owing to an increase in its glandular component, is known as gynecomastia (see also CIBA COLLECTION, Vol. 2, page 251). The *degree of enlargement* is very variable, ranging from a barely visible, small, central, subareolar disk of mammary tissue to the proportions of a normal female adolescent breast. It may be unilateral or bilateral, is frequently painful and tender, and, occasionally, emits a secretion. Its presence is sometimes difficult to ascertain in obese males, since their breast enlargement may be due entirely, or in large part, to fat deposition (pseudogynecomastia).

The *histopathology* is characterized by stimulation of ducts and proliferation of stroma. The ducts undergo lengthening and branching, with budding and formation of new ducts but no alveoli. Epithelial hyperplasia occurs. Simultaneously, there is an increase in the bulk of the stromal tissue, which is often hyalinized. Stromal replacement of adipose tissue and periductal infiltrations with round cells are common. Since these changes may be induced by the administration of estrogen to males or to unstimulated females, it is logical to seek a similar explanation in patients with gynecomastia, but efforts in this direction have been only partly successful, especially because the condition is encountered in a great variety of apparently unrelated pathological disorders. Easier to explain is its occurrence in certain physiologic states.

PHYSIOLOGIC STATES. *Neonatally,* slight transitory breast enlargement is common in both sexes. This is presumably due primarily to high levels of *maternal estrogens.* Gynecomastia, often slight, bilateral, and frequently painful, occurs in about two thirds of boys during *puberty.* It subsides spontaneously within 2 to 4 years in over 90 per cent of cases. *Involutional* enlargement occurs in some men later in life.

PATHOLOGICAL CONDITIONS. Superficially, these appear to be divisible into *endocrine* and *nonendocrine disorders.* Analysis of the clinicopathological features of large series of cases reported in the literature provides a unitary concept for a pathogenetic mechanism which is applicable in most, if not all, patients. Chronic hyperestrogenism, possibly synergized by the action of one or more anterior pituitary hormones (*i.e.*, growth hormone) appears to be the principal etiologic factor. Estrogenic preponderance (without overt feminization) may arise by increased estrogen production, impaired estrogen inactivation, and reduced androgen elaboration, or even increased androgen production by virtue of the conversion of androgens to estrogens. Augmented mammary sensitivity to circulating estrogens may explain certain innocuous familial cases, among others.

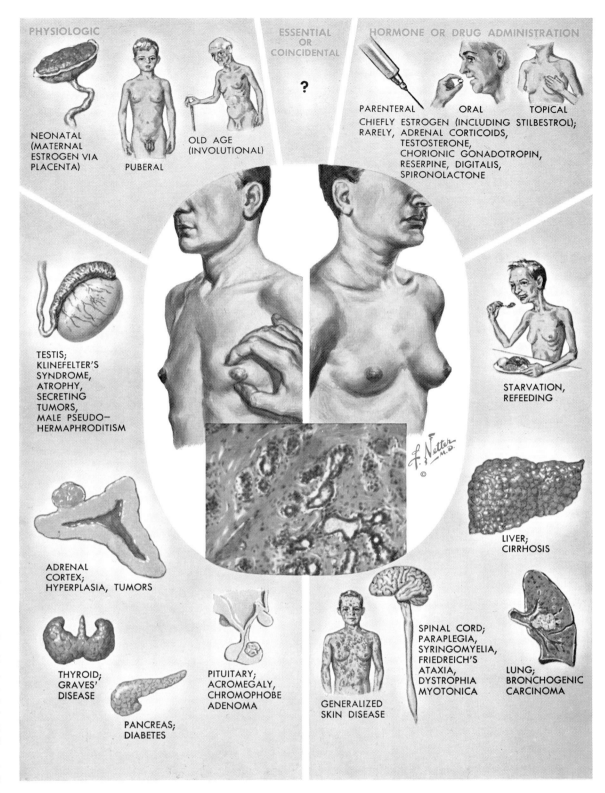

In most pathological conditions involving the endocrine glands (as well as in the aforementioned physiologic states), hypothetical or actual hyperestrogenism (absolute or relative) is readily and rationally invoked. It is much more difficult to demonstrate evidence of endocrine imbalance in the large variety of nonendocrine pathological disorders accompanied by gynecomastia. Besides, the association in some of these may be entirely fortuitous. Urinary hormonal assays are usually of little diagnostic help.

In general, gynecomastia appearing in or after the third decade of life is most often a manifestation of a serious underlying disease. Examples are *disorders of the testis* (tumors, hypogonadism, *male pseudohermaphroditism*), *adrenal cortex* (tumor, hyperplasia), *thyroid* (hyperthyroidism) and *pituitary* (acromegaly, chromophobe adenoma). Other disorders, not originating in endocrine glands, include *liver cirrhosis,*

malnutrition, *refeeding after starvation, bronchogenic carcinoma,* traumatic *paraplegia,* and *generalized* exfoliative *dermatitis.* Furthermore, gynecomastia readily develops after the prolonged *administration of estrogens* and estrogen-contaminated *drugs.* It also occurs infrequently after treatment with *testosterone* (in hypogonadism), *chorionic gonadotropin, digitalis, spironolactone,* and *reserpine. Diabetes mellitus* and many other miscellaneous conditions are, very seldom, accompanied by gynecomastia.

A prerequisite for treatment is thorough diagnostic investigation. Hormonal therapy is of no avail. Mammoplasty is indicated exclusively for cosmetic reasons and only when spontaneous regression has not taken place. This surgical procedure usually improves the patient's ability to carry on a normal social life as a male, preventing recurrent embarrassment due to the feminine breast development.

GALACTORRHEA

Galactorrhea (abnormal lactation) refers to the mammary secretion of milky fluid, which is nonphysiological in that it may be *persistent,* excessive, and *unrelated to a recent pregnancy.* (The onset may date back to a normal postpartum lactation which failed to stop.) *Amenorrhea* (which may or may not precede the lactation), genital atrophy, and other evidences of *estrogen deficiency* are frequent but not invariable. Pathological lactation occurs very seldom in females and extremely rarely in males.

For *normal lactation* and galactopoiesis (maintenance of lactation), the basic requirements include optimal amounts of hormones: from the anterior pituitary gland, *prolactin* and *somatotropic* (growth) *hormone;* from the adrenals, *adrenal corticoids;* from the ovaries, *estrogens* for duct formation and *progesterone* for lobule-alveolar development; and thyroid in a permissive fashion. *Suckling* apparently has a dual action — one in stimulating the release of prolactin, the other in promoting the secretion, by the neurohypophysis, of *oxytocin* (see page 32). The latter presumably leads to the contraction of the myo-epithelial cells of the mammary acini, thereby providing for the free flow of milk into the larger ducts.

The factors operative in abnormal lactation are much less clear, especially in view of the large variety of clinical conditions with which it is associated. In most instances the galactorrhea can be traced to an organic functional intracranial disorder, involving particularly the pituitary-hypothalamic structures. The final and effective link in the various pathogenetic mechanisms appears to be an unphysiological production of one or more adenohypophysial tropic hormones, *i.e., prolactin* or *somatotropin* (growth hormone), the latter having well-defined galactopoietic properties.

By further analogy with normal lactation, mechanical and psychic as well as humoral components seem to play a rôle. On the other hand, abnormal lactation is relatively rare in the various disease states occasionally associated with lactation, many of which are quite common. It is thus necessary to postulate increased end-organ sensitiveness or an intangible predisposition to lactation to explain it in connection with the various predisposing conditions.

Among the better-known and more frequent causes of galactorrhea are *pituitary tumors,* with or without *acromegaly.* Eosinophilic, chromophobe, or basophilic neoplasms may be present. Galactorrhea and amenorrhea may be the first symptoms, so that, even when no tumor can be demonstrated, it is advisable to suspect this lesion in an incipient form. Other organic brain lesions include encephalitis, meningitis, and trauma. *Dysfunctional pituitary disorders*

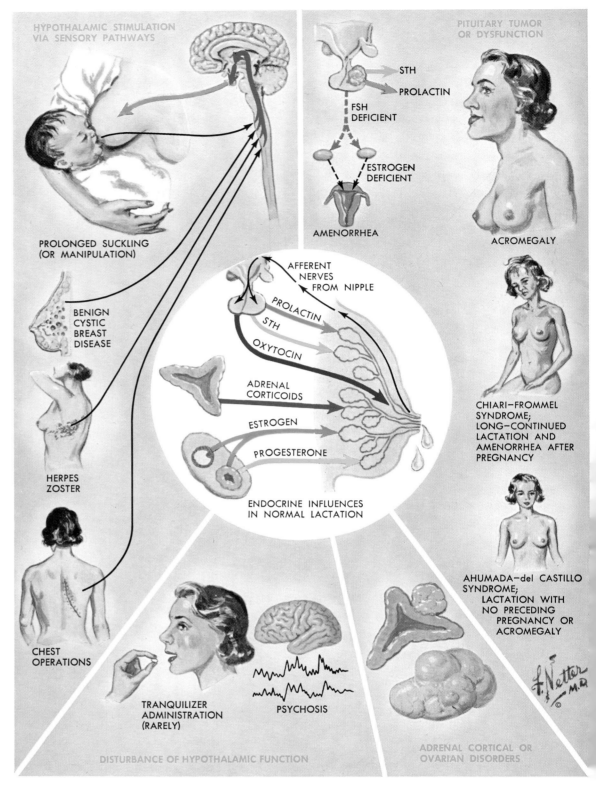

include the rare *Chiari-Frommel syndrome* (follows pregnancy, some cases due to unrecognized pituitary tumor, others to primary ovarian failure), the *Ahumada-del Castillo syndrome* (not related to pregnancy or acromegaly, some due to pituitary neoplasm, others to selective hyperpituitarism), Sheehan's syndrome (selective hypopituitarism), and juvenile hypothyroidism with precocious menstruation (Van Wyk and Grumbach). The possibility of compensatory pituitary adenoma cannot be excluded in these cases.

Galactorrhea also occurs in some *psychoses* and in certain patients receiving large doses of *tranquilizers* (phenothiazine derivatives, Rauwolfia alkaloids or meprobamate), suggesting *hypothalamic involvement.* The pathogenetic mechanisms in *prolonged suckling, benign cystic breast disease,* dorsal *herpes zoster,* or *chest operations* presumably involve stimulation of the sensory reflex arc from the chest region to the

hypothalamus. Other associated conditions include *adrenal cortical* or *ovarian disorders,* such as adrenal cortical hyperfunction (tumor, hyperplasia), menopause (physiological and precocious), castration, and *ovarian tumors.* Sparse cyclic premenstrual lactation has been noted.

Galactorrhea has been recorded in males with adrenal, testicular, and pituitary tumors, the last with or without acromegaly. Gynecomastia need not be present. In some instances, evidences of malfunction of the pituitary, adrenals, or testes could not be demonstrated. Scant lactation has been induced in a male transvestite by intensive hormonal and manipulative treatment (Foss).

Therapy is quite unsatisfactory, except when the cause is found and removed. Manipulation of the breast should be avoided as much as possible so as not to induce lactation.

Section V

THE PANCREAS
(ENDOCRINE FUNCTION)
CARBOHYDRATE METABOLISM

by

FRANK H. NETTER, M.D.

in collaboration with

RACHMIEL LEVINE, M.D.
Plates 1-31

NORMAL HISTOLOGY OF PANCREATIC ISLETS

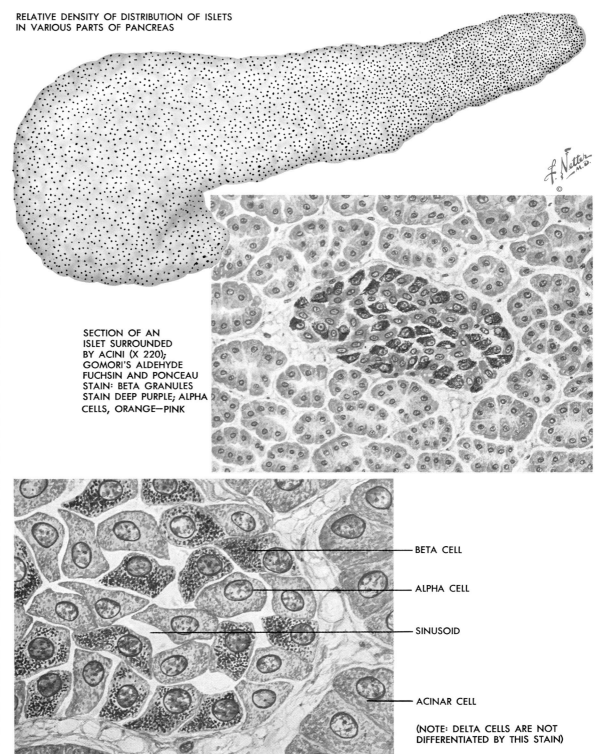

SECTION OF AN
ISLET SURROUNDED
BY ACINI (X 220);
GOMORI'S ALDEHYDE
FUCHSIN AND PONCEAU
STAIN: BETA GRANULES
STAIN DEEP PURPLE; ALPHA
CELLS, ORANGE—PINK

BETA CELL

ALPHA CELL

SINUSOID

ACINAR CELL

(NOTE: DELTA CELLS ARE NOT
DIFFERENTIATED BY THIS STAIN)

PORTION OF ISLET GREATLY MAGNIFIED (X 1200); GOMORI'S ALDEHYDE FUCHSIN AND PONCEAU STAIN

In 1682 Brunner, after removing nearly all the pancreas from a number of dogs, described resulting symptoms (polydipsia and polyuria) which were suggestive of diabetes mellitus. Cawley, 100 years later (1788), reported finding multiple pancreatic calculi and general destruction of the pancreas at autopsy of a diabetic. No correlation of these isolated findings was made, however, until the time was ripe for the consideration of humoral regulating "messengers". In 1869 Paul Langerhans described the existence, within the pancreas, of islets of cells unconnected to the pancreatic ducts, but he did not assign any specific function to them. At the same time, the physiological studies of Hedon established these islets as a "scattered" gland of internal secretion. Laguesse, in 1883, suggested the secretion of some hypoglycemic factor by the islets of Langerhans, but the definitive relationship of the pancreas to diabetes mellitus was not established until 1889, when Minkowski produced the syndrome, in dogs, by total extirpation of the gland. He then drew renewed attention to the findings of Langerhans, linking them with the cause of diabetes.

The normal *adult human pancreas* contains about 1,000,000 *islets,* which are scattered about the *acini* and are nearly twice as numerous in the *tail* of the gland as in the *neck* and *body*. The total weight is from 60 to 100 gm, of which the islets represent about 1.5 per cent, or about 0.9 to 1.5 gm. Individual islets measure about 75 by 150 microns, but, occasionally, islets with a diameter up to 300 microns are seen. The polygonal islets contain several types of cells: *alpha cells,* which are probably the seat of glucagon production; C cells and delta cells, of unknown function; and *beta cells,* which manufacture, store, and secrete insulin and which constitute 60 to 80 per cent of the total cells of each islet. The Gomori aldehyde fuchsin and Ponceau technique stains the insulin-containing granules a deep bluish-purple, whereas the alpha cells appear pink or red.

The pancreas arises, from the anlage of the duodenum, in two portions which normally fuse (see CIBA COLLECTION, Vol. 3/III, page 25). In man, the islets appear by the end of the third month of fetal life. The specific secretory cells arise from the epithelium of the small ducts of the pancreas. The islets are surrounded by loops of capillaries and sinusoids, but few lymphatics. Thus, a direct route for the hormones into the blood stream is provided.

The fact that the BETA CELL is the seat of insulin synthesis, storage, and secretion is attested to by (1) the strict parallelism between the abundance of granules and the content of insulin; (2) the observation that beta granules are the only cellular structures of the islet to which specific insulin antibodies can be attached (see page 145); and (3) the effect of alloxan, which produces diabetes by injuring the beta cells without visible changes in the alpha cell system.

The composition and intimate molecular architecture of the beta cell granule are not known. Obviously, aggregating forces and substances are present, which hold many insulin molecules together in an insoluble, packaged form, demonstrable (in a variety of shapes, in different species) by electron microscopy (see page 144).

Zinc is present, in islet tissue, in comparatively large amounts. Studies suggest that this metal may be the complexing agent which maintains the beta granule in aggregated form. Zinc seems to be released from the cells by the same stimulants and at the same time as insulin. However, zinc is not a necessary, integral part of the insulin molecule for the exercise of its hormonal actions.

The relationship of ALPHA CELLS to glucagon production rests on fairly good general evidence. The distribution of extractable glucagon, from various portions of the pancreas, parallels the relative abundance of alpha cells, and these cells stain with fluorescent antibodies specific to glucagon (see page 145). Their selective damage by cobalt salts and by synthalin A (decamethylenediguanidine) is not as specific a procedure as is the alloxan effect on the beta system.

ELECTRON MICROSCOPY OF THE BETA CELL

In recent years, advances in the techniques of histochemistry and electron microscopy have provided a clearer picture of the relationship between cell structure and the chemical events linked to it.

After insulin is synthesized in the *beta cell*, it is stored in distinct secretory *granules,* each of which is enclosed in a little *sac* with a double membrane. The *shapes* of the *granules* are characteristic for particular *animal species; e.g.,* those in *man* are spherical, in contrast to the rod-shaped structures in the *dog.* Direct evidence for the presence of insulin in the secretory granules is provided by the demonstration that these structures combine with the fluorescent antibody specific to the hormone (see page 145). It must be assumed that the synthesis of insulin, from the constituent amino acids (see page 146), takes place along the endoplasmic reticulum of the cell through the synthetic activity of the ribosomes, which are attached to the reticulum (see pages 218 and 219). The resulting insulin granule is enclosed in a *capsular sac* derived from the reticulum. The *mitochondria* and the *Golgi apparatus* comprise the powerhouse of the cell, providing highly organized loci for enzyme-controlled oxidative processes leading to the formation of adenosine triphosphate (ATP), which is the ultimate source of energy for the synthesis of insulin. The sausage-shaped mitochondria measure 15,000 by 5,000 Å (one angstrom unit equals a ten millionth of a millimeter), and the insulin granules are considerably smaller.

Under normal circumstances the *membranous capsules* containing the insulin, which are situated close to the cell membrane, coalesce with it, leading to a *discharge* of the granules *into the extracellular spaces.* When the blood sugar level rises, it stimulates, by an as yet unknown mechanism, the migration and solubilization of the secretory granules, which migrate from the cell interior toward the cell membrane, leading to a more rapid rate of extrusion of insulin from the cell. Characteristic changes may be demonstrated in the Golgi apparatus during insulin secretion. Glucose

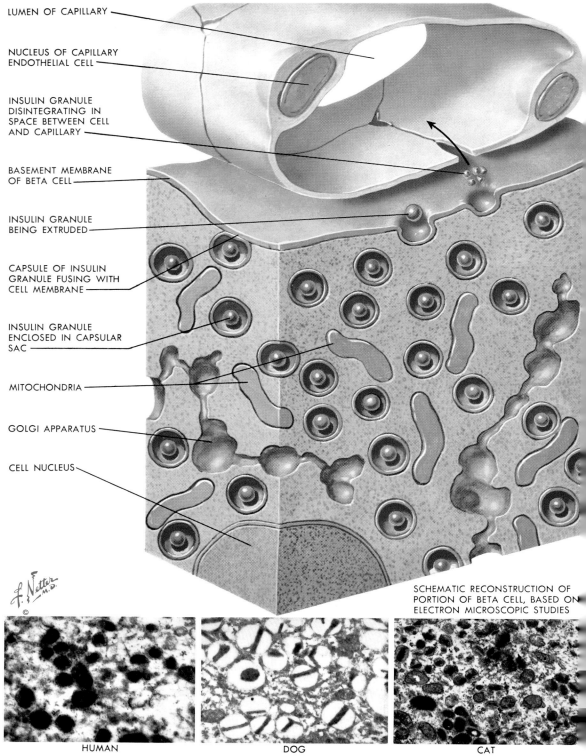

LUMEN OF CAPILLARY

NUCLEUS OF CAPILLARY ENDOTHELIAL CELL

INSULIN GRANULE DISINTEGRATING IN SPACE BETWEEN CELL AND CAPILLARY

BASEMENT MEMBRANE OF BETA CELL

INSULIN GRANULE BEING EXTRUDED

CAPSULE OF INSULIN GRANULE FUSING WITH CELL MEMBRANE

INSULIN GRANULE ENCLOSED IN CAPSULAR SAC

MITOCHONDRIA

GOLGI APPARATUS

CELL NUCLEUS

SCHEMATIC RECONSTRUCTION OF PORTION OF BETA CELL, BASED ON ELECTRON MICROSCOPIC STUDIES

HUMAN   DOG   CAT

ELECTRON MICROSCOPIC APPEARANCE OF INSULIN GRANULES OF VARIOUS SPECIES

seems to be the specific hexose which exerts a significant insulin-discharging activity. Closely related mannose acts similarly. One group of oral antidiabetic drugs, the sulfonylureas, exerts an action similar to that of glucose. The hypoglycemic effect of these drugs depends primarily on their ability to cause a moderate insulin discharge, but they also appear to have a tropic effect on the proliferation of islets.

In sensitive infants, the amino acid leucine and some of its derivatives produce hypoglycemia by accelerating insulin extrusion from the beta cells. The islets of certain fish have been shown to respond to leucine rather than to glucose. In individuals who are normally not sensitive to leucine, pretreatment with one of the sulfonylureas induces a brief period of leucine sensitivity.

Within a very short time after the administration of alloxan, accelerated insulin discharge is seen. This

is soon obscured by its specific toxic effect, which causes irreversible degeneration of the beta cells.

Recently, it has been found that individuals possessing the genetic traits for diabetes (close relatives of overly hyperglycemic patients) may suffer from hypoglycemia 3 to 4 hours after the ingestion of a carbohydrate meal. Nearly all obese subjects exhibit an exaggerated insulin response to glucose, and overweight is now considered one of the most important prediabetic conditions. Rats, artificially overfed, have been shown to have grossly enlarged islets of Langerhans. These observations suggest that the prediabetic patient may, for a time, manifest a compensatory hyperplasia of the islets and may possess beta cells which are hyperreactive (for varying periods prior to eventual decompensation and the onset of frank clinical diabetes) to the normal stimulus for insulin discharge.

Demonstration of Insulin in the Pancreatic Islets

The biosynthesis of insulin and its control are not yet fully understood (see page 144). Since the insulin molecule consists of 2 peptide chains, one may assume, by analogy with the 2-chain molecule of hemoglobin, that two genetic loci dictate its assembly. The visible *granule*, seen by light microscopy, consists of a large number of insulin molecules, held together in unknown fashion. Also unknown are the other materials associated with the hormone in its storage form.

The presence of *insulin* can be unequivocally demonstrated by the technique of the *fluorescent antibody* (Coons). The accompanying illustration, based on the work of Lacy, shows a *normal islet* of a *rabbit pancreas* to which has been added insulin antibody produced in the serum of a properly immunized guinea pig. The combination of antibody with insulin, in the beta cells, leads to localization of the fluorescence exclusively in the beta cells. Normal human islets show the same type of reaction. Curiously, however, sections made from most human insulinomas do not react with fluorescent antibody. The reason may be that the cell membranes of such tumor cells are not penetrated by the antibody molecules. Equally possible is that the insulin molecule produced by an adenoma or carcinoma may actually show a somewhat different amino acid sequence or spatial configuration (compared with the normal one) which would abolish the antibody-binding capacity without changing its usual biological effects.

The beta cell does not seem to depend on outside trophic support, at least to any significant degree. Interruption of the vagal nerve supply does not lead to histological or secretory changes. Removal of the anterior pituitary does not cause atrophic changes in the islets. Some evidence shows that, after hypophysectomy, the amount of stored and secreted insulin is diminished, but no specific trophic factor can be demonstrated in pituitary extracts. An excess of growth hormone, glucocorticoids, or thyroid hormones stimulates and, eventually, may exhaust the beta cells. The most likely explanation of the effects of these substances is that they lead to hyperglycemia (which has been shown to be a potent stimulus to insulin secretion in isolated preparations of pancreas) and not that they act directly on the beta cell.

The physiological stimulus to insulin secretion is undoubtedly the level of the blood sugar itself. It is interesting that the two endocrine glands which are in-

INSULIN DEMONSTRATED IN BETA CELLS OF RABBIT ISLET BY MEANS OF INSULIN—SPECIFIC ANTIBODIES WHICH HAVE BEEN MADE FLUORESCENT BY ADDITION OF FLUORESCIN

DEXTROSE INJECTED (5 g/kg BODY WEIGHT). THIS STIMULATES OUTPUT OF INSULIN

½   1   2   3   4   5   6   HOURS

½ HOUR AFTER INTRAPERITONEAL DEXTROSE INJECTION: BETA CELLS DEPLETED OF INSULIN GRANULES

6 HOURS AFTER INJECTION: INSULIN GRANULES RESTORED IN BETA CELLS; ISLET SECTION HAS RESTING STAGE APPEARANCE

dependent of neurotrophic or pituitary influence are regulated by the substrates on which they act. These are the parathyroid, in relation to ionized calcium, and the beta cells, in relation to glucose. A rise in blood *glucose* stimulates insulin output and raises its level in the blood. In the *beta cell* the *insulin granules disappear*. When the glucose level is brought down again to a normal value, *restitution of granules* becomes evident. A lowered blood sugar (fasting, phlorhizin, insulin) is associated with a lessened insulin release, and the beta cell is said to be in a resting stage.

The hyperplastic and hypertrophic islets found in newborn infants of diabetic mothers are, presumably, the result of the hyperglycemic environment during fetal life.

Other substances (metabolites and drugs) are known to influence insulin secretion. Thus, in some

children, the amino acid leucine and its related compounds evoke insulin release. They raise insulin secretion in many hyperfunctioning tumors, but not in the vast majority of normal human beings.

The sulfonylureas, employed in the treatment of some cases of adult-onset diabetes, exert their effect by causing insulin release from the beta cell granules, whether the blood sugar is high or low. Some evidence indicates that these drugs may also lead to beta cell proliferation, or that they may stimulate the formation of new beta cells from the epithelium of the small pancreatic ducts.

Alloxan seems directly cytotoxic to the beta cell. Recent evidence indicates that it may interfere with normal insulin release, perhaps by inactivating the active release mechanism, at low dosage, after which the cell and its insulin content are completely destroyed as the dosage is increased.

CHEMICAL STRUCTURE OF INSULIN AND GLUCAGON

As early as 1909, De Meyer suggested the name "insuline" for the hormone produced by the islets of Langerhans. In 1921 Banting and Best extracted the first consistently potent insulin, which was used almost immediately in the therapy of human diabetes. Its chemical behavior, during further purification, was that of a simple protein. It contained the usual array of *amino acids,* with an uncommonly high percentage of cystine. In 1956 Frederick Sanger, completing a brilliant 10-year study, elucidated the amino acid sequence of insulin.

The hormone has a molecular weight of about 6000 and consists of 2 *polypeptide chains (A and B).* The *A chain,* of *21 amino acids,* contains an *internal S-S bridge.* The *B chain* contains *30 amino acids.* The A and B chains are linked by *2 S-S bridges.* A number of models of the tridimensional structure have been proposed.

The structure shown here is that of beef insulin. It is evident that some chemical differences exist between the insulins of various species, since interspecies antibodies can be produced. This is borne out by amino acid analyses, showing small differences in the number of certain amino acid residues in insulins of the various species examined. These variations seem to be confined mainly to the components of the *intrachain ring* lying between the *sixth* and the *eleventh residues* of the A chain. The known differences are:

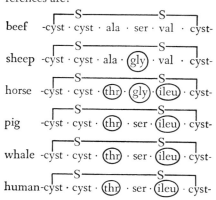

In the foregoing table the amino acid residues which are ringed indicate differences as compared with beef insulin. Note the chemical identity of pig and whale to human insulin within the S-S ring.

Based on this evidence, one would expect antibody formation to parallel the extent of differences in amino acid composition of the insulins of the various species. This, however, is only partly the case; it appears that different molecular configurations may also play a rôle. The hormone obtained from the whale pancreas is identical in composition to human insulin, but it gives rise to antibodies in man. Hog insulin has the same amino acids, at positions 8, 9, and 10 of the A chain, as does that obtained

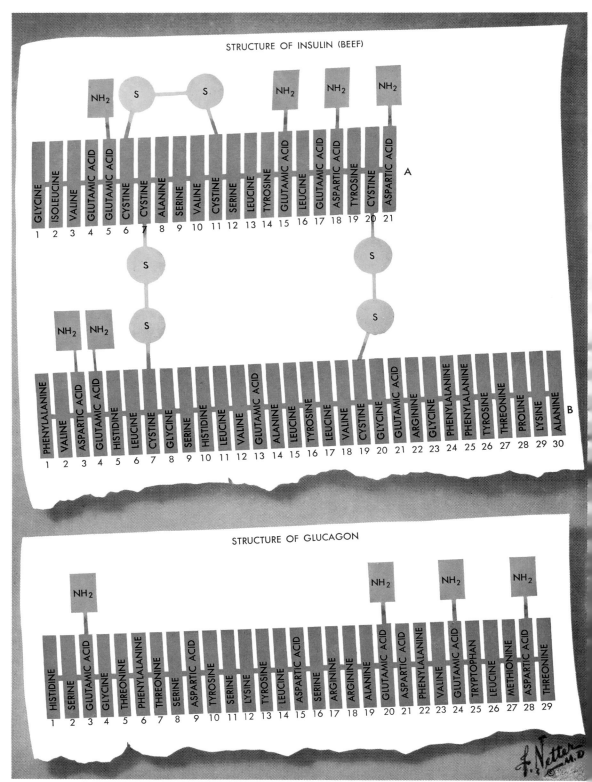

from human beings. However, the terminal amino acid (30) of the B chain in man is threonine, whereas that of pig insulin is *alanine.* Possibly, pig insulin with the terminal alanine removed would then not produce antibodies in man. This is a feasible procedure, since it has been shown that the terminal 4 to 6 amino acids of the B chain are not necessary for the physiological actions of insulin. In fact, "dealaninated" pork insulin has caused hypoglycemic activity in human subjects resistant to beef insulin because of high specific antibody titers. This activity, however, was not as good as might have been expected in a previously untreated case. Thus, it appears that differences between the chemically isolated insulin molecule and that of native insulin may preclude the preparation of any type of insulin which would not give rise to some antibodies. In fact, recently, antibodies were demonstrated in cows after the admin-

istration of cow insulin and in pigs after pig insulin.

It was noted, some years ago, that incompletely pure insulin preparations, when given intravenously, caused a short-lived rise in blood sugar before the occurrence of the expected hypoglycemia. This was more marked when given intraportally than when administered through a systemic vein. Between 1945 and 1952, the work of De Duve, Sutherland, and others showed that a polypeptide, distinct from insulin, could be extracted from islet tissue. It was named *glucagon,* and it most probably is produced by the alpha cells. Behrens showed that pure glucagon consists of a single *polypeptide chain of 29 amino acids.* The molecular weight is 3485. Unlike insulin, it does not contain cystine. Its pharmacological effects on carbohydrate turnover are nearly identical to those of epinephrine, *i.e.,* promotion of glycogen breakdown.

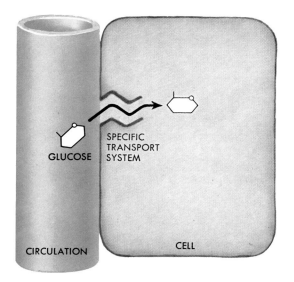

RED BLOOD CELLS; NEURONS
TRANSPORT (ENTRY) SYSTEM SPECIFIC
FOR CERTAIN SUGARS:
INSULIN HAS <u>NO</u> EFFECT ON RATE OF UPTAKE

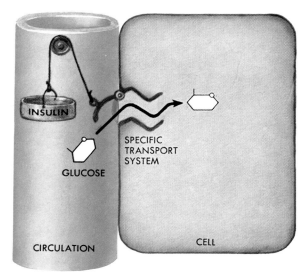

FAT CELLS; MUSCLE CELLS
SPECIFIC TRANSPORT SYSTEM KEPT
INHIBITED OR COVERED:
INSULIN REMOVES COVER AND THUS
<u>PROMOTES</u> UPTAKE

UPTAKE OF GLUCOSE BY DIFFERENT CELLS

INTESTINAL EPITHELIUM (AND POSSIBLY RENAL TUBULAR EPITHELIUM)
SPECIFIC TRANSPORT SYSTEM <u>WITHOUT</u>
COVER; ALSO ACCUMULATOR MECHANISM
FOR TRANSPORT AGAINST GRADIENT:
INSULIN HAS <u>NO</u> EFFECT ON RATE OF UPTAKE

LIVER CELL
NO SPECIFIC SUGAR TRANSPORT SYSTEM:
RELATION OF INSULIN TO SUGAR UPTAKE
AND RELEASE BY LIVER NOT YET
CLEARLY DETERMINED

For many years it was assumed that the metabolic turnover of glucose in the cell interior determined the rate at which sugar entered the cell from the extracellular fluids. As a matter of fáct, it was thought that the rate of entry of glucose depended on its rate of phosphorylation. It has now been shown conclusively that most mammalian cells do not permit the rapid free entry of sugars in an indiscriminate fashion. The cell membrane possesses a specific transport system which carries certain sugars into the cell interior at a rate greater than can be explained by diffusion. The exact biochemical mechanism of this transport event is not yet known. It behaves kinetically as if it were operating by means of a saturable carrier system. The transport system will operate on sugars of particular chemical structure, e.g., glucose, mannose, galactose, D-xylose, 2-deoxyglucose, etc., but not on closely related materials such as L-xylose, glucuronic acid, fructose, etc., whether or not such substances can be further metabolized by the intracellular enzyme systems. If they are not utilized, they accumulate until the equilibrium concentration is reached between the inside and the outside, and further entry of glucose ceases.

The accompanying diagrams illustrate the operation of such transport systems in various cells and demonstrate certain differences between tissues. Thus, the *red blood cells* and the *neurons* exhibit the full activity of sugar transport, whether or not insulin is present in the body. Therefore, in the diabetic, both the rate of glycolysis in the red

blood cell and the rate of sugar metabolism of the central nervous system are normal, in spite of the virtual absence of insulin in depancreatized animals and in some diabetics.

The absorption of glucose by the *intestinal epithelium* and reabsorption by the *renal tubular epithelium* are also independent of insulin. In the intestinal cells, transport is followed by intracellular glucose accumulation, which permits unloading of glucose into the blood stream against a gradient. Thus, in diabetes, carbohydrate absorption in the gut and glucose handling by the kidney are normal in rate and extent. Glycosuria in diabetes results from overloading of the kidney tubules with high concentrations of glucose in the glomerular filtrate and not from their functional inadequacy.

The *fat cells* of adipose tissue (see pages 202 and 203), the *muscle cells* (whether skeletal or cardiac),

and the fibroblasts exhibit a low rate of glucose transport in the absence of insulin, as if their transport system were "inhibited" or "covered". This has been shown diagrammatically, as though the hormone lifted the cover and permitted transportation to go on. Those are the tissues which are TRULY diabetic in an organism deprived of insulin.

The *liver cell* demonstrates unique behavior in this respect. There seems to be no hindrance to the free exchange of sugars across its membrane. However, the diabetic liver is deficient in glycogen storage. Apparently, there is a direct action by insulin on the carbohydrate metabolism of the liver cell, but this does not seem to be related to cell membrane transport. Insulin acts, perhaps, on one or more of a number of phosphorylating systems in the liver. The details of this subject are now under concerted inquiry in many laboratories.

GLYCOLYSIS

The term *glycolysis* refers to the series of enzyme reactions by which a molecule of *glucose-6-phosphate* is transformed to *pyruvic* and/or *lactic acid*. The source of this phosphate ester may be either a molecule of *free glucose* phosphorylated intracellularly in the presence of *hexokinase,* or glucose-1-phosphate derived from *glycogen* by phosphorolysis — a splitting off of glucose molecules by the interposition of phosphoric acid residues through the catalytic action of phosphorylase.

The first step of the transformation undergone by glucose-6-phosphate consists of an intramolecular rearrangement to *fructose-6-phosphate* by a specific mutase. This intermediate is then phosphorylated to yield *fructose-1,6-diphosphate.* At this stage the hexose molecule is cleaved to two 3-carbon compounds—dihydroxyacetone phosphate (DHA-P) and *glyceraldehyde phosphate* (G ald-P) by an aldolase. Since the DHA-P is quickly converted to G ald-P, only the fate of the latter need be considered. In the presence of a complex enzyme system, the aldehyde group (CHO) of glyceraldehyde phosphate is oxidized, and a phosphate group is attached, yielding 1,3-diphosphoglyceric acid. The energy of this oxidative step now rests in the phosphate bond at position 1. This energy is transferred to a molecule of adenosine diphosphate (ADP), forming adenosine triphosphate (ATP). The oxidative step is aided by the coenzyme DPN (diphosphopyridine nucleotide), which becomes reduced, DPNH. The net result may be summarized as follows: 3-glyceraldehyde phosphate + inorganic phosphate + DPN + ADP → *3-phosphoglyceric acid* + DPNH + ATP

The above reaction yields energy which is not immediately given off as heat but is stored in the form of ATP, capable of doing work. In the ensuing transformation of 3-phosphoglyceric to *3-phosphopyruvic acid,* another energy-yielding step occurs, which gives rise to another ATP:

phosphopyruvic + ADP → pyruvic + ATP

When a tissue possesses the systems for further oxidation of pyruvate, and, provided oxygen is present, pyruvic acid is cleaved to *acetyl coenzyme A (CoA).* This is an activated form of acetate. In it, the 5'-phosphoryl group of adenosine-3'-5'-diphosphate is linked by pyrophosphate to phosphopantotheine, a derivate of the vitamin pantothenic acid. This may then proceed to form aceto-acetic acid or fatty acids and triglycerides, eventually. However, when the oxidative systems are absent (*e.g.,* in the mature nonnucleated erythrocyte), or if oxygen is excluded or is present in

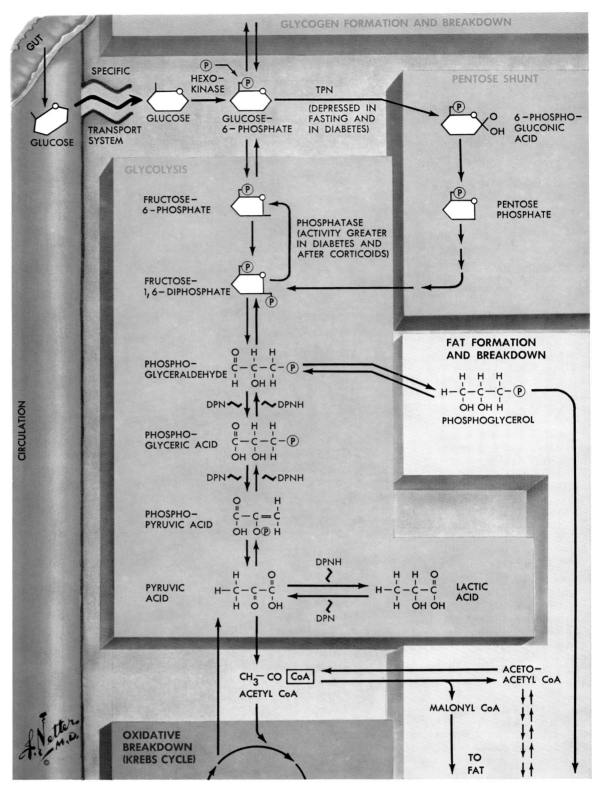

insufficient amounts, as under anaerobic conditions, pyruvic acid is reduced to *lactic acid* by the enzyme, lactic dehydrogenase, in the presence of reduced DPN. This system provides for the reoxidation of DPNH and thus enables its participation again in oxidizing 3-glyceraldehyde phosphate; otherwise, the latter reaction would stop as soon as all the molecules of DPN were reduced.

(1) glyceraldehyde phosphate + DPN
→ phosphoglyceric acid + DPNH

(2) pyruvic acid + DPNH → lactic acid + DPN
The coupling of these two reactions allows the glycolytic process to go on; *i.e.,* it allows the provision of energy by carbohydrates in the absence of oxygen, albeit at the expense of considerable amounts of carbohydrate.

Oxygen lack has other regulatory effects which aid the glycolytic system. Anoxia stimulates, in some manner, the glucose transport system through the membranes of such cells as those of muscle. More glucose can, therefore, come into the cell interior. At the same time, the activity of hexokinase is also increased. Thus, a large amount of glucose-6-phosphate is provided for the operation of the glycolytic pathway. This is needed for cell preservation, especially during anaerobic conditions, because the net energy yield of the transformation of glucose to lactate is only about one fourth that of a similar sequence in the presence of oxygen, and only one eighteenth that provided by the complete breakdown of the glucose to CO_2 and H_2O with oxygen present. Thus, oxygen regulates the rate of carbohydrate breakdown in many tissues, reducing it markedly as compared to carbohydrate utilization in the absence of oxygen. This phenomenon, first described for yeast and then for muscle, is known as the Pasteur effect.

Glycogen Metabolism

Glycogen, a polymer of glucose, is found primarily in animal cells and is the analogue of the starch of plants. It is a highly branched molecule, built up in tiers. The predominant linkage is between the first carbon and the fourth carbon of adjacent glucose units (1:4). At the branch points, the linkage is a 1:6 glycosidic link.

The polymer grows by the addition of more glucose units to its outer branches. As isolated from tissues, it has no set molecular weight; the particle weights range from 1,000,000 to 30,000,000.

The synthesis of glycogen begins with *glucose-6-phosphate,* which undergoes phosphate transfer within the molecule, to become *glucose-1-phosphate.* This reaction is catalyzed by the reversible system—phosphoglucomutase. Under the influence of another enzyme, glucose-1-phosphate reacts with uridine triphosphate. The products are *uridine diphosphoglucose* (UDPG) and pyrophosphate. The UDPG reacts with the free end of a terminal glucose unit of a glycogen particle and becomes incorporated in it, liberating the coenzyme. The two reactions just described are not reversible. The last step, catalyzed by *glycogen synthetase,* may be activated by *insulin,* although the evidence for this effect is not firmly established.

Glycogen synthetase explains only the formation of 1:4 linkages. Another system — the branching enzyme — catalyzes the formation of 1:6 linkages.

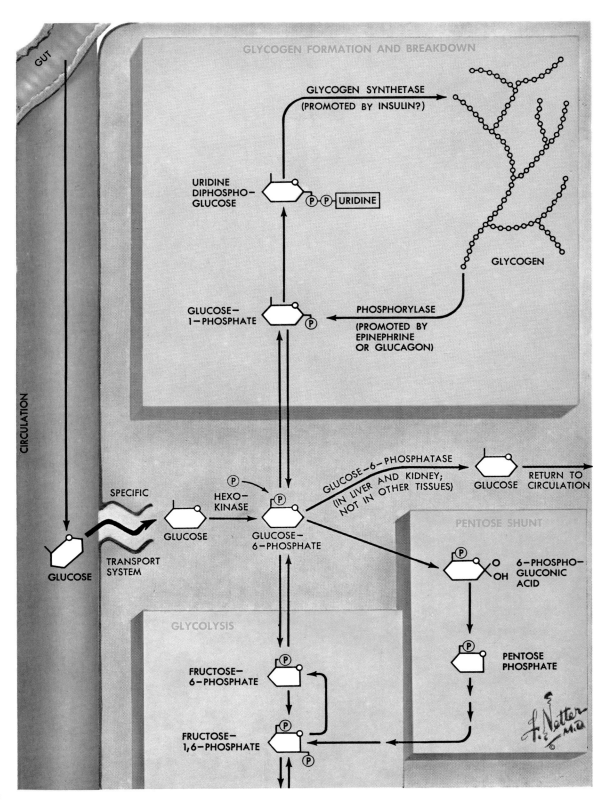

The breakdown of glycogen to glucose-1-phosphate proceeds via the enzyme *phosphorylase,* which is present in tissues in both the active and inactive forms. *Epinephrine* and *glucagon* have been shown to aid the activation of inactive phosphorylase. Therefore, these hormones promote glycogen breakdown. Since phosphorylase is specific for promoting the dissolution of the 1:4 linkages, glycogen breakdown stops as soon as a branch point is reached. The branched glucose unit is hydrolyzed by the enzyme amylo-1:6-glucosidase and is liberated as a free glucose molecule. After this occurs, the phosphorylase can proceed again to the next branch point.

The significance of the fact that glycogen formation and glycogen breakdown are catalyzed by two different sets of enzyme systems, not reversible in vivo, lies in the possibility of delicate control of the two events by hormonal and other regulating factors.

Normally, tissues differ in their quantitative capacity of glycogen synthesis. In a well-fed animal the liver may contain about 6 per cent of stored glycogen per unit wet weight of the organ, whereas the brain or the kidney will have only about 0.1 to 0.2 per cent, and skeletal muscle 1 to 1.5 per cent.

In the liver the glucose-1-phosphate derived from glycogen is transformed to glucose-6-phosphate, which can be hydrolyzed to free sugar by the specific *glucose-6-phosphatase.*

Muscle, however, lacks the specific phosphatase, and thus glycogen breakdown in muscle supplies only glucose-6-phosphate as material for glycolysis, the end product of which is pyruvic or lactic acid. Therefore, the administration of epinephrine raises the blood sugar by promoting glycogenolysis in the liver, and increases the blood lactate level by promoting the same process in muscle.

THE OXIDATIVE TRICARBOXYLIC ACID CYCLE

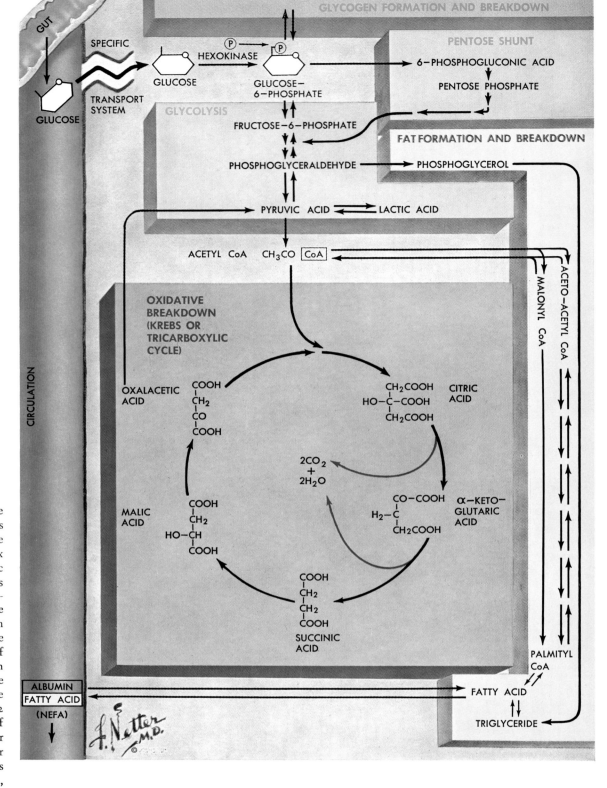

The *glycolytic breakdown* of glucose results in the formation of 2 molecules of *pyruvic acid* from 1 molecule of the sugar. In the presence of a complex enzyme system aided by thiamine, lipoic acid, and coenzyme A, the pyruvate is split to CO_2 and *acetyl CoA*. A condensation reaction next occurs, by which the 4-carbon *oxalacetic acid* combines with acetyl-CoA (2 carbons) to form the 6-carbon tricarboxylic *citric acid*. Each of two successive enzymatic steps results in the production of CO_2 and water. The net result is the appearance of the 4-carbon compound, *succinic acid,* 2 molecules of CO_2, and 2 molecules of water. The decarboxylations and water formation are quite complex. They occur with the aid of electron transfer systems (DPN [diphosphopyridine nucleotide], TPN [triphosphopyridine nucleotide], and the cytochromes) interacting between the substrates and oxygen. By further rearrangement, oxalacetate is re-formed from succinate. Another molecule of acetyl CoA can now be condensed. It is evident that one revolution of the cycle, as described, leads to the complete dissimilation of the acetate. In animal tissues, acetate cannot give rise directly to pyruvate. Regeneration of pyruvate occurs from *malic acid* or oxalacetic acid, from which phosphopyruvate can be formed.

The acetate which serves as the fuel for the cycle is derived either from *car-bohydrate* or from *fatty acids*. Since each revolution gives rise to an amount of CO_2 equivalent to the total carbon of the acetate, the latter cannot serve as the net carbon source for glucose. Net glucose formation can come only from the dicarboxylic acids of the cycle itself or from pyruvate.

The enzyme systems of the oxidative cycle are located within the mitochondria of the cells. They are "packaged" together with the electron transfer machinery, so that the hydrogens, removed from metabolites during the operation of the cycle, are carried in an orderly fashion by various coenzymes, until, finally, they form water with the oxygen "activated" by the respiratory ferment, cytochrome oxidase. In recent years, it has been clearly demonstrated that the mitochondrion is a precisely ordered organelle, in which the catalytic systems form a fully co-ordinated, spatially ordered, multi-enzyme system.

Within the mitochondrion as well, linked to the electron transfer steps, occurs a series of phosphorylations by which adenosine triphosphate is generated at the expense of the oxidative energy. In this way this energy can be used by the cell to promote synthetic reactions or to do mechanical or electrical work (see page 251).

When 1 molecule of glucose is broken down to pyruvic or lactic acid, it gives rise to 2 molecules of ATP (adenosine triphosphate). However, if the sugar is oxidized completely, 38 molecules of ATP are formed by 1 molecule of glucose. It is evident, then, that anaerobic sugar breakdown is, energetically, quite inefficient.

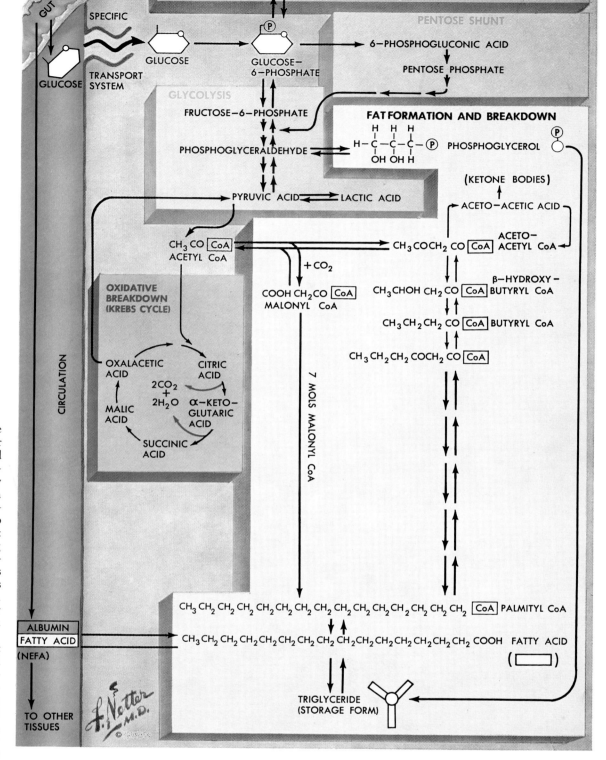

FAT METABOLISM

The capacity of bodily cells for the storage of a *glucose* load as *glycogen,* or for its total dissimilation to CO₂ and H₂O, is comparatively limited. In contrast, the storage capacity for fat is very large and hence, in those tissues which possess the requisite enzymatic equipment, the transformation of glucose to fat represents the quantitatively most important avenue for its disposal. During the postabsorptive phase, or during more-prolonged fasting, the stored fat is broken down to *fatty acids* and used as fuel by most of the tissues of the body, yielding 9 as opposed to 4 calories per gram of carbohydrate. Thus, fat is a superior source of storage fuel.

On its way to form fat, glucose is first broken down to *acetyl coenzyme A* (*CoA*). Each molecule of the sugar provides 2 molecules of acetate and 2 molecules of CO₂. There appear to be at least two distinct pathways by which acetyl CoA is condensed to the long-chain, even-numbered, fatty acids. These separate pathways may exist in two distinct portions of the cell.

1. In the first pathway, 2 molecules of acetyl CoA condense to form 1 molecule of *aceto-acetyl CoA.* The keto group on the β-carbon atom is reduced, and the result is 1 molecule of *β-hydroxybutyryl CoA.* A further reduction of the β-carbon produces the 4-carbon *butyryl CoA.* The next step is the condensation of butyryl CoA with another molecule of acetyl CoA. Succeeding reductions and condensations follow each other, until the 16-carbon *palmitic acid* is formed.

2. The second pathway begins with the addition of CO₂ to 1 molecule of acetyl CoA to form *malonyl CoA;* then 7 molecules of this intermediate plus 1 molecule of acetyl CoA in the presence of ATP (adenosine triphosphate) and

reduced coenzymes condense to form 1 molecule of palmitic acid. The CO₂ is liberated for re-use.

Both pathways require a ready supply of hydrogen-carrying reduced coenzymes (reduced diphosphopyridine nucleotide + reduced triphosphopyridine nucleotide). A major portion of the required TPNH is probably generated by the oxidation of *glucose-6-phosphate* to *6-phosphogluconic acid* in the *pentose shunt.* It is thus evident that the glucose molecule supplies all the carbon, hydrogen, and oxygen of the resulting fatty acid.

The fatty acids are not stored as such. Their acid groups are neutralized by combination with *phosphoglycerol,* a substance derived from the intermediates of glycolysis. The result is 1 molecule of *triglyceride,* or *neutral fat.*

The breakdown of neutral fat is catalyzed by a distinct enzyme (a lipase) which liberates 3 fatty

acids and 1 glycerol for each molecule of neutral fat. The *free fatty acids* (FFA or NEFA) (see pages 202 and 203) are carried in the blood in combination with *serum albumin.* In this form they reach the tissues, where they are rapidly utilized. The half-life of the free fatty acids is measured in minutes. The glycerol is carried to the liver via the blood stream and is broken down there. It cannot be reutilized in the synthesis of neutral fat in adipose tissue, unlike glycerophosphate arising during glycolysis.

Insulin promotes the rate of glucose penetration into the cell interior of adipose tissue. Thereby, all pathways of glucose disposal are stimulated, notably lipogenesis and the formation of triglycerides, through the provision of glycerophosphate. The hormonal materials which promote fat mobilization include the catecholamines, the growth hormone of the pituitary, and the glucocorticoids of the adrenal cortex.

PROTEIN-CARBOHYDRATE INTERRELATIONSHIPS

Free *amino acids* are present in the *circulation,* in the extracellular fluids, and in the cell interior. They are derived from food *proteins* by digestion and from the breakdown, by cell proteases, of *tissue and circulating (plasma) proteins.* In all cells, protein synthesis occurs from amino acids by a complex process centered in the ribosomes. In most tissues there exists a set of enzymes known as amino transferases. Aided by coenzymes derived from the vitamin pyridoxine, they catalyze a transfer of the α-amino group of a specific amino acid to the α-carbon of a keto acid. Thus, a keto acid is transformed to an amino acid. An example will illustrate such a process:

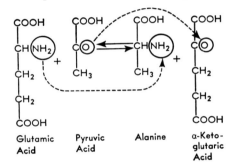

| Glutamic Acid | Pyruvic Acid | Alanine | α-Keto-glutaric Acid |

In this way, a specific amino acid required for a synthetic reaction, but unavailable, may be provided in place of another one available at the moment.

Essentially, the amino acids in extra-hepatic tissues provide the building blocks for the synthesis of protein. Protein formation is favored by a ready supply of carbohydrate, by insulin, by pituitary growth hormone, and by the sex hormones. Insulin and growth hormone (GH) seem to operate in concert, since, in the absence of insulin, GH does not stimulate synthesis, and, in the absence of GH, insulin does not lead to normal growth. The precise mechanisms of these effects are not yet understood, but, whereas GH and insulin both increase nuclear mass in tissue culture (hyperplasia), gonadal hormones merely increase cytoplasm (hypertrophy) in tissue culture of liver.

Only certain cells possess enzymes (deaminases) which deaminate by removing the α-amino group irreversibly as *ammonia* (NH_3). For the most part NH_3 is combined with CO_2, through the so-called ornithine cycle in the *liver,* to form the end product, *urea.* Ammonia may also be used to neutralize acids for excretion in the kidney, having previously formed glutamine.

The keto acids produced by deamination can enter the oxidative phase of metabolism through several portals, as indicated in the accompanying diagram. By transformation to *pyruvate, oxalacetate,* and *α-ketoglutarate,* the deaminated residues may be used to provide energy

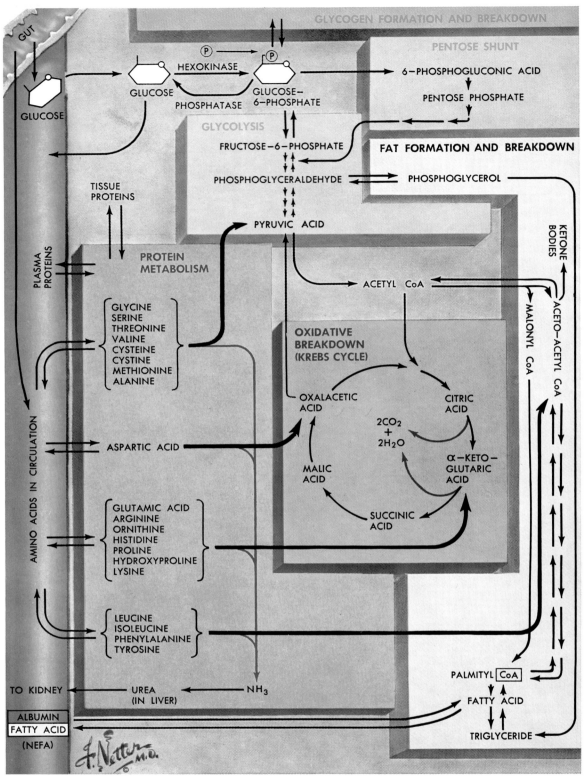

in the tricarboxylic acid (*Krebs*) *cycle.* This will occur when the liver is deprived of carbohydrate fuel for its needs. It can also be seen that these keto acids may form *glucose* or *glycogen* by going upward from pyruvate in the *glycolytic scheme.* This is the pathway of gluconeogenesis from protein. It is favored in the presence of increased activity of two specific phosphatases, which lead to wastage of intracellular glucose; these are the phosphatase which removes the phosphate group on carbon 1 of fructose-1,6-diphosphate, and *glucose-6-phosphatase* which produces free *glucose* from *glucose-6-phosphate.* Fasting, diabetes, and glucocorticoids increase these phosphatase activities.

The keto residues of certain ketogenic amino acids, notably *leucine, isoleucine, phenylalanine,* and *tyrosine,* bypass the Krebs cycle. They are transformed to *aceto-acetyl coenzyme A* and thence to aceto-

acetate, partaking of its further fate.

Starvation or the absence of insulin leads to a net breakdown of proteins in the tissue. The resulting amino acids are then irreversibly deaminated, primarily in the liver but, to a small extent, in the kidneys. The resulting keto acids yield *glucose* or aceto-acetate and *ketone bodies.* The rôle of the liver appears passive, in the sense that the extent of deamination depends only on the rate with which amino acids are brought to the organ. This is analogous to ketone body production, which is regulated by the supply of fatty acids to the liver.

Many of the amino acids have special functions, *e.g., phenylalanine* is converted to epinephrine and norepinephrine; *tyrosine* to thyroxine; *histidine* is decarboxylated to histamine; and *glycine* serves as starting material for the purines, the pyrimidines, and the pyrroles.

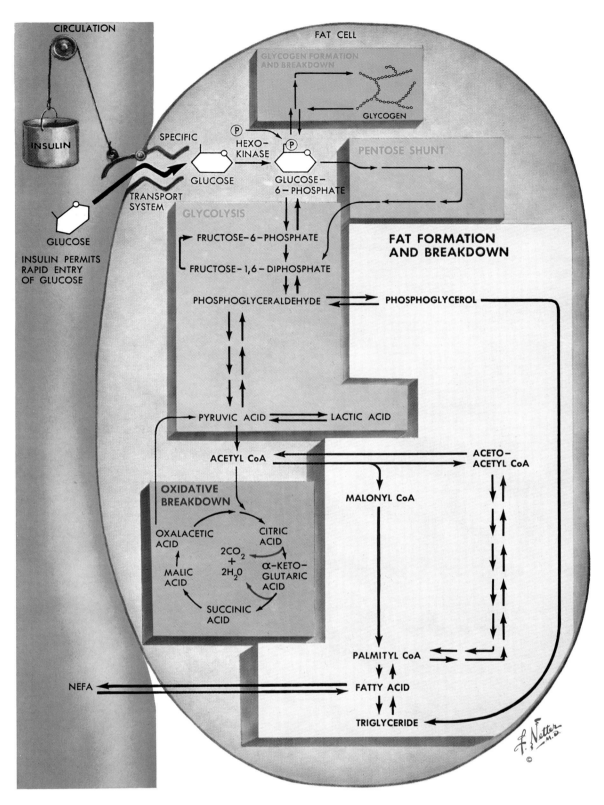

nucleotide and reduced triphosphopyridine nucleotide. The latter is provided by the first reaction of the *pentose shunt*. It is evident, therefore, that a high rate of glucose intake and of pentose shunt activity provides the conditions for a high rate of formation of *fatty acids* and of *triglycerides*.

The fatty acids are not stored as such. They are neutralized by combination with *phosphoglycerol*, which is formed from the trioses arising during glycolysis. The result is a neutral fat, or triglyceride. *Free*, or nonesterified, *fatty acids* (NEFA), carried by serum albumin to the fat depots or to the liver, can be stored by the fat cell in a similar fashion. The stored fat is broken down by a lipase into FREE fatty acids and FREE glycerol, which goes to the liver for further transformation but cannot itself function in

the triglyceride synthesis (see pages 202 and 203).

It is thus evident that insulin, by ensuring a rapid entry of glucose into the fat cell, provides the necessary conditions for the formation and storage of fat. On the other hand, the catecholamines (secreted either by the sympathetic nerve endings in adipose tissue or by the adrenal medulla), the glucocorticoids, ACTH, and growth hormone favor lipolysis, or the liberation of fatty acids from adipose tissue. The uncontrolled, insulin-deficient diabetic is characteristically very thin, because of decreased lipogenesis and increased lipolysis resulting from glucose deprivation of the adipose tissue. Patients with a catecholamine-producing pheochromocytoma are always thin, whereas those suffering from an insulin-producing islet cell adenoma are nearly always obese.

CARBOHYDRATE METABOLISM OF THE MUSCLE CELL

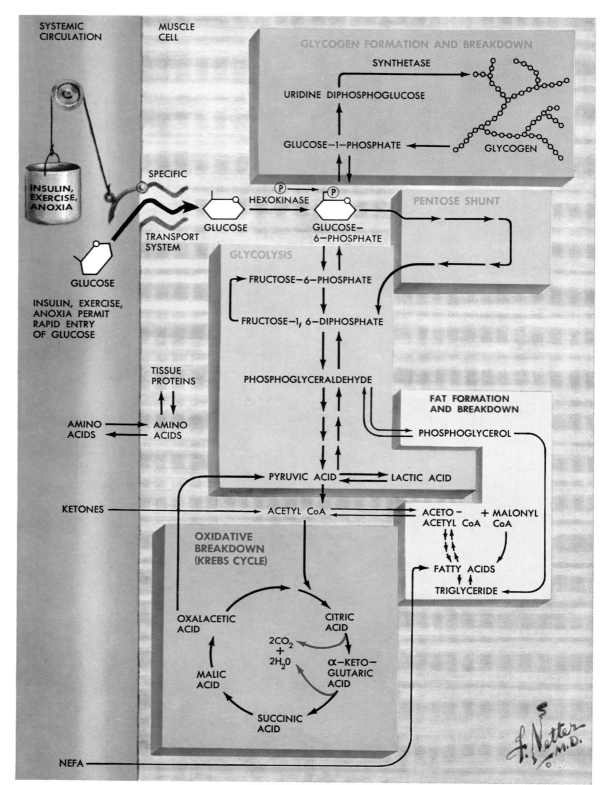

The characteristics of the intermediary metabolism of skeletal and cardiac muscle are (1) an insulin-sensitive sugar transport system, (2) considerable glycogen storage capacity, (3) a high rate of glycolysis, (4) a highly developed oxidative capacity, (5) a moderate pentose shunt, and (6) relatively poor fat formation.

The *membrane transport system* is "opened" by *insulin,* by *muscular exercise,* and by *tissue anoxia.* The activity of muscle *hexokinase* is of a very high order, permitting rapid utilization of glucose when the demand is great. The initial stages of severe muscular work utilize the stores of *glycogen* until the rate of sugar entry is adjusted to a higher level. During a period of relative anoxia, glycogen and glucose break down to the stage of *lactic acid,* permitting some muscular contraction even under an unfavorable oxygen supply. As oxygenation improves, oxidative processes favor the resynthesis of glycogen. Muscle can also utilize *free fatty acids (NEFA)* and the *ketones,* both of which break down to *acetyl coenzyme A (CoA),* which is oxidized via the *Krebs cycle.* Cardiac

muscle, particularly, thrives on fatty acids and is not at all dependent on glucose; this is in contrast to brain tissue, which cannot exist without it. Cardiac muscle shows extensive lactic dehydrogenase activity and therefore can use lactate, derived from other tissues, for its energy expenditure. *Amino acids* can be transaminated, but no significant deamination occurs.

There exists in the muscle cell a basic biochemical mechanism for the regulation of glucose utilization, known as the glucose–fatty acid cycle (P. O. Randle). Whenever an excess of fatty acids reaches the muscle, the increase in acetyl CoA inhibits the citric acid cycle and some phases of the glycolytic cycle, and glucose utilization falls. The converse is true when an excess of glucose is being utilized. This fundamental mechanism serves to prevent serious hypoglyce-

mia in a fasted organism undergoing severe exercise.

The exact molecular mechanisms by which insulin, exercise, and anoxia open up the glucose transport system are not known. Some workers believe that muscular exercise does this by a combination of increasing the effective blood supply and causing some degree of relative anoxia, which favors more rapid phosphorylation of glucose, intracellularly. Other investigators have adduced evidence that the effect of muscular work is exerted via the release of a humoral material with actions similar to insulin. This product is released in the completely depancreatized animal as well as in the normal one. The old clinical observation that physical work has an insulinlike effect in the diabetic is consonant with these experimental data.

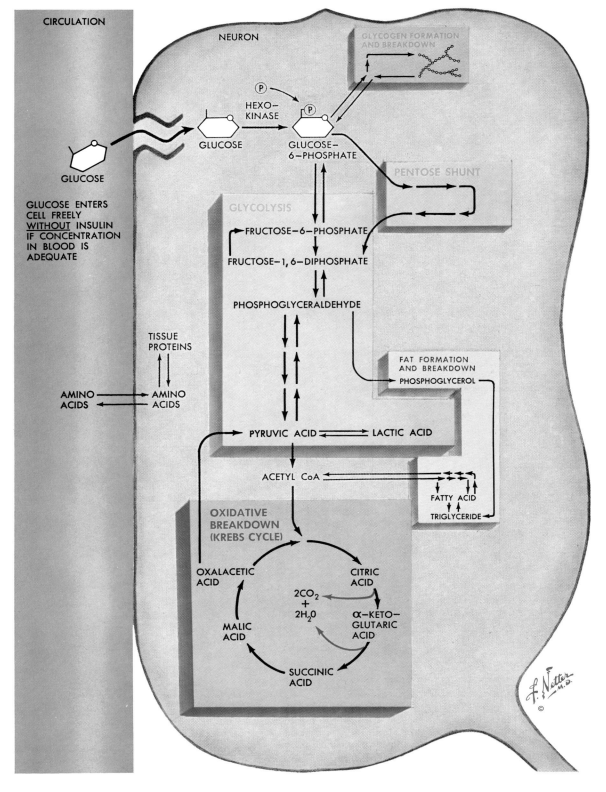

CIRCULATION

NEURON

GLYCOGEN FORMATION AND BREAKDOWN

HEXO-KINASE

GLUCOSE → GLUCOSE-6-PHOSPHATE

GLUCOSE

GLUCOSE ENTERS CELL FREELY **WITHOUT** INSULIN IF CONCENTRATION IN BLOOD IS ADEQUATE

PENTOSE SHUNT

GLYCOLYSIS

FRUCTOSE-6-PHOSPHATE

FRUCTOSE-1,6-DIPHOSPHATE

PHOSPHOGLYCERALDEHYDE

TISSUE PROTEINS

AMINO ACIDS ⇌ AMINO ACIDS

FAT FORMATION AND BREAKDOWN

PHOSPHOGLYCEROL

PYRUVIC ACID ⇌ LACTIC ACID

ACETYL CoA

FATTY ACID

TRIGLYCERIDE

OXIDATIVE BREAKDOWN (KREBS CYCLE)

OXALACETIC ACID

CITRIC ACID

$2CO_2 + 2H_2O$

MALIC ACID

α-KETO-GLUTARIC ACID

SUCCINIC ACID

F. Netter M.D. ©

aliza-
the
ative
ergy

rans-
un-
rate
the
cose
ıase,
of a
y to
The
able
rom
y of
ove
ron
glu-
tely
the
; to
era-
ons,
om-
and
ced
en.
ize
ifi-
ter
ust
.est
the
the
ter
uc-

tion or degeneration of many of the cells in the cortical areas is noted at autopsy, whereas the lower centers are only moderately affected cytologically.

In man, only glucose, mannose, and fructose relieve the acute stages of a hypoglycemic reaction, fructose being transformed into glucose by the liver. Thus, the neurons of the brain exhibit a high degree of substrate specificity.

The feedback system which protects the brain against loss of its vital fuel, glucose, resides in the sensitivity of the neuro-endocrine system of the anterior pituitary, the adrenal medulla, and the response to hypoglycemia by the α-cells of the pancreas. A decline in the blood sugar level, especially if rapid, leads to the release of growth hormone, of epinephrine, and of glucagon. Whereas discharges

from hypothalamic centers account for the first two, glucagon secretion appears to respond to hypoglycemia directly. Growth hormone blocks the action of insulin, whereas epinephrine and glucagon stimulate glycogen breakdown in the liver, attempting thus to restore the blood sugar to normal levels.

It is noteworthy that there may be no significant disturbances in central nervous system (CNS) function when the blood sugar level is lowered very gradually over a long period of time. It should also be added that CNS disturbance may be encountered at blood sugar levels ordinarily considered normal. This may occur in the depancreatized animal when there is a rapid descent from pronounced hyperglycemia to levels of about 150 mg per 100 ml and in patients with uncontrolled Addison's disease.

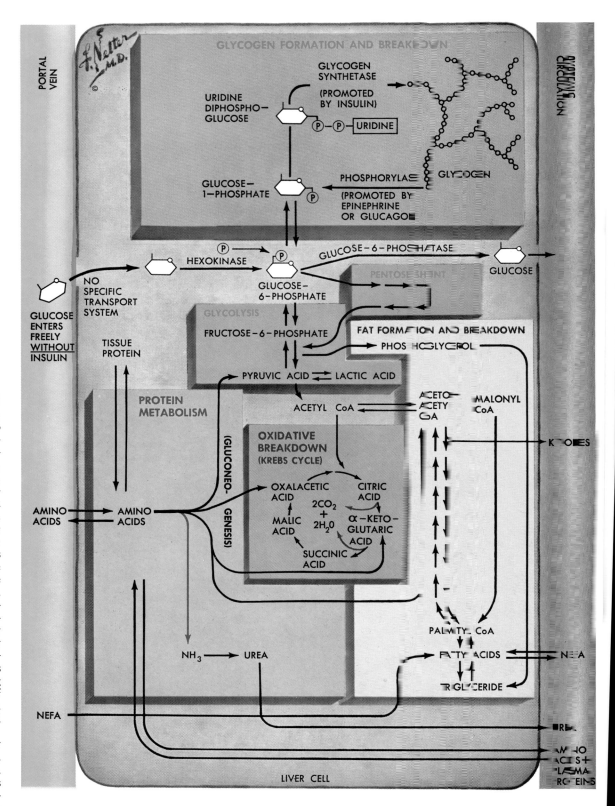

INTERMEDIARY METABOLISM OF THE LIVER CELL

The specialized functions of many cell systems, such as muscle, brain, fat, etc., show parallel metabolic adaptation, so that one or another aspect of intermediary metabolism is developed out of proportion to other pathways. The *liver cell,* however, which is a specialist, so to speak, in metabolism, exhibits intense development of all phases of most pathways. In regard to the handling of carbohydrate, the liver cell shows *no cell barrier to glucose entry.* Unlike muscle or fat, the free sugar content of its cell interior is almost identical to the level in the extracellular fluid. This is so because the capacity to phosphorylate glucose, thereby reducing intracellular free glucose and thus enhancing the extracellular-intracellular gradient, is relatively weak. In addition, the liver has a very active enzyme system, namely *glucose-6-phosphatase,* which specifically breaks down *glucose-6-phosphate,* liberating free *glucose* for delivery to the rest of the body. The liver, thus, is an organ which supplies the blood sugar and guards its level.

When sugar is not being actively absorbed from the gastro-intestinal tract, the liver cell manufactures glucose from noncarbohydrate sources, by a process known as *gluconeogenesis.* The raw material is primarily composed of *amino acids.* After deamination, the *ammonia nitrogen* is incorporated into *urea* and is excreted, while the carbon skeleton is transformed, via the *Krebs cycle* intermediates, into *pyruvate* and thence to glucose. The degree of activity of glucose-6-phosphatase determines the glucose output of the liver. It is increased by an adaptive mechanism in the presence of hypoglycemia, and it is gradually reduced by hyperglycemia. Any glucose-6-phosphate which escapes breakdown to free glucose can be temporarily stored in the form of *glycogen.* The synthesis of glycogen, or glycogenesis, via *glucose-1-phosphate* is catalyzed by uridine phosphate in a step entirely different from any involved in glycogen breakdown, or

glycogenolysis. Glycogenesis may be definitely enhanced by insulin. When the blood sugar is lowered, *glycogen phosphorylase* is *activated by epinephrine* or *glucagon,* thus increasing glucose-1-phosphate by enhancing the phosphorolysis of glycogen. This leads to a subsequent accumulation of glucose-6-phosphate, which provides a ready source of glucose after hydrolysis, allowing it to diffuse out of the cell to sustain or increase the level in the blood.

The liver cell readily forms *fat* from glucose and has a large capacity for the uptake of *nonesterified fatty acids (NEFA)* from plasma. These either are stored as *triglycerides* (neutral fat) or are broken down rapidly to *acetyl CoA.* Whenever the influx of fat to the liver exceeds the capacity of its machinery to dispose oxidatively of acetyl CoA, condensation to *aceto-acetate* occurs. Together with its immediate precursor, β-hydroxybutyric acid, aceto-acetate repre-

sents the first water-soluble stage in the breakdown products of fat catabolism and, thus, diffuses into the blood stream as part of the *ketones.* Acetone, the spontaneous breakdown product of aceto-acetic acid, is the third member of this group and, in contrast to the others, is not utilized by the liver or by muscle.

It is not possible, at present, to give a definitive picture of the hormonal control of the above described reactions in the liver cell. Under certain experimental circumstances, insulin seems to exert a restraining effect on sugar output by the liver, but it enhances normal glycogen deposition. The glucocorticoids favor new formation of sugar, and ketone production seems to be under joint control by pituitary and adrenal cortical factors. Whether or not these influences are exerted by the hormones directly on the liver cell or by their general effects on substrate concentration is still a debatable issue.

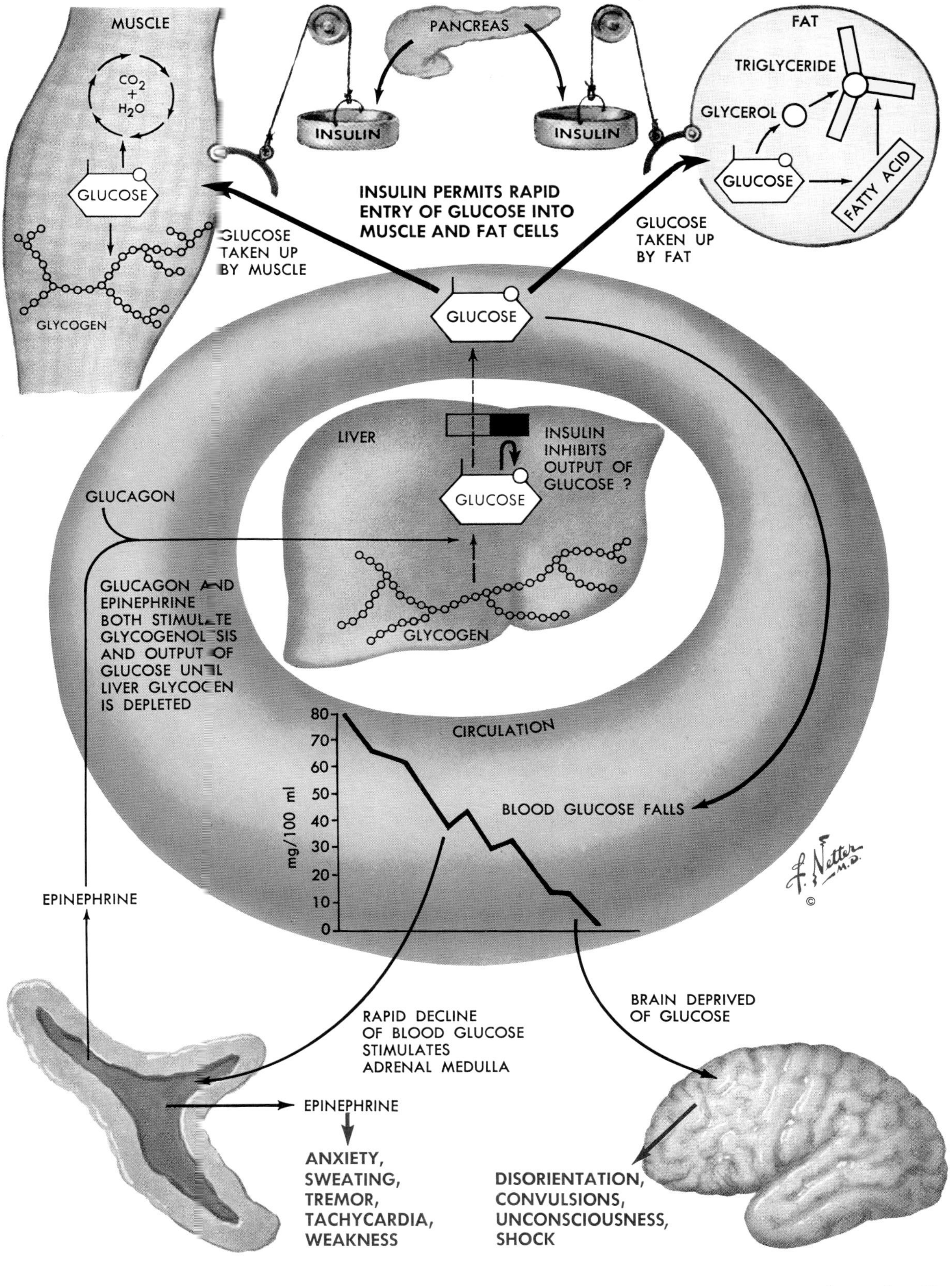

MUSCLE

$CO_2 + H_2O$

GLUCOSE

GLYCOGEN

GLUCOSE TAKEN UP BY MUSCLE

PANCREAS

INSULIN

INSULIN

FAT

TRIGLYCERIDE

GLYCEROL

GLUCOSE

FATTY ACID

GLUCOSE TAKEN UP BY FAT

INSULIN PERMITS RAPID ENTRY OF GLUCOSE INTO MUSCLE AND FAT CELLS

GLUCOSE

LIVER

INSULIN INHIBITS OUTPUT OF GLUCOSE ?

GLUCOSE

GLUCAGON

GLYCOGEN

GLUCAGON AND EPINEPHRINE BOTH STIMULATE GLYCOGENOLYSIS AND OUTPUT OF GLUCOSE UNTIL LIVER GLYCOGEN IS DEPLETED

CIRCULATION

BLOOD GLUCOSE FALLS

mg/100 ml — 80 70 60 50 40 30 20 10 0

EPINEPHRINE

RAPID DECLINE OF BLOOD GLUCOSE STIMULATES ADRENAL MEDULLA

EPINEPHRINE

ANXIETY, SWEATING, TREMOR, TACHYCARDIA, WEAKNESS

BRAIN DEPRIVED OF GLUCOSE

DISORIENTATION, CONVULSIONS, UNCONSCIOUSNESS, SHOCK

F. Netter M.D.

istration of glucose, in severe cases; in milder instances, oral intake of readily absorbable sugar solutions may suffice. However, repeated and/or prolonged attacks produce irreversible neuronal damage, with their consequences: paresis, paralysis, rigidity, and mental deficiency. Especially is this true of infants and young children, in whom the intellectual functions may be severely and permanently affected.

The symptoms, signs, and effects of hypoglycemia seem to depend not only on the depth of the blood sugar level but also on the rate at which it falls. Thus, the slowly absorbable insulins (protamine zinc, NPH,® Lente®) cause a slow descent of blood glucose. Since the release of epinephrine is slowed, the symptoms and signs of anxiety, agitation, tachycardia, and sweating may be absent. This is true also in diabetics with autonomic insufficiency due to dia-

betic neuropathy. The brain seems, also, to be able to adapt its energy metabolism; thus, convulsions and coma may not occur even at blood sugar levels close to zero. Headaches and personality changes may be the only evident phenomena.

Typical "hypoglycemic" attacks occur, under certain circumstances, when there has been a rapid descent of the blood glucose from hyperglycemic values (e.g., 300 to 400 mg per 100 ml) to lower levels, even if these are still above the normal range (100 to 150 mg per 100 ml). This phenomenon is seen in depancreatized animals, in some diabetics, and in Addisonian patients following the cessation of glucose infusions.

All available data point to the conclusion that all the consequences of insulin excess are due to the effects of hypoglycemia and not to an immediate, direct action of the insulin molecule on brain tissue.

157

Hypoglycemia with Functional Tumors of the B-Cells

Within 2 years following the discovery (1921) of insulin and the appreciation of the symptoms and signs of a rapid decline in blood sugar due to overdosage, Seale Harris related the clinical picture of spontaneous *hypoglycemia* to excess insulin. Previously, however, because of the neurological and emotional aspects of the symptomatology (hunger, anxiety, perspiration, tremors, and convulsions, see page 157), diagnoses of neurasthenia, epilepsy, and psychosis had generally been made. Such clinical findings, with a fasting true blood sugar below 40 mg per 100 ml during an attack and with rapid improvement after glucose administration, usually prove diagnostic of hypoglycemia (Whipple's triad), though low blood sugar values are found in other conditions which exhibit more or less the same symptom complex.

When hypoglycemia is pancreatic in origin, the lesions of the islets vary; there may be functional hypersensitivity to the usual stimulus to insulin secretion (*viz.*, hyperglycemia), hyperplasia or adenoma formation, and, more rarely, carcinomatous transformation with metastases. Individuals exist whose β-cells are more than normally sensitive to rises in blood sugar; in them, insulin secretion seems to continue for some time after the blood sugar has returned to normal values. It may be that others lack a brisk epinephrine, glucagon, or growth hormone response to hypoglycemia, rather than that they have an oversensitive β-cell, and these are said to suffer from reactive hypoglycemia (after a carbohydrate meal).

Rarely, children become hypoglycemic after a meal containing leucine. The β-cells in these patients are overly sensitive and secrete insulin in response to this and related amino acids. Normal subjects, following tolbutamide administration, show a similar response.

Equally rarely, hypoglycemia follows the blocking of glycogenolysis by an accumulation of hexosephosphate in the liver, in galactose or fructose intolerance, both of the latter being hereditary conditions (see page 247).

In other patients the hypoglycemic episodes are associated with a more or less generalized hyperplasia of the islets, so that hyperglycemia, following food intake, evokes an abnormally large insulin secretion. For the most part, such episodes occur from 1 to 2 hours after meals and are not encountered early in the morning, after a night's fast.

Tumors of the islets, like functional

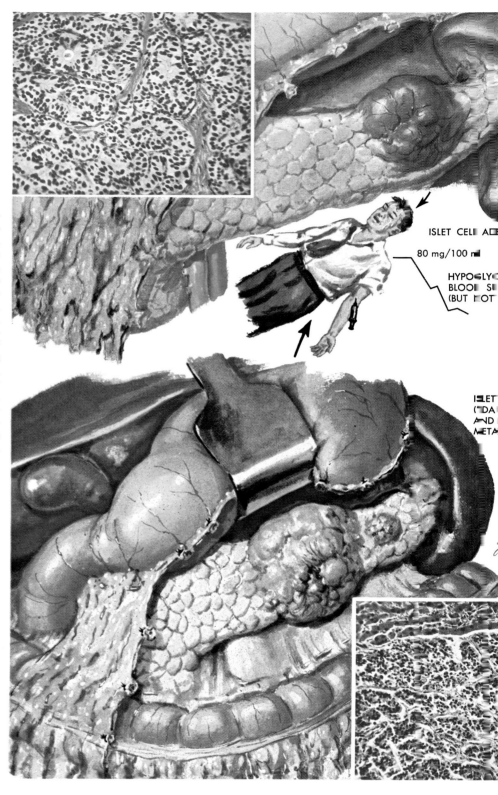

tumors of other endocrine glands, are generally more independent of control than are the normal structures. Thus, a large output of insulin may occur without a previous rise in blood sugar, and, usually, during fasting. The amount of insulin released is generally larger than in instances of hyperplasia. The symptomatology is more intense, with convulsions.

Benign tumors or *adenomas* may occur anywhere in the gland, or in aberrant tissue located in the wall of the duodenum or deep in the porta hepatis. They are generally small (0.5 to 2.0 cm in diameter). Occasionally, more than one is present.

The stored insulin in islet cell tumors, unlike that in normal islets, often fails to show stainable insulin granules, although the insulin content of the tumor is high.

The *islet cell carcinoma* (malignant insulinoma) is usually larger than the average adenoma, and it

metastasizes early, f[r]equently to [th]e [metas]tases are often func[t]ional, contin[uing] [to] secrete insulin.

With the clinica[l] history and th[e pro]cedures employed [at] present, it [is pos]s[ible] to differentiate hype[r]plasia from [tumor:] the attacks are mor[e] severe, less d[ependent on car]bohydrate ingestion[,] and more fr[equent dur]ing. The blood insu[l]in level is us[ually high in] attacks. Following a[d]ministration [of tolbuta]mide (1 gm intraven[o]usly), blood [s]u[gar is] depressed for many [h]ours (in con[trast to the] return to control leve[l]s within 1 h[our, and] plasma insulin is mu[c]h greater than [normal. It] often evokes a bloo[d] sugar fall [in affected] individuals. In contr[a]st, the insuli[n rise in hypo]glycemia may be red[u]ced, and, occ[asionally, a flat] blood sugar curve is [f]ound.

DYSFUNCTION OF THE ISLET CELLS

Diffuse hyperplasia of the beta cells of the islets of Langerhans has been noted, almost invariably, in offspring of diabetic mothers. The increase in islet cell mass appears to follow lack of control in the mother, but some hypertrophy is present even when control is satisfactory. Rarely, hyperplasia of the beta cells is found in infants of normal mothers. In either case, spontaneous *hypoglycemia* is the result. Typically, in infants, *convulsions* are the presenting symptom, and temporary relief is obtained by feeding carbohydrate. At all times, but particularly after birth, hypoxia aggravates the sensitivity of the cerebral cortex to hypoglycemia, the higher centers being dependent, to a critical extent, on both oxygen and glucose. Most children with this disease have done well on frequent feedings and administration of pituitary corticotropin; some have shown spontaneous improvement with advancing age.

McQuarrie has described several instances of hypoglycemia, in which the pathological lesion consisted of the virtual *absence of alpha cells* but with a seemingly normal complement of beta cells. He postulated that the hypoglycemia resulted from the action of normal amounts of secreted insulin without counteraction by glucagon. These cases seem to be unique, and the interpretation is dubious, since it has not been established that a lack of glucagon, in the face of a good epinephrine and growth hormone mechanism, will lead to hypoglycemia.

Tumors (benign or malignant) of certain organs and tissues may produce and secrete materials which imitate the actions of several known hormones. Among these have been found tumors of mesenchymal origin, fibromas and fibrosarcomas, located in the thorax and behind the peritoneum, which generally attain a large size. The clinical picture is indistinguishable from that of hyperinsulinism.

At least three different mechanisms have been postulated to explain the hypoglycemia caused by such tumors: A markedly increased utilization of glucose by the tumor may overtax the hepatic glycogen reserve in some debilitated patients, thus producing hypoglycemia. The fibrosarcoma, often made up of spindle-shaped cells, may be an atypical metastasis of a small, primary islet cell adenocarcinoma. One such case has been demonstrated beyond doubt. Finally, such tumors may secrete compounds with a hypoglycemic potential. Resected tumors frequently contain an insulinlike

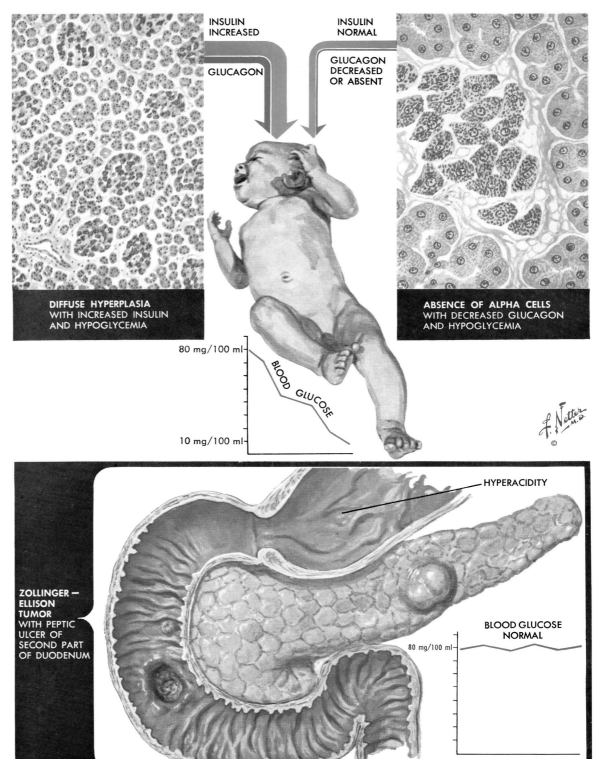

material which yields a positive hypoglycemic assay. To date, however, no direct molecular identification with insulin has been made by showing that the material reacts with specific insulin antibody.

Zollinger and Ellison, in 1955, drew attention to the occurrence of islet cell tumors which do not secrete insulin or glucagon but which are found in association with a definite syndrome consisting of the following clinical triad:

1. There is marked *gastric hyperacidity* with abdominal pain. The 12-hour nocturnal acid production may exceed 2000 ml and, typically, is not affected by vagotomy, subtotal gastric resection, or gastric irradiation.

2. Multiple, atypically located, often recurrent *peptic ulcerations* are found in the gastro-intestinal tract, in the second or third portion of the duodenum or in the jejunum. They are most recalcitrant to the

usual therapy. Not infrequently, the hyperacidity precedes by years the overt ulcerations.

3. A noninsulin-producing *tumor of the pancreas* is often located outside it, *e.g.*, in the wall of the small intestine or of the stomach. Its histology consists of spindle-shaped cells, bearing no relation to either alpha or beta cells, but resembling the argentophil cells normally scattered throughout the small intestine. An increased secretion of gastrin from such tumors has been postulated, and this might account for the excessive secretion of gastric juice. A polyadenomatosis, with coexistence of hypophysial, adrenal cortical, or parathyroid tumors, has been noted in some 25 per cent of reported cases. Even with tumors located in the islets, a *normal blood sugar level* is found. The only means of alleviating the progressive gastro-intestinal ulcerations is the early and complete removal of the tumor.

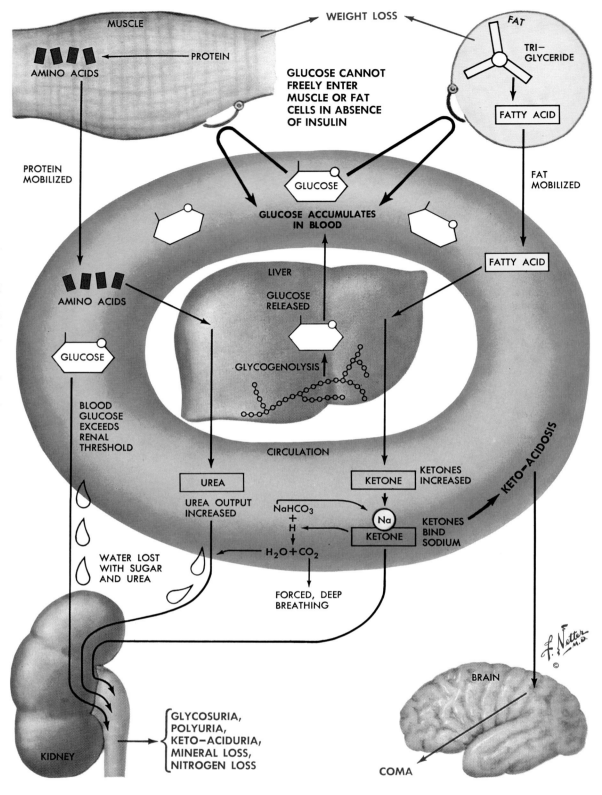

CONSEQUENCES OF INSULIN DEPRIVATION

Insulin deprivation can occur in many ways, both experimentally and clinically. Pancreatectomy, alloxan administration, and destruction of β-cells (by prolonged hyperglycemia due to growth hormone and adrenal corticoids or thyroxine excess) lead to severe curtailment or absence of insulin production and release. Insulin antibodies arising naturally in an organism, or administered to it, and various cellular antagonists either bind the insulin molecule, forming an inactive complex, or interfere peripherally with the proper reaction of insulin at the receptor site.

In all such cases the insulin-sensitive tissues (skeletal muscle, heart, adipose tissue, fibroblasts, etc.) are effectively deprived of hormone. The *transit of glucose* from the blood into the interior of their cells is markedly slowed. At the same time, the *liver* increases its rate of *glucose release by glycogenolysis.* Therefore, *glucose accumulates in the blood,* and the level of the circulating glucose of the blood rises. At this stage, glucose derived from a meal or an administered glucose load cannot be disposed of at a rapid rate. The tolerance for glucose is diminished. When the blood sugar level rises further, the concentration of glucose presented to the *kidney* tubule begins to exceed its capacity for glucose reabsorption (*renal threshold*). Sugar is lost in the urine, "dragging" *water* and salts with it.

Many of the cardinal features of the metabolic phase of diabetes — decreased glucose tolerance, *hyperglycemia, glycosuria, polyuria,* and *loss of minerals,* especially sodium chloride—are thus already accounted for. *Weight loss,* thirst, and hunger occur, depending on the degree of glycosuria causing polyuria.

In the insulin-sensitive tissues, metabolic adjustments occur as a consequence of the lessened sugar supply. *Proteins* are broken down faster than they can be resynthesized; hence, *amino acids* are liberated from *muscle,* brought to the *liver,* and transformed to *urea.* The nonprotein nitrogen of the urine rises, and, with the *nitrogen loss,* a negative nitrogen balance results. The carbon residues of the amino acids form glucose, for the most part, and some are transformed into aceto-acetate, the major *ketone.*

In the *fat tissues* the slow rate of sugar metabolism leads to extreme depression of *fatty acid* formation. This is because of (1) a lack of building stones

(acetate); (2) a lowered supply of reduced coenzymes (especially TPNH); and (3) the fact that the newly formed fatty acids, or those resulting from the breakdown of stored *triglyceride,* are not resynthesized into neutral fat because glycerophosphate, normally derived from the glycolytic breakdown of sugar, is lacking. All these phenomena result in a net liberation of stored fat, as free fatty acids. These are conveyed by the blood and utilized by many tissues for energy production. A large amount of such fatty acids reaches the liver. Because of the particular enzyme equipment of the liver, *ketones* (aceto-acetate and β-OH-butyrate) are produced. These substances are strong organic acids, thus leading to keto-acidosis. They are excreted readily by the kidney, accompanied by base, so fixed base is lost. The β-OH-butyric and the aceto-acetic acids circulating in the blood obtain their sodium from $NaHCO_3$, thus leading to *acidosis.*

The metabolic events just described account for the (1) negative nitrogen balance, (2) additional loss of weight, (3) ketosis, and (4) acidosis. These are the earmarks of the severest state of metabolic decompensation characteristic of diabetes.

Acidosis, when not compensated, exerts its major effect on *brain* function. Lethargy and, eventually, *coma* supervene. In addition, acidosis affects the contractile responses of the small blood vessels throughout the body. This, coupled with loss of fluids and consequent reduction in blood volume, results in vascular shock. Thus, diabetic coma and death comprise the end result of an uncompensated insulin deficiency. Before the advent of insulin, it was the eventual fate of all juvenile diabetics and of most adult cases afflicted with complicating diseases. Today, death from diabetic coma is, fortunately, very rare indeed.

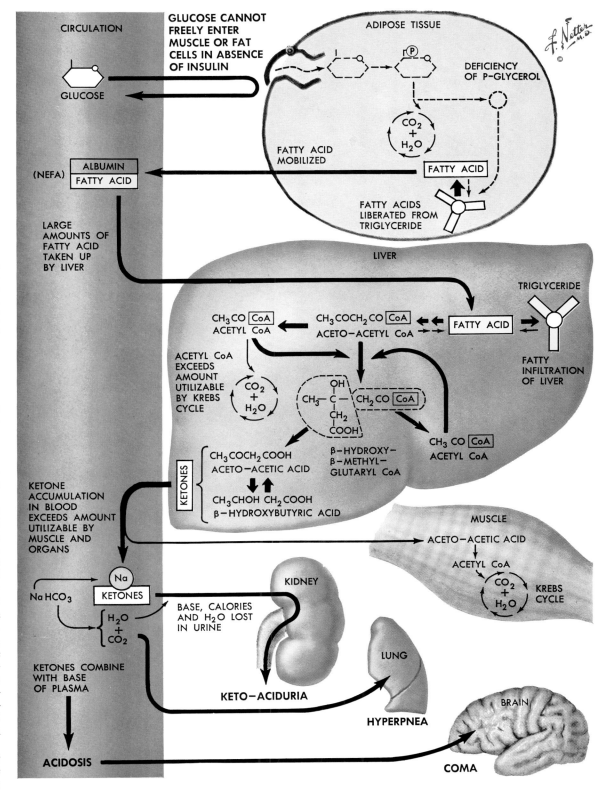

KETO-ACIDOSIS

The term ketone bodies refers to three substances: *aceto-acetic acid, β-hydroxy-butyric acid,* and acetone. The primary material produced in the tissues is aceto-acetic acid. This keto acid can be reduced by a specific enzyme to β-hydroxybutyric acid, with which it soon equilibrates:

$$CH_3CO\ CH_2COOH + 2H$$
(aceto-acetic acid)
$$\rightleftharpoons CH_3CHOH\ CH_2\ COOH$$
(β-hydroxybutyric acid)

In the lung and bladder, aceto-acetic acid can be spontaneously decarboxylated to acetone:

$$CH_3CO\ CH_2\ COOH \rightarrow CH_3CO\ CH_3$$
$$+ CO_2 \quad \text{(acetone)}$$

The latter material is volatile and accounts for the fruity odor of the breath of a patient in keto-acidosis.

Aceto-acetic acid is a normal product of the metabolism of fatty acids and of other foodstuffs which give rise to acetyl CoA. As pictured, a long-chain *fatty acid* is broken down gradually to the stage of *aceto-acetyl CoA* and/or *acetyl CoA*. These 2 molecules condense, forming β-hydroxy-β-methyl-glutaryl CoA (liberating 1 molecule of CoA). This 6-carbon compound splits into free aceto-acetic acid and 1 molecule of acetyl CoA, which can again condense as before. The liver possesses a limited capacity to transform the free water-soluble aceto-acetate to aceto-acetyl CoA. Therefore, aceto-acetate and its reduction product, β-hydroxybutyric acid, leave this organ and are conveyed by the blood stream throughout the body.

Under most normal circumstances the amount of acetyl CoA formed in the liver cell from the primary foodstuffs is largely oxidized via the *Krebs cycle*. Some aceto-acetate is always being released by the liver, so that the plasma level of ketone bodies is generally of the order of 1 to 2 mg per 100 ml. When fatty acids come to the liver in greater abundance than usual (because of an increased release rate of free fatty acids from adipose tissue), the release of ketone bodies rises markedly. Thus, one finds *increased blood ketone levels* during fasting or reduced food intake, in gastro-intestinal disturbances, after epinephrine stimulation, etc. — all events which cause an initial increase in blood *nonesterified fatty acids (NEFA)*.

In the absence of an adequate insulin supply, the *triglycerides* of *adipose tissue* are broken down more rapidly to free fatty acids and free glycerol, and lipogenesis is at a minimum. The breakdown of triglycerides is largely irreversible, since, because of impaired intracellular glucose metabolism, sufficient *glycerolphosphate* is lacking to provide for resynthesis to neutral fat. The *liver* is overwhelmed by the *excess of fatty acids, fatty infiltration of the liver* results, and, thus, ketone body production and release may reach tremendous heights. Although the ketone bodies can normally be used by the extrahepatic tissues (notably *muscle*) for energy purposes, in ketosis the rate of their production exceeds the capacity for their utilization, so they accumulate.

The ketone bodies are strong organic acids, displacing sodium from the bicarbonate of the *plasma*. They are readily excreted by the *kidney*, together with *base*. This leads to *keto-aciduria*, polyuria, and a shift toward acidosis. When the body's compensatory mechanisms fail, *acidosis* increases, respirations become deep (*hyperpnea*) and frequent (stimulated by the fall in pH), and, finally, the activity of the higher *brain* centers is depressed, leading to *coma*. The continuous *loss of water and salts* reduces the circulating blood volume, causing the symptoms and signs of shock. The lowered pH diminishes the contractility of the small blood vessels, thereby aggravating the shock state.

An abnormal globulin becomes evident in the serum, opposing insulin action and thereby making therapy with ordinary doses of insulin largely ineffective.

Keto-acidosis and the resulting coma are the end results of a general metabolic decompensation which begins with the relative, or absolute, lack of insulin, leading to an inability of the glucose molecule to penetrate adipose tissue cells fast enough to slow down the rapid release of fatty acids.

ISLET CELL PATHOLOGY IN EXPERIMENTAL ANIMALS

By their secretion of insulin, the beta cells of the pancreatic islets respond rapidly to changes in food intake, as these lead to varying degrees of hyperglycemia. Many chemical agents, such as *alloxan* and dehydro-ascorbic acid, *decrease beta cell secretion* of insulin. Indirectly, the pituitary growth hormone (GH), the glucocorticoids, and thyroxine have the same effect by blocking peripheral glucose utilization, by increasing gluconeogenesis, or by mobilizing liver glycogen, respectively.

Early work by Evans and by Houssay showed that crude pituitary extracts (rich in growth factor) could produce hyperglycemia and could aggravate the mild diabetes of hypophysectomized and depancreatized animals. In 1937 Young demonstrated the production of a permanent *diabetes in dogs* by means of the injection of crude pituitary extracts.

Many studies have subsequently clarified the events leading to these types of diabetes. The potent factor is the *growth hormone,* or somatotropin (STH). During the first period of GH administration, the beta cells show signs of heightened activity, associated with signs of insulin release (*degranulation*). Increased numbers of *mitoses* and cell proliferation occur. (The histological changes in the *spontaneous diabetes* of the *Chinese hamster* resemble the changes seen in the reversible stage of marked degeneration just discussed.) With further doses of GH, *vacuolization, fibrosis,* and, eventually, *hyalinization* of the islets take place. This state is irreversible, and the diabetes becomes permanent.

Several mechanisms are responsible for the irreversible state. First, GH reduces peripheral glucose uptake by muscle and adipose tissue and, thereby, raises the blood sugar level. This, in turn, acts to stimulate insulin release and synthesis by the beta cells. In addition, GH in some manner, gives rise to a factor (or factors) which opposes insulin action in tissues. The insulin resistance produces a "demand" for more insulin. This multipronged attack leads to overwork and consequent cellular damage within the islets.

Production of permanent diabetes by GH depends on the animal species and its physiological state. Thus, a young, growing puppy shows the proliferative phase but not the beta cell destruction; similar resistance to beta cell destruction is shown by a pregnant or lactating animal. In the cat, partial pancreatectomy sensitizes the islets to the destructive effects of GH. The rat pancreas is wholly resistant to the diabetogenic effects of growth hormone. Though occurring in the *Chinese hamster,* as mentioned above, only lately have some strains of dogs been found to have spontaneous diabetes.

Other hormones which stimulate gluconeogenesis and produce hyperglycemia have also been shown to produce pancreatic pathology and permanent

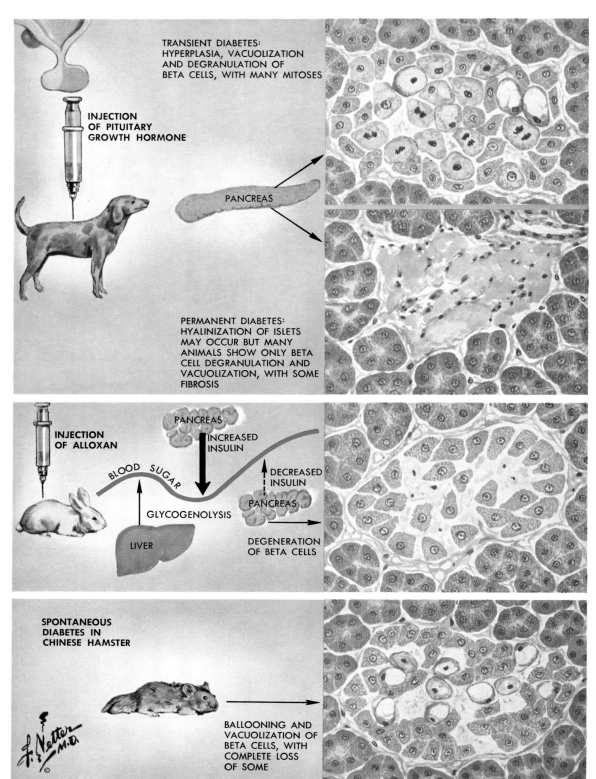

INJECTION OF PITUITARY GROWTH HORMONE

TRANSIENT DIABETES: HYPERPLASIA, VACUOLIZATION AND DEGRANULATION OF BETA CELLS, WITH MANY MITOSES

PANCREAS

PERMANENT DIABETES: HYALINIZATION OF ISLETS MAY OCCUR BUT MANY ANIMALS SHOW ONLY BETA CELL DEGRANULATION AND VACUOLIZATION, WITH SOME FIBROSIS

INJECTION OF ALLOXAN

PANCREAS

INCREASED INSULIN

BLOOD SUGAR

DECREASED INSULIN

PANCREAS

GLYCOGENOLYSIS

LIVER

DEGENERATION OF BETA CELLS

SPONTANEOUS DIABETES IN CHINESE HAMSTER

BALLOONING AND VACUOLIZATION OF BETA CELLS, WITH COMPLETE LOSS OF SOME

diabetes. Such irreversible diabetic states are known as metadiabetes (metahypophysial, meta-adrenal, metathyroid).

Alloxan, a strong oxidizing agent, which combines readily with zinc and with sulfhydryl groups, can cause damage to many types of living cells. However, the beta cells seem particularly sensitive. The sequence of events, following alloxan injection, begins with hyperglycemia mediated by a temporarily excessive epinephrine secretion. This is followed quickly by stimulation of insulin release and a consequent fall in the blood sugar level. Then beta cell damage ensues, insulin disappears, and the cells degenerate. The alpha cells of the islets remain undamaged. Excessive amounts of the drug lead to wider cytotoxic activity in the liver, the kidney, and the adrenal cortex.

Alloxan is a most valuable agent for the induction of pancreatic diabetes in small animals, since pan-

createctomy in such species is a very difficult surgical feat. Also, unlike total pancreatectomy, alloxan leaves the alpha cells and glucagon secretion intact, and it favors ketosis.

The thought has been expressed that perhaps a naturally occurring derivative of pyrimidine metabolism (chemically related to alloxan) could be an etiologic factor in human diabetes. However, the search for such substances has proved fruitless thus far.

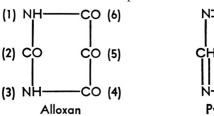

Alloxan

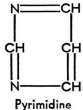

Pyrimidine

ISLET CELL PATHOLOGY IN HUMAN DIABETES

Correlation of the histological state of the islets of Langerhans with the nature and severity of the clinical state of chemical diabetes has been unsatisfactory. Utilizing available routine staining methods, definite abnormalities in the islets could be demonstrated in few more than 50 per cent of diabetics coming to autopsy. Even with improved methodology, there was no significant increase in this figure. With the advent of electron microscopy, abnormalities could be demonstrated in nearly every islet derived from a diabetic, but this is not a routine method. In determining quantitative values, the scattered nature of the "insular organ" made it ordinarily impossible to judge its total weight and/or volume without laborious, specialized study.

Only after the assay for insulin became available was it possible, as in the studies of Wrenshall, to demonstrate that, whereas there was practically no insulin in most pancreases derived from juvenile-onset diabetics, there usually were close to normal amounts in those of adult-onset diabetics. Even the most severe case had some normally functioning cells and produced a small amount of effective hormone. Recent assays of blood insulin tend to show normal values in most adult-onset, nonketonic diabetics and lower values only in the chronic juvenile-onset, keto-acidosis-prone diabetic. It is important to realize that the reserve capacity of the pancreas is, normally, extremely high. In animals about seven eighths of the pancreas must be removed to produce metabolic diabetes, and, in some species such as the rat, a remnant of about 5 per cent of the gland prevents the full expression of the syndrome. Thus, the histopathology of the islets cannot bear an important quantitative relation to the severity of the diabetic syndrome.

In stillborn infants of diabetic mothers, and in some early stages of severe juvenile diabetes, hypertrophy of the islands of Langerhans is seen. Presumably, this is the result of stimulation induced by the hyperglycemia. This hyperplasia, in the face of an elevated glucose level in the blood (the most potent known stimulus to insulin secretion), does, in fact, precede eventual exhaustion of the insulinogenic reserve.

Hydropic changes (vacuolization) are the first step in the destruction of the islet, but they still are reversible. This change is due to infiltration with *glycogen,* and the clear, "watery" areas, which give the change its name, are artifacts. It is surmised that the continual

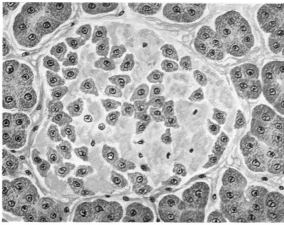

PARTIAL HYALINIZATION
(MALLORY'S ANILINE BLUE STAIN)

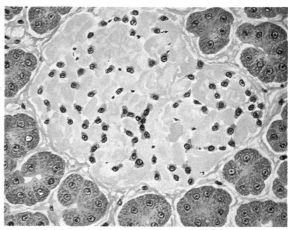

COMPLETE HYALINIZATION
(MALLORY'S ANILINE BLUE STAIN)

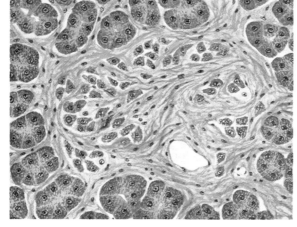

FIBROSIS
(MALLORY'S ANILINE BLUE STAIN)

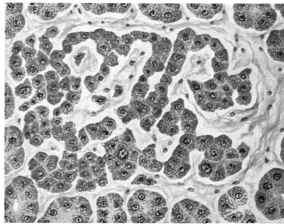

CORDLIKE FORMATION
(MALLORY'S ANILINE BLUE STAIN)

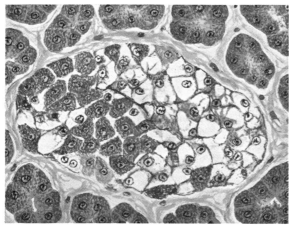

HYDROPIC CHANGE (VACUOLIZATION)
(GOMORI'S ALDEHYDE FUCHSIN AND PONCEAU STAIN)

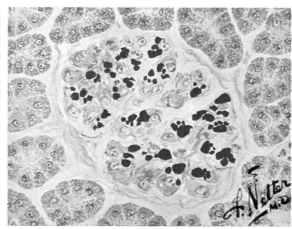

GLYCOGEN DEMONSTRATED IN VACUOLES
BY PERIODIC ACID SCHIFF REAGENT

demand on such islets leads, in time, to atrophy of the β-cells (leaving groups of α-cells undamaged) and to *hyalinization, i.e.,* a deposition of homogeneous, subendothelial substance, which partially or completely replaces an islet. The nature of this deposit is presumably that of a glycoprotein. In the juvenile group, an infiltration of the islet with small round cells sometimes occurs; this process is termed "insulinitis". Comparatively rare even in the juvenile group, it is hardly ever found in adults. *Fibrosis,* a late reparative state, may presumably follow any one of those mentioned above. An earlier phase is the *cordlike formation.*

The work of MacLean and Ogilvie and that of Gepts has concentrated on the number of β-cells remaining in the pancreas of diabetics. Their data point to a significant reduction from normal numbers and to a consequent shift in the β-cell:α-cell ratio.

These results agree with Wrenshall's data on the amounts of extractable insulin in the pancreas at autopsy.

Despite the great variety of histopathological data and the difficulties encountered in interpreting them, they are consistent with the view that an extrapancreatic agent may be concerned with the initiation of islet cell lesions, presumably because of a secondary rise in blood sugar and an overstimulation of insulin secretion. This is nearly always true in obesity. The delayed insulin response of diabetics is due to a relative sluggishness of the damaged β-cells with regard to a prompt release of insulin. The inhibitory "serum" as well as "tissue factors", having initiated the sequence, will tend to keep up the raised demand for insulin, so that, in the end, those patients who carry an inherited diabetic trait may exhaust their insulinogenic reserve.

DIABETIC
MICRO-ANGIOPATHY

Electron microscopic study of normal and diabetic microvasculature has advanced our understanding of the deposits previously found, in many sites, by light microscopy. It is now quite well established that the *glomerular capillaries* in the kidney are the seat of characteristic changes rather early in the course of overt chemical diabetes and very probably also in the genetic diabetic, prior to the onset of hyperglycemia. These early changes consist of *thickening* of the *basement membrane* (*BM*) lying between the *endothelium* and the foot processes of the *epithelium*. In the non-diabetic the BM is about 2500 to 3000 Å in thickness; early in diabetes, even before any signs of kidney dysfunction appear, it may be two to three times the normal thickness. As far as we now know, the material that makes up the BM is of the same nature as that of the PAS-positive deposits in glomerulosclerosis (see page 166). It appears most probable that the nodular deposits are formed by the coiling and lengthening of BM material, together with deposits from the blood stream, and constitute a late phase of the diffuse, thickening process.

The material deposited in the renal glomeruli, in nodular glomerulosclerosis (see page 166), stains red with the periodic acid Schiff reagent (PAS). It is thus said to be *PAS-positive*. After fixation and staining, the material which reacts is probably a polymeric substance with high OH content, most particularly a polysugar. More recent chemical analyses of isolated glomeruli have demonstrated that these deposits consist of a collagenous type of protein (or proteins) and polysaccharide(s), i.e., glycoprotein.

The vascular changes in the *retina* of the human diabetic, when studied by a like technique, show striking resemblances, in that the accumulation of PAS-positive material in the walls of the smallest blood vessels is the characteristic, seemingly specific, change in the early stages of retinopathy. The BM thickening, followed by cell proliferation, has recently been demonstrated in the microcirculation of many organs and tissues of the diabetic. Consider the simi-

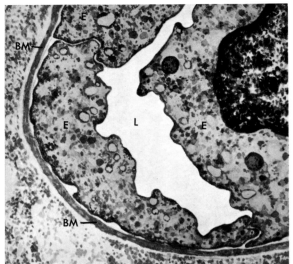

NORMAL CAPILLARY FROM SKIN PAPILLA (ELECTRON MICROSCOPIC VIEW). BM=BASEMENT MEMBRANE; E=ENDOTHELIAL CELL; L=CAPILLARY LUMEN

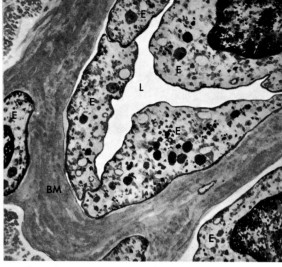

SKIN CAPILLARY IN DIABETES: MARKED THICKENING OF BASEMENT MEMBRANE BY DEPOSITION OF HOMOGENEOUS MATERIAL

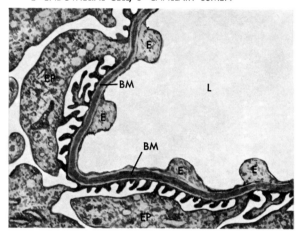

PORTION OF NORMAL RENAL GLOMERULUS: BM=BASEMENT MEMBRANE; E=ENDOTHELIUM; L=CAPILLARY LUMEN; EP=EPITHELIAL CELL

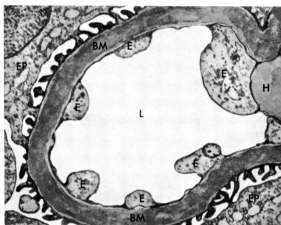

CHARACTERISTIC CHANGES IN DIABETIC GLOMERULO-SCLEROSIS: MARKED THICKENING OF BASEMENT MEMBRANE AND HYALIN DEPOSITION (H)

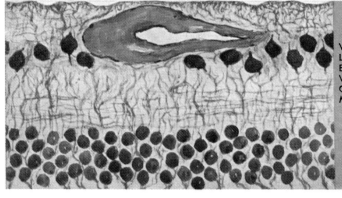

VENULE IN SUPERFICIAL LAYER OF RETINA OF DIABETIC; ECCENTRIC THICKENING OF VENULE WALL BY DEPOSITION OF PAS-POSITIVE STAINING MATERIAL AND NARROWING OF LUMEN

larities of the changes in a *skin capillary* with those of the *glomerular vessel*, as illustrated here. The heart muscle, the tissues of amputated extremities, and the brain — all are seats of such changes. The most recent finding concerns changes in the capillary walls in needle biopsies of the earlobes in early juvenile diabetics, as well as in prediabetics in whom both parents or one twin show overt chemical diabetes, and early thickening of muscle capillaries in non-glycosuric relatives of diabetics.

These studies are still fragmentary, but they do indicate that the syndrome diabetes mellitus consists, in part at least, of a micro-angiopathy of characteristic type, which, in most instances, is progressive over the years, ends in nephropathy and retinopathy, and probably forms favorable conditions for arteriolo- and arteriosclerosis.

The relation of micro-angiopathy to the genetic factor (or factors) of diabetes is unknown. The interdependence between these blood vessel disturbances and abnormalities in intermediary metabolism is, at present, unclear. The origin of the deposited glycoproteins is itself a mystery. Are they the result of local overproduction, or does a circulating serum protein get caught in transit between the blood and the tissue spaces?

Most intriguing are recent reports that insulin and/or insulin antibodies can be demonstrated, by immunohistochemistry, within the BM of glomerular and retinal capillaries. Speculations concerning the possible rôle of insulin in these lesions have arisen but seem, as yet, premature. Further detailed study of the capillary basement membrane, by histochemical and analytical means, is in the forefront of concern on the part of scientific workers throughout the world.

DIABETIC RETINOPATHY AND CATARACT

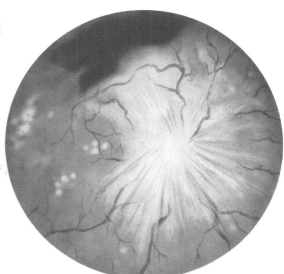

VENOUS DILATATION, MICRO—ANEURYSMS, MINUTE HEMORRHAGES AND YELLOWISH SPOTS IN OCULAR FUNDUS

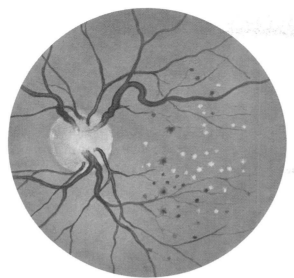

RETINITIS PROLIFERANS AND MASSIVE HEMORRHAGE

The presence of high blood sugar levels and, more particularly, sudden large swings in such values are often accompanied by changes in the refraction and accommodation of the eyes. In the main, such changes are due to osmotic effects on the lens. The muscles of the ciliary body may also be affected by changes in glucose metabolism. All these effects are clearly due to insulin lack and the resulting hyperglycemia, and they can be reversed by good control.

In former years, *cataracts* of the metabolic type were seen frequently in severe diabetics. These begin in the subcapsular portions of the lens and have the so-called snowflake appearance. Their incidence has decreased steadily since the advent of insulin, and experimental data suggest that their formation is due directly to long-standing hyperglycemia.

In contrast, the incidence of progressive diabetic retinopathy has steadily increased, mainly, perhaps, because of the lengthening of the diabetic's lifespan. The exact pathogenesis of these lesions remains unknown. Even though there are indications that frequent bouts of diabetic acidosis are associated with severe eye lesions in some diabetics, progressive retinopathy is seen also in well-controlled diabetics, in those whose metabolic deficit is mild, or even in a few patients whose only abnormality may be a slight decrease in carbohydrate tolerance. There is some correlation with the duration of known hyperglycemia, but this relationship may indicate only that the vascular lesions require a long period of years to become clinically significant rather than that they are causally related to blood sugar deviations.

Characteristically, micro-aneurysms in crops are the first specific lesions to become evident. The outcroppings may persist, regress, or be complicated by hemorrhages. Ophthalmoscopic examination of the *ocular fundus* reveals the *hemorrhages* around *micro-aneurysms* as dark dots and the *exudates* as *yellowish spots*. At first *thin-walled*, the aneurysms subsequently become *hyalinized* and *thrombosed*. The walls are thickened by a PAS-positive staining material (glycoprotein?). These lesions bear a histochemical similarity to the basement membrane deposits of the glomerulosclerotic kidney and of other capillaries throughout the body of the diabetic.

Waxy deposits may appear between

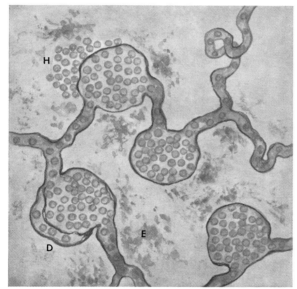

THIN—WALLED MICRO—ANEURYSMS AND CAPILLARY KINKING IN FLAT PREPARATION OF RETINA (X 500)
H=HEMORRHAGE; D=DISSECTING ANEURYSM; E=EXUDATE

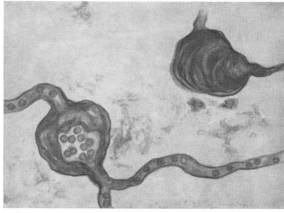

PARTIALLY HYALINIZED AND COMPLETELY HYALINIZED (THROMBOSED) MICRO—ANEURYSMS (X 500)

CATARACT

the areas of aneurysms and of hemorrhage. These are probably related to the level of blood lipids and lipoproteins, and clearing of such deposits has followed the rigid dietary restriction of fat intake. Such a regimen, however, does not affect the course of events related to aneurysm and hemorrhage.

In time, weakening of the walls of many blood vessels occurs, with *hemorrhage* into the vitreous. This is followed by neovascularization and fibrosis (*retinitis proliferans*), both arising from the optic disk; eventually, retinal detachment ensues.

For a number of years it has been suspected that some factor (or factors) which favors progression of the retinal lesion depends, for full expression, on intact pituitary function. Thus arose the therapeutic attempts to arrest diabetic retinopathy by means of pituitary ablation by surgery or radiation, or by section of the pituitary stalk. Less successful has been

the suppression of pituitary function by estrogens or glucocorticoids. Adrenalectomy has not brought much benefit. Some successful arrests (about 35 to 45 per cent) have been obtained by pituitary suppression. No firm foundation for the involvement of a particular known factor of the pituitary in pathogenesis has as yet been achieved, though growth hormone is the favored suspect.

In most instances, retinopathy and diabetic nephropathy coexist, even though the lesions of one organ may be more advanced than those of the other. Clinically significant kidney dysfunction in the diabetic, especially of the nephrotic type, is almost always associated with retinopathy. Retinopathy may progress, however, before kidney function is noticeably diminished. Hypophysial ablation, radiation, or stalk section are generally not attempted if kidney function is noticeably impaired.

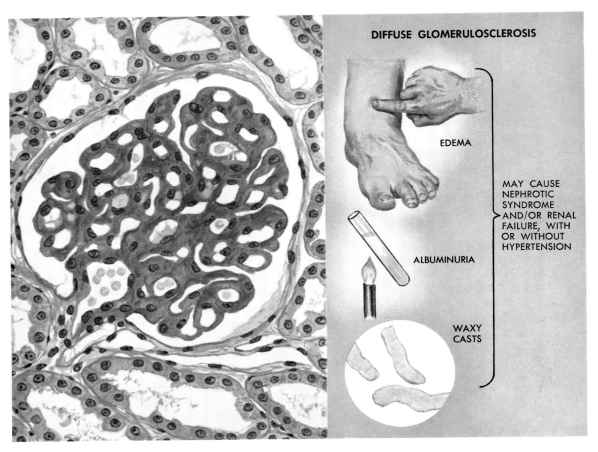

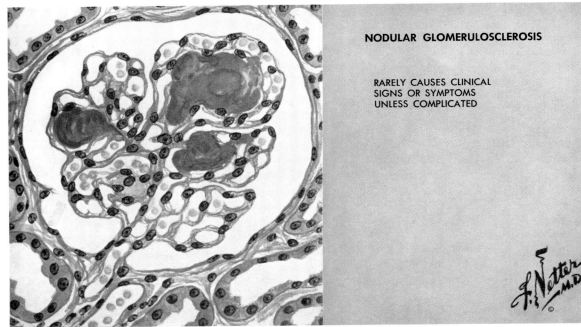

INTERCAPILLARY GLOMERULOSCLEROSIS

In 1936 Kimmelstiel and Wilson described a renal lesion, seemingly specific for and characteristic of diabetes, named *nodular intercapillary glomerulosclerosis.* It consists of spherical or oval nodules, measuring about 20 to 100 microns at their greatest diameter, located at the peripheral aspect of the glomerular tufts. These stain red with the periodic acid Schiff reagent and consist principally of reticulin fibers with high polysaccharide content (glycoproteins).

The *diffuse* form of *glomerulosclerosis* was first described by Fahr in 1942. It consists of diffuse deposition of PAS-positive material in the walls of the glomerular capillaries, leading, first, to pronounced thickening of the basement membrane. Later, the deposit engulfs the endothelial and, lastly, the epithelial cell layers, and the capillary lumina become narrowed and finally disappear by occlusion.

It would seem probable, from serial biopsy studies, that these two types of lesions originate from diffuse basement membrane thickening, which begins early in the course of diabetes, even before the appearance of overt hyperglycemia. As time goes on, the lesion progresses, and, in some cases, the deposition of basement membrane material is so great that convolutions of the membranes appear as *nodular deposits.* Chemical analysis reveals that the membrane material consists of protein of a collagenous type (rich in hydroxyproline) and of polysaccharides of unknown structure. It seems plausible that such glycoprotein deposits characterize diabetic micro-angiopathy in almost all organs.

In the kidneys, the effect of capillary closure, together with the vascular lesions of arteriosclerosis and the inflammatory cell collections of pyelonephritis, leads eventually to the signs and symptoms of irreversible kidney insufficiency. Not infrequently, a nephrotic state supervenes, with *edema,* profuse *albuminuria, waxy*

urinary casts, and *hypertension,* with nitrogen retention. More often, chronic progressive uremia with proteinuria is the grim clinical outcome. It is difficult to ascribe to any one lesion the clinical kidney insufficiency of the diabetic of long duration. For this reason the mixed picture often seen at autopsy, consisting of glomerulosclerosis, arteriosclerosis, and patchy pyelonephritis, has been considered as a triad—diabetic nephropathy.

In association with glomerulosclerosis one may see eosinophilic deposits or "drops" in Bowman's space, usually attached to the glomerular capsule. The material resembles fibrinoid; it does not contain a collagenlike protein but does contain some sugars and lipids.

The origins of glomerulosclerosis are obscure, the speculations many. Is the glycoprotein deposit a material filtered from the plasma, or is it manufac-

tured in situ? Are these renal lesions or, for that matter, are the other angiopathic deviations, such as waxy deposits and aneurysms, the results of an autoimmune phenomenon? Is typical glomerulosclerosis regularly found in acquired diabetes (pancreatectomy, hemochromatosis, acromegaly, Cushing's disease)? Even though the severity of the diabetic state does not bear a direct relationship to the degree of glomerulosclerosis, do long-standing, wide fluctuations of the blood sugar affect the lesion? Does insulin therapy with the hormone derived from beef or pork aggravate angiopathy because of antibody formation? Are the pituitary and adrenal hormones necessary for the full expression of angiopathy?

These are some of the major, incompletely resolved problems under discussion at present. Precise answers will require continued painstaking and imaginative research.

DIABETIC NEPHROPATHY AND NECROTIZING PAPILLITIS

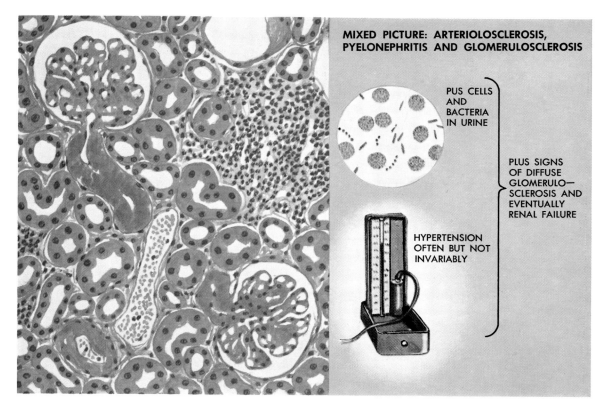

MIXED PICTURE: ARTERIOLOSCLEROSIS, PYELONEPHRITIS AND GLOMERULOSCLEROSIS

PUS CELLS AND BACTERIA IN URINE

PLUS SIGNS OF DIFFUSE GLOMERULO-SCLEROSIS AND EVENTUALLY RENAL FAILURE

HYPERTENSION OFTEN BUT NOT INVARIABLY

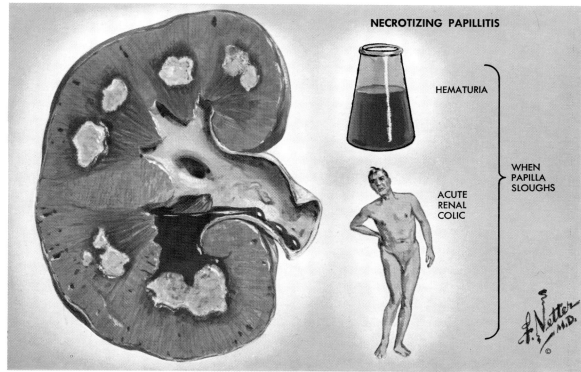

NECROTIZING PAPILLITIS

HEMATURIA

ACUTE RENAL COLIC

WHEN PAPILLA SLOUGHS

The overwhelming majority of renal lesions found at autopsy, in long-standing cases of diabetes, affect the circulatory apparatus of the kidney, the glomerular and peritubular capillaries, the arterioles of the glomerulus, and the small muscular arteries as well as the renal artery and its immediate branches. A significant percentage of such kidneys also exhibit the cellular infiltrations characteristic of both acute and chronic pyelonephritis. Occasionally, one encounters necrosis of the renal papillae and, more rarely, glycogen and fat infiltration of the tubular epithelium. Usually, several types of histological change are found simultaneously; and the relationship between the clinical and laboratory pictures of renal dysfunction and the totality of the lesions found post mortem is often confusing.

It is the hope of workers in the field that recent studies of in vivo kidney biopsies, by electron microscopy and associated chemical procedures, will, in time, give a dynamic picture of the evolution of several of the late renal lesions characteristic of diabetes of long duration. Tantalizing beginnings have been made which already offer a tempting field for speculation.

Arterio- and Arteriolonephrosclerosis

As is the case in many regions of the vascular tree, the arteriosclerotic process occurs more frequently, and at an earlier age, in the medium and small arteries of the kidney in the diabetic. Histologically, the lesions are not distinguishable from those found in the nondiabetic population. However, it is common to find hyalinization of both the afferent and efferent arterioles of the *glomerulus,* whereas in the nondiabetic group the afferent arteriole is more frequently affected. These lesions account for some of the *reduction of kidney function* during life, as well as for some degree of *hypertension.*

Pyelonephritis (Acute and Chronic)

At the autopsy table, evidence of pyelonephritis is quite frequently seen in diabetics. The incidence of pyelonephritis during life, in the population of diabetics, has declined during the past 10 to 15 years, possibly because of the increased use of antibiotics. Random renal biopsies demonstrate less pyelonephritic lesions than would be anticipated from autopsy material. It is possible, therefore, that the inflammatory foci found post mortem are a late, preterminal development, in many instances. In any case, one may still safely state that focal pyelonephritis is more frequent in the diabetic than in the nondiabetic human being, especially in women.

Although rare, *necrotizing papillitis* is a most serious complication of pyelonephritis. The combination of vascular obstruction and overwhelming infection may lead to necrosis of the renal papillae already severely compromised by an endarteritis of the small vessels supplying the tips. This presents as *hematuria, renal colic,* azotemia, and fever. The urine may contain shed portions of renal papillae and a large number of bacteria but, on occasion, none at all. The appearance of an intravenous urogram may be diagnostic, revealing small, lifesaverlike negative shadows in the papillae, representing shed papillary tips. This dread condition is more frequent in diabetic females than in diabetic males.

DIABETIC NEUROPATHY

The lesions of diabetic neuropathy affect both the *motor* and *sensory systems* and the *voluntary* as well as the *autonomic systems*. Pathogenetic mechanisms include, to varying degrees, a direct affection of the peripheral nervous system by metabolic inadequacies or by interference with its intimate blood supply through either micro-angiopathy or atherosclerosis. Damage to nuclei in the central nervous system or in the cord, to ganglia, or to nerve fibers is found. Many diabetics with minimal glycosuria and hyperglycemia may show neuropathy, which may be the presenting symptom in an unsuspected case of diabetes and may also precede the onset of hyperglycemia. Pain in the leg muscles, especially at night, is found in diabetics with frequent episodes of hyperglycemia. This is related to water and electrolyte shifts and may be readily improved by better control. However, generally, the signs and symptoms of diabetic neuropathy become considerably worse for a period of 2 to 3 weeks after good diabetic control has been re-established in a previously uncontrolled diabetic, after which any improvement depends on how much of the neuropathy results from an acute neuritis, occasioned by lack of vitamin B complex (especially B_{12}), or is due to irreversible micro-angiopathy and endarteritis in the nervous system.

Peripheral nerve involvement is often mixed, usually sensory, and less frequently motor. *Paresthesia, hyperalgesia,* and *hypesthesia* occur predominantly in the lower extremities, and most often there is involvement of the peroneal more than of the posterior tibial nerve and of the femoral more than of the sciatic. The pain is deep and burning. Cutaneous hyperalgesia may be severe. Tingling and stabbing paresthesias are common, yet pain and touch sensation are usually fairly normal, whereas *decreased vibratory sense* is very common. With loss of position sense, patients are prone to injure their extremities. When pain sensation has finally been lost, *neuropathic (painless) ulcers* may develop. The motor involvement may lead to *wrist drop* or *ankle drop,* often spotty in distribution and unilateral, in contrast to what might be found in lead poisoning.

Cranial nerve damage is not uncommon, involving control of facial expression and of extra-ocular movements. Thus, *extra-ocular muscle paralysis,* most often affecting the third, fourth, and sixth nerves, may lead to *strabismus* and *diplopia,* most frequently in older patients with diabetes of long duration. *Ptosis* is frequently present, with severe retrobulbar pain extending upward and involving much of the affected side. Unilateral ptosis, without pupillary or

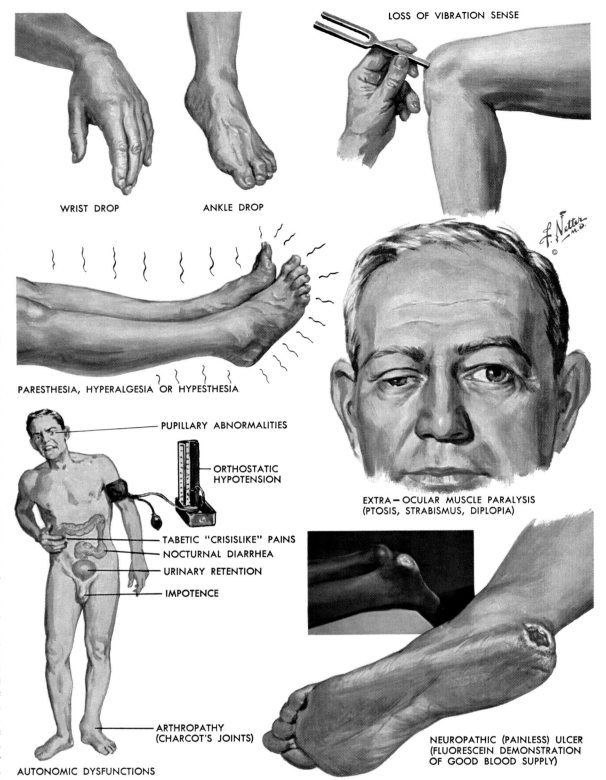

WRIST DROP

ANKLE DROP

LOSS OF VIBRATION SENSE

PARESTHESIA, HYPERALGESIA OR HYPESTHESIA

PUPILLARY ABNORMALITIES

ORTHOSTATIC HYPOTENSION

TABETIC "CRISISLIKE" PAINS

NOCTURNAL DIARRHEA

URINARY RETENTION

IMPOTENCE

ARTHROPATHY (CHARCOT'S JOINTS)

AUTONOMIC DYSFUNCTIONS

EXTRA—OCULAR MUSCLE PARALYSIS (PTOSIS, STRABISMUS, DIPLOPIA)

NEUROPATHIC (PAINLESS) ULCER (FLUORESCEIN DEMONSTRATION OF GOOD BLOOD SUPPLY)

extra-ocular involvement, is absolutely pathognomonic of diabetic neuropathy. Symptoms usually disappear in a matter of months as secondary centers take over from those damaged by micro-angiopathy.

Autonomic involvement and dysfunction are insidious. *Pupillary abnormalities* include miosis, irregularities of diameter and shape, and, rarely, lack of contraction to light but with normal contraction with accommodation. This type of *Argyll Robertson pupil* must be distinguished from that due to lues. Such patients may also suffer from *crisislike,* stabbing *abdominal pains* resembling tabes, which shares the absence of vibration and position senses. Rarely, *arthropathy* resembling *Charcot's joints* enforces the simile further, though distal rather than proximal joints are most often affected in the diabetic.

Gastro-intestinal involvement is common. Constipation is enhanced by dehydration; diarrhea often occurs alternatingly. Most disturbing is the *nocturnal diarrhea,* which interferes with sleep and is very characteristic of diabetic neuropathy. *Orthostatic hypotension* is quite common and when, added to this, the nephrotic phase of the Kimmelstiel-Wilson syndrome depletes the plasma volume, the patient's incapacity may make him bedridden unless a regimen of elastic stocking and tight abdominal support is established. The genito-urinary tract is involved early and with increasing severity. *Urinary retention* follows parasympathetic involvement of bladder innervation, and *impotence* in males is related to both sympathetic and parasympathetic innervation of the erectile tissue of the penis. Some 70 per cent of diabetic patients with neuropathy show an elevation of the cerebrospinal fluid protein levels up to 100 mg per 100 ml, or more, which is not found in diabetics without this complication.

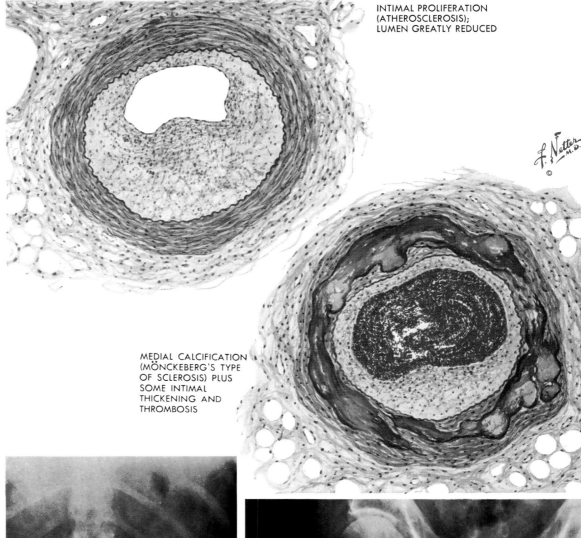

INTIMAL PROLIFERATION
(ATHEROSCLEROSIS);
LUMEN GREATLY REDUCED

MEDIAL CALCIFICATION
(MÖNCKEBERG'S TYPE
OF SCLEROSIS) PLUS
SOME INTIMAL
THICKENING AND
THROMBOSIS

ATHEROSCLEROSIS IN DIABETES

The problems attending long-term diabetes mellitus are primarily centered around the vascular system. The term diabetic angiopathy has been coined for the picture as a whole. Some aspects of it have been called nonspecific, because the lesions are seemingly indistinguishable from similar ones occurring in the nondiabetic population. Some of these consist primarily of typical *intimal proliferation,* associated with atheroma formation (atherosclerosis), and of *medial calcification* (arteriosclerosis). The clinical expression of such lesions is seen in the *obstruction* of peripheral *arteries,* associated with intermittent claudication of the legs, poor nutrition and pallor of the lower extremities, loss of peripheral pulsations, and dry and wet gangrene. Angina pectoris, coronary insufficiency, and coronary occlusions often coexist with moderate hypertension.

In the population of diabetic patients, 70 per cent of all deaths are due to vascular disease. This figure is about two and one half times the death rate from the same causes among nondiabetic individuals of all ages. The vascular lesions range from thickening of capillary basement membranes and endothelial proliferation of small blood vessels, through medial calcification and atherosclerosis of medium vessels, to enhanced atheroma and plaque formation in the aorta. The coronary vessels are involved very frequently, and to a similar extent in females and males. This is in contrast to the favorable ratio, in respect to females under 55, among the nondiabetic group. The over-all incidence of myocardial infarction in all diabetics is approximately four times that found in the normal population.

Calcification of pelvic arteries and of the *femoral artery* is often seen in middle-aged diabetics. Obstruction, which occurs more rarely, is shown typically in the *aortogram* of the *left iliac artery,* which nowadays would have been done by a retrograde femoral arteriogram.

Although, seemingly, the arterial lesions are not of specific character, they nevertheless occur, in diabetics, at much

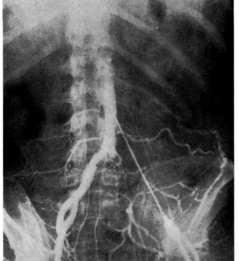

AORTOGRAM: OBSTRUCTION OF LEFT
ILIAC ARTERY IN A DIABETIC

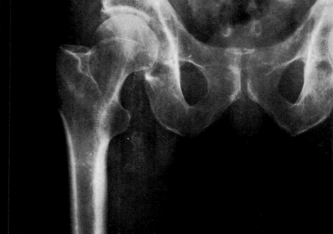

CALCIFIED FEMORAL ARTERY IN A DIABETIC
DEMONSTRATED BY X-RAY

younger age periods, with greater incidence, and with a faster rate of progression. These phenomena remain unexplained. The known disturbances in intermediary metabolism do not throw any light on the diabetic propensity toward arteriosclerosis; neither do the data concerning cholesterol, triglyceride, and lipoprotein levels. Experimentally, it is less easy to produce atheroma by high cholesterol diets in the diabetic rabbit than in the nondiabetic control animal.

Perhaps the arterial lesions are actually more specific for diabetes than they appear to be by conventional histologic techniques. Some recent findings by Diezel indicate that the vessel wall may be infiltrated heavily with a variety of polysaccharides in the diabetic, but, much less so in the nondiabetic individual. Since thickening of the capillary basement membranes seems so universal and early a lesion in diabetes, is it possible that the microcirculation is

functionally affected early, producing the immediate environment which favors plaque formation and calcification in the larger vessels? Not enough work has yet been done on the state of the vasa vasorum, in early diabetes, to know whether disturbances in the supply of the medium and larger blood vessels are, in fact, predisposing them to arterio- and atherosclerosis.

Since young patients with Cushing's disease, who remain untreated, develop arteriosclerosis and coronary disease in a few years, one may ask whether, in diabetes mellitus, much evidence of hyperadrenocorticalism can be found. The available data speak against such a concept. Urinary steroid levels are high only in stressful situations such as ketosis, acidosis, or major infections. In the reasonably controlled diabetic (even though glycosuric), the adrenal cortex is not hyperactive; in fact, it is often hypo-active.

VASCULAR INSUFFICIENCY IN DIABETES

Long before insulin was introduced as a therapeutic agent, it was noted by clinicians that the diabetic individual seemed much more prone to cardiovascular degenerative disease than did the nondiabetic person of the same age. Coronary thrombosis and arteriosclerosis of the larger vessels are very prevalent in the population of diabetics, and the usually expected advantage of the female sex, with regard to coronary thrombosis, is almost completely lost. In the limbs the arteriosclerotic process advances very rapidly and leads, in many instances, to occlusions and to gangrenous lesions.

Dependent rubor and the *absence of dorsalis pedis* or posterior tibial *pulsations* suggest arterial insufficiency in the diabetic. At this point, extreme cleanliness of the feet and the prevention, by the use of soft socks and protective boots, of any trauma are all that stand between a normal extremity and *diabetic ulcers*. Occasionally, these are accompanied by *lymphedema,* which enhances the spread of infection to the ulcer. *Gangrene of a toe* is a consequence of an endarteritis and poor development of collateral circulation. Both wet and dry types occur, the latter being far less likely to spread to *extensive gangrene.* In the dry type, particularly, the extremities are quite likely to detach spontaneously, with little or no bleeding. Gangrene can be minimized by adequate diabetic control and the consumption of little saturated fat, and it can be delayed or prevented by scrupulous foot care throughout life, avoiding trauma at all cost.

The incidence of gangrene of the lower extremities is some sixty times greater in the diabetic population over the age of 50 years than among normal subjects.

The arteriosclerosis itself does not completely explain the frequency of gangrene in the diabetic, since an equally advanced vascular lesion in the nondiabetic is associated much less frequently with this calamity. It must be realized that although arteriosclerosis of the larger vessels is the more obvious lesion, the diabetic leg suffers simultaneously from two other pathological processes: The small blood vessels are the seat of a diffuse proliferative, obliterating lesion— a part of diabetic micro-angiopathy. Thus, the possibilities for the development of a collateral blood supply are meager indeed. In addition, loss of sensory input, owing to a coexistent neuropathy, may provide the background for poorly perceived injuries. A combination of these three types of lesion explains

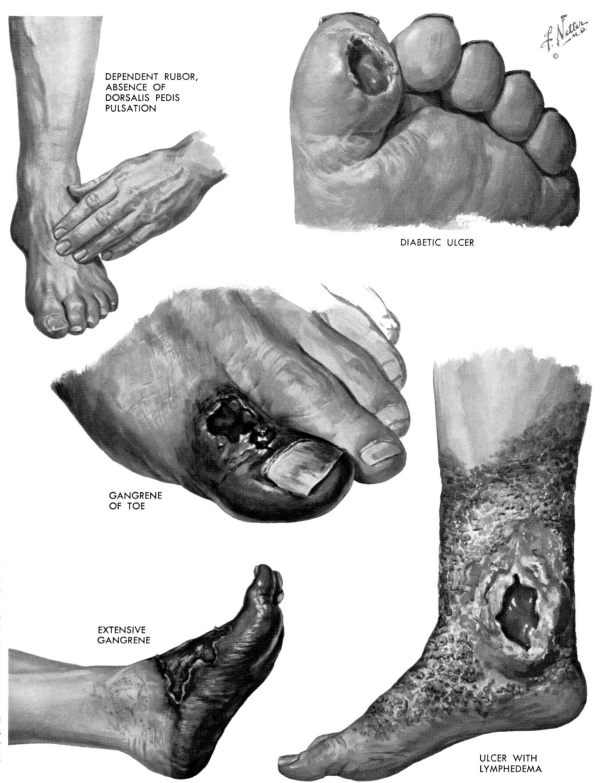

DEPENDENT RUBOR, ABSENCE OF DORSALIS PEDIS PULSATION

DIABETIC ULCER

GANGRENE OF TOE

EXTENSIVE GANGRENE

ULCER WITH LYMPHEDEMA

fully the appalling frequency of gangrene with its aftermath of amputation.

Surprisingly, the frequency of cerebrovascular disease (hemorrhage and thrombosis) is no greater in the diabetic than it is in the nondiabetic population of the same age range.

Recent histological and histochemical studies have demonstrated that, even in the larger vessels, the arteriosclerotic process in the diabetic shows certain distinguishing characteristics. There is a distinct and pronounced infiltration of the vessel wall with mucopolysaccharide material, which can be brought into view only by special stains. As in the case of micro-angiopathy, there is a relation between diabetes and an increase in deposition of the carbohydrate and protein complexes of the ground substance and connective tissue. Although this is of vital importance, its biochemical mechanisms of origin and mainte-

nance remain poorly understood.

The influence of genetic and of dietary factors on the development of the progression of atherosclerosis in the diabetic deserves intensive study. For example, it is known that, in Japan, diabetes is more frequently associated with hypertension and cerebrovascular accidents and less frequently with arterial occlusive disease of the heart and the lower extremities. Amputation for gangrene is a comparatively rare occurrence in that environment. The usual Japanese diet is high in carbohydrate (rice) and low in protein and saturated fats. The salt intake is, however, very high. Do these factors explain the above-mentioned differences in incidence, or are we dealing with a difference in genetic constitution (perhaps with regard to anterior pituitary function)? Only further comparative studies will, perhaps, bring some insight concerning this problem.

Tests for Diabetes and Prediabetes

In the distant past, diagnosis of the metabolic phase of diabetes was made only in individuals who exhibited glycosuria. Since the renal threshold for glucose may vary from about 160 to 250 mg per 100 ml of blood sugar, glycosuria reveals only the moderate or severe cases.

Determinations of *fasting blood sugar* levels widened the area of correct diagnosis by including those diabetics whose elevated blood sugar values did not exceed their renal threshold. A group of individuals whose fasting blood sugar values fall within normal range, but who fail to handle an orally administered load of glucose as efficiently as do a control normal group, may be detected by a *2-hour postprandial blood sugar* value after a standard meal. This requires only one 2-hour blood sugar determination and the administration of a high-carbohydrate meal, with approximately 100 gm of mostly rapidly absorbable carbohydrate. However, since this is not all glucose, the results are not completely reliable.

The *oral glucose tolerance test* is a more stringent test of glucose intolerance, although it is dependent on the rate of gastric emptying and of sugar absorption by the intestinal tract. With pylorospasm a flat glucose tolerance curve is found. In contrast, with hyperthyroidism or following partial gastrectomy, an excessive hyperglycemic response is noted. To avoid these factors the test dose may be given intravenously, as indicated in the *rapid intravenous glucose tolerance test*. When the logarithm of the *excess* of the *blood sugar level* above the fasting level is plotted against time, the result is a straight line. Its slope expresses the rate of sugar utilization. K in the chart is the blood sugar fall per minute which may be calculated from the half disappearance time ($\frac{1}{2}Co$) found at the one half point of the peak (Co) of blood sugar excess.

Cortisone increases gluconeogenesis by the liver and leads to a higher blood sugar level with a glucose load. Thus, coupled with an oral dose of glucose in the *cortisone glucose tolerance test*, it represents an additional load and a more severe test of the reserve capacity of the β-cells. According to the data of Conn and Fajans, almost 25 per cent of individuals, who are members of families with one or more overt diabetics, show an abnormal cortisone glucose tolerance test, even though the standard oral test lies within normal limits. This test is thus adapted to detect prediabetics or "premellitic" diabetics.

Since the sulfonylureas (tolbutamide, chlorpropamide, acetohexamide) stimulate insulin discharge from β-cells, they

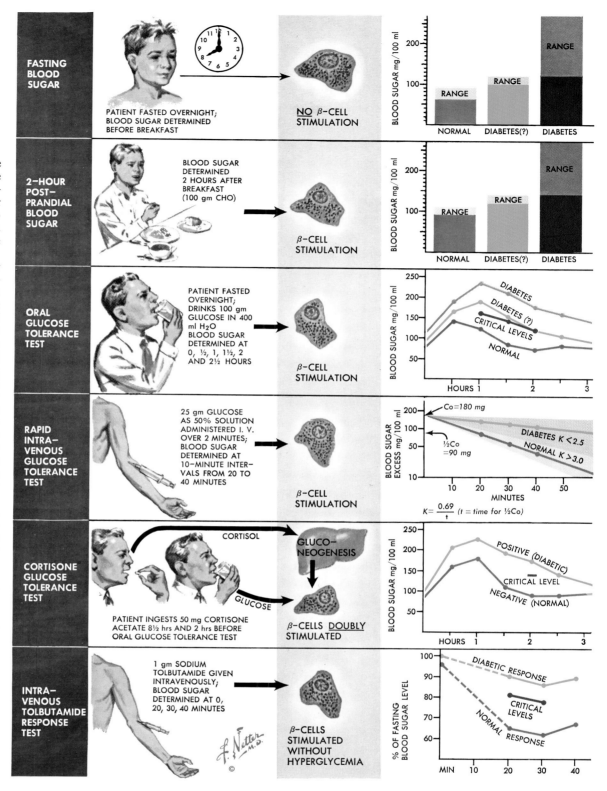

can be used to measure insulin reserve, indirectly, by recording the rate of blood sugar fall after their administration. The accompanying chart shows the curves obtained in normal individuals and in diabetic patients, using 1 gm of *sodium tolbutamide*, given intravenously. With concurrent oral administration of sodium carbonate, an oral tolbutamide test may be carried out with 3 gm of tolbutamide. The rapidity of these tests is an advantage. They are useful in differentiating between diabetes and the hyperglycemic response to glucose which is found in some patients with obesity and those afflicted with certain types of hepatic insufficiency, notably biliary cirrhosis, as tolbutamide produces a good fall in blood sugar in either case.

The refinements of all the tests mentioned require that the preparation of the patient and the quality of laboratory technique be meticulous. Thus, it is neces-

sary to be sure that the carbohydrate intake, prior to the day of the test, consisted of at least 150 gm of carbohydrate per day, and that the blood sampling was accurate as to timing. The blood sugar method used should determine true blood glucose, rather than "reducing" substances, using techniques such as the Somogyi-Nelson or the glucose oxidase method. When the various types of tolerance tests are used in the same patient, the results, unfortunately, do not coincide in all subjects. The immunochemical assay of insulin (see page 172), in conjunction with a glucose load, promises to become ever more important diagnostically.

At present, we do not know precisely whether early diagnosis of the metabolic phase of diabetes should be followed by such regimens as dietary modifications, sulfonylureas, etc.; initial attempts to preserve insulinogenic reserve are promising.

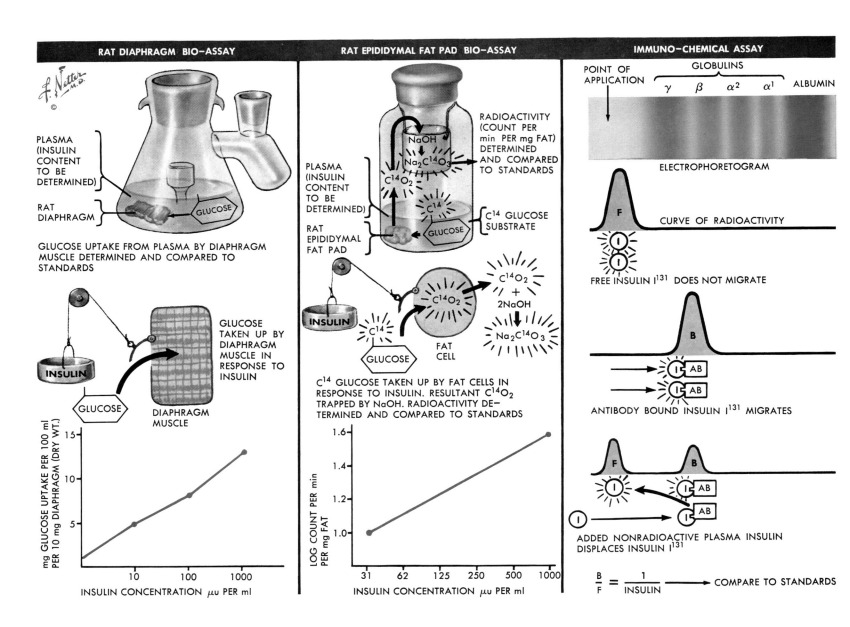

PLASMA (INSULIN CONTENT TO BE DETERMINED)

RAT DIAPHRAGM

GLUCOSE

GLUCOSE UPTAKE FROM PLASMA BY DIAPHRAGM MUSCLE DETERMINED AND COMPARED TO STANDARDS

INSULIN

GLUCOSE

GLUCOSE TAKEN UP BY DIAPHRAGM MUSCLE IN RESPONSE TO INSULIN

DIAPHRAGM MUSCLE

GLUCOSE UPTAKE PER 100 ml PER 10 mg DIAPHRAGM (DRY WT.)

INSULIN CONCENTRATION μu PER ml

NaOH

Na₂C¹⁴O₃

C¹⁴O₂

C¹⁴

RADIOACTIVITY (COUNT PER min PER mg FAT) DETERMINED AND COMPARED TO STANDARDS

PLASMA (INSULIN CONTENT TO BE DETERMINED)

RAT EPIDIDYMAL FAT PAD

C¹⁴ GLUCOSE SUBSTRATE

GLUCOSE

INSULIN

$C^{14}O_2$

$C^{14}O_2 + 2NaOH$

$Na_2C^{14}O_3$

GLUCOSE

C^{14}

FAT CELL

C¹⁴ GLUCOSE TAKEN UP BY FAT CELLS IN RESPONSE TO INSULIN. RESULTANT C¹⁴O₂ TRAPPED BY NaOH. RADIOACTIVITY DETERMINED AND COMPARED TO STANDARDS

LOG COUNT PER min PER mg FAT

INSULIN CONCENTRATION μu PER ml

POINT OF APPLICATION

GLOBULINS
γ β α² α¹ ALBUMIN

ELECTROPHORETOGRAM

CURVE OF RADIOACTIVITY

F

FREE INSULIN I¹³¹ DOES NOT MIGRATE

B

I AB

I AB

ANTIBODY BOUND INSULIN I¹³¹ MIGRATES

F

I

B

I AB

I AB

I

ADDED NONRADIOACTIVE PLASMA INSULIN DISPLACES INSULIN I¹³¹

$$\frac{B}{F} = \frac{1}{INSULIN} \longrightarrow \text{COMPARE TO STANDARDS}$$

SECTION V—PLATE 30

INSULIN ASSAYS

Because insulin is a protein, direct and specific chemical quantitative determination is impossible. The amounts present in the circulation at any one time are extremely small. According to the best estimates, normal fasting man has an insulin concentration of about 1/10,000 of a microgram of insulin per milliliter of plasma. In molar terms this is 10^{-9} M. Insulin assays are, therefore, performed with biological techniques; they are, as a rule, more sensitive but are inherently less accurate than are quantitative chemical techniques.

The oldest methods for blood insulin assay were those using the hypoglycemic reaction of mice as the end point. Of these, the most sensitive method was to prepare the experimental animals by adrenalectomy, hypophysectomy, and alloxan administration, and to record the time that elapsed between injection of the serum to be tested and the moment when the animal, in insulin shock, dropped off a wire screen above some water. Comparing this with dilute standards of insulin, an extremely rough quantitative measurement was obtained. Modern methods are far more sensitive.

The *rat diaphragm* and *epididymal fat pad*

assays depend on the fact that these tissues take up glucose at a faster rate when insulin is added to the medium in which they are incubated, and that, within certain ranges of insulin concentrations, there is a reproducible quantitative dependence of the sugar uptake on the insulin content. In the diaphragm assay the usual measurement is glucose uptake; in the case of the fat pad, glucose uptake, the appearance of $C^{14}O_2$ from C^{14}-labeled glucose, or total CO_2 output can be measured. In the fat pad, CO_2 output depends linearly on the amount of glucose entering the tissue.

In plasma there are, in addition to insulin, other substances which may influence glucose uptake. Also, some of the protein fractions of plasma may either form a complex with insulin or interfere with its proper action at effector sites of the cell. Vallance-Owen has described an antagonist which appears to be the B chain of insulin attached to albumin. This constituent, synalbumin, is, apparently, formed in the liver. A higher-than-normal titer is found in relatives of diabetics who themselves do not have the disease. It is evident that the bio-assays measure glucose-uptake-promoting activity which is the resultant of insulin and of the factors that aid or interfere with its action. Most careful workers in the field refer, therefore, to the determinations as "insulinlike activity" (ILA).

The *immuno-assay* of Berson and Yalow measures immunologically intact insulin and is not affected by insulin antagonists or insulinlike sub-

stances, yet biologically inactive insulin may react in the test. It depends on the fact that *free insulin* (F in the chart) stays at the point of application on the paper in an *electrophoretic procedure,* but, when forming a complex with guinea pig *anti-insulin antibody,* the *hormone* (B in the chart) migrates with it. If the insulin is labeled (with I¹³¹), it can be localized on the paper. The "unknown" plasma contains non-labeled insulin, which will compete with and displace some of the I¹³¹ insulin. Using suitable standards, one can arrive at quantitative values by this procedure.

In general, the immuno-assay gives the lowest and most reliable values for blood insulin, often exceeded greatly by the fat pad procedure. The diaphragm assay may give lower values, because interfering peptides and proteins exert their actions unhampered.

Although much that is confusing still pervades this area of investigation, it is reasonably certain that (1) most adult-onset diabetics, as well as freshly discovered juveniles, have normal ranges of plasma insulin in the fasting state; (2) any rise in plasma insulin, following glucose ingestion, may be delayed in onset and prolonged in the diabetic, and abnormally high levels of insulin are especially common in obese diabetics; (3) severe, established juvenile cases and thin adults have low blood insulin levels; and (4) many adult-onset diabetics have, in their plasma, peptides and/or proteins which either bind insulin or interfere with its cellular action.

ORAL ANTIDIABETIC AGENTS

Insulin, being a protein, is inactivated by the acid and enzyme secretions of the gastro-intestinal tract. An ideal oral substitute for insulin should be a freely absorbable, nontoxic substance which acts at the cellular level by the same biochemical mechanism as does the hormone. As yet, such agents are not available. The substances presently in use as oral antidiabetic agents require, for their effectiveness, either insulin-producing β-cells or the presence of some exogenously introduced insulin.

Many chemical materials may, under some circumstances, lower the blood sugar, yet they are useless in therapy because of their toxic side effects. Thus, an amino acid extracted from the fruit of the akee tree (Blighia sapida), named hypoglycin, leads to a blood sugar fall, but it is a powerful emetic. Salicylates can lower the blood sugar, but only in doses which also provoke the signs of salicylism, i.e., tinnitus, vomiting, and acidosis. Some guanidines are hypoglycemic but have been known, on occasion, to produce liver necrosis.

The modern era in this field was ushered in by Janbon and Loubatières, who, between 1942 and 1946, studied the blood-sugar-lowering action of sulfonamide derivatives. The initial clinical testing began in Germany in 1951 and has been continued in the United States and in other countries since 1955.

Thus far, the four widely used compounds are *tolbutamide, chlorpropamide, acetohexamide,* and *tolazamide*. They belong to the chemical family of *sulfonylureas*. It is well established that the primary mechanism of action of these agents is the *stimulation of insulin secretion from β-cells*. It is possible, but has not been proved, that the sulfonylureas may directly inhibit the liver's output of sugar. *Blood glucose falls as a rise in plasma insulin levels occurs.* Because of their mode of action, the sulfonylureas are therapeutically useful only in those diabetics who have a significant pancreatic reserve of β-cells, i.e., in the milder, nonketonic adult-onset type of patient. Established juvenile-onset patients with a marked elevation of fasting blood sugar, as well as the severe adult-onset group, do not respond to sulfonylureas.

At present, investigations are being pursued to determine the possible usefulness of sulfonylureas in delaying the onset of frank chemical diabetes in individuals with prediabetes who exhibit moderate and early deviations of glucose

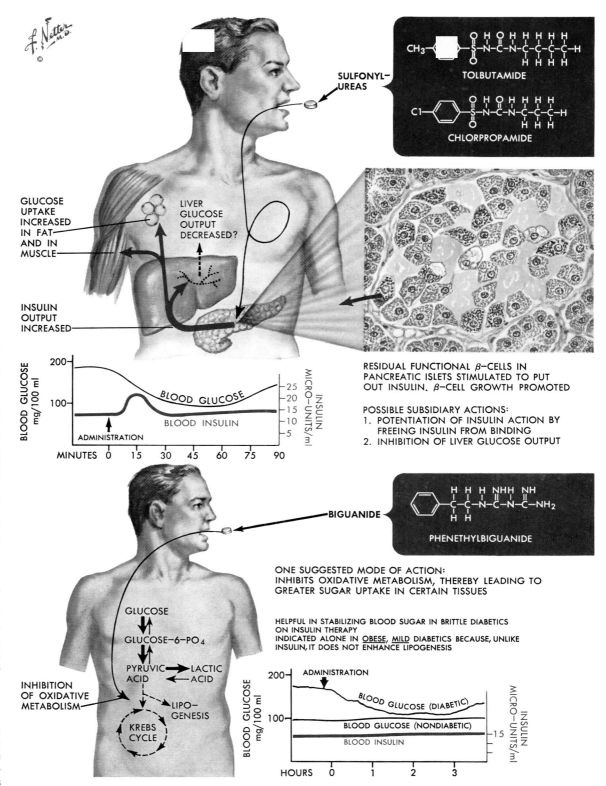

SULFONYL-UREAS

TOLBUTAMIDE

CHLORPROPAMIDE

GLUCOSE UPTAKE INCREASED IN FAT AND IN MUSCLE

LIVER GLUCOSE OUTPUT DECREASED?

INSULIN OUTPUT INCREASED

RESIDUAL FUNCTIONAL β–CELLS IN PANCREATIC ISLETS STIMULATED TO PUT OUT INSULIN. β–CELL GROWTH PROMOTED

POSSIBLE SUBSIDIARY ACTIONS:
1. POTENTIATION OF INSULIN ACTION BY FREEING INSULIN FROM BINDING
2. INHIBITION OF LIVER GLUCOSE OUTPUT

BLOOD GLUCOSE

BLOOD INSULIN

ADMINISTRATION

MINUTES 0 15 30 45 60 75 90

BIGUANIDE

PHENETHYLBIGUANIDE

ONE SUGGESTED MODE OF ACTION:
INHIBITS OXIDATIVE METABOLISM, THEREBY LEADING TO GREATER SUGAR UPTAKE IN CERTAIN TISSUES

HELPFUL IN STABILIZING BLOOD SUGAR IN BRITTLE DIABETICS ON INSULIN THERAPY
INDICATED ALONE IN OBESE, MILD DIABETICS BECAUSE, UNLIKE INSULIN, IT DOES NOT ENHANCE LIPOGENESIS

GLUCOSE

GLUCOSE-6-PO₄

PYRUVIC ACID → LACTIC ACID

INHIBITION OF OXIDATIVE METABOLISM

LIPO-GENESIS

KREBS CYCLE

ADMINISTRATION

BLOOD GLUCOSE (DIABETIC)

BLOOD GLUCOSE (NONDIABETIC)

BLOOD INSULIN

HOURS 0 1 2 3

tolerance, especially when stressed with corticosteroids. These research attempts are based on experimental data that sulfonylureas, under certain circumstances, stimulate the formation of new β-cells in laboratory animals.

The second group of oral agents now in use is composed of the *biguanides,* such as *phenethylbiguanide*. This substance does not act by stimulating β-cells, for there is *hypoglycemia* without any change in measurable *plasma insulin*. For efficacy, it requires the presence of some endogenous or exogenous insulin. Irritation of the gastro-intestinal tract limits the usefulness of this drug in some patients. The mechanisms of action in vivo are not known. In vitro experiments have suggested that the biguanides *inhibit oxidative metabolism,* thus leading to enhanced glucose uptake for anaerobic breakdown to *lactic acid*. Recent in vivo work points to a possible effect on

reducing both insulin binding to plasma proteins and its inactivation.

Therapeutic usefulness seems more restricted than is that of the sulfonylureas. In older, obese diabetics, who often show high insulin responses to glucose loads, phenethylbiguanide will produce hypoglycemia, reduce the excessive insulin response, and thus decrease lipogenesis from glucose. In the brittle diabetic phenethylbiguanide, together with insulin as a stabilizing agent, has been helpful occasionally.

It should be emphasized that proper dietary control, especially the reduction of weight, remains the most helpful and least toxic mode of treatment of the mild diabetic, and that oral hypoglycemic agents should be used only after such control has been established. Whenever they fail to control the diabetic state, especially in the presence of keto-acidosis, insulin therapy must be promptly started.

Section VI

PARATHYROID DISORDERS AND
METABOLIC BONE DISEASES

by

FRANK H. NETTER, M.D.

in collaboration with

FELIX O. KOLB, M.D.
Plates 2-6, 8-19

SANFORD I. ROTH, M.D.
Plates 1 and 7

HISTOLOGY OF THE NORMAL PARATHYROID GLANDS

Human parathyroid tissue is divided into two to six portions (glands), though four is the usual number. In the adult, each of these glands measures 4 to 6 mm by 2 to 4 mm by 0.5 to 2 mm and weighs approximately 35 mg.

The gland, in the infant and child, is composed of sheets of closely packed *chief cells,* with little intervening stroma. *Oxyphil cells* first make their appearance at the time of puberty. Fat cells begin to appear in the stroma in late childhood. Both the oxyphil cells and the fat cells increase in number until they may occupy more than 50 per cent of the volume of the glands during the fifth and sixth decades. The adult gland is composed of cords, sheets, and acini of two forms of chief cells (light and dark) in a loose areolar stroma containing numerous mature fat cells. Scattered individually or in groups among these chief cells are the oxyphil cells.

The *light chief cell* (inactive cell) measures approximately 8 microns in diameter. It has a well-defined cell membrane and a 4- to 5-micron centrally located nucleus. The chromatin is densely packed, appearing almost pyknotic, or it is finely fibrillar with peripheral margination. Nucleoli are rare. The cell cytoplasm is clear and amphophilic in *hematoxylin and eosin (H. and E.)* preparations. The *periodic acid Schiff (PAS)* reaction reveals abundant *glycogen* in these cells. The *dark chief cell* (active cell) is approximately 6 microns in diameter. It has a less-well-defined cell membrane than has the light chief cell, probably due to closer packing of the cells. The nucleus is identical with that of the light chief cell. The cell cytoplasm is somewhat basophilic with H. and E., and some glycogen is present in PAS preparations.

Identification of the secretory product by light microscopic preparation of the parathyroid glands has never been completely satisfactory. Seen with the electron microscope, the *secretory granules* correspond to the argyrophilic granules in Bodian-stained preparations, and to the hematoxylin-positive bodies seen in preparations stained with chrome alum or iron hematoxylin. These stains show secretory granules largely limited to the small dark chief cell. Unfortunately, these reactions are valid only on optimally fixed (within seconds after removal) tissue. The *Bodian stain* is especially difficult, since most of the Protargol® presently available leaves a precipitate on the slide which is impossible to distinguish from secretory granules.

The oxyphil cell is polygonal and 10 to 15 microns in diameter. The cell mem-

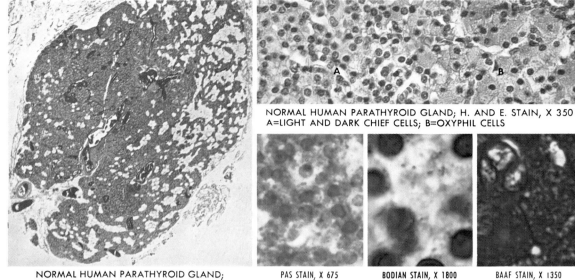

NORMAL HUMAN PARATHYROID GLAND; H. AND E. STAIN, X 350
A=LIGHT AND DARK CHIEF CELLS; B=OXYPHIL CELLS

NORMAL HUMAN PARATHYROID GLAND; H. AND E. STAIN, X 17½

PAS STAIN, X 675 GLYCOGEN IN CHIEF CELLS

BODIAN STAIN, X 1800 SECRETORY GRANULES IN CHIEF CELLS

BAAF STAIN, X 1350 MITOCHONDRIA IN OXYPHIL CELLS

ULTRASTRUCTURE OF PARATHYROID GLAND

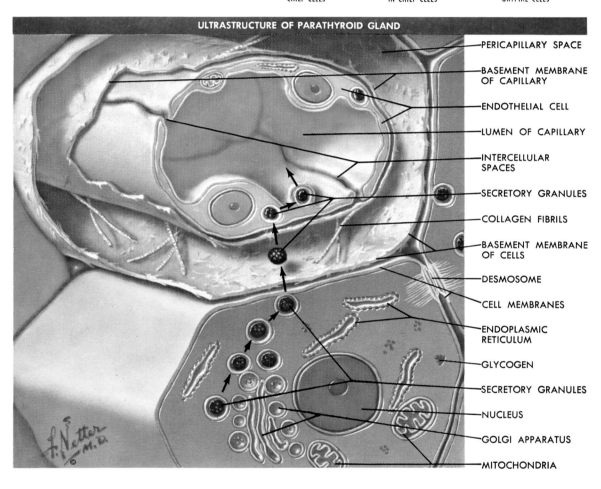

- PERICAPILLARY SPACE
- BASEMENT MEMBRANE OF CAPILLARY
- ENDOTHELIAL CELL
- LUMEN OF CAPILLARY
- INTERCELLULAR SPACES
- SECRETORY GRANULES
- COLLAGEN FIBRILS
- BASEMENT MEMBRANE OF CELLS
- DESMOSOME
- CELL MEMBRANES
- ENDOPLASMIC RETICULUM
- GLYCOGEN
- SECRETORY GRANULES
- NUCLEUS
- GOLGI APPARATUS
- MITOCHONDRIA

branes are usually clear, and the nucleus is identical to that of the chief cell. The cytoplasm is composed of highly eosinophilic fine granules, which stain carmine with *Bensley's acid aniline fuchsin (BAAF)* and dark blue with phosphotungstic acid hematoxylin, after mordanting. Electron microscopy has confirmed the histochemical and light microscopic studies, indicating that these granules are tightly packed *mitochondria* filling the cytoplasm. Only a very rare secretory granule is identifiable in the cell by either light or electron microscopy, and, in the normal parathyroid gland, this cell has no significant rôle in the production of parathyroid hormone. It is believed that the oxyphil cell represents a degenerative form of the chief cell.

The *ultrastructure* of the active form of the chief cell (small, dark) and the mode of secretion are schematized in the illustration. In addition to the usual organelles, during the active phase the Golgi apparatus enlarges, numerous vacuoles and vesicles appear in the *Golgi apparatus,* and many mature *secretory granules* appear in the cell. The mature secretory granule in the human is oval to dumbbell-shaped and has a single membrane surrounding a thin clear space inside of which is a dense area composed of short rodlike profiles. The granule migrates out of the cell through the *basement membrane* into the wide *pericapillary space.* It then goes through the *capillary basement membrane* and into the *endothelial cell,* from which it is presumably liberated into the blood stream. The active cell is relatively sparse in *glycogen.*

The inactive form of the chief cell, on the other hand, has a small Golgi apparatus, few secretory granules, abundant glycogen, and, often, arrayed granular ergastoplasm.

PHYSIOLOGY OF THE PARATHYROID GLANDS

The *four parathyroid glands* secrete a protein hormone (*parathyroid hormone*), which recently has been isolated in fairly pure form. There is no evidence for a parathyrotropic hormone which stimulates the parathyroid glands. The falling level of ionized serum calcium is the primary *stimulus* for parathyroid hormone secretion. A rise in serum calcium level *inhibits* parathyroid hormone. The principal action of parathyroid hormone is the regulation and maintenance of a *normal serum calcium level* approximately between 9 and 11 mg per 100 ml. Recent evidence from animal experiments suggests that a second parathyroid hormone, "calcitonin", which lowers the serum calcium level, helps in this regulation. A similarly acting hormone has been isolated, is secreted by the parafollicular ("C") cells of the thyroid gland, and is often referred to as "thyrocalcitonin". It is also found in the ultimobranchial bodies in certain animal species. The calcium-lowering effect is probably due to an inhibition of the action of parathormone on bone resorption. There is a reciprocal relationship between serum calcium and *serum phosphorus,* so that the product of calcium times phosphorus is maintained at a fairly constant level with a constant, K, of 40 mg per 100 ml of plasma. As the serum calcium level rises, the serum phosphorus level falls, and vice versa.

Under normal circumstances it appears that there is only one parathyroid hormone with several actions rather than several parathyroid hormones. The principal actions are (1) inhibition of *phosphate reabsorption* (or enhanced phosphate secretion) by the renal tubule, and phosphaturia; and (2) *resorption of calcium and phosphate from bone,* presumably by stimulating the action of the *osteoclasts.* Secondary actions are (1) *increased calcium absorption from the gastro-intestinal tract,* similar to the action of vitamin D; and (2) an action on the renal tubule *enhancing calcium reabsorption,* usually overshadowed by the calcium-mobilizing activity of the hormone. The net effect of the four actions of parathyroid hormone is a rise of the serum calcium level and an increase in the urinary calcium level exceeding the *normal of 100 to 300 mg per 24 hours.* At the same time, there is a tendency for the serum phosphorus level to fall, with a rise in the urinary phosphorus level exceeding the *normal of 500 to 1000 mg per 24 hours.* If the serum calcium level tends to fall, *e.g.,* with excessive fecal losses, the parathyroid glands become stimulated and mobilize calcium from bone. They also tend to raise the serum calcium level by promoting the excretion of phosphate via the kidney tubule.

If the parathyroid glands are not functioning properly or are absent, this readjustment does not occur; the serum calcium level will fall, usually below

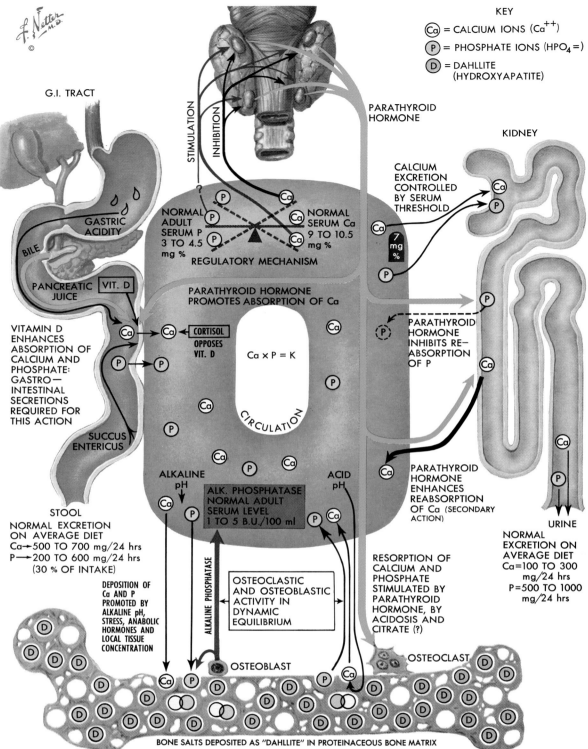

the normal serum threshold of 7 mg per 100 ml, and urine calcium will be absent. The presence of a large reservoir of calcium in the skeleton as lime salts (*dahllite or hydroxyapatite*), however, will prevent the serum calcium from falling below 5 mg per 100 ml, even in the absence of the parathyroid glands. In states of excessive parathyroid hormone secretion, there is resorption of calcium and phosphate from bone matrix, probably through stimulation of the *osteoclasts;* this action may be mediated by an increased production of *citric acid,* which solubilizes calcium. The osteoclastic overresponse will then evoke a tendency for the *osteoblasts* to become overactive and lead to bone repair, with the subsequent rise of the *alkaline phosphatase level in the serum* above the normal of 1 to 5 Bodansky units (B.U.) per 100 ml. Bone repair will be promoted by *enhanced absorption of calcium and phosphate from*

the gastro-intestinal tract, by changes in the local tissue pH, by anabolic hormones, and by *factors which tend to raise the local tissue concentration of calcium and phosphate.* Although the urinary calcium excretion is rather constant, the *excretion of calcium in the stool* depends greatly on the body's need and the dietary intake; *normally, 500 to 700 mg are excreted per 24 hours.* The *fecal excretion of phosphate is roughly 30 per cent* of the dietary intake, whereas the urinary phosphate excretion varies widely with the intake.

Vitamin D greatly enhances the absorption of calcium (and phosphate) from the gastro-intestinal tract. *Cortisol* has an action on calcium metabolism which appears to *oppose* this action of vitamin D. Parathyroid hormone seems to play an important rôle in the regulation of magnesium metabolism as well, increasing its excretion.

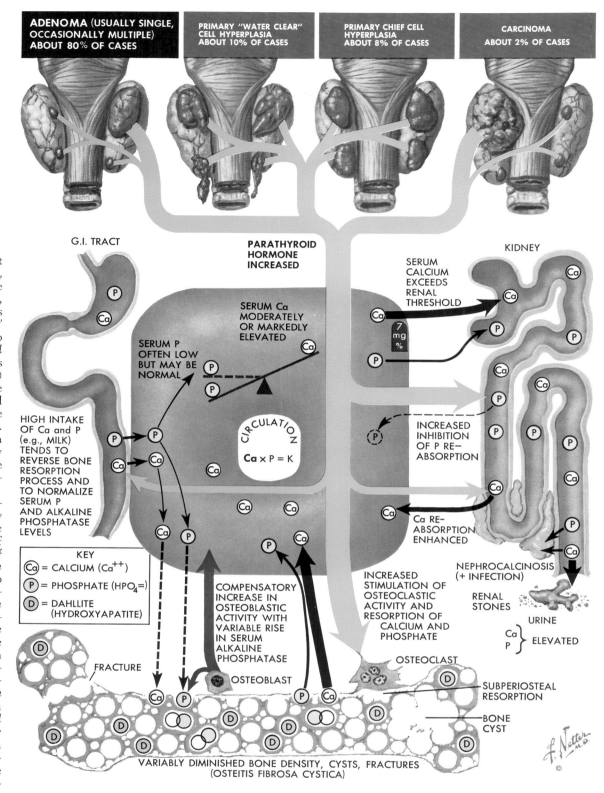

ADENOMA (USUALLY SINGLE, OCCASIONALLY MULTIPLE) ABOUT 80% OF CASES

PRIMARY "WATER CLEAR" CELL HYPERPLASIA ABOUT 10% OF CASES

PRIMARY CHIEF CELL HYPERPLASIA ABOUT 8% OF CASES

CARCINOMA ABOUT 2% OF CASES

PATHOLOGIC PHYSIOLOGY OF PRIMARY HYPERPARATHYROIDISM

Primary hyperparathyroidism is most commonly due to a *single adenoma,* which is the cause in roughly 80 or more per cent of the cases. Occasionally, *multiple adenomas* are found. A less common cause is *primary "water clear" cell hyperplasia* of all four glands (10 per cent or less) or *primary chief cell hyperplasia* of all four glands, which is even less common (8 per cent or less) and, at times, is mistaken for multiple adenomas. *Carcinoma* of one parathyroid gland is the rarest form of this disease (2 per cent) and is usually incurable. Although most commonly located within the neck, ectopic parathyroid tumors may occur (10 per cent) anywhere in the anterior or even in the posterior mediastinum.

An *excessive production of parathyroid hormone* leads to *hypercalcemia by increased stimulation of the osteoclastic activity of bone,* with the release of calcium and phosphate. *Absorption of calcium from the gut and reabsorption of calcium by the renal tubule* are also *enhanced.* Likewise, parathyroid hormone *inhibits the tubular reabsorption of phosphate* (or promotes tubular secretion of phosphate), causing an *excessive loss of phosphate in the urine.* By the reciprocal action, the lowered serum phosphorus level raises the serum calcium level. The net effect of these chemical changes is a *rise in serum calcium and a fall in serum phosphate,* with increasing amounts of both *calcium and phosphate being excreted in the urinary tract.* This predisposes to the formation of calcium phosphate and calcium oxalate *renal stones.* At times, there may be precipitation of calcium in the soft tissues of the *kidneys,* producing *nephrocalcinosis,* which is often associated with *infection.*

In roughly 25 per cent of the cases of primary hyperparathyroidism, clinical evidence of bone disease, with marked bone resorption and a *compensatory increase in osteoblastic activity* and *increases in the serum alkaline phosphatase level,* is present. This may be seen as *subperiosteal resorptive changes, diminished bone density, cyst formation,* and, at times, even *fractures (osteitis fibrosa cystica).*

The principal physiologic events, therefore, lead to stone formation in about 70 per cent or more of the cases and to bone disease in only about 25 per cent of them. Recent evidence sug-

gests that dietary intakes of calcium and phosphate may not be the only factors responsible for the distribution of cases, *i.e.,* patients who have primarily bone disease and those who have primarily stone disease. It has been suggested that, in abnormal states of hyperparathyroidism, the tumorous or hyperplastic glands may secrete different types of hormones, either attacking bone primarily or primarily causing renal stones. A small percentage of patients show neither bone disease nor stone disease but suffer primarily from the physiologic manifestations of the hypercalcemic state (see page 180). There is an increased tendency to peptic ulcer formation and calcific pancreatitis. A prolonged low-phosphate intake in the diet will tend to produce a more classical chemical picture, *i.e.,* a low phosphate level and a high calcium level in the blood. A *high-calcium and high-phosphate intake* will have a

tendency to heal or lessen the trend toward bone disease and will usually *restore the phosphate and alkaline phosphatase levels to normal.* However, increased losses of phosphate and calcium in the urine will still be evident. Hypercalciuria may, however, not be manifested in patients who have progressive renal damage with nephrocalcinosis.

The diagnosis of primary hyperparathyroidism is essentially a chemical one. A serum calcium above the normal range for the particular laboratory, occurring on three occasions, establishes hypercalcemia. Sometimes low-phosphorus intake will bring this out. States of hypercalcemia other than that caused by primary hyperparathyroidism must be ruled out by appropriate tests (see page 181). The type of parathyroid disease present must be established, at the time of surgery, by histological examination of the tumor or by the finding of hyperplastic glands.

PATHOLOGY AND CLINICAL MANIFESTATIONS OF HYPERPARATHYROIDISM

Regardless of type, the most common manifestation of primary hyperparathyroidism is *nephrolithiasis.* It has been estimated that 5 per cent of all renal stones may be associated with this disease. While single or recurrent calculi or the passage of sand or gravel may be present, the more serious type of diffuse *nephrocalcinosis,* involving both kidneys and often associated with chronic pyelonephritis, is occasionally found with primary hyperparathyroidism. This type may go on to irreversible renal damage, *hypertension,* and eventual death from *cardiorenal failure.*

Clinical or radiologic evidence of bone disease occurs in less than 25 per cent of the cases, but *focal resorption* may be seen on *bone biopsy* in many more patients. There may be *absence of the lamina dura* around the teeth, although this is not a constant finding. More specific is the X-ray finding of *subperiosteal resorption of the bone,* especially around the radial margins of the phalanges, the sternal end of the clavicle, and along the margins of other bones. Diffuse *"salt and pepper"* decalcification of the skull, resembling multiple myeloma, is sometimes present. There may be fractures of the terminal phalanges, with telescoping, giving the appearance of *pseudoclubbing.* The joints show *increased flexibility;* the *nails* are often exceptionally *strong.* At times, large *bone cysts* have been observed in various locations, and fractures through these cysts, or *fractures* through rarefied bone, may occur. There also may be diffuse demineralization of the skeleton, especially of the spine, with *"codfishing"* of the vertebral bodies.

One of the presenting signs of the disease may be a *giant cell tumor (epulis* or *osteoclastoma)* of the jaw, protruding through the gums (see CIBA COLLECTION, Vol. 3/1, page 124). Calcium may deposit diffusely throughout the body, *e.g.,* in *blood vessels;* it may be seen, by careful examination of the eye with a slit lamp, in a semicircular form around the limbus of the cornea, the so-called *"limbus keratopathy"* (or band keratitis). The patient may show, primarily, manifestations of the hypercalcemic state, such as polyuria, excessive thirst, nausea, anorexia, and vomiting, at times associated with stubborn constipation. Unexplained anemia, weakness, and weight loss may also be present. Not infrequently, *peptic ulcer* is associated with primary hyperparathyroidism, possibly owing to increased gastric secretion, and there may be associated recurrent *pancreatitis.* Other symptoms of hypercalcemia, such as mental confusion and even psychosis, may be seen. The elec-

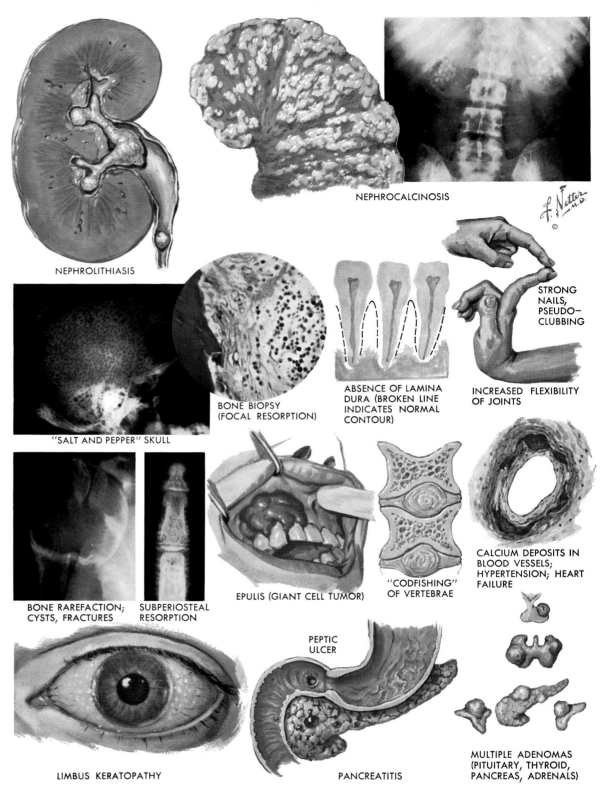

NEPHROLITHIASIS

NEPHROCALCINOSIS

f. Netter M.D.

"SALT AND PEPPER" SKULL

BONE BIOPSY (FOCAL RESORPTION)

ABSENCE OF LAMINA DURA (BROKEN LINE INDICATES NORMAL CONTOUR)

STRONG NAILS, PSEUDO-CLUBBING

INCREASED FLEXIBILITY OF JOINTS

BONE RAREFACTION; CYSTS, FRACTURES

SUBPERIOSTEAL RESORPTION

EPULIS (GIANT CELL TUMOR)

"CODFISHING" OF VERTEBRAE

CALCIUM DEPOSITS IN BLOOD VESSELS; HYPERTENSION; HEART FAILURE

PEPTIC ULCER

LIMBUS KERATOPATHY

PANCREATITIS

MULTIPLE ADENOMAS (PITUITARY, THYROID, PANCREAS, ADRENALS)

trocardiogram may show a shortened Q-T interval. The chemical findings typical of the disease are described on page 182. Rarely, the disease may be familial, and *multiple adenomas* (including *pituitary* tumors and *thyroid, pancreatic,* and *adrenal adenomas*) may be present. There is a greater incidence of associated thyroid carcinoma and hyperthyroidism.

The only treatment of single or multiple parathyroid adenomas is surgical removal, or removal of three glands and a subtotal resection of the fourth gland if primary hyperplasia of all glands is present. Spontaneous improvement due to necrosis of a tumor is exceedingly rare. The prognosis is related directly to the degree of renal impairment, which may become irreversible. The patient may succumb to the manifestations of acute hypercalcemia with cardiac arrest, especially while on digitalis (there being increased digitalis toxicity), or to irreversible renal failure

before the tumor can be successfully removed ("parathyroid poisoning"). Postoperatively, the serum calcium falls to subnormal levels, with transient tetany, but it gradually returns to normal if sufficient parathyroid tissue remains. An occasional patient may show marked weakness, tremors, and even seizures, in the postoperative state, because of magnesium deficiency requiring magnesium therapy. The serum phosphate may remain low, and the alkaline phosphatase level often even rises if bone disease is present, which tends to heal rapidly ("hungry bones") postoperatively. This may require treatment with calcium and vitamin D for prolonged periods of time. Some of the cysts may remain permanently. The prognosis of parathyroid carcinoma, fortunately rare, is usually hopeless, since these tumors are, as a rule, inoperable and metastasize widely, leading to calcification of all tissues of the body.

TESTS FOR THE DIFFERENTIAL DIAGNOSIS OF THE CAUSES OF HYPERCALCEMIA

A variety of disorders which exhibit hypercalcemia may give rise to the signs and symptoms of hyperparathyroidism and must be considered in the differential diagnosis of this disease. Some of these causes, *e.g., metastatic carcinoma* of the breast to bone are obvious; others, such as *carcinoma of the lung,* not involving bone but producing hypercalcemia, may be more occult. Likewise, *multiple myeloma* and *sarcoidosis* may be in a stage that is difficult to diagnose. Hypercalcemia is shared by all the disorders illustrated here, as well as by a few other conditions, such as acute Addison's disease (especially in childhood). Only a few of these disorders have the combination of a high *serum calcium* as well as a depressed *serum phosphorus* level in common with hyperparathyroidism. Low serum phosphate and elevated *alkaline phosphatase* levels are not by themselves constant findings in hyperparathyroidism. The *urinary calcium excretion,* although variable, is increased in practically all the disorders noted on the chart. For this reason, more subtle tests must be employed, especially involving the phosphate dynamics, to serve in the differential diagnosis of these disorders.

The *percentage of tubular reabsorption of phosphate (TRP) test* is a measurement of *renal tubular phosphate reabsorption.* The test, in essence, is a *phosphate clearance* compared to the *creatinine clearance.* A 12-hour urine is collected, in the postprandial state, from 8 p.m. to 8 a.m., and the *urinary phosphate* and *creatinine* are determined. A morning fasting *specimen of blood* is examined for *creatinine* and *phosphate.* The *normal TRP,* on an average diet, is 80 to 90 per cent. On a low-phosphate diet, most normal people will show a TRP closer to 95 per cent, and, on a high-phosphate intake, closer to 75 per cent. The patient with hyperparathyroidism will tend toward an inability to conserve phosphate; his percentage of TRP will, therefore, be lower than normal, on both a high- and a low-phosphate intake. By and large, most disorders exhibiting hypercalcemia will have a normal percentage of TRP, with the exception of the extraparathyroid tumors not involving bone, such as carcinoma of the lung, hypernephroma, etc., which apparently secrete a parathyroidlike substance. However, the TRP test is not invariably helpful, and it depends on control of the dietary intake

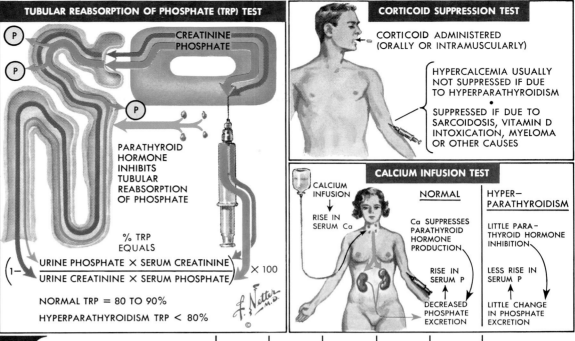

$$\% \text{ TRP EQUALS } \left(1 - \frac{\text{URINE PHOSPHATE} \times \text{SERUM CREATININE}}{\text{URINE CREATININE} \times \text{SERUM PHOSPHATE}}\right) \times 100$$

NORMAL TRP = 80 TO 90%
HYPERPARATHYROIDISM TRP < 80%

DIFFERENTIAL DIAGNOSIS OF HYPERCALCEMIC STATES

CONDITION	SERUM Ca	SERUM P	ALK.P'ASE	URINE Ca	TRP	MISC. FINDINGS
HYPER-PARATHYROIDISM	↑	↓	N OR ↑	↑	↓	SUBPERIOSTEAL RESORPTION
MILK–ALKALI SYNDROME	↑	N	N	N OR ↓	N	ULCER HISTORY, SUBCUTANEOUS CALCIFICATION, ALKALOSIS
VITAMIN D INTOXICATION	↑	N OR ↑	N	N OR ↑	N	HISTORY OF VITAMIN D INTAKE
SARCOIDOSIS	↑	N OR ↑	N OR ↑	N OR ↑	N	SERUM GLOBULIN ELEVATED
MULTIPLE MYELOMA	↑	N	N	N OR ↑	N	BENCE JONES PROTEIN IN URINE; SERUM GLOBULIN ELEVATED
METASTATIC CARCINOMA	↑	N	N OR ↑	↑	N	DESTRUCTIVE LESION ON X–RAY
PRIMARY CARCINOMA, NOT INVOLVING BONE	↑	N OR ↓	N	N OR ↑	N OR ↓	PRIMARY LESION, X–RAY, BRONCHOSCOPY
DISUSE ATROPHY (OSTEO-POROSIS)	↑	N OR ↑	N	↑	N	HISTORY OF IMMOBILIZATION
THYROTOXICOSIS	↑	N	N OR ↑	↑	N	LONG–STANDING HYPERTHYROIDISM

of phosphorus for critical evaluation. It is invalidated if the creatinine clearance is subnormal.

The *corticoid suppression test* is used in the differential diagnosis of states of hypercalcemia not due to hyperparathyroidism, especially *sarcoidosis, vitamin D intoxication, myeloma,* and, at times, *carcinoma metastatic to bone.* In these disorders *cortisol,* administered in large doses (*i.e.,* 100 to 120 mg daily for 10 days), or any of the anti-inflammatory synthetic derivatives in equivalent amounts, will lead to a fall of the elevated serum calcium level. Only a *rare* case of *hyperparathyroidism will show suppression of hypercalcemia.*

The *calcium infusion* test is based on the principle that *parathyroid hormone can be "shut off",* if under physiologic control, by *raising the serum calcium* level, whereas an autonomous parathyroid tumor cannot be *shut off.* If, after *infusing calcium* (12.5

mg per kg body weight) intravenously over a short period (usually 4 hours), a *diminished phosphate excretion* and a *rise in serum phosphate* are noted, a *normal* physiologic state of the parathyroids exists; if primary *hyperparathyroidism* is present, *little parathyroid inhibition* and only a *slight rise, if any, in serum phosphorus,* with *little change in the urinary phosphate excretion,* will occur.

Although all these tests (with many refinements and modifications) are of value in differential diagnosis, there are sufficient exceptions so that the ultimate diagnosis will depend on carefully ruling out, clinically, all the other disorders noted on the plate. In doubtful cases, bone or tissue biopsy may help to settle the diagnosis. In the future, the availability of direct parathyroid hormone assay in blood and urine should facilitate the differential diagnosis.

SECONDARY (RENAL) HYPERPARATHYROIDISM (RENAL OSTEODYSTROPHY)

Although primary hyperparathyroidism is a relatively rare disease, secondary (renal) hyperparathyroidism (renal osteodystrophy, renal rickets) is the usual event in any patient showing chronic renal insufficiency of any kind, with *diminished glomerular filtration.* Aside from retaining nonprotein nitrogen (*NPN*), including waste products such as creatinine, which rise in the serum, there is also *inability to filter phosphate,* which is retained, causing marked hyperphosphatemia. The *high serum phosphate level depresses the serum calcium level.* The low *level of ionized calcium* (and possibly also the high serum phosphate level itself) stimulates the *parathyroid glands,* which become *secondarily hyperplastic* and may enlarge considerably. *Excessive amounts of parathyroid hormone are secreted,* but this hyperparathyroidism is ineffective in promoting phosphate diuresis, since *little is filtering through the glomerulus.* Likewise, only a small amount of calcium can filter through, so that the *urinary calcium and phosphate are both low.*

While unable to act on the renal tubules, excessive amounts of parathyroid hormone act on bone, causing an *increased stimulation of the osteoclastic activity* and excessive resorption of *calcium* and *phosphate* from the bone minerals (dahllite or hydroxyapatite). The presence of *chronic acidosis* in renal failure *enhances this bone resorptive* activity. The resulting *subperiosteal resorption, cyst formation,* and variably *diminished bone density (osteitis fibrosa cystica)* lead to deformity and, at times, even to *fractures.* In children, there is also marked irregularity at the margins of the epiphyses (resembling rickets) and, at times, slipping of the epiphyses. Some areas of the skeleton, *e.g.,* the vertebral plates, may show increased density on X-ray examination.

The calcium released from bone fails to raise the ionized serum calcium level adequately, since the serum phosphate level is maintained in the high range. In addition, there is evidence that the *high phosphate level* in the tissues of the intestinal tract *binds the calcium* that enters through this route (from dietary sources), and, therefore, less calcium is absorbed. It has also been demonstrated that *vitamin D,* which usually promotes the absorption of both calcium and phosphate, is less effective in chronic renal failure with acidosis.

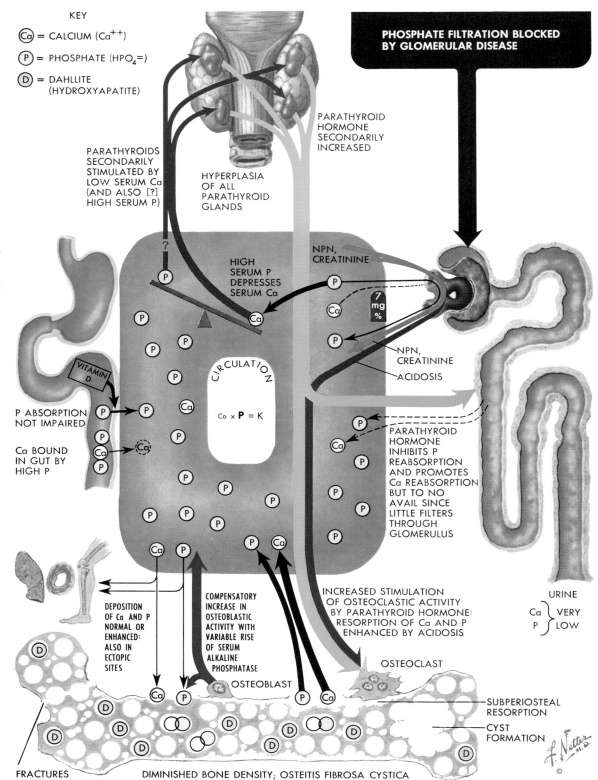

KEY
- Ca = CALCIUM (Ca⁺⁺)
- P = PHOSPHATE (HPO₄=)
- D = DAHLLITE (HYDROXYAPATITE)

PHOSPHATE FILTRATION BLOCKED BY GLOMERULAR DISEASE

PARATHYROIDS SECONDARILY STIMULATED BY LOW SERUM Ca (AND ALSO [?] HIGH SERUM P)

HYPERPLASIA OF ALL PARATHYROID GLANDS

PARATHYROID HORMONE SECONDARILY INCREASED

HIGH SERUM P DEPRESSES SERUM Ca

NPN, CREATININE

$Ca \times P = K$

VITAMIN D

P ABSORPTION NOT IMPAIRED

Ca BOUND IN GUT BY HIGH P

NPN, CREATININE ACIDOSIS

PARATHYROID HORMONE INHIBITS P REABSORPTION AND PROMOTES Ca REABSORPTION BUT TO NO AVAIL SINCE LITTLE FILTERS THROUGH GLOMERULUS

DEPOSITION OF Ca AND P NORMAL OR ENHANCED: ALSO IN ECTOPIC SITES

COMPENSATORY INCREASE IN OSTEOBLASTIC ACTIVITY WITH VARIABLE RISE OF SERUM ALKALINE PHOSPHATASE

INCREASED STIMULATION OF OSTEOCLASTIC ACTIVITY BY PARATHYROID HORMONE: RESORPTION OF Ca AND P ENHANCED BY ACIDOSIS

OSTEOBLAST

OSTEOCLAST

URINE
Ca VERY
P LOW

SUBPERIOSTEAL RESORPTION

CYST FORMATION

FRACTURES

DIMINISHED BONE DENSITY; OSTEITIS FIBROSA CYSTICA

Therefore, calcium absorption, which depends more on vitamin D, is lessened, while *phosphate absorption proceeds relatively unimpaired.*

As the disease progresses, the skeleton becomes unstable, and there is an *increase in the osteoblastic activity* of bone in an attempt to repair the destroyed bone; the *serum alkaline phosphatase level shows progressive rises.* In spite of very low serum calcium levels, the patient exhibits few of the manifestations of tetany, since systemic acidosis is present, increasing the ionized calcium fraction. The solubility product of calcium and phosphate is exceeded, resulting in *calcium-phosphate deposits* in soft *tissues,* especially in organs which secrete acid (such as the stomach, the *lungs,* and the kidneys); deposits are also noted in other *ectopic sites* such as the *media of blood vessels* and the *subcutaneous tissue.*

Treatment is usually directed toward lessening the

phosphate intake by a low-phosphate diet and the use of aluminum hydroxide gel, as well as by correction of the acidosis. Vitamin D is required to correct hypocalcemia and to heal the demineralized bones, but it must be used cautiously in order to avoid enhancement of a tendency to ectopic calcification. Most recently, surgical subtotal resection of the hyperplastic parathyroid glands has been suggested to promote healing of the bones, since the hyperparathyroidism is a harmful, rather than a beneficial, compensatory phenomenon.

The term renal rickets has been applied to this form of bone disease, since the X-ray and histologic appearance of bone may resemble that of rickets. However, this expression should be reserved for renal tubular disorders with or without secondary hyperparathyroidism (see page 191). Here, the more general wording—renal osteodystrophy—is preferable.

HISTOLOGY OF THE PARATHYROID GLANDS IN HYPERPARATHYROIDISM

There are three basic causes of primary hyperparathyroidism: adenoma, carcinoma, and hyperplasia of the parathyroid glands. The incidence of these diseases, as seen at the Massachusetts General Hospital over a period of some 40 years, has been:

Adenoma 253 (84%)
  Single . 240 (80%)
  Double
  (involving
  2 glands) 13 (4%)
Carcinoma 11 (4%)
Hyperplasia 36 (12%)
  Clear Cell 15 (5%)
  Chief Cell 21 (7%)
_____
Total 300 (100%)

Adenoma

The adenoma, single or double, is statistically the most frequent cause of primary hyperparathyroidism. The adenoma is composed of tightly packed sheets, cords, and acini of predominantly *chief cells*. Clear cells and *oxyphil cells,* singly and in groups, are often present, and some adenomas may be composed entirely of oxyphil cells. The tumor may be homogeneous or nodular. The chief cell of an adenoma is usually somewhat larger than a normal chief cell. The *nuclei* are variable in size, and *mononuclear giant cells with hyperchromatic nuclei,* not indicative of malignancy, are often present. *Multinuclear giant cells* are frequently seen in adenomas. The most important criterion for differentiating an adenoma from chief cell hyperplasia is the identification, in the patient with an adenoma, of *normal parathyroid tissue,* which may occur either as a *rim* outside the capsule of the adenoma or in another gland. This "normal" parathyroid in the presence of an adenoma is seen, by either light or electron microscopy, to be composed almost entirely of large, light, inactive chief cells, with abundant glycogen, small Golgi apparatuses, and rare secretory granules. Ultrastructural studies of the adenoma have shown that the cells lack the clear distinction present between the active and inactive forms of the normal glands. Secretory granules are frequent in the cells of the adenoma.

Chief Cell Hyperplasia

In hyperplasia, all four glands are invariably involved. Each gland is composed of cords, sheets, and acini of tightly packed chief, oxyphil, and clear cells. The cells are similar or slightly enlarged, compared to normal cells. The gland is often nodular, owing to separation of the cells by stroma or to aggregation of cell types. In primary chief cell

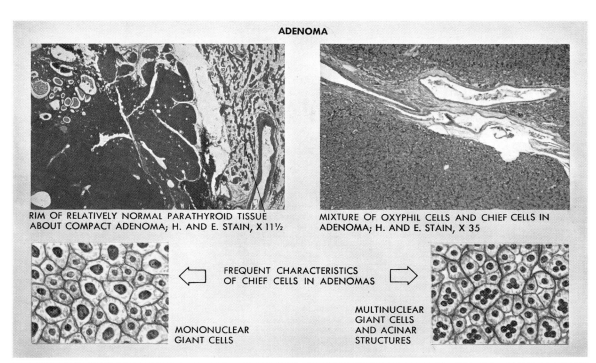

ADENOMA

RIM OF RELATIVELY NORMAL PARATHYROID TISSUE ABOUT COMPACT ADENOMA; H. AND E. STAIN, X 11½

MIXTURE OF OXYPHIL CELLS AND CHIEF CELLS IN ADENOMA; H. AND E. STAIN, X 35

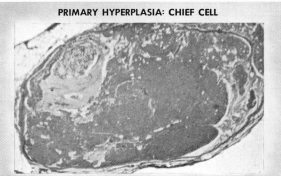

FREQUENT CHARACTERISTICS OF CHIEF CELLS IN ADENOMAS

MONONUCLEAR GIANT CELLS

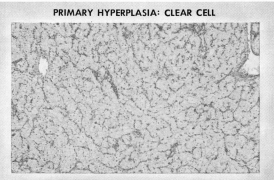

MULTINUCLEAR GIANT CELLS AND ACINAR STRUCTURES

PRIMARY HYPERPLASIA: CHIEF CELL

PRIMARY HYPERPLASIA: CLEAR CELL

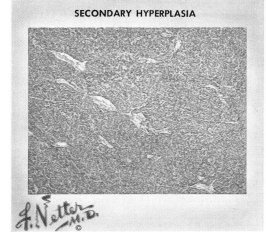

SECONDARY HYPERPLASIA

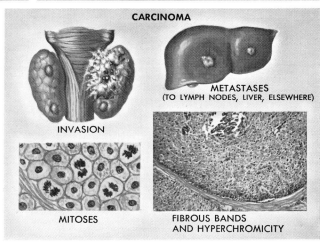

CARCINOMA

METASTASES (TO LYMPH NODES, LIVER, ELSEWHERE)

INVASION

MITOSES

FIBROUS BANDS AND HYPERCHROMICITY

hyperplasia, the appearance of each gland may be identical to that of an adenoma, except for the absence of normal parathyroid tissue.

Secondary Hyperplasia

This is often indistinguishable from primary chief cell hyperplasia, though nodularity is somewhat less frequent in secondary hyperplasia and each gland is often composed of uniform sheets of small, dark chief cells. Oxyphil cells and clear cells are occasionally seen.

Clear Cell Hyperplasia

The four glands are composed of sheets, cords, and acini of uniform, large (10 to 40 microns) cells, with distinct cell membranes and empty-appearing cytoplasm. The nuclei are small and densely stained. There is a tendency for palisading of the nuclei, and

giant nuclear forms may be seen. Secretory granules are present in these glands.

Carcinoma

Owing to the difficulty in distinguishing parathyroid carcinomas from thyroid and other carcinomas in the same region, the absolute diagnosis of parathyroid carcinoma cannot be made on histological grounds in the absence of proved hyperfunction. A large, dense fibrous capsule (with *invasion* of the capsule) and broad, dense *fibrous bands* traversing the tumor are present. The cells are large and uniform and have distinct cell membranes. The nuclei are large, regular, and *hyperchromatic. Mitotic figures* are almost invariably seen. A rim of normal parathyroid tissue may rarely be noted. However, in many cases local invasion, recurrence, and *metastases* are the only absolute criteria for the diagnosis of parathyroid carcinoma.

PATHOLOGIC PHYSIOLOGY OF HYPOPARATHYROIDISM

A deficiency of parathyroid hormone is most commonly seen following *subtotal or total thyroidectomy*. Less commonly, it may occur after surgery for parathyroid tumors. It very seldom follows massive radioactive iodine administration for cancer of the thyroid gland. *Idiopathic hypoparathyroidism*, by contrast, is rare. It is usually a disease that starts in childhood, but adult cases have been described. There may be an association with moniliasis and with Addison's disease (at times familial). It has been suggested that an auto-immune mechanism is involved in this type of hypoparathyroidism. Transient hypoparathyroidism may be seen in the neonatal period, presumably due to the relative underactivity of the parathyroid glands and their inability to handle the excessive phosphate content in the diet (cow's milk). Neonatal tetany may also indicate maternal *hyperparathyroidism*.

The chemical picture of hypoparathyroidism is a *low serum calcium,* usually below 7 mg per 100 ml, a *high serum phosphorus*, above 5 mg per 100 ml, and a *low excretion of calcium and phosphorus in the urine*; the *alkaline phosphatase is usually normal*. These chemical features can be explained by the absence of the major actions of parathyroid hormone. The calcium level is low because of *little stimulation of the osteoclastic activity of bone*, causing little resorption of calcium. There is also *diminished absorption of calcium from the gut*. Since the serum calcium level is usually below the kidney *threshold of 7 mg per 100 ml*, little urine calcium is found and the *Sulkowitch test* is usually *negative*. By contrast, the serum phosphorus is elevated because there is *excessive reabsorption of phosphate by the renal tubules*, which is not blocked by parathyroid hormone. The high serum phosphorus level has the additional effect of depressing the serum calcium level. A great deal of *calcium is "bound" in the gut* by the high phosphate concentration, and recent evidence has shown that the action of vitamin D on calcium absorption is less effective in the presence of high phosphate concentrations. In spite of the low calcium level, the very high level of phosphate in tissues, especially in bone tissue, prevents bone dissolution, and, as a rule, normal or even *increased bone density* is present. The combination of a low serum calcium, a high serum phosphorus level, and a normal alkaline phosphatase, in the absence of renal failure or malabsorption,

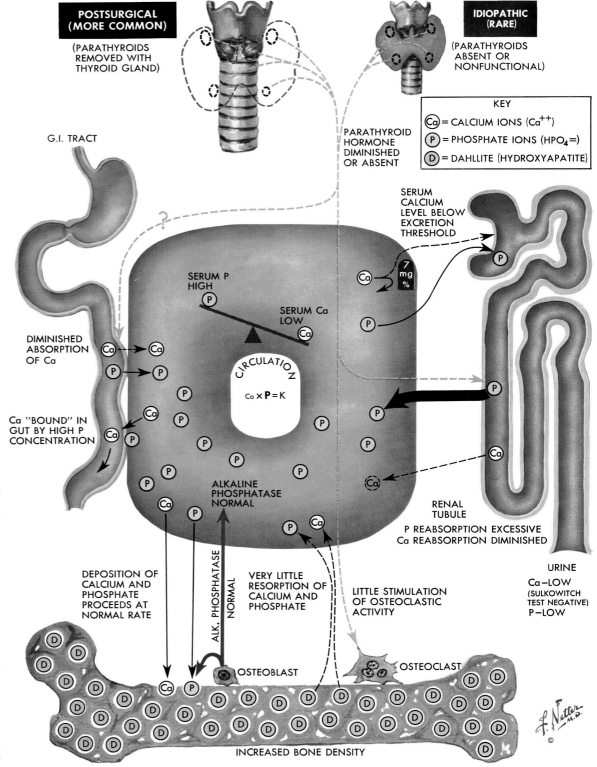

is pathognomonic of a state of hypoparathyroidism.

Although classic hypoparathyroidism is a relatively rare disease, recent studies have shown that a latent, mild or incomplete hypoparathyroidism may exist far more frequently. This can be brought to light by a number of stress tests, which include restricting the calcium intake severely by diet and sodium phytate, or by the administration of cortisone, an antagonist to the action of vitamin D, or EDTA (Versenate®), which may precipitate hypoparathyroidism in patients who have latent underfunction. Studies of the renal tubular handling of phosphate are valuable adjuncts to the study of minor parathyroid changes. Excessive tubular reabsorption of phosphorus, in the presence of normal glomerular function with falling urine phosphorus, would indicate hypoparathyroidism (high per cent TRP) (see page 181). These tests are affected, to a large extent, by the dietary intake of phosphorus,

which must be controlled during the test period.

Vitamin D in very large amounts, *i.e.,* over 100,000 to 150,000 units per day, simulates, to some degree, the action of parathyroid hormone, but it is less effective in eliminating phosphorus through the renal tubules. Dihydrotachysterol (A.T. 10) has a better phosphaturic action than does vitamin D. The action of vitamin D in regard to phosphate elimination is, in part, conditioned by the absence or presence of the parathyroid glands. (In hypoparathyroidism vitamin D, in large amounts, will produce phosphaturia, whereas it will reduce phosphaturia in disorders associated with secondary hyperparathyroidism, *e.g.,* rickets.) A chemical picture quite similar to idiopathic hypoparathyroidism can occur when the parathyroid glands are present but their action at the periphery is ineffective, a syndrome known as pseudohypoparathyroidism (see pages 187 and 188).

CLINICAL MANIFESTATIONS OF ACUTE HYPOCALCEMIA

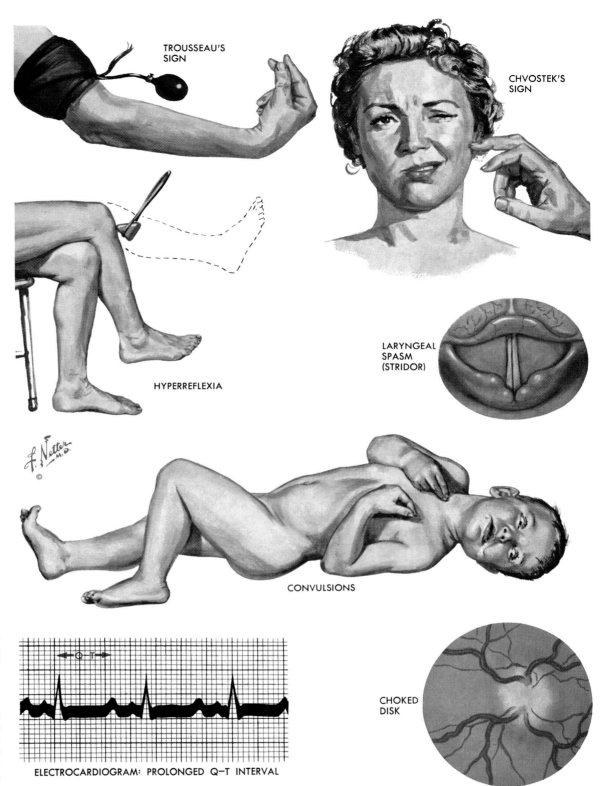

TROUSSEAU'S SIGN

CHVOSTEK'S SIGN

HYPERREFLEXIA

LARYNGEAL SPASM (STRIDOR)

CONVULSIONS

ELECTROCARDIOGRAM: PROLONGED Q–T INTERVAL

CHOKED DISK

The classic manifestation of acute hypocalcemia is tetany, which may be very dramatic if the calcium level falls rapidly, *e.g.*, after the removal of a parathyroid tumor or after the accidental removal of parathyroid glands during thyroid surgery. Symptoms are quite variable, however, from case to case, and manifestations of tetany may not be present clinically in spite of a marked fall in serum calcium level. Patients may develop latent or chronic manifestations of hypocalcemia (see page 186) insidiously. Recurrent signs and symptoms of acute tetany may occur in this state sporadically.

The two outstanding signs of hypocalcemic tetany are the *Trousseau* and the *Chvostek signs.* The former is elicited by the application of a blood-pressure cuff, to slightly above the systolic level, for a few minutes. The resulting *carpopedal spasm,* with contractions of the fingers and *inability to open the hand,* stems from the increased muscle irritability in hypocalcemic states, aggravated by the ischemia produced by the blood-pressure cuff. The Chvostek sign is a *contracture of the facial muscles, produced by tapping the facial nerves at the angle of the jaw.* Mild twitching of the face may occur, but in severe hypocalcemic states contracture of the orbicularis oculi and even contraction of the contralateral facial muscles may be seen. These two tests do not always indicate hypocalcemia or hypoparathyroidism; the signs may also be seen in states of alkalosis as, *e.g.*, in the hyperventilation syndrome or in primary aldosteronism. The deep *tendon reflexes are usually hyperactive. Laryngeal spasm* will lead to *stridor* and to labored respiration. This is the most serious complication of postoperative hypoparathyroidism, especially if the recurrent laryngeal nerve has been damaged, since it may lead to respiratory insufficiency. Some patients simply complain of anxiety and irritability; others may show marked personality changes or may become frankly psychotic. Photophobia and diplopia may be seen. In children, *convulsions* may occur instead of the other manifestations of hypocalcemia, and any patient with idiopathic epilepsy should be screened for the possibility of hypocalcemic tetany. The electro-encephalogram may reveal a generalized dysrhythmia. One of the unusual manifestations of hypocalcemia is *choking of the disks,* with elevation of spinal-fluid pressure (pseudotumor cerebri). This does not usually lead to visual loss, but, on rare occasions, it may involve the macular area and interfere with vision. Other signs are abdominal cramps, urinary frequency, and, on occa-

sion, intestinal ileus due to partial obstruction of segments of the small bowel. Cardiac abnormalities have been noted, *varying from prolongation of the Q-T interval* in the electrocardiogram, to tachycardia and actual cardiac dilatation.

These signs and symptoms subside with the administration of calcium, but they may recur when the calcium level falls again. The presence of alkalosis will markedly enhance the signs and symptoms, whereas acidosis may completely suppress the manifestations. Since some patients exhibit only a very few signs and symptoms of hypocalcemia, serum levels of calcium and phosphorus should be determined periodically in patients who (*e.g.*, following thyroidectomy) show peculiar symptoms or personality changes. Latent hypoparathyroidism can be revealed by the measures described on page 189. Although acute intravenous administration of cal-

cium will give relief of symptoms, other measures, designed to lower the serum phosphorus level and to maintain adequate calcium absorption by the administration of calcium products, will be necessary to prevent recurrence. Parathyroid hormone is practically never used for the treatment of acute hypoparathyroidism, but A.T. 10 (dihydrotachysterol) or vitamin D in large doses is effective in maintaining serum calcium. Though the acute manifestations of hypoparathyroidism are alarming, they are not of serious consequence unless laryngeal obstruction or uncontrollable convulsions are present. Follow-up treatment, to prevent the far more serious and disabling manifestations of chronic hypoparathyroidism (see page 186), is imperative. The patient may lose practically all of the acute manifestations in spite of continued hypocalcemia, only to show some of the chronic signs and symptoms years later.

CLINICAL MANIFESTATIONS OF CHRONIC HYPOPARATHYROIDISM

Although manifestations of acute hypocalcemia, as seen in hypoparathyroidism, are often dramatic and striking and are usually not missed, chronic hypocalcemia may be very subtle in most of its clinical signs and symptoms and, often, is diagnosed accidentally after permanent damage has already occurred. The manifestations are more serious if the state of hypoparathyroidism occurred in childhood, and the prognosis for ultimate recovery is worse. The patient with chronic hypocalcemic tetany may lose many of the signs and symptoms outlined on page 185, but he may still show a mildly positive Chvostek sign and, occasionally, also a Trousseau sign.

The outstanding symptoms may be, primarily, mental lassitude, personality changes, sleepiness, or blurring of vision. Careful examination of the eye with a slit lamp will show *spiculate opacities in the posterior subcapsular area* of the lens, which may progress to *cataract* formation and blindness. Mental sluggishness or *mental retardation* would indicate that hypocalcemia has persisted for many years. It is for this reason that these complications are far more commonly seen in idiopathic hypoparathyroidism, but they also occur in patients who have had untreated hypoparathyroidism for many years following thyroid surgery. Cutaneous manifestations occur primarily in patients who have idiopathic hypoparathyroidism. *A spotty alopecia* progressing to almost complete loss of hair, including the eyebrows, is seen, at times associated with moniliasis. Hypoparathyroidism may occur in families and may be associated with Addison's disease and also with sprue. The presence of steatorrhea makes the diagnosis of hypoparathyroidism difficult, since it also causes hypocalcemia, but the serum phosphate level is usually low. *Moniliasis of the nails* and also of the *mucous membranes of the mouth* may be present. The exact relationship of this fungus infection to hypoparathyroidism is not clear. In many patients with chronic hypoparathyroidism, brittle nails are found. The status of the teeth may give a clue as to the onset of the disease. If it occurred before the age of 6 years, *dental hypoplasia,* with poor dental root formation, is usually present. If it began during childhood, there will be crumbling of the teeth because of poor enamel structure. The *lamina dura* is often rather *dense,* in contrast to hyperparathyroidism in which the lamina dura is frequently resorbed. In the majority of patients seen in adult life, the teeth are not involved. The skeleton is usually not demineralized; at times, very dense bones have been noted in

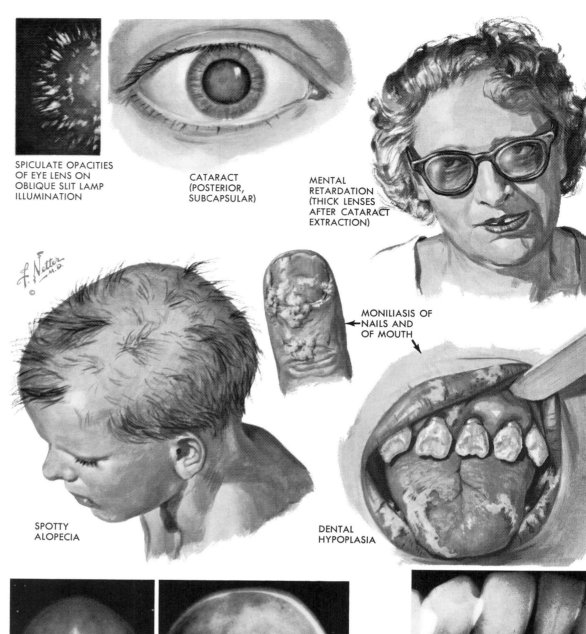

SPICULATE OPACITIES OF EYE LENS ON OBLIQUE SLIT LAMP ILLUMINATION

CATARACT (POSTERIOR, SUBCAPSULAR)

MENTAL RETARDATION (THICK LENSES AFTER CATARACT EXTRACTION)

MONILIASIS OF NAILS AND OF MOUTH

SPOTTY ALOPECIA

DENTAL HYPOPLASIA

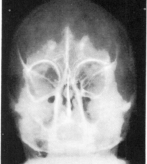

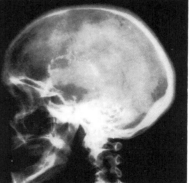

CALCIFICATION OF BASAL GANGLIA

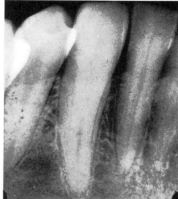

INCREASED DENSITY OF LAMINA DURA

patients with hypoparathyroidism. If the disease has been lifelong, a general stunting of growth may take place. X-rays of the skull may show the typical *calcification of the basal ganglia.* Tomograms will demonstrate this quite well. Not all instances of basal ganglia calcification are due to hypocalcemia and hypoparathyroidism. Recent evidence suggests that this calcification of the basal ganglia may not be due to chronic hypocalcemia per se but may be an associated genetic defect. Calcification of the falx and other intracranial structures may also be noted.

Treatment consists of a high-calcium, low-phosphate diet, which usually demands the elimination of cow's milk and dairy products; the administration of some type of calcium salt, to provide 1 to 2 gm of calcium per day; and the administration of vitamin D, usually 50,000 to 200,000 units per day. As an alternative, A.T. 10 (dihydrotachysterol) may be

used, but it is far more expensive. Parathyroid hormone has no place in the treatment of chronic hypoparathyroidism. Since vitamin D accumulates in the system, treatment must be carefully followed with accurate determinations of serum calcium levels. The urinary Sulkowitch test (see page 189), which initially indicates the presence or absence of normal or excessive amounts of calcium in the urine, unfortunately is not of great value following chronic treatment with vitamin D, since practically all patients develop hypercalciuria on vitamin D, regardless of whether their serum calcium level is high or low. Attempts to transplant parathyroid tissue have been generally unsuccessful even after an initial take.

Though many of the manifestations of chronic hypocalcemia will improve with appropriate treatment, the dental pathology, cataract formation, and brain changes are usually permanent and irreversible.

PATHOLOGIC PHYSIOLOGY OF PSEUDOHYPOPARATHYROIDISM

The syndrome resembling idiopathic hypoparathyroidism, but having *associated genetic defects* such as *short stature, round face, short metacarpals,* and *ectopic bone formation,* is called pseudohypoparathyroidism. In this syndrome the *parathyroid glands* are not absent, but their hormone fails to act on the *renal tubule;* therefore, there is *little inhibition of phosphate reabsorption, phosphate excretion* by the *kidneys* is diminished, and the *serum phosphorus level* is kept *high.* Because of the *reciprocal relationship of phosphorus and calcium,* the *serum calcium is low.* The chemical picture, i.e., a *high serum phosphorus and low serum calcium* level, resembles that of idiopathic hypoparathyroidism.

However, since the parathyroid glands are present in this syndrome, the falling level of serum calcium may lead to *secondary stimulation of the parathyroid glands* and to *increased production of parathyroid hormone.* This secondary hyperparathyroidism is ineffective in producing phosphaturia, since the *renal tubule* is relatively *unresponsive,* but in some instances the other end-organ, bone, may show *overstimulation of the osteoclasts,* and *bone resorptive changes may be seen.* If this secondary hyperparathyroidism occurs, the *alkaline phosphatase is elevated,* and the bone picture resembles that of hyperparathyroidism. Similar to other types of renal osteitis fibrosa, this bone resorption is ineffective in restoring the calcium level to normal, as this is opposed by the serum phosphorus level which is maintained in the high range. Since bone resorption is found in only a few patients with this syndrome, resistance at the level of bone may be an additional feature of the disease. The calcium that is mobilized is *"bound"* in soft tissues and also in the *gastro-intestinal tract* by the high phosphate level. More recently, it has been demonstrated that, in the presence of a high tissue phosphate level, the action of vitamin D on calcium absorption is less effective, which further enhances the hypocalcemia seen in this syndrome. The essential chemical features of this syndrome, then, are *low calcium, high serum phosphorus,* and *normal or sometimes elevated alkaline phosphatase.* The *urinary calcium and phosphorus are low.*

The term "Seabright Bantam syndrome" was applied by Albright *et al.* to this syndrome, since the Seabright Bantam rooster has testes but has the plumage of the female bird, thus also showing end-organ resistance to the action of a hormone. The additional sex reversal would correspond to the occasional hyperparathyroidism found in pseudohypoparathyroidism. The patient with pseudohypoparathyroidism has the chemical features of hypoparathyroidism,

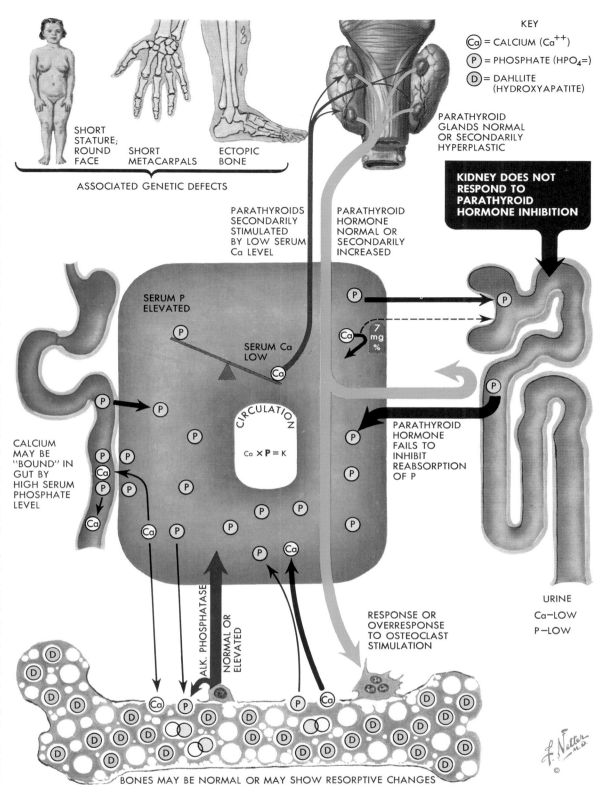

KEY
Ca = CALCIUM (Ca^{++})
P = PHOSPHATE (HPO$_4$=)
D = DAHLLITE (HYDROXYAPATITE)

SHORT STATURE; ROUND FACE — SHORT METACARPALS — ECTOPIC BONE

ASSOCIATED GENETIC DEFECTS

PARATHYROID GLANDS NORMAL OR SECONDARILY HYPERPLASTIC

PARATHYROIDS SECONDARILY STIMULATED BY LOW SERUM Ca LEVEL

PARATHYROID HORMONE NORMAL OR SECONDARILY INCREASED

KIDNEY DOES NOT RESPOND TO PARATHYROID HORMONE INHIBITION

SERUM P ELEVATED

SERUM Ca LOW

7 mg %

CALCIUM MAY BE "BOUND" IN GUT BY HIGH SERUM PHOSPHATE LEVEL

CIRCULATION

Ca × P = K

PARATHYROID HORMONE FAILS TO INHIBIT REABSORPTION OF P

URINE
Ca—LOW
P—LOW

ALK. PHOSPHATASE NORMAL OR ELEVATED

RESPONSE OR OVERRESPONSE TO OSTEOCLAST STIMULATION

BONES MAY BE NORMAL OR MAY SHOW RESORPTIVE CHANGES

but, physiologically, has those resembling secondary hyperparathyroidism.

The inability of the kidneys to respond to parathyroid hormone is demonstrated by the Ellsworth-Howard test (see page 189), which consists of the intravenous administration of 200 units of parathyroid hormone and of measuring the hourly phosphate excretion. In contrast to idiopathic hypoparathyroidism, which shows a prompt response with phosphaturia, the patient with pseudohypoparathyroidism fails to show significant rises of the urinary phosphorus. Continued administration of parathyroid hormone may also demonstrate resistance to its calcium-mobilizing action.

Treatment with A.T. 10 (dihydrotachysterol) or vitamin D and calcium and a low-phosphorus diet will raise the serum calcium and lower the serum phosphorus and also will reduce secondary hyperpara-

thyroidism by restoring the chemical picture to normal. The manifestations of secondary hyperparathyroidism on bone (osteitis fibrosa) also are readily reversible by this treatment.

Although this syndrome is almost always a genetic congenital disorder, there have been descriptions of isolated cases which apparently were acquired and failed to manifest some of the associated genetic defects. An excess of thyrocalcitonin has been recently suggested in this disorder. Whereas many of the signs and symptoms are due to hypocalcemia and hyperphosphatemia, other findings, such as the short stature, the short metacarpals, and, especially, the ectopic bone formation, appear to be genetic rather than biochemical defects, since they are also found in a related syndrome lacking the chemical abnormalities of calcium and phosphorus metabolism, the so-called "pseudo-pseudohypoparathyroidism".

CLINICAL MANIFESTATIONS OF PSEUDOHYPO-PARATHYROIDISM

The clinical manifestations of pseudo-hypoparathyroidism are, in many respects, similar to those found in idiopathic or postsurgical hypoparathyroidism. All the manifestations of acute hypocalcemic tetany and of chronic hypocalcemia may be found in this syndrome (see pages 185 and 186).

In addition, a number of characteristic physical features are diagnostic, *e.g.*, a strikingly *short, thickset figure*, a tendency to *generalized obesity*, and, especially, *rounding of the face*. Typically, these patients have a *dull appearance*, and, at times, mental retardation is associated with this disease. The most outstanding distinguishing features are *shortening of the* first, *fourth*, and *fifth* (and, at times, also of the third) *metacarpal* and *metatarsal* bones. This can be demonstrated not only on X-rays but also by having the patient make a fist which will demonstrate the so-called *"knuckle, knuckle, dimple, dimple" sign*, first pointed out by Albright. Instead of a proper knuckle appearing, the short metacarpal will lead to a depression. Recent surveys of serial X-rays have shown that the reasons for the short metacarpals are (1) premature fusion of the epiphyses and (2) failure of the proper appearance of some of the epiphyses, not only of the metacarpals but also of the phalanges, which will, therefore, be short. Other long bones also may be short. In addition to these features, there may be multiple exostoses, resembling a dyschondroplasia, and striking *subcutaneous calcification and ossification*, at times in the form of *osseous plaques* or *nodules*, which may be seen and felt in *soft tissues*. Biopsy shows actual ectopic bone formation in these nodules. Occasionally, nodules in soft tissue *ulcerate*.

As discussed on page 187, it has been shown that the parathyroid glands are present in this syndrome and may become secondarily overstimulated, leading to secondary hyperparathyroidism. Therefore, all the manifestations of secondary hyperparathyroidism may be seen at times, especially if the skeleton responds to this stimulation. *Subperiosteal resorptive changes* in the digits have been observed, as have been changes in the epiphyses which are indistinguishable from renal osteitis fibrosa (renal rickets) (see page 182). The subcutaneous ossification is often quite extensive and resembles that of myositis ossificans, a disease in which the first metacarpal bones may be short but which is not associated with abnormalities of the serum calcium and phosphorus metabolism.

A syndrome known as "pseudo-pseudo-hypoparathyroidism" shares many of the

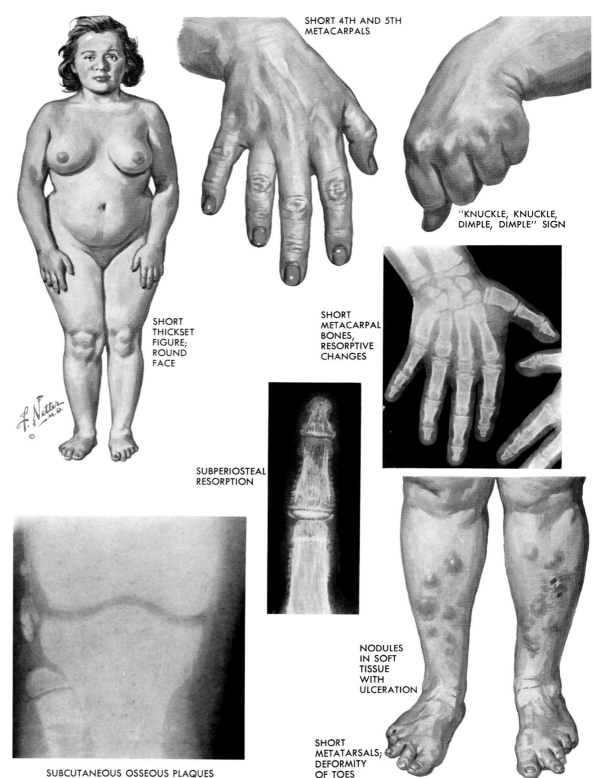

SHORT 4TH AND 5TH METACARPALS

"KNUCKLE, KNUCKLE, DIMPLE, DIMPLE" SIGN

SHORT THICKSET FIGURE; ROUND FACE

SHORT METACARPAL BONES, RESORPTIVE CHANGES

SUBPERIOSTEAL RESORPTION

NODULES IN SOFT TISSUE WITH ULCERATION

SHORT METATARSALS; DEFORMITY OF TOES

SUBCUTANEOUS OSSEOUS PLAQUES

physical features of pseudohypoparathyroidism, including short stature, short metacarpals, and even subcutaneous ossification, yet does not show either a low serum calcium or a high serum phosphorus level. It has recently been demonstrated that members of the families of patients with pseudo-pseudohypoparathyroidism may show cataract formation and also basal ganglia calcification without exhibiting any chemical abnormalities. For that reason the current thought is that these latter abnormalities may be due not to chronic hypocalcemia but, instead, to genetic aberrations.

The treatment of acute hypocalcemia and of the chronic hypocalcemic state is in no way different from that of idiopathic or postsurgical hypoparathyroidism (A.T. 10 may be more effective in some cases). If bone disease is present, it heals promptly, with the return of the alkaline phosphatase to normal and the

filling in of the bone resorption; epiphysial changes are promptly reversed. Vitamin D and A.T. 10 are capable of healing bones as well as reversing the hypocalcemia of this syndrome. The osseous plaques may require surgical removal. Although many of the features of the syndrome are thus successfully treated, others, *e.g.*, short stature, may remain or progress in spite of adequate treatment. The patient must be followed up by periodic determinations of serum calcium and phosphorus levels during therapy, in order to avoid the danger of hypercalcemia, which will enhance the problem of subcutaneous calcification. The outlook for rehabilitation is only fair, since many features of the syndrome are of the nature of a dyschondroplasia rather than being due to a metabolic defect. Spontaneous reversal from pseudohypoparathyroidism to pseudo-pseudohypoparathyroidism (with normal serum calcium level) may occur.

COMMONLY USED TESTS FOR DIAGNOSIS OF ABNORMALITIES IN CALCIUM METABOLISM

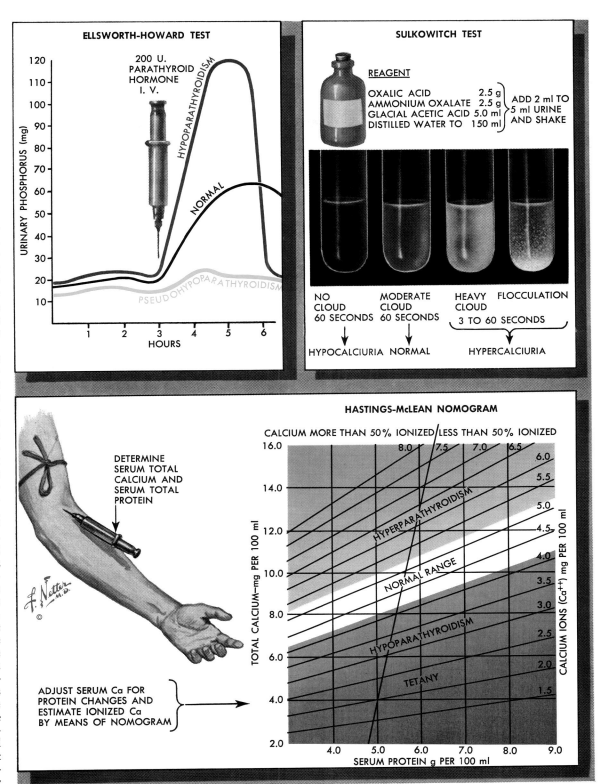

The direct measurement of parathyroid hormone in blood and urine is still in the investigative state; but immuno-chemical methods appear very promising as highly purified hormonal peptides are becoming available. One must still rely clinically on indirect tests of calcium abnormalities and phosphate dynamics to reach a conclusion concerning the status of the parathyroid glands.

The *Ellsworth-Howard test* depends on the phosphaturic action of parathyroid hormone, which appears to block the reabsorption of phosphorus by the renal tubule, leading to enhanced phosphate excretion in the urine. This is a rather rapid action, occurring within a matter of several hours. The test is performed by having the fasting subject force fluids and collect hourly urine specimens, which are assayed for phosphorus and creatinine (the latter to ensure that the specimens are comparable). After two control periods, 200 *units of parathyroid hormone are injected intravenously.* Urine specimens are collected for the next 4 hours. If the patient's renal tubules are able to respond *normally* to parathyroid hormone, the urinary phosphorus excretion will double or triple over the next several hours. In a patient who has either idiopathic or postsurgical *hypoparathyroidism* (see page 184), a marked rise in phosphate excretion usually takes place, with a subsequent lowering of the serum phosphorus. The patient whose renal tubules are unresponsive to parathyroid hormone (*pseudohypoparathyroidism*) (see page 187) will show little, if any, rise of phosphate in the urine. Some parathyroid preparations of animal origin have not been potent, and it is, therefore, advisable to use a normal subject (preferably a subject of comparable age) as a control before a diagnosis of pseudohypoparathyroidism is made. A very rare patient shows anaphylaxis, and the test should probably not be performed if there is known allergy.

The *Sulkowitch test* is a rapid, semiquantitative screening test for urinary calcium concentration. In principle, it involves the addition, in a dropwise fashion, of an *oxalic acid solution in glacial acetic acid* to 5 ml of *urine.* If no cloud appears even after standing for 60 seconds, then a state of *hypocalciuria* is present, indicating that the serum calcium level is usually below 7 mg per 100 ml, which is the normal kidney threshold. It would also indicate that less than 50 mg of calcium are present in the urine per 24 hours. *Normal* urine

specimens, especially in the fasting state, usually do not contain more than a small trace, occurring after several seconds of standing. A heavy *flocculent* precipitate ordinarily indicates *hypercalciuria* and, often, hypercalcemia also. Although quite reliable as a simple screening test, it is only semiquantitative, and the correlation between quantitative urine calcium and the degree of precipitation is not good, owing to the great variation in urine volume. The Sulkowitch reagent is highly toxic and must be labeled "POISON".

The accurate *determination of the total serum calcium* is still the most reliable single measure to evaluate parathyroid function, since hyper- and hypocalcemia are the prime manifestations of abnormalities of the parathyroid glands. About 45 per cent of the serum calcium is protein-bound; 55 per cent is diffusible and mostly ionized. Since only the ionized

calcium is biologically important, it should, ideally, be determined directly. However, since this test is not generally available, the level of the *ionized calcium* may be roughly estimated by the *Hastings-McLean nomogram.* Whenever a serum calcium is determined, measurement of the *total protein* should also be made in order to estimate the ionized calcium level by means of the nomogram. In drawing blood for this determination, it is important to have calcium-free glassware. It is also important that the tourniquet not be left on too long, because this may give rise to falsely high values, since the total serum protein will be raised.

Other tests, *i.e.*, the TRP test, a measurement of the percentage of tubular reabsorption of phosphorus, and the calcium infusion test, designed to demonstrate if phosphaturia can be shut off, are discussed on page 181.

Osteomalacia (Rickets) of Alimentary Origin

The bone disorder primarily concerned with insufficient deposition of lime salts, in an otherwise normal matrix, is called RICKETS if it occurs in childhood and OSTEOMALACIA if in the adult. This disease is comprised of two broad groups: in one there is insufficient entry of calcium and/or phosphate from the gastro-intestinal tract; in the other, although lime salts reach the circulation, excessive losses occur through the urinary tract (renal rickets) (see page 191). The former may be due simply to *dietary lack of calcium* or of *vitamin D,* or a *deficiency of endogenous vitamin D synthesis* may arise because of *insufficient* exposure to *sunlight*.

Calciferol, or vitamin D₂, one of a family of steroids, is the most potent of the series in man. It is derived from a steroid precursor, ergosterol, which is activated in the skin by ultraviolet light to form the biologically active vitamin. The liver of animals feeding on fish is a good source of vitamin D, but, in practice, irradiated milk provides the bulk of vitamin D. Daily requirements vary from 400 to 800 international units (I.U.). Overdosage of vitamin D (at least 200,000 I.U. daily) may lead to widespread metastatic calcifications.

Rather than true dietary lack of vitamin D, there may be *resistance to the normal action of vitamin D on intestinal calcium absorption. A high dietary intake of phosphate* or *phytate* will *impair calcium absorption.* Since normal *alimentary secretions* are necessary for the proper absorption of vitamin D and calcium, an insufficiency of gastric acid, bile, and pancreatic and intestinal juices leads to improper absorption of vitamin D, fats, and fatty acids and to their precipitation as calcium soaps in the gastro-intestinal tract (*malabsorption, sprue* syndrome). Likewise, during stress, *e.g., pregnancy* and *lactation,* the excessive demands for calcium may not be met by the usual dietary intake. *Excessive sweating* has also been considered a cause of calcium deficiency.

On poor calcium intake or if inadequate amounts of calcium reach the circulation, the *serum calcium tends to fall,* its lowered level giving rise to *secondary parathyroid stimulation* and *secondary physiologic hyperparathyroidism.* This will tend to compensate for the hypocalcemia by *increased osteoclastic stimulation* and *acceleration of resorption of calcium and of phosphate,* from the skeleton and will lead to *inhibition of phosphate reabsorption* and a *lowering of the serum phosphorus level. Initially,*

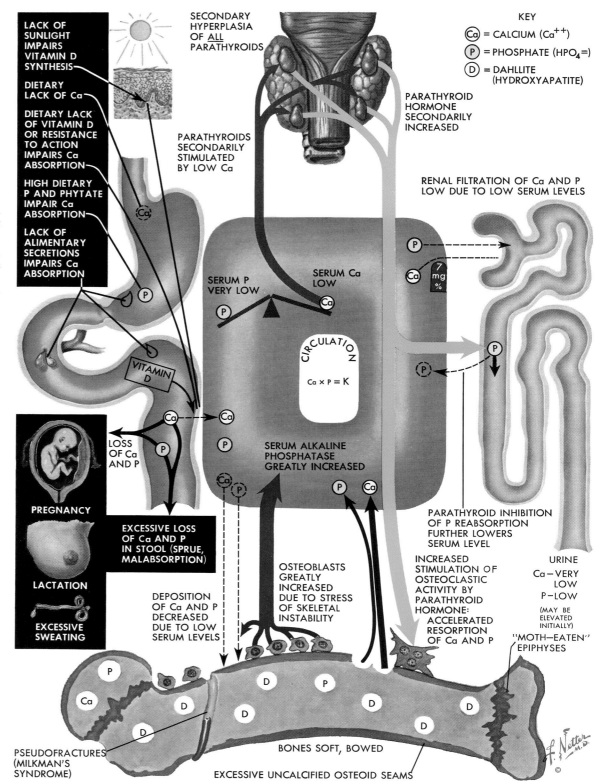

there will be a *rise in the urinary phosphate,* but this will *eventually* become *low,* just as the *calcium excretion is very low* in this type of osteomalacia or rickets. By contrast, *fecal losses of calcium and of phosphate may remain excessive.*

The *increased osteoclastic activity* on bone leads to *skeletal instability* and *compensatory rise of osteoblastic activity,* with *marked increase in the serum alkaline phosphatase* levels. Stimulation of *osteoid production,* which is *poorly calcified,* is enhanced. The typical lesions in bone are widened, *"moth-eaten", irregularly calcified epiphyses* in the child and, in the adult, primarily uncalcified bone with *large uncalcified osteoid seams.* The bones become *soft* and *bowed.* Fractures are rare, but the appearance of so-called *pseudofractures,* which are bilateral, symmetric lesions (often in association with circumflex arterial blood vessels) appearing as incomplete

fractures or incompletely calcified callus (Looser's zones) in the so-called *Milkman's syndrome,* are pathognomonic of osteomalacia. Tetany may occur initially in rickets when the serum calcium level drops rather acutely, but then the parathyroid stimulation usually restores the calcium level to normal. In all but elderly patients, the serum alkaline phosphatase level is usually markedly elevated in osteomalacia, in contrast to that in osteoporosis.

A most unusual form of rickets or osteomalacia is the disease HYPOPHOSPHATASIA, the only form of rickets in which the alkaline phosphatase level is low rather than high, with a characteristically high urinary phospho-ethanolamine titer and, in severe cases, elevated serum calcium levels. Any disorder of rapid bone healing ("hungry bones"), *e.g.,* the state after removal of parathyroid tumor, will give rise to a picture quite similar to osteomalacia or rickets.

OSTEOMALACIA (RICKETS) OF RENAL ORIGIN

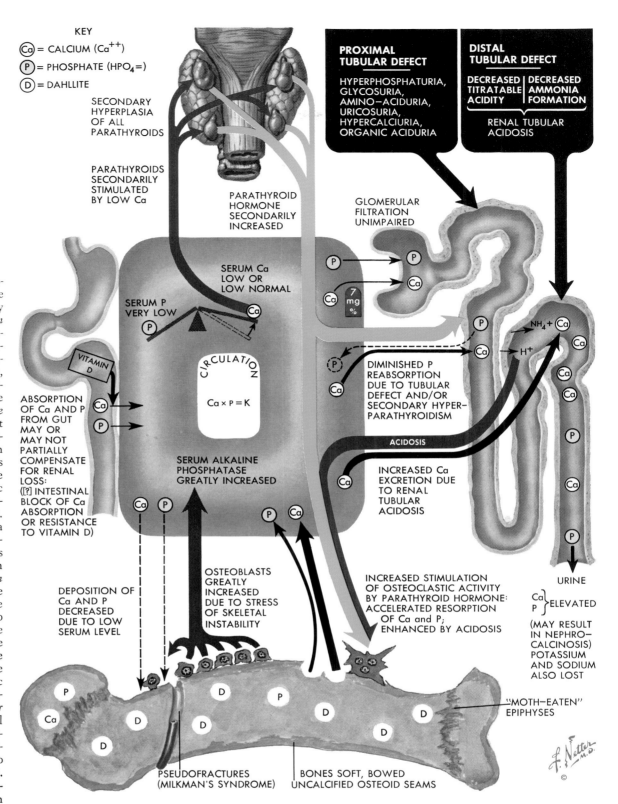

The second large category in osteomalacia or rickets (referred to on page 190) appears to be associated primarily with excessive *renal losses of calcium and/or phosphate* (renal rickets, vitamin-D-resistant rickets, de Toni-Fanconi syndrome, renal tubular acidosis). In contrast to the alimentary forms of rickets, in which both serum calcium and phosphorus are often low, in this variety the *hypophosphatemia* and *elevated alkaline phosphatase* level often give the first indication of a basic bone disorder. Frequently, the serum calcium level is in the normal range. Several types of this disorder are congenital in origin and are most likely associated with an intrinsic *renal tubular defect* involving *reabsorption of phosphate* and other electrolytes. The adult form of hypophosphatemia may actually be due to *secondary hyperparathyroidism*. Recent evidence suggests that in this disorder there may be an *intestinal absorptive defect of calcium and phosphate* or a resistance to the normal action of *vitamin D*. This type of rickets has been frequently referred to as vitamin-D-resistant rickets, since tremendous amounts of vitamin D are necessary to restore the serum phosphate (and calcium) levels to normal. The classic form of the renal tubular intrinsic disorders is the de Toni-Fanconi syndrome, which shows *multiple tubular defects* (see also page 243). Proximal tubular defects comprise *hyperphosphaturia, glycosuria, generalized amino-aciduria, uricosuria,* and, at times, also *hypercalciuria* and *organic aciduria*. There may also be associated *distal tubular defects* concerned with preservation of normal acid-base balance, *i.e., inability to form adequate amounts of titratable acidity* and *ammonia,* leading to acidosis with *increased losses of calcium* (and also, at times, of *potassium* and *sodium*) and nephrogenic diabetes insipidus.

Another form of renal rickets is primarily concerned with distal tubular inability to conserve acid-base balance. This is often seen in adults, sometimes after pyelonephritis, but also, at times, in a familial form, which is probably congenital. This so-called *renal tubular acidosis* is manifested primarily by *nephrocalcinosis,* secondary to the excessive losses of calcium and phosphate in the urine. At times, the hypokalemia of this syndrome simulates periodic paralysis.

The physiologic effect of these various disorders will be a tendency toward a *lowering of the serum calcium,* which appears to cause *secondary hyperparathyroidism* with *hyperplasia of all the parathyroid glands.* The increased parathyroid hormone production will cause *increased stimulation of osteoclastic activity* on bone with *resorptive changes.* The presence of *acidosis* in some of these disorders may *enhance this bone resorption.* Likewise, secondary hyperparathyroidism will cause *diminished tubular reabsorption of phosphate* and *enhance the urinary phosphate losses.* The resulting bone disease is that of classical rickets or osteomalacia, with *softening* and *bowing of the bones, uncalcified osteoid seams,* "moth-eaten" epiphyses, and pseudofractures quite similar to those found in any type of rickets. The *osteoblastic overresponse due to the skeletal stress of instability* will cause *elevation of the serum alkaline phosphatase level.*

A calcium infusion test will usually demonstrate the presence or absence of secondary hyperparathyroidism. If it raises the serum phosphate level and diminishes the urinary phosphate losses, it can be assumed that secondary hyperparathyroidism is present; if it fails to do so, the primary lesion may be in the renal tubule itself. Glomerular function is usually unimpaired initially; however, in the end stages of the renal disease (often due to pyelonephritis), glomerular filtration of phosphate becomes impaired. In contrast to treatment of the simple types of rickets of alimentary origin, very large amounts of vitamin D, sometimes in the toxic range, are often required to reverse the chemical and clinical picture. Apparent healing of the rickets will be seen with a progressive rise in the serum phosphate level, but, eventually, this will lead to secondary renal osteitis fibrosa (see page 182).

CLINICAL MANIFESTATIONS OF OSTEOMALACIA (RICKETS)

The clinical manifestations vary considerably if onset of the disease takes place in childhood or infancy (*rickets*), or if it occurs in the adult (*osteomalacia*), in which case it is often a mild and clinically unsuspected disorder. Hypocalcemia and hypophosphatemia produce relatively few symptoms; tetany, except in the initial stages of rickets, is rare. There may be muscular weakness and listlessness, irritability, and inability to grow normally. The outstanding features of *childhood rickets* are the grossly visible deformities such as generalized *dwarfing, prominence of the forehead,* and *craniotabes.* The peculiar shape of the skull (*dolichocephaly*) is due to premature closure of the sagittal suture. A pronounced *"pigeon" breast* and prominence of the rachitic cartilages of the ribs, producing the so-called *rachitic rosary,* are common characteristics. A groove at the insertion of the diaphragm (*Harrison's groove*), with flaring of the angles of the rib cage, may be seen. *Widening of the epiphyses* at the wrists is often observed. Slipping of the larger epiphyses, especially of the femoral heads, may occur. The lower limbs show definite *bowing,* and a tendency to *knock knees* is quite common.

X-rays of the joints show "moth-eaten", ragged, *saucer-shaped,* and widened epiphysial lines. A bone biopsy will reveal a *wide, irregular zone of proliferative cartilage invaded by perichondral and marrow vessels.* The *normal line of calcification is irregular,* and a great deal of *uncalcified osteoid* is noticeable *about the trabeculae.*

In milder forms, the changes may be confined to the weight-bearing joints, especially the knees and the hip joints. In certain forms of rickets, premature loss of the teeth takes place. *Pseudofractures* of bones may be seen, but true fractures are uncommon.

The *adult form of osteomalacia* is often subtle in appearance. It may be suspected primarily because of some *bowing of the limbs* or *short stature,* or a peculiar appearance of the skull. Symptoms are few, but extreme weakness and listlessness may be present, especially in the disorders associated with malabsorption and severe calcium depletion (*e.g.,* sprue syndrome). Many patients complain primarily of long-bone or rib pains or of "arthritic pains" which are disabling, and, typically, the affected bones are sore to touch. There may be muscular weakness and paralysis if there is a renal potassium-wasting disorder.

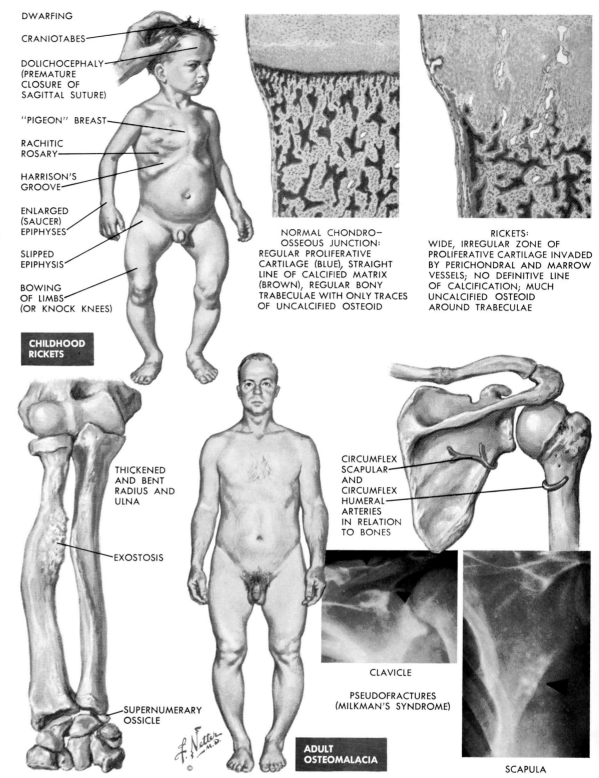

DWARFING

CRANIOTABES

DOLICHOCEPHALY (PREMATURE CLOSURE OF SAGITTAL SUTURE)

"PIGEON" BREAST

RACHITIC ROSARY

HARRISON'S GROOVE

ENLARGED (SAUCER) EPIPHYSES

SLIPPED EPIPHYSIS

BOWING OF LIMBS (OR KNOCK KNEES)

CHILDHOOD RICKETS

NORMAL CHONDRO—OSSEOUS JUNCTION: REGULAR PROLIFERATIVE CARTILAGE (BLUE), STRAIGHT LINE OF CALCIFIED MATRIX (BROWN), REGULAR BONY TRABECULAE WITH ONLY TRACES OF UNCALCIFIED OSTEOID

RICKETS: WIDE, IRREGULAR ZONE OF PROLIFERATIVE CARTILAGE INVADED BY PERICHONDRAL AND MARROW VESSELS; NO DEFINITIVE LINE OF CALCIFICATION; MUCH UNCALCIFIED OSTEOID AROUND TRABECULAE

THICKENED AND BENT RADIUS AND ULNA

EXOSTOSIS

SUPERNUMERARY OSSICLE

CIRCUMFLEX SCAPULAR AND CIRCUMFLEX HUMERAL ARTERIES IN RELATION TO BONES

CLAVICLE

PSEUDOFRACTURES (MILKMAN'S SYNDROME)

SCAPULA

ADULT OSTEOMALACIA

F. Netter M.D.

Nephrocalcinosis or the passage of stones may be the prominent feature of renal tubular acidosis.

Some types of *familial hypophosphatemic osteomalacia* (often sex-linked to males) are associated with *thickening of the bones* and with *exostoses* and *supernumerary ossicles* resembling dyschondroplasia. In most renal forms of rickets as well as in the malabsorption types, diffuse bony demineralization takes place. The pathognomonic lesion of osteomalacia in the adult form is the *pseudofracture,* typically seen in a symmetric bilateral position along the *axillary borders of the scapulae,* around the *midportions of the clavicles,* and also at other sites, such as around the femoral heads and along the rami of the ischium (*Milkman's syndrome*). Some evidence exists that these pseudofractures may be due to the pulsatile stress of *circumflex arterial vessels* on the softened bone, producing an excessive amount of

callus which is uncalcified, but some authors claim that they are due simply to unusual mechanical stresses on the uncalcified bone.

In the malabsorption types of osteomalacia, increased bone avidity for calcium can be demonstrated by an intravenous calcium infusion test (see page 181), which shows a great tendency for calcium to be retained. The hypophosphatemic renal form of the disease does not exhibit such an avidity, but rises of the serum phosphate may be thus produced. In these cases, much larger amounts of vitamin D are required than are needed to correct the simple types of rickets, hence the term vitamin-D-resistant rickets. This poses the risk of vitamin D intoxication, with hypercalcemia, so serial serum calcium determinations are required following treatment. The associated disorders, *e.g.,* acidosis, hypokalemia, and malabsorption, must be treated as well.

OSTEOPOROSIS

Osteoporosis is the metabolic bone disease seen most commonly in the United States. In the classical sense it is considered to be, primarily, a disorder of *bone matrix formation* with *deficient sites for the deposition of calcium salts*. However, most types of osteoporosis are most likely due to excessive bone resorption rather than lack of bone formation, and some recent evidence indicates that chronic calcium depletion may be another cause. *Postmenopausal osteoporosis,* the most commonly encountered form of the disease, is in some way related to *estrogen deficiency*. It is seen in roughly one third or more of the female population within 10 to 20 years after a *natural menopause,* but it may occur much sooner after an *artificial menopause* or in states of congenital *hypogonadism*. By contrast, hypogonadal states associated with *testosterone deficiency* cause osteoporosis less frequently. Osteoporosis of disuse is seen, at times, for prolonged periods following trauma and *immobilization in casts*. Osteoporosis of *old age* may be considered to be a physiologic phenomenon in the nature of bone atrophy. Among the more unusual causes of osteoporosis is congenital *osteogenesis imperfecta,* with association of blue sclerae, brittle bones, and deafness. *Adrenal cortical glucocorticoid excess,* either in the form of naturally occurring *Cushing's syndrome,* or, more frequently seen nowadays, with the excessive administration of *cortisol and its derivatives or ACTH,* leads to a severe osteoporosis, presumably due to *excessive bone catabolism*. Long-standing *hyperthyroidism* may, at times, cause osteoporosis on much the same basis. *Vitamin C depletion* with *scurvy* used to be a common cause of nutritional osteoporosis. Severe *protein starvation* has been said to lead to osteoporosis ("hunger osteopathy") and *chronic dietary calcium deficiency* may be another cause. *Multiple myeloma* and *leukemia,* aside from localized bone invasion, may give rise to a diffuse type of osteoporosis. Among the rare causes of osteoporosis are *achlorhydria, cirrhosis of the liver,* and *long-standing diabetes with acidosis*. The cause of osteoporosis in *acromegaly* is unexplained, but it may be due to the associated hypogonadism. A progressive severe type of osteoporosis due to unknown causes (*idiopathic osteoporosis*) is found in young females, often following pregnancy, and, more rarely, in young males.

There are only a few signs or symptoms, and osteoporosis is often found accidentally, on X-ray survey, only after 30 per cent or more of the *mineral content of bone* has been lost. A partial collapse

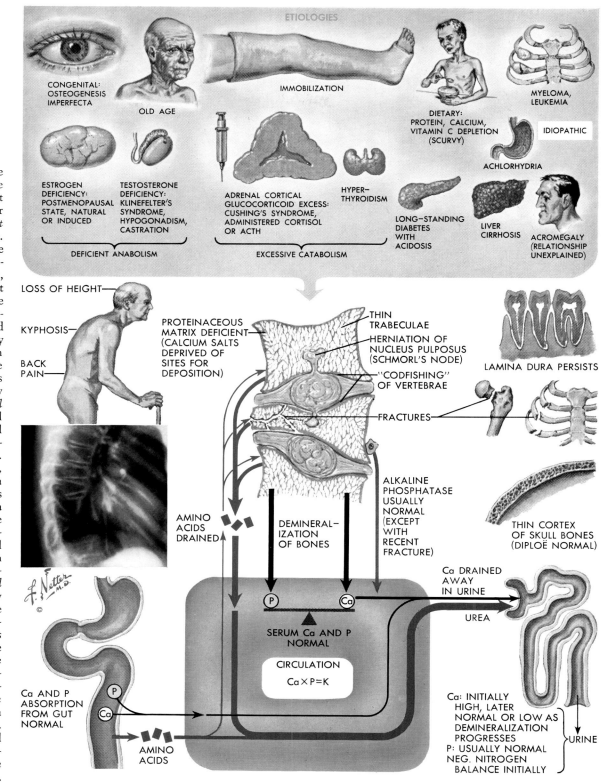

("codfishing") of the vertebral bodies, with *herniation of the nucleus pulposus,* may be the only evidence of the disease. The principal involvement in postmenopausal osteoporosis is usually confined to the *spine* and pelvis and, rarely, to the skull bones, which show *thinning of the cortex*. The *diploë* are normal, and the *lamina dura of the teeth* is usually *preserved*. However, in idiopathic and senile osteoporosis, *fractures of long bones* and *ribs* may occur. The principal signs and symptoms are *back pain,* with moderate *kyphosis* and *progressive loss of height*. There may also be associated atrophy of skin, nails, and hair, and other signs of the postmenopausal or senile state.

Ordinarily, *normal calcium and phosphate absorption from the gut* takes place, and the *serum calcium and phosphate levels are normal*. In acute osteoporosis, especially in young patients, hypercalcemia

may be seen. The *serum alkaline phosphatase level,* except when there has been a recent fracture, is usually *normal*. As a rule, the *urinary calcium is high in the initial stages* of the disease, but *normal or low in chronic or late stages*. The patients are often in *negative nitrogen balance*.

Treatment, designed to improve the bone matrix and to force its calcification, includes a high-protein and an adequate- to high-calcium intake, with anabolic hormonal therapy. The latter relieves symptoms and forestalls the progression of the disease. The use of sodium fluoride is experimental at present. To date, no therapy has effectively produced remineralization of the depleted skeleton in most cases of postmenopausal or senile osteoporosis. Although adequate support to the involved skeleton is necessary, excessive immobilization must be avoided, as this may aggravate rather than benefit the existing bone disease.

OSTEITIS DEFORMANS (PAGET'S DISEASE)

The most common nonmetabolic bone disease, which must be differentiated from hyperparathyroidism, is *osteitis deformans* (*Paget's disease* of bone). It is a disease of unknown etiology, which increases in incidence with every decade of life. It has been estimated that 3 per cent of persons over the age of 50 years will show lesions of Paget's disease. The incidence of clinically important manifestations, however, is far less.

The initial stimulus in the disease seems to be bone destruction of a rapid and irregular type, which may attack any bone but most commonly involves the lower extremities, the pelvis, or the skull. The *osteoclastic overactivity* causes erosion of bone, with skeletal instability, which is compensated for by an *osteoblastic overresponse*. The clinical picture depends on the stage of the disease when the lesions are first discovered. Initially, when the disease is primarily one of destruction, the blood chemistries will be fairly normal, but the *urine calcium will be elevated.* However, when bone repair starts taking over, there usually is a marked *increase in the serum alkaline phosphatase* which, at times, reaches very high levels. If a fracture occurs and an involved part is immobilized, the tendency to bone healing is lessened, while bone destruction continues unabated and hypercalcemia and *hypercalciuria* may occur. Calcification within the renal tract may be a consequence of the marked hypercalciuria, and *renal stones* are reported in up to *20 per cent of the cases.* In long-standing Paget's disease, depletion of lime salts may take place, and the *urinary calcium* may actually be quite low. Bone biopsy usually shows evidence of both excessive osteoclastic activity and osteoblastic activity. The osteoid is deposited on irregular trabeculae in a disorganized fashion, the so-called *"mosaic bone",* which is typical of Paget's disease.

The clinical features of the disease are variable. An isolated lesion (monostotic Paget's disease) may be present; it consists of either a destructive lesion or an isolated expanding hyperplastic lesion of bone. Sarcomatous degeneration, usually toward a fibrosarcoma, occurs in 1 to 3 per cent of cases. Solitary benign lesions are especially common in one of the vertebral bodies, which is usually larger than the surrounding vertebrae. Because of its more usual multiple bone involvement, Paget's disease can mimic any type of primary or metastatic bone disease as well as hyperparathyroidism, which may coexist with it. Lesions in the skull are common, and *enlargement of the head* is a prominent feature, often

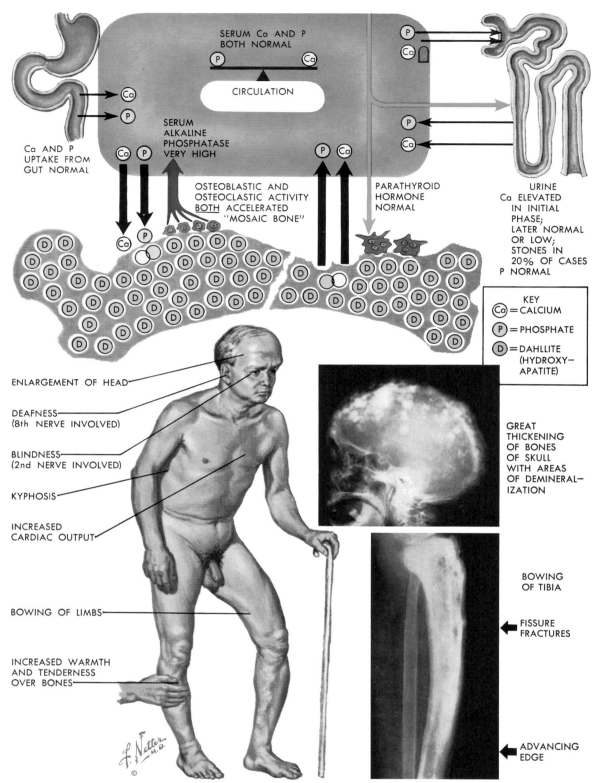

making it impossible for the patient to obtain a properly fitting hat. Dense overgrowth may impinge on nerve structures, causing severe headaches, *deafness,* and even *blindness. Kyphosis* is often found, and, if the lower spine and pelvis are involved, backache is a frequent complaint. The involved bone is usually expanded and often *bowed,* and an *increased warmth* and, at times, *tenderness over the areas* are noticeable. Prominent blood vessels are noted. In advanced cases the increased vascularity will lead to a rise in *cardiac output, with high-output heart failure.*

Serial X-rays will often reveal the progression of the disease, which usually moves slowly down an extremity, with an *advancing edge* of the disease process visible on serial X-ray studies. Although *punched-out lesions* may occur initially, they are frequently replaced by dense, coarse *overgrowth of bone,* with expansion of the involved structures. With

advancing bowing of an extremity, which is especially noted in the upper regions of the femur or of the tibia, *fissure fractures* occur, which may resemble the pseudofractures of osteomalacia. Pathologic fractures through involved bone occur, and healing is usually uneventful. If immobilization is required, it must be minimized in order to avoid hypercalcemia.

No specific treatment is known. Anabolic hormones and a high-protein diet, with calcium, vitamin D, and ascorbic acid, promote healing. Corticosteroid therapy has been shown to shut off the destructive bone process, but the high doses required lead to undesirable complications. Recently, high-dosage salicylate therapy has been reported to show both symptomatic and chemical remission of the disease as has sodium fluoride. The disease usually has a good prognosis, but it may be rather malignant in young people.

POLYOSTOTIC FIBROUS DYSPLASIA (OSTEITIS FIBROSA DISSEMINATA), ALBRIGHT'S SYNDROME

NEUROFIBROMATOSIS (VON RECKLINGHAUSEN'S DISEASE)

FIBROUS DYSPLASIA OF BONE, a disease of unknown etiology, must be differentiated from osteitis fibrosa cystica among the nonmetabolic bone diseases. It causes dense overgrowth of bone and cystic transformation, most commonly involving several areas of the skeleton, the so-called polyostotic variety. The disease may present as a single lesion in the monostotic type of fibrous dysplasia. Occasionally, there are only isolated *rib lesions* or lesions in the *digits*. A more unusual variety causes primarily *dense overgrowth of the bones of the base of the skull* (the craniofacial variety), giving rise to proptosis, and, at times, to *leontiasis ossea.* The more *typical distribution* of the lesions is unilateral.

In the disease, bone is transformed into fibrous tissue (osteitis fibrosa), with islets of cartilage and cyst formation. Fractures occur, which usually heal fairly promptly, but pseudo-arthrosis is not rare. When bone lesions are present in association with *pigment spots of the skin,* which show a ragged margin (the so-called *"coast of Maine"* contour), and with *sexual precocity,* principally *in females,* the condition is named *"Albright's syndrome".* True *isosexual precocity* is present with early menstruation, often with precocious *breast development.* This must be differentiated from other types of isosexual precocity (see page 120), and from pseudoprecocity (see CIBA COLLECTION, Vol. 2, page 202).

The chemical picture is normal, except for some elevation of the serum alkaline phosphatase level.

The greatest disability arises with lesions in the upper end of the *femur,* which becomes gradually enlarged and loses its normal contour, assuming the so-called *"shepherd's crook" deformity,* making weight-bearing difficult. Surgical correction is often required. Most of the bone lesions heal readily. Due to advancement of the bone age, girls with this disease may, occasionally, be of short stature.

NEUROFIBROMATOSIS must be differentiated from osteitis fibrosa cystica. Neurofibromatosis involves neuro-ectodermal structures throughout the body. In bone, the typical clean, punched-out lesions are usually *multiple* and are located, most commonly, in a *symmetric fashion* in areas *close to joints,* especially at the *lower ends of the femurs* and the

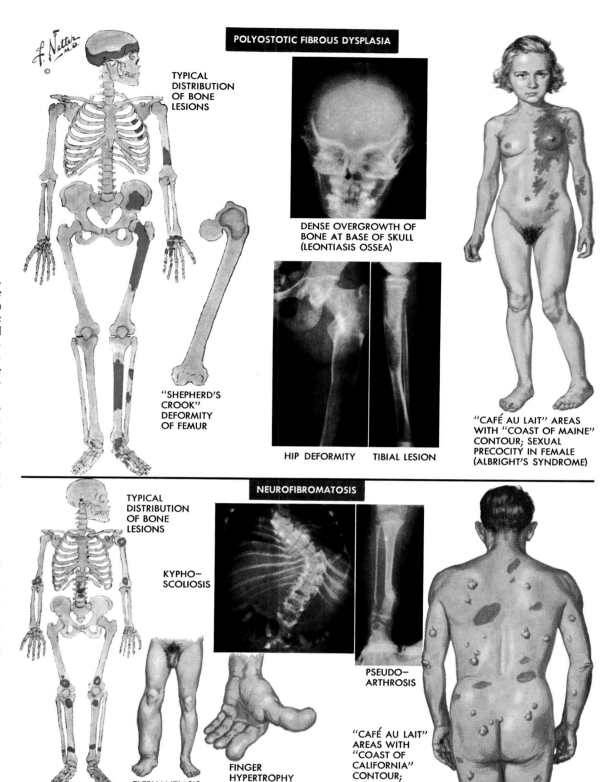

POLYOSTOTIC FIBROUS DYSPLASIA

TYPICAL DISTRIBUTION OF BONE LESIONS

DENSE OVERGROWTH OF BONE AT BASE OF SKULL (LEONTIASIS OSSEA)

"SHEPHERD'S CROOK" DEFORMITY OF FEMUR

HIP DEFORMITY   TIBIAL LESION

"CAFÉ AU LAIT" AREAS WITH "COAST OF MAINE" CONTOUR; SEXUAL PRECOCITY IN FEMALE (ALBRIGHT'S SYNDROME)

NEUROFIBROMATOSIS

TYPICAL DISTRIBUTION OF BONE LESIONS

KYPHO-SCOLIOSIS

ELEPHANTIASIS

FINGER HYPERTROPHY

PSEUDO-ARTHROSIS

"CAFÉ AU LAIT" AREAS WITH "COAST OF CALIFORNIA" CONTOUR; CUTANEOUS TUMORS

upper ends of the tibias. Biopsy shows replacement of bone by neurofibromatous tissue. In the tibia, non-healing or nonunion, with *pseudo-arthrosis,* may be observed. An unusual lesion is marked *kyphoscoliosis,* which may lead to gross deformity and short stature, especially in young children. This is not due to direct involvement of bone by neurofibromatous tissue but, probably, is caused by a neurogenic spinal-cord lesion. At times, the posterior vertebral foramina are eroded by dumbbell tumors. Rarely, there may be isosexual precocity in males owing to lesions near the hypothalamus (pineal syndrome). Pheochromocytoma (at times familial and also bilateral) may be associated with this disease.

The telltale of neurofibromatosis is the presence of fibromatous *nodular lesions* throughout areas of the skin, at times along trunks of nerves. The other typical lesion of the skin is the *"café au lait" pigment*

spot with smooth borders (the so-called *"coast of California" contour*). Sometimes "Mollusca-like" lesions are noted. Extensive plexiform neuromas may develop, which obstruct the lymphatic supply, causing *elephantiasis* of one of the extremities. In addition, there may be *hypertrophy of a single digit,* such as the finger, or there may be *hemihypertrophy of the entire lower or upper extremity.* Fracture through the cystic bone lesions may occur, and healing, in contrast to that of hyperparathyroidism and fibrous dysplasia, is rather poor. The blood and urine chemistries are entirely normal, but association with renal rickets has been reported. Malignant degeneration of some of the involved neurofibromatous areas may occur, especially after surgical interference. The great familial incidence of this disease makes rewarding a search for lesions in other members of the patient's family.

Section VII

LIPID METABOLISM
LIPIDOSES
ATHEROSCLEROSIS
OBESITY

by

FRANK H. NETTER, M.D.

in collaboration with

DONALD S. FREDRICKSON, M.D.
Plates 1-4, 9

ROBERT E. OLSON, Ph.D., M.D.
Plates 12-15

S. J. THANNHAUSER, M.D., Ph.D.
Plates 5-8, 10 and 11

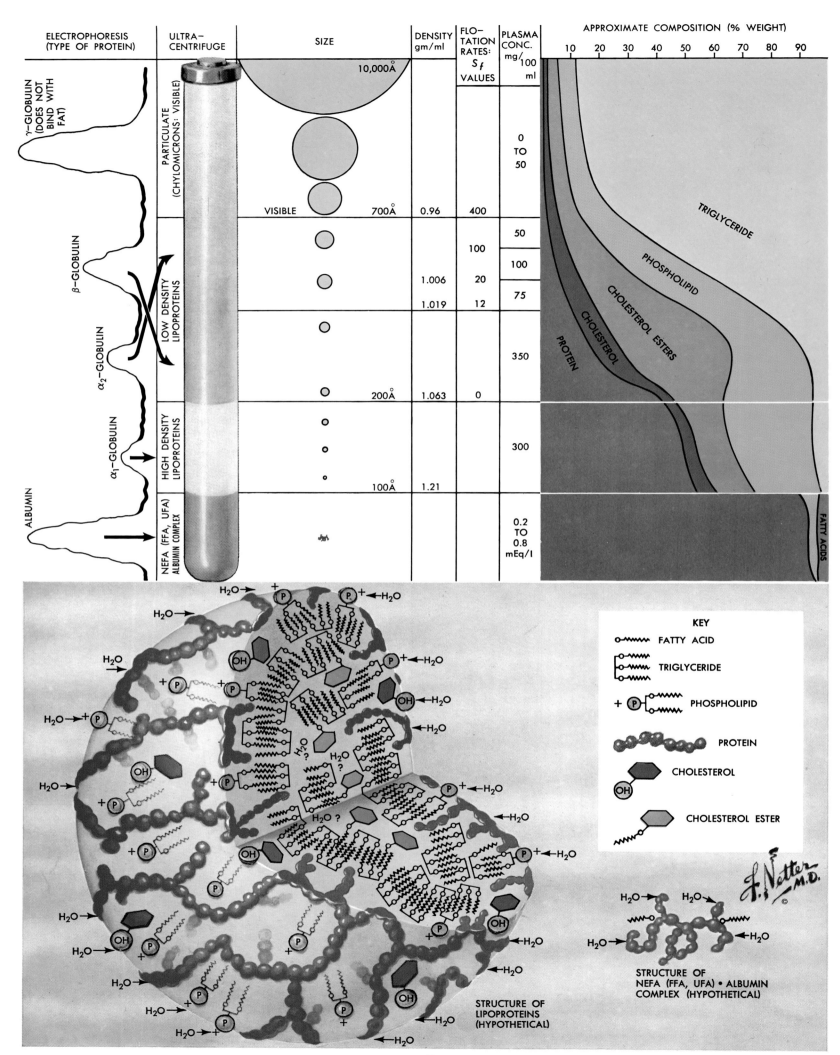

ELECTROPHORESIS (TYPE OF PROTEIN)	ULTRA-CENTRIFUGE	SIZE	DENSITY gm/ml	FLO-TATION RATES: S_f VALUES	PLASMA CONC. mg/100 ml
γ-GLOBULIN (DOES NOT BIND WITH FAT)	PARTICULATE (CHYLOMICRONS: VISIBLE)	10,000Å			0 TO 50
		VISIBLE 700Å	0.96	400	
β-GLOBULIN	LOW DENSITY LIPOPROTEINS			100	50
			1.006	20	100
			1.019	12	75
α₂-GLOBULIN					350
		200Å	1.063	0	
α₁-GLOBULIN	HIGH DENSITY LIPOPROTEINS				300
		100Å	1.21		
ALBUMIN	NEFA (FFA, UFA) ALBUMIN COMPLEX				0.2 TO 0.8 mEq/l

APPROXIMATE COMPOSITION (% WEIGHT)

TRIGLYCERIDE

PHOSPHOLIPID

CHOLESTEROL ESTERS

CHOLESTEROL

PROTEIN

FATTY ACIDS

KEY

—◦〜〜〜 FATTY ACID

TRIGLYCERIDE

+ ⓟ PHOSPHOLIPID

PROTEIN

(OH) CHOLESTEROL

CHOLESTEROL ESTER

STRUCTURE OF LIPOPROTEINS (HYPOTHETICAL)

STRUCTURE OF NEFA (FFA, UFA) • ALBUMIN COMPLEX (HYPOTHETICAL)

198

MEDIA OF FAT TRANSPORT

Although lipids are water-insoluble, from 5 to 10 gm are normally carried in 1 liter of plasma. A variety of compounds are represented; they reside in the plasma for varying lengths of time, so that some are more obviously in transit through this extracellular waterway than are others. *Cholesterol, cholesterol esters,* and the *phospholipids* — phosphatidyl choline and sphingomyelin — make up more than half of the total lipids. Their concentrations are relatively stable, and their turnover is sufficiently slow to suggest that part of their function in plasma may be as vehicles to help transport other lipids. *Triglycerides* and unesterified fatty acids *(UFA),* also known as nonesterified fatty acids *(NEFA)* or free fatty acids *(FFA),* on the other hand, undergo two- to fivefold changes in concentration during the day, consistent with considerable net transport of these lipids. On a smaller scale there also occurs movement, from tissue to tissue, of fat-soluble vitamins, hydrocarbons, and glycolipids, such as transport of carotenoids from the gut to the liver or vitamin A from the liver to the eye.

To solubilize all these hydrophobic materials in plasma, lipid-lipid interactions are important, but the successful transport of most fats also depends on interaction with *proteins.* Four major fat transport systems exist, and, for several of these, two special proteins are synthesized in the liver (and possibly other sites) for the purpose of carrying fat.

1. *Free fatty acids,* or *FFA,* have metabolic importance quite out of proportion to their low *plasma concentrations* of only 5 to 20 mg per 100 ml (usually expressed as 0.2 to 0.8 *mEq/l,* since they are measured as acids by titration with alkali after suitable organic extraction from the plasma). Their *carrier protein* is *albumin,* which has a number of cationic binding sites for the fatty acid anions. The sites of strongest binding number 2 per albumin molecule, which, in view of the large amount of albumin present, supply more than is required for the carriage of the usual amounts of FFA in plasma. This *complex* is not a lipoprotein. Ordinary amounts of FFA do not alter the density or charge of albumin. The FFA molecules readily leave their carrier at the vascular wall and pass into the tissues, after spending only a few minutes in circulation. Although the plasma FFA pool may be only 20 mg, its half-life of about 2 minutes permits the transport of over 1000 calories per day without requiring extra cations or much expenditure of energy in the process. This system is remarkably well adapted for moving stored fat to sites where it is utilized to supply caloric demands.

2. *"Chylomicrons"* afford *bulk transport* of large quantities of fatty acids, such as are provided in the diet, and represent glyceride *particles.* The chylomicrons (formed, for the most part, when dietary fat embarks from intestinal mucosa cells for various tissues) are the prime physiological example of such particles. Glycerides have very low affinity for water and are packed in emulsions. These tend to be of large particle size, economically reducing the relative surface area in contact with water at which they must be stabilized by micelles of phospholipids, cholesterol, and, possibly, small amounts of protein. These particles scatter light and produce cloudiness or, in pathologically high amounts, even a creamy appearance in plasma. Being practically all lipid, they have a density less than water and float to the top of plasma after standing overnight, or within a few minutes when centrifuged. With zone *electrophoresis* on paper or on other media, chylomicrons do not migrate from the origin.

Light-scattering particles may also be formed in sites other than the intestine. Often, these have greater density and more protein than chylomicrons and migrate, on electrophoresis, in the region of the α_2-*globulins.* They fail to rise completely to the top of the tube after standing overnight.

As chylomicrons are hydrolyzed in various tissues or at vascular walls during clearing of absorbed fat, progressively smaller particles seem to recycle in the circulation until all lactescence disappears. In their wake are left small increases in lipoprotein, cholesterol, and phospholipid, which recede over a period of hours and are the last vestiges of previous heavy glyceride transport.

In abnormal states, endogenous particles and lipoproteins of very low density also appear in the plasma in the absence of fat ingestion. These usually represent triglyceride secreted by the liver in response to very heavy intake of carbohydrate or alcohol and, perhaps, to heavy previous flux of FFA from adipose tissue.

Practically all the lipid in plasma in the postabsorptive state, other than FFA, is contained in two major lipoprotein systems. They are readily separated from each other, since each has a specific protein moiety and other distinctive chemical or physical behavior. They appear to have evolved independently, under separate genetic control, and, presumably, they serve different functions.

3. *Low-density lipoprotein,* or *LDL,* normally includes all the lipid floating to the top when postabsorptive plasma is adjusted to a *density* of 1.063 and centrifuged at high speeds in a preparative *ultracentrifuge.* A broad density spectrum is represented, which can be quantified, in the analytical ultracentrifuge, into discrete classes defined by their *flotation rates* (Sf values). As a useful clinical rule, all abnormal increases in plasma lipids involve one or more of the LDL classes, except for unusual instances in which disproportionately increased glycerides may be carried in chylomicrons or other particles. The Sf 0 to 12 class is β-lipoprotein, according to its electrophoretic migration. When this class of lipoproteins is discretely elevated, as in familial hypercholesterolemia, the plasma glyceride is normal and cholesterol is markedly increased over phospholipid, consonant with its composition. The plasma is clear, but dark orange, owing to the increased carotene carried in this lipoprotein class. When less-dense LDL classes are increased, glyceride more accurately reflects the changes in lipoprotein concentrations than does cholesterol. These $Sf > 20$ lipoproteins usually migrate as α_2-lipoproteins.

4. *High-density lipoproteins,* or *HDL,* are isolated in the *ultracentrifuge* between the *density* limits of 1.063 and 1.21 and are the α_1-lipoproteins on electrophoresis. Further subfractionation of HDL does not have clinical usefulness at present. Their concentration is normally quite stable but may be decreased in severe hyperglyceridemia and may be negligible in obstructive liver disease or Tangier disease (see page 200). Females have higher HDL concentrations than do males, HDL being increased by estrogens and decreased by testosterone.

An average high-density *lipoprotein* contains over 100 molecules each of cholesterol and phospholipid to 1 molecule of protein. Knowledge of how these components are combined to form such stable *structures* of reproducible composition is currently quite limited. The important features are surmised to be the presence of protein at the surface, in limited amount, where it is needed to establish mixing between the fat and water phases. It is abetted in this by phospholipids, whose combination of polar and nonpolar groups makes them good "physiological detergents". Very little of the lipid is attached to the protein by covalent bonds, and cohesion is provided by electrostatic bonds and weaker "dispersion" forces existing between the hydrophobic fatty acid chains of the several lipids and probably between them and parts of the protein chain. The state of hydration of the molecules is important, for they are readily denatured by freeze-drying and can be disrupted by freezing alone. An interesting feature of lipoproteins is the free exchangeability of their lipid components, whereas the peptide portions of HDL and LDL are not interchangeable.

Clinical assessment of hyperlipidemia can be simplified if one keeps in mind the plural nature of lipoprotein composition. Changes in plasma concentration of a single type of lipid are, therefore, rarely seen. Thus, an aberration in glyceride metabolism will also produce some hypercholesterolemia. The nature of the various lipoprotein peptides no doubt affects over-all lipid levels in plasma. These peptides are made in the liver (and perhaps in other tissues) and, rarely, if ever, circulate in plasma without being associated with lipid. They have a half-life, in extracellular fluid, of 3 to 5 days — shorter than that of most other serum proteins.

A-Beta-Lipoproteinemia, Tangier Disease

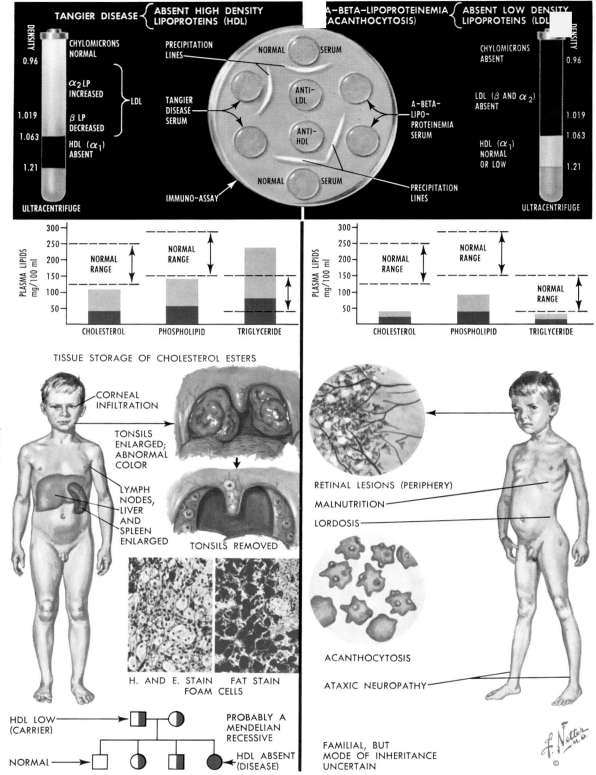

Two familial syndromes are characterized by severe deficiency or absence of specific lipoproteins. A comparison of their clinical features reveals important differences in the apparent biological functions of these lipid-carrying systems.

A-BETA-LIPOPROTEINEMIA has, as a unique feature, the *absence of all plasma low-density lipoproteins (LDL)* and lighter particles, including *chylomicrons.* The syndrome follows a fairly uniform course, beginning before the age of 1 year, with *malnutrition* and growth retardation, *lordosis,* abdominal distention, and steatorrhea. *Ataxia,* nystagmus, weakness and areflexia, and other signs of progressive neurological dysfunction, particularly involving the posterolateral columns and spinocerebellar tracts, then appear. *Pigmentary retinal degeneration* develops during adolescence. The erythrocytes have a crenated appearance *(acanthocytosis),* which is possibly related to decreased lecithin and linoleic acid in the esterified lipids of the cells. It is not known whether similar lipid abnormalities might be the basis for dysfunction in the nervous system.

The primary defect may be malabsorption of fat. Chylomicrons are not formed. Dietary fat remains in the intestinal mucosal cells, creating a pathognomonic picture detectable by peroral biopsy. Some fat is absorbed, possibly through direct passage via the portal system into the liver. An obvious interrelationship between low-density lipoproteins and chylomicron metabolism is suggested by this syndrome, and this still must be clarified.

The disease may occur in siblings, and the consanguinity rate, in affected families, is high. Probably the disease is due to a double dose of a mutant autosomal gene. With possible rare exceptions, the relatives of these patients have normal concentrations of plasma lipoproteins.

FAMILIAL HIGH-DENSITY LIPOPROTEIN DEFICIENCY is also called TANGIER DISEASE, after the island home of the first known cases — two siblings who had *low serum cholesterol, peculiar tonsils,* and practically *no plasma high-density lipoprotein (HDL).* The disease has been detected in other children and adults, and it must be suspected when hypocholesterolemia is associated with orange or yellowish-gray discoloration of the pharyngeal or rectal mucosa or *enlargement of spleen, liver,* or *lymph nodes.*

Reticulo-endothelial *tissues* are infiltrated with *foam cells* containing huge amounts of *cholesterol esters.* In adults, corneal infiltration (lipid?), hypersplenism, and, possibly, advanced coronary artery disease have been seen as complications. There are no abnormalities in absorption, in neurological function, or in erythrocytes.

Parents and other relatives of patients with Tangier disease have lower than normal amounts of plasma high-density lipoproteins (HDL). Probably the propositi are *homozygous* for a mutation at a gene locus which regulates the formation of HDL and, possibly, has some lesser influence on low-density lipoproteins *(LDL)* as well, since these lipoproteins are also not completely normal. This syndrome suggests that HDL has some rôle, as yet undefined, in maintaining equilibrium between tissue and plasma cholesterol, but HDL does not appear to be essential for chylomicron formation or fat absorption.

Diagnosis of either Tangier disease or a-beta-lipoproteinemia must be established by *immunochemical analyses.* The latter disease appears to be the less benign of the two, but there has been too little experience, thus far, to make an accurate forecast regarding the prognosis in either case. No specific treatment is known.

CHOLESTEROL METABOLISM

The average plasma cholesterol concentration is 75 mg per 100 ml in the newborn. By the first year this has approximately doubled. There follows a period of relative constancy, until, in early adulthood, a slow rise of 2 to 3 mg per 100 ml per year begins, which continues until the age of 50 years or older. More than 5 per cent of apparently healthy, middle-aged Americans have cholesterol concentrations higher than 300 mg per 100 ml and a comparable percentage below 150. The variation in any individual from month to month is negligible compared to the great spread in the population. The causes of the latter are of special interest in regard to the association of higher cholesterol levels with greater incidence of coronary artery disease.

Cholesterol is a *facultative precursor* of *adrenal cortical, ovarian,* and *testicular steroid hormones.* Most of the plasma cholesterol comes from the *liver,* and its concentration is primarily a resultant of the balance between *synthesis* and *catabolism* in this organ. Isotopic studies indicate that cholesterol molecules in *plasma, liver,* and *erythrocytes* exchange freely and turn over at the same rate. The greater flexibility of cholesterol concentrations in the plasma compartment of this "common pool" is related to availability of a vehicle for solubilization and, thus, is secondarily dependent on many factors controlling over-all lipoprotein metabolism.

The 2-carbon precursors from which cholesterol is synthesized are widely available from fat, protein, or carbohydrate. The formation of *mevalonic acid* is one of the rate-limiting steps in this pathway. Condensation and cyclization of 6 molecules of this acid are required to form cholesterol. Recent experience has indicated that attempts to depress synthesis pharmacologically can best be directed at steps in the pathway prior to the formation of sterols that are very similar to cholesterol. An important negative *"feed-back" control* of hepatic synthesis is the amount of cholesterol in the liver. Practically all hepatic cholesterol is in the nonesterified form. *Esterification* takes place in the gut and in the blood, as well as in the liver, but the latter organ probably excretes most of the esters found in plasma.

The cholesterol ring cannot be broken down in the body, and such catabolism as is achieved is mainly carried out by the liver through formation of *bile acids.* The side chain is shortened and carboxylated, and the ring is altered with the addition of 2 or 3 hydroxyl groups to make chenodeoxycholic or *cholic acid,* respectively.

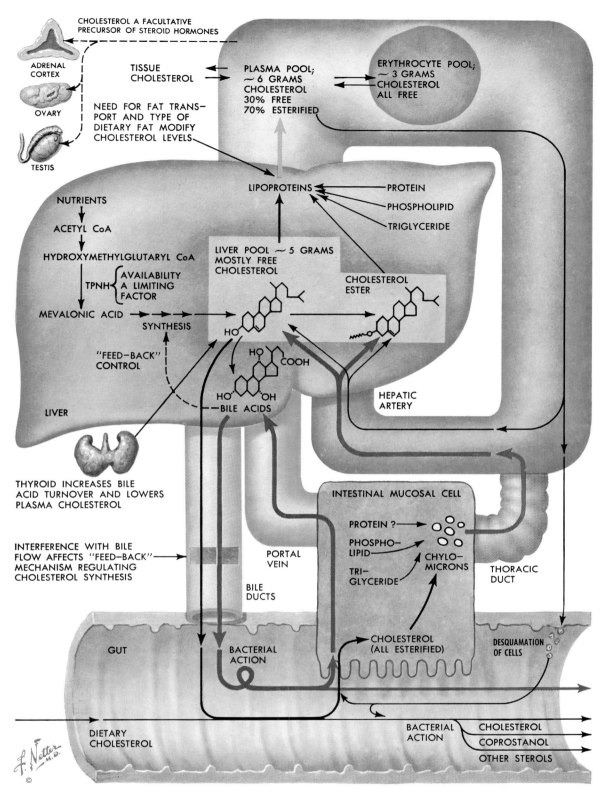

These are conjugated with taurine or glycine, and at least 95 per cent are excreted by way of the bile. The production of bile acids is 500 to 700 mg per day, or about twice that excreted in the stool. The balance is recycled, and any interference with this *enterohepatic circulation* will affect the amount of bile acids in the liver. This, in turn, regulates the conversion of cholesterol to bile acids. Bile acid production is thus increased by decreased return of cholic acid from the gut, which may occur with a biliary fistula, increased bacterial degradation, or binding of acids with certain resins. Concomitantly, cholesterol synthesis accelerates up to 25 times as the sterol is removed faster by its stepped-up catabolism.

Cholesterol participates in a similar *cycle* between the *gut* and the liver. This can also be unbalanced by changes in *bacterial flora* in the gut, in fat absorption and *chylomicron formation,* and at other points.

Decreasing *cholesterol* in the *diet* (which usually ranges from 250 to 1000 mg per day) produces a modest decrease in the plasma level.

The feed-back mechanisms regulating cholesterol metabolism are many and compensatory in design. An alteration at any one locus does not produce easily predictable changes in the plasma concentration. Malabsorption is associated with decreased cholesterol uptake from the gut. The immediate effect is, no doubt, increased hepatic synthesis, but the net effect is a decreased plasma level. In *hyperthyroidism* bile acid production is increased, while plasma cholesterol falls. In hypothyroidism bile acid production and hepatic synthesis of cholesterol are both diminished, but the plasma concentration is increased. The explanation of such resultant effects, including mechanisms by which plasma cholesterol is lowered by unsaturated dietary fats, awaits biochemical clarification.

TRIGLYCERIDE METABOLISM

Fatty acids supply nearly half the calories burned in the body and are utilized by all tissues, with the possible exceptions of the brain and red blood cells. They are broken down to 2-carbon fragments, which are oxidized in the *Krebs,* or tricarboxylic acid, *cycle,* thus providing formation of high-energy *phosphate bonds* as the immediate form of usable energy. Practically all cells are also able to convert *acetyl CoA* to *long-chain fatty acids.* The synthetic pathway is not simply the reverse of the catabolic one. It involves stepwise elongation by the addition of 3 carbon units of malonyl CoA, which are then decarboxylated, 1 molecule of carbon dioxide being taken up and released with each step. The usual length of the fatty acids thus synthesized is 14 to 18 carbons. Other enzymes catalyze the elongation or shortening of the chains or the insertion of double bonds. Some "essential" fatty acids — linoleic and linolenic acids — are not synthesized and must be obtained from the diet. Their absolute requirement for man has never been accurately assessed.

In a real sense, the ubiquity in the body cells of mechanisms for the metabolism of fatty acids is due to the uncertainty of supply of the preferred fuel, *glucose.* The latter is in scant supply during postabsorptive periods and can be stored as *glycogen* in only limited amounts. Appreciable excesses of glucose must be converted to fatty acids if they are to be retained and stored in optimal form as a source of energy with the lowest relative weight.

An over-all view of the rôle of fatty acids in the body economy should include the site of intake of preformed acids, the *gut;* the major location of storage, the *adipose tissue;* and at least two major sites of utilization, the *liver* and *muscle.*

Glycerides are the chemical form of the bulk of ingested fat. They are hydrolyzed (most of them completely so) in the upper portion of the small intestine. Hydrolysis is catalyzed by pancreatic lipase, *bile salts* being essential emulsifiers in the process. Short-chain fatty acids enter the liver via the portal circulation. The long-chain fatty acids are resynthesized into *chylomicron glycerides* in the *mucosal cells* and move into the *systemic circulation* via the *thoracic duct.* The chylomicrons normally are taken up quite rapidly from the circulation. Within 6 hours after ingestion, as much as 100 gm of fat can be entirely absorbed and

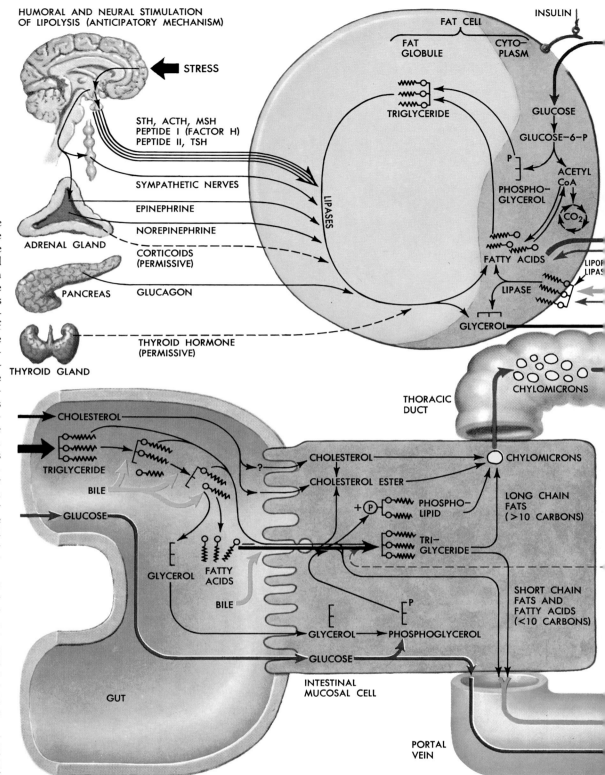

removed from the blood in a normal subject. As they enter cells, or immediately thereafter, the glycerides are quickly broken down to *free fatty acids* and *glycerol,* or at least to partial glycerides. The fatty acids are redistributed to new glycerides or other esterified lipids, and some may be oxidized with little delay. Deficiency of the enzyme *lipoprotein lipase* is thought to be associated with retarded clearance of chylomicrons from the blood in states of hyperlipemia. The importance of this enzyme is still uncertain, however. Its site of action may be in, or very near, capillary walls, since it is so readily released into the circulation by heparin.

Adipose tissue has great metabolic activity and plays a major rôle in ensuring the body of a supply of fuel at all times. Within the narrow *cytoplasmic segment* of the fat cell, fat from the adjacent *globule* is constantly being broken down and resynthesized.

When adequate *glucose* is available to the cell, it is also converted to *fatty acids* and then to *triglyceride.* This is the ideal "packaging" for fuel storage, since it has a higher caloric equivalent per weight than glycogen has, does not increase weight by a tendency to take on water as does carbohydrate, and its formation and breakdown involve low-energy ester bonds.

When glucose is in short supply, either because the blood level has dropped or the "gate" has closed from lack of *insulin* activity (see page 147), the synthesis of new glyceride stops. The re-formation of glyceride also ceases, because the adipose tissue cell cannot form the essential intermediate, *phosphoglycerol,* from glycerol, but only through glucose degradation (see page 153).

In addition to glucose supply, the lipolytic cycle is controlled by a variety of *humoral* and *neurogenic factors,* all of which can accelerate glyceride breakdown

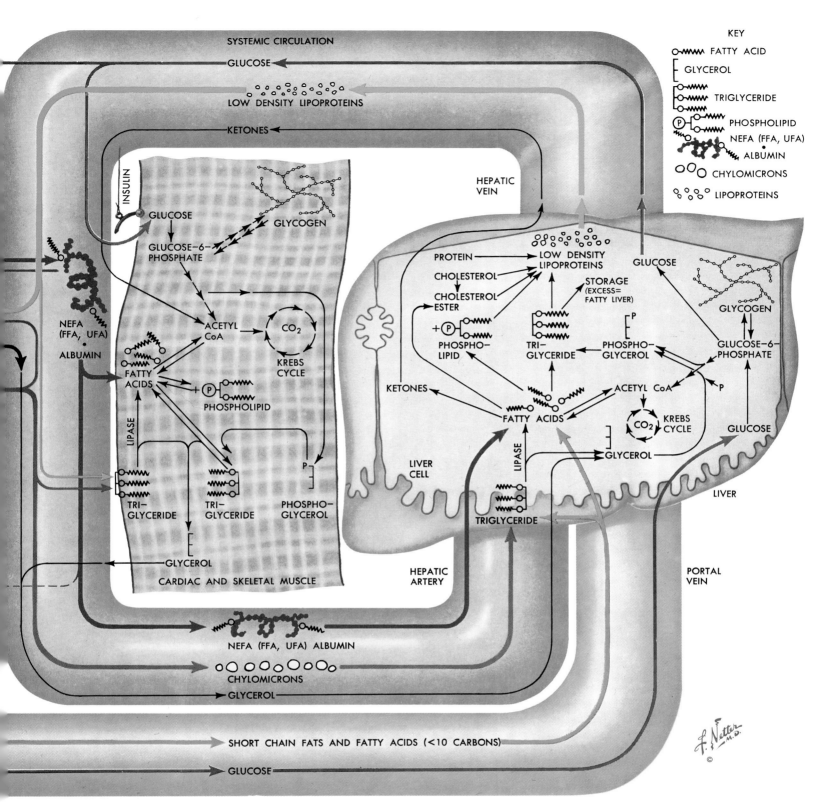

in excess of resynthesis. It is notable that many of these are associated with "alarm" reactions designed to provide extra energy quickly for an anticipated need. Tonic activity of the *sympathetic nerves,* or, perhaps more specifically, availability of *norepinephrine* at nerve endings within the cell, appears to be very important in conditioning the responses to other humoral agents such as a number of lipolytic factors isolated from the anterior pituitary, including growth hormone (*STH*) (see page 9). At least one posterior pituitary factor, vasopressin (see page 33), also promotes lipolysis. The exact mechanism by which any of these agents control lipolysis has not been established. *Glucocorticoids* and *thyroid hormone* play a *permissive* rôle in lipolysis.

Once released, *free fatty acids* (*FFA*) do not accumulate in the adipose tissue but move into the circulation, bound to *albumin,* and are quickly taken up by other tissues. In the *liver* they enter pools indistinguishable from those entered by glyceride fatty acids. If glucose utilization is diminished, a large percentage will be oxidized rapidly. The liver converts much of an FFA load to *ketones,* which are transported to muscle for complete oxidation. Heavy egress of FFA during starvation or diabetic acidosis, for example, is associated with ketonemia. When glucose is in short supply, both *skeletal and cardiac muscle* depend heavily on both FFA uptake and utilization of their own endogenous glyceride stores. The FFA pathway relieves such active organs from on-site storage of all the fat they may require for fuel. Glyceride is not released, as such, from adipose tissue.

Excessive amounts of fat coming to the liver from adipose tissue as FFA, or synthesized in that organ from glucose, may threaten that organ's function if not removed. Fat is secreted for distribution to adipose tissue and other organs, but FFA does not appear to be employed for this purpose. Glyceride is dispatched either in *low-density lipoproteins* or as particles, if the amounts are quite large. Endogenous hyperlipemia may arise from the overloading of this compensatory pathway.

Fatty acids are also required by many tissues for the synthesis of *phospholipid* and other complex lipids whose functions are still obscure but include maintaining the stability of membranes and other intracellular structures. The transport of fatty acids for this purpose is less critical than that required for meeting energy demands, since many of these structural lipids are made in situ.

HYPERTRIGLYCERIDEMIA

Reference to the term "hypertriglyceridemia" implies the presence of an opalescent serum which has lost the usual transparency.

The *creamy serum* of essential, or idiopathic, hyperlipemia is occasionally mentioned in the old literature as "white blood". Buerger and Grütz are credited with having described, in 1932, *hepatosplenomegalic lipidosis* with milky serum and eruptive xanthoma. The first familial case of idiopathic hyperlipemia was reported by Holt and co-workers in 1939. Chapman and Kinney later described the autopsy of a child with idiopathic hyperlipemia, which had been clinically

observed by Thannhauser and Goodman. The outstanding feature of this autopsy was the observation that in spite of the enormous increase of neutral fat in the serum, neither the liver nor other organs showed any considerable accumulation of triglycerides in the tissue. The designation "hyperlipemia" should be used only for a substantial increase of glycerides in serum. The more specific term, "hypertriglyceridemia", is now commonly used. The skin lesion of *eruptive xanthoma,* observed in cases with hyperlipemia, is different in appearance from that of tuberous and plain xanthomata. Eruptive xanthoma appears more like vesicles with *umbilicated tops.* During an acute onset, the situation may be confused with chickenpox. However, the lesions of eruptive xanthoma are solid. Most of these lesions have, at the base, a fine *reddish*

halo, which gives them an inflammatory appearance. The histology of the eruptive skin xanthoma in idiopathic hyperlipemia shows, mainly, elements of *inflammation* interspersed with scattered *foam cells.* *Hyperlipemia retinalis* (milky retinal vessels) affords direct evidence, by inspection, for the existence of hyperlipemia.

It is very important to remember that a moderate increase in serum glycerides may occur also in familial hypercholesterolemic xanthomatosis. A distinction between it and hyperlipemia can be made by placing the patient on a fat-free diet for several weeks. In cases of idiopathic hyperlipemia, the glycerides will fall to nearly normal levels in a few days; thus, the current term of "familial fat-induced hypertriglyceri-

(Continued on page 205)

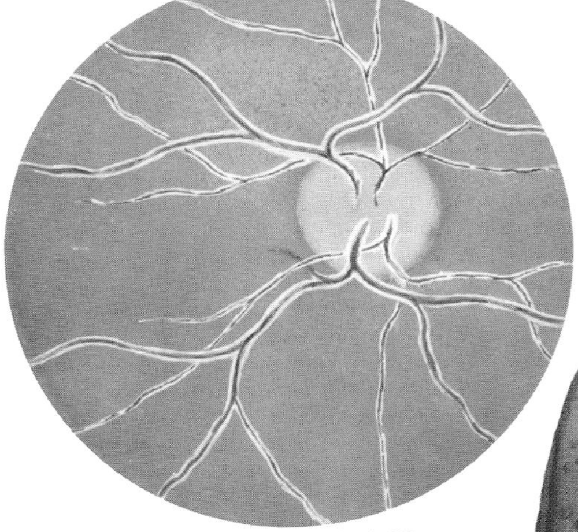

HYPERLIPEMIA RETINALIS

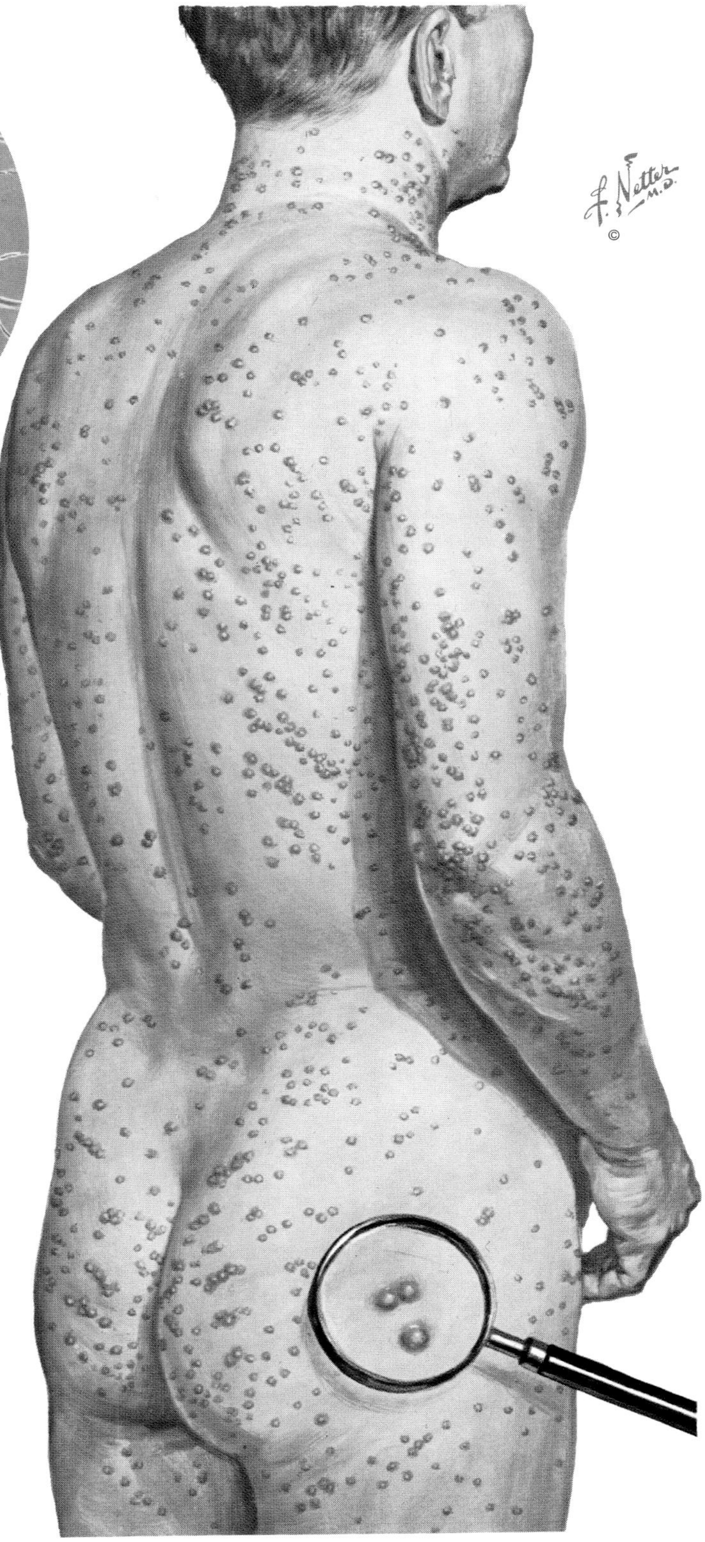

HYPERTRIGLYCERIDEMIA

(Continued from page 204)

ERUPTIVE
XANTHOMATOSIS
IN ADULT
WITH IDIOPATHIC
HYPERLIPEMIA

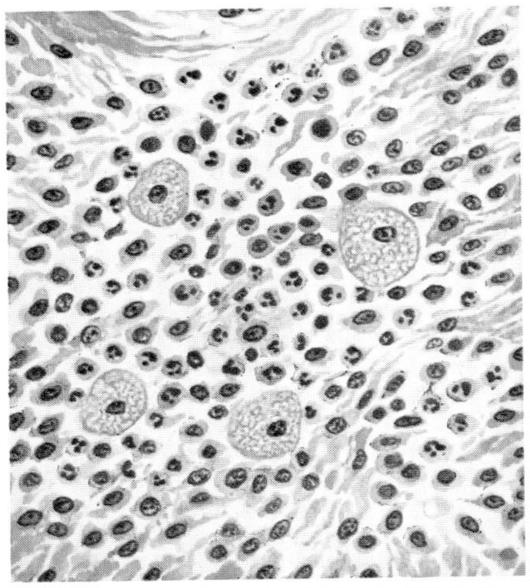

HYPERLIPEMIC XANTHOMATOUS NODULE
(HIGH MAGNIFICATION): FEW FOAM
CELLS AMID INFLAMMATORY EXUDATE

emia" for this syndrome. Most of these patients also have subnormal amounts of lipolytic activity (lipoprotein lipase) in the plasma, following heparin injection.

The etiology of primary hyperlipemia is not known. However, a slowed removal of chylomicrons from the circulation is well established in the fat-induced variety. The existence of a so-called "carbohydrate-induced hypertriglyceridemia" in some patients indicates that abnormal clearance of exogenous fat is not the sole cause of all types of hypertriglyceridemia.

Patients with essential hyperlipemia do not usually suffer from early angina pectoris and myocardial infarction, in contrast to the early and constant occurrence of these diseases in familial hypercholesterolemic xanthomatosis.

Hypertriglyceridemia may be found at all ages, but in *children* it is almost always either the fat-induced type or else secondary to untreated biliary disease or diabetes. Very often, *adult* patients with *idiopathic hyperlipemia* show traces of sugar in the urine and a slight elevation of fasting blood sugars. Such a moderate tendency to glycosuria should not be confused with severe diabetes accompanied by secondary hyperlipemia, in which atheromatous lesions of the blood vessels and eruptive xanthoma are complications of the diabetic state.

Secondary hyperlipemia is considered to be a transport hyperlipemia; *i.e.*, there is increased mobilization of free fatty acids from the peripheral fat depots, with subsequent esterification and incorporation into circulating lipoproteins of very low density. It may occur as a result of various primary disorders, with and without eruptive xanthoma, (1) in diabetes mellitus; (2) in chronic pancreatitis [However, rarely, early cases are observed in which hyperlipemia occurs before and appears to induce pancreatitis, so that pancreatitis is not invariably the cause of hyperlipemia.]; (3) in the nephrotic syndrome, especially in children; (4) in biliary cirrhosis with biliary stasis; (5) in glycogen storage disease, in which increased fat mobilization accompanies a deficit in available calories from glucose; and (6) in rare cases of neoplastic or cystic involvement of the hypothalamus and pituitary.

Fasting Total Serum Cholesterol mg/100 ml chart — NORMAL RANGE

Fasting Total Serum Phospholipid mg/100 ml chart — NORMAL RANGE

Fasting Total Serum Neutral Fat mg/100 ml chart — NORMAL RANGE

HYPERCHOLESTEROLEMIC XANTHOMATOSIS
Plain and Tuberous Xanthoma

XANTHELASMA OF EYELIDS

CLEAR SERUM

PLAIN AND TUBEROUS XANTHOMATA OF BUTTOCKS

f. Netter M.D. ©

PLAIN AND TUBEROUS XANTHOMATA OF ELBOWS AND KNEES

Hypercholesterolemic xanthomatosis is one of a number of conditions grouped under the hypercholesterolemias, the majority of which are familial. The primary type, manifested by plain and tuberous xanthomata, should not be confused with those sometimes found with xanthomatous biliary cirrhosis, the nephrotic syndrome, or diabetes. The term "essential familial hypercholesterolemia" comprises a syndrome characterized by abnormally high concentrations of *cholesterol*, sometimes of *phospholipid* and, rarely, of *neutral fat* in the *serum*, accompanied by *cutaneous* and also *tendinous xanthomata*, depending on the severity and duration of the hypercholesterolemia and on the nature of abnormal lipid and lipoprotein patterns. An early corneal arcus is seen and, in varying degrees, a very serious tendency toward accelerated development of atherosclerosis. The disease results from an abnormality in the homeostatic mechanisms for the regulation of plasma-cholesterol concentration, but the specific defect is, as yet, not fully understood. This hypercholesterolemic trait is apparently inherited as an autosomal dominant, and the expression of the trait is influenced by the generic make-up of the individual, the diet, and the age, occurring early in the more severe type of disease and later in life in the milder cases as a forme fruste, in which only an elevation in serum cholesterol is found, without any xanthoma.

Cutaneous and tendinous xanthomata were first reported in 1836 by Rayer, and again in 1851 by Addison and Gull. Not until 1908 was evidence provided by Pick and Pinkus that the double refractile lipid in the involved foam cells consisted mainly of cholesterol and cholesterol esters, thereby establishing the connection between hypercholesterolemia and the xanthomata. These foam cells are large histiocytes, 10 to 20 microns in diameter, containing droplets of lipid,

which account for the finely reticulated or foamy appearance. They occur among the reticulo-endothelial cells of the spleen, liver, and lymph nodes. They stain with Sudan III, and the Schultz reaction reveals the presence of cholesterol. They represent the phagocytic reaction to elevated lipid levels in the blood. They do not, as once assumed, represent increased synthesis of cholesterol in situ. In 1910 hypercholesterolemia with xanthoma was noted by Chauffard and LaRoche in patients with obstructive liver disease, and the observation was made that "what the tophus is to gout the xanthoma is to hypercholesterolemia". In 1920 a case was published by Burns, in which the xanthoma was associated with hypercholesterolemia in the absence of any other demonstrable disease. Finally, in 1938, xanthoma of the skin and organs was clinically demonstrated (Thannhauser and Magendantz) in patients with normal as well as

elevated cholesterol levels in the serum. The conclusion was reached that not all xanthomata arise as a direct consequence of elevated serum cholesterol levels, although the majority do, the former being termed normocholesterolemic and the latter, hypercholesterolemic xanthomatosis; these differ etiologically, histologically, and clinically.

The clinical types of essential familial hypercholesterolemia comprise any number of cutaneous and tendinous forms. *Xanthelasma of the eyelids* is frequently accompanied by an early arcus senilis surrounding the cornea. *Plain* and *tuberous xanthomata* are most frequently found over the *elbows*, *knees*, and on the *buttocks*, possibly related to continuous irritation by garments. Tuberous xanthoma is seen most frequently in cases with elevated S_f (20 to 400 lipoproteins) and hence is not characteristic of the

(Continued on page 207)

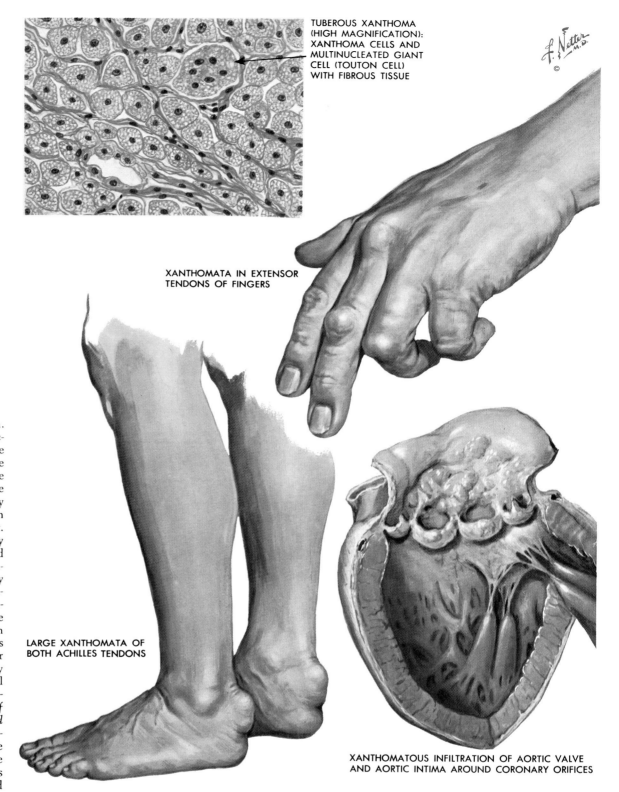

TUBEROUS XANTHOMA
(HIGH MAGNIFICATION):
XANTHOMA CELLS AND
MULTINUCLEATED GIANT
CELL (TOUTON CELL)
WITH FIBROUS TISSUE

XANTHOMATA IN EXTENSOR
TENDONS OF FINGERS

LARGE XANTHOMATA OF
BOTH ACHILLES TENDONS

XANTHOMATOUS INFILTRATION OF AORTIC VALVE
AND AORTIC INTIMA AROUND CORONARY ORIFICES

HYPERCHOLESTEROLEMIC XANTHOMATOSIS

Plain and Tuberous Xanthoma

(Continued from page 206)

"pure" familial hypercholesterolemia. The characteristic lesions of *tendinous xanthoma* are actually part of the tendon, from which they cannot be mechanically separated. The nodules are found, typically, in the tendons of the fingers and knuckles, and, especially characteristically, in the Achilles tendon and the tendon below the knee joint. This type of nodular lesion may be easily confused with the nodules of rheumatoid arthritis, but it can readily be differentiated histologically and chemically by the fact that, usually, no marked elevation of cholesterol is present in rheumatoid arthritis. Characteristically, the xanthomata are not painful. There is an increase in lipoproteins, with S_f values from 0 to 20, as a rule. Usually, a greater propensity for clinically evident coronary artery disease exists than for cerebral vascular or peripheral vascular involvement. Fortunately rare is *involvement of the aortic valve* and *aortic intima around the coronary orifices*. These lesions consist, in the first phase, of cushionlike elevations of foam cells beneath the intima; later, they become sclerotic. This is part of the advanced, generalized atherosclerosis so commonly found, which leads to death from coronary infarction in the very young (including children) afflicted with this disease. The xanthoma of the arterial intima is, clinically, the most dangerous feature of familial hypercholesterolemic xanthomatosis, because of its frequent occurrence in the coronary vessels, causing angina and myocardial infarction at an early age.

The diagnosis of essential familial hypercholesterolemia rests on the finding of cutaneous and tendinous manifestations and early coronary insufficiency or coronary infarction in an individual with a family history. Laboratory diagnosis is established by a marked elevation of serum cholesterol, without any significant abnormality in phospholipids or total neutral fat. Mono-aminophosphatides do increase; hence, the total lipid phosphorus increases, but this is not proportionate to the increase in serum cholesterol. As a result, the *serum* of these subjects is characteristically *clear,* which decisively sets off the hypercholesterolemias from the hyperlipemias often accompanied by eruptive xanthoma (see page 204). The upper limit of normal serum cholesterol is very difficult to define, but, in the American population, it is probably not higher than about 250 mg per 100 ml. The upper limit of distribution tends to rise with increasing age. To confirm the diagnosis of a "familial type", it is not enough to note hypercholesterolemia with atherosclerosis, but the tracing of hypercholesterolemia to at least one other family member has been required to define the presence of the trait (Adlersberg). A history of coronary artery disease at an early age, in other family members, is also helpful in differentiating the diagnosis from other causes. The earlier the age of onset, the more likely will be the familial type. Most patients with essential familial hypercholesterolemia have an elevated concentration primarily of low-density lipoproteins with an S_f from 0 to 20, and this would correspond to a high cholesterol, a normal to only slightly elevated phospholipid, and a relatively normal glyceride level. The most frequently observed xanthomata are xanthelasma of the eyelids and involvement of the tendons. When an elevation of neutral fats occurs as well, then elevated concentrations of lipoproteins of high S_f values are present, ranging from 20 upward, and the disease is characterized by having a tendency to tuberous xanthoma. The serum uric acid levels (often checked because the involvement of tendons simulates tophi) are frequently elevated to levels found in gout, but the lesions do not contain uric acid.

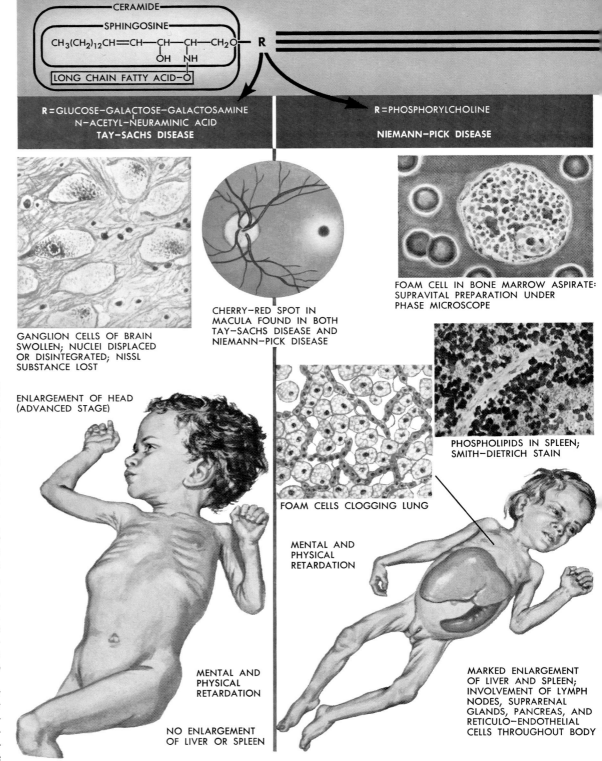

CERAMIDE
SPHINGOSINE
$CH_3(CH_2)_{12}CH=CH-CH-CH-CH_2O-$ **R**
OH NH
LONG CHAIN FATTY ACID-O

R = GLUCOSE-GALACTOSE-GALACTOSAMINE
N-ACETYL-NEURAMINIC ACID
TAY-SACHS DISEASE

R = PHOSPHORYLCHOLINE
NIEMANN-PICK DISEASE

GANGLION CELLS OF BRAIN SWOLLEN; NUCLEI DISPLACED OR DISINTEGRATED; NISSL SUBSTANCE LOST

CHERRY-RED SPOT IN MACULA FOUND IN BOTH TAY-SACHS DISEASE AND NIEMANN-PICK DISEASE

FOAM CELL IN BONE MARROW ASPIRATE: SUPRAVITAL PREPARATION UNDER PHASE MICROSCOPE

PHOSPHOLIPIDS IN SPLEEN; SMITH-DIETRICH STAIN

ENLARGEMENT OF HEAD (ADVANCED STAGE)

FOAM CELLS CLOGGING LUNG

MENTAL AND PHYSICAL RETARDATION

MENTAL AND PHYSICAL RETARDATION

NO ENLARGEMENT OF LIVER OR SPLEEN

MARKED ENLARGEMENT OF LIVER AND SPLEEN; INVOLVEMENT OF LYMPH NODES, SUPRARENAL GLANDS, PANCREAS, AND RETICULO-ENDOTHELIAL CELLS THROUGHOUT BODY

THE SPHINGOLIPIDOSES

Five inheritable disease entities are characterized by the accumulation of sphingolipids, so called because they contain *sphingosine,* an 18-carbon amino alcohol synthesized in the body from palmitic acid and serine. A *long-chain fatty acid* is bound in peptide linkage to the amide group of sphingosine to form *ceramide.* The sphingolipids are distinguished by the polar group linked to the C-1 hydroxyl of their ceramide moiety (R). Some are concentrated in nervous tissue, either in ganglion cells (gangliosides) or in myelin (cerebrosides, cerebroside sulfatides); others are distributed more widely in cell membranes (globosides, various glycolipids); and sphingomyelin, the *phosphorylcholine* ester of ceramide, is found in almost every type of cell. In the sphingolipidoses, changes in the normally small concentration of sphingolipids in plasma are not dramatic, the abnormalities being mainly confined to tissues.

Tay-Sachs disease, gangliosidosis or infantile amaurotic familial idiocy (AFI), is characterized by the accumulation of excessive amounts of gangliosides, neurolipids containing *n-acetylneuraminic acid* (sialic acid), which are the most complex of the sphingolipids, although water-soluble because of their high carbohydrate content. This is an inherited autosomal recessive disease, found most commonly in children of Eastern European Hebrew ancestry. It is usually detected by the age of 6 months, and it runs a gamut of progressive neurologic deficits to fatal termination by the age of 3 years. Destructive *swelling of ganglion cells* and gliosis are so widespread that the *cranium* becomes abnormally *enlarged.* The "Tay-Sachs gangliosides" differ in composition from those normally present in gray matter. Lesser increases in gangliosides have been found in milder forms of AFI, which appear later in life. These syndromes have different population distributions and may represent mutations at different loci.

Niemann-Pick disease, or sphingomyelinosis, is rare (less than 200 reported cases). Its manifestations appear in nearly every tissue, and early *neurological damage* is characteristic. Massive amounts not only of sphingomyelin but also of cholesterol accumulate in *large,* nonspecific *foam cells.* Marked enlargement of the *liver, spleen, lymph nodes, suprarenal glands,* and of the total *reticulo-endothelial system* is found. The disease is most often rapidly fatal by the age of 2 years, but "chronic" forms (perhaps due to different mutants) exist. The disease frequently occurs in Hebrews but is not limited to any ethnic group and is inherited as an autosomal recessive gene.

In *Gaucher's disease,* or cerebrosidosis, reticulo-endothelial cells throughout the body accumulate cerebrosides and take on a unique appearance. A *bone marrow aspirate,* after suitable analysis, is diagnostic. The cerebroside in visceral tissues is *ceramide-glucose* instead of the normal ceramide-galactose. Although chemical differences have not been detected, Gaucher's disease appears in at least two clinically distinct forms. In the *"acute" infantile form, hepatosplenomegaly,* general lymphadenitis, and severe neurological deficits appear a few months after birth. Bulbar signs, *strabismus,* and spasticity leading to *retroflexion of the head* and *laryngospasm* are common. Death from inanition often occurs within the first year. The more common *"chronic" form* in the *adult* may also be manifest by *hepatosplenomegaly* early, or it may not be detected for years. The nervous system is not affected, and the disease takes its toll through relentless expansion of masses of typical storage cells, with severe bone pain. The *bone marrow* and surrounding *bone,* the *liver, lungs,* and, especially, the *spleen* are particularly affected. Secondary

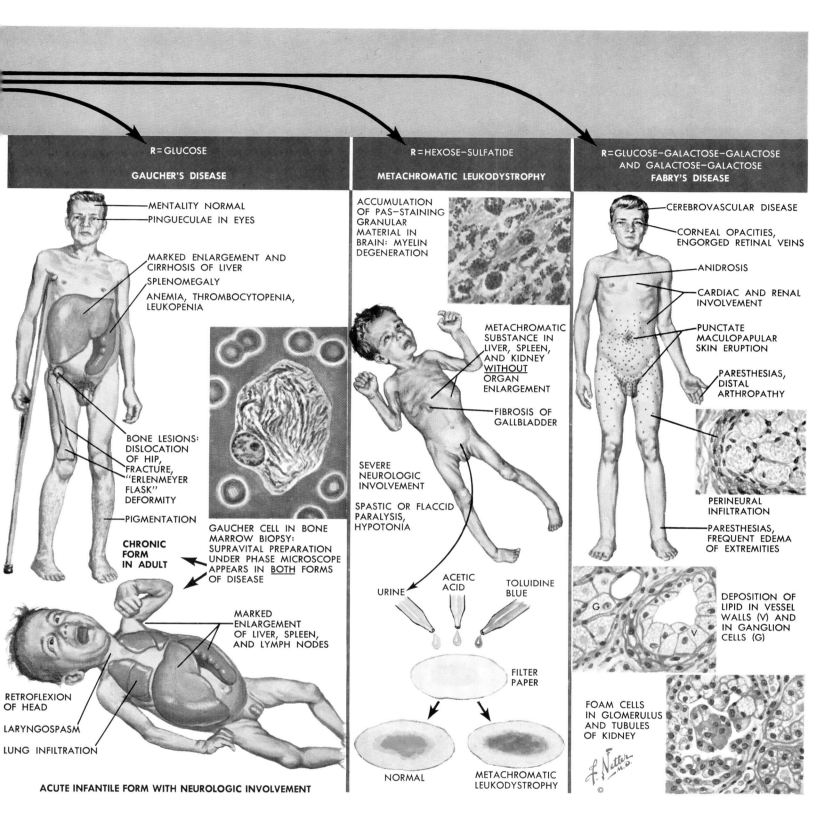

R = GLUCOSE
GAUCHER'S DISEASE

R = HEXOSE–SULFATIDE
METACHROMATIC LEUKODYSTROPHY

R = GLUCOSE–GALACTOSE–GALACTOSE AND GALACTOSE–GALACTOSE
FABRY'S DISEASE

MENTALITY NORMAL
PINGUECULAE IN EYES
MARKED ENLARGEMENT AND CIRRHOSIS OF LIVER
SPLENOMEGALY
ANEMIA, THROMBOCYTOPENIA, LEUKOPENIA
BONE LESIONS: DISLOCATION OF HIP, FRACTURE, "ERLENMEYER FLASK" DEFORMITY
PIGMENTATION
CHRONIC FORM IN ADULT
GAUCHER CELL IN BONE MARROW BIOPSY: SUPRAVITAL PREPARATION UNDER PHASE MICROSCOPE APPEARS IN BOTH FORMS OF DISEASE
MARKED ENLARGEMENT OF LIVER, SPLEEN, AND LYMPH NODES
RETROFLEXION OF HEAD
LARYNGOSPASM
LUNG INFILTRATION
ACUTE INFANTILE FORM WITH NEUROLOGIC INVOLVEMENT

ACCUMULATION OF PAS–STAINING GRANULAR MATERIAL IN BRAIN: MYELIN DEGENERATION
METACHROMATIC SUBSTANCE IN LIVER, SPLEEN, AND KIDNEY WITHOUT ORGAN ENLARGEMENT
FIBROSIS OF GALLBLADDER
SEVERE NEUROLOGIC INVOLVEMENT
SPASTIC OR FLACCID PARALYSIS, HYPOTONIA
URINE
ACETIC ACID
TOLUIDINE BLUE
FILTER PAPER
NORMAL
METACHROMATIC LEUKODYSTROPHY

CEREBROVASCULAR DISEASE
CORNEAL OPACITIES, ENGORGED RETINAL VEINS
ANIDROSIS
CARDIAC AND RENAL INVOLVEMENT
PUNCTATE MACULOPAPULAR SKIN ERUPTION
PARESTHESIAS, DISTAL ARTHROPATHY
PERINEURAL INFILTRATION
PARESTHESIAS, FREQUENT EDEMA OF EXTREMITIES
DEPOSITION OF LIPID IN VESSEL WALLS (V) AND IN GANGLION CELLS (G)
FOAM CELLS IN GLOMERULUS AND TUBULES OF KIDNEY

to hypersplenism, *thrombocytopenia* occurs. The characteristic *"Erlenmeyer flask" deformity* of the *femur* is often present. *Pingueculae* (single yellow nodules that may occur on either side of the cornea, but more commonly on the nasal aspect) are found frequently on the conjunctiva in Gaucher's disease but are not, in themselves, pathognomonic. All involved members of a sibship usually have the same clinical form of Gaucher's disease. Transmission from a single involved parent to an offspring has also been reported, and mutations at three or more different genetic loci may be involved in Gaucher's disease. There is no certain test for detection of the subclinical trait.

In *metachromatic leukodystrophy*, or *sulfatidosis*, *degeneration of myelin* becomes clinically manifest by the age of 1 or 2 years, progressing through *hypotonia* and *paralysis* to a vegetative state by 5 to 6 years of age, with death from pulmonary or other infections. Cerebroside sulfates accumulate in granular deposits both within and outside the nerve cells. Like other acidic polysaccharides, the sulfatides may be detected by the *metachromasia* they produce with certain dyes. Visceral involvement is not prominent, but sulfatides are detectable in the *liver, kidney,* and *spleen.* Apparent increase in the biliary excretion of sulfatides results in *fibrosis* and poor function of the *gallbladder. Metachromatic material* also appears in *urine,* permitting a *diagnostic test.* This must be carefully interpreted, since similar material is excreted in other conditions such as Hurler's syndrome (see page 229) and, in smaller amounts, in normal individuals.

Fabry's disease is transmitted as an X-linked recessive gene and is found in serious forms only in *males,* although female carriers may have similar mild abnormalities. The *glycosides, deposited* in widely spread *vascular* and *neural lesions,* probably represent greatly increased amounts of normal constituents. The disease can be diagnosed from the striking *diffuse angiokeratoma* in the *skin.* The life span is limited mainly by attendant *dysfunction* in the *kidneys, brain,* or *heart.*

The inheritable biochemical "lesions" in the sphingolipidoses remain speculative.

The most advanced techniques for lipid analyses must be utilized in the diagnosis, and tissues should be preserved by freezing, not by fixation, for later chemical and enzymatic study. There is currently no specific therapy for any of the sphingolipidoses.

NORMOCHOLESTEROLEMIC EOSINOPHILIC XANTHOMATOUS GRANULOMA

HAND-SCHÜLLER-CHRISTIAN SYNDROME (EXOPHTHALMOS, DIABETES INSIPIDUS, BONE LESIONS) INVOLVEMENT OF SKIN, LIVER, SPLEEN AND LUNGS MAY ALSO OCCUR. THESE DIVERSE MANIFESTATIONS MAY APPEAR INDIVIDUALLY OR IN VARIOUS COMBINATIONS

DIMINISHED ANTIDIURETIC HORMONE

XANTHOMATOUS LESION OF DURA IN REGION OF HYPOTHALAMUS AND PITUITARY STALK RESULTING IN DIABETES INSIPIDUS. XANTHOMATA OF HYPOTHALAMUS OR OF ANTERIOR PITUITARY MAY ALSO CAUSE THIS SYNDROME

INCREASED URINE

OSTEOLYTIC LESIONS OF BONES

OSTEOLYTIC XANTHOMATOUS LESIONS OF SKULL (GEOGRAPHIC SKULL)

LUNG INVOLVEMENT

This entity variously presents as eosinophilic xanthomatous granuloma or lipid granuloma, or in the form of Hand-Schüller-Christian syndrome. In the older literature the skin manifestations were designated as xanthoma multiplex. Schüller, as well as Christian, described children with the defects of membranous bones, exophthalmos, and diabetes insipidus (1920). Similar cases were published by Hand, suggesting tuberculosis as the etiology. Finally, Rowland (1928) showed that the lesions of the bones, lymph glands, and liver contained cells of the reticulo-endothelial system, which were filled with lipids. Chester (1930), as well as Fraser (1935), in studies of the lesions, described their detailed histological pathogenesis as a lipid granuloma. Thannhauser and Magendantz (1938) demonstrated first in a clinical study that normal cholesterol values in the serum are found in this lipogranulomatous disease, whether it involves the skin, meninges, bones, liver, or spleen. They showed that lipid granuloma is, histologically, a generalized disease, whether it occurs only in one or in more organs. It has four developmental phases. An early proliferative stage consists mainly of *reticulum cells*; clusters of *eosinophils* appear in the second phase; in the third, numerous *multinucleated giant cells* develop; in the fourth (*xanthomatous*) phase, the *reticulum cells* form *lipid substances* (especially cholesterol) within the cells and become foamy in structure, i.e., *foam*, or xanthoma, *cells*; this lipid granuloma later becomes fibrous but still contains some scattered foam cells. The four phases are not considered, by all authors, as one disease in different stages.

The mechanism underlying xanthoma cell formation in lipid granuloma differs from that in familial hypercholesterolemic xanthomatosis (FHX), wherein the foam cells are the secondary result of hypercholesterolemia. In lipid granuloma the foam cells develop independently of the normal cholesterol content of the serum. *Normal serum levels of cholesterol, phospholipids,* and *neutral fat* characterize this disease. Thus, the marked cholesterol accumulation in the reticulum cell of granuloma occurs with-

out an increased supply from the blood stream. Cholesterol infiltration from the blood stream, as it occurs in the hypercholesterolemic group, is, therefore, unacceptable as the mechanism of foam cell formation in lipid granuloma. Chemical analysis of tissue in the xanthomatous phase of lipid granuloma shows an increase of cholesterol 10 to 20 times over that of normal tissue, predominantly cholesterol esters as opposed to free cholesterol, which, normally, is the major intracellular sterol. Phospholipid is also increased. Such an enormous increase cannot be attributed to cholesterol infiltration from the detritus of a small area of focal necrosis. Thus, the cholesterol originates intrinsically in cells of the granuloma. During the course of the disease, undifferentiated reticulum cells in the primary proliferative phase develop gradually into xanthoma (foam) cells, while the formation of lipid material within the cells

increases. These cells of reticular and histiocytic origin maintain the functional possibilities of undifferentiated reticulum cells to form various kinds of lipids, including cholesterol.

A well-known allergist coined the words: "Not every patient has asthma who wheezes". Analogously, foam cells do not always indicate systemic xanthomatosis. Foam cells may originate in inflammatory tissue (xanthoma of the breast), in old necrotic scar tissue (sclerosing lipogranuloma), in necrotizing areas of large rheumatic nodules beneath the elbow, or in xanthomatous transformation of the mesentery (Whipple's disease) (see CIBA COLLECTION, Vol 3/II, page 138). Occasionally, scattered foam cells may originate in sarcomatous or carcinomatous tissue. The cholesterol content of the serum, in all these instances, is normal.

(Continued on page 211)

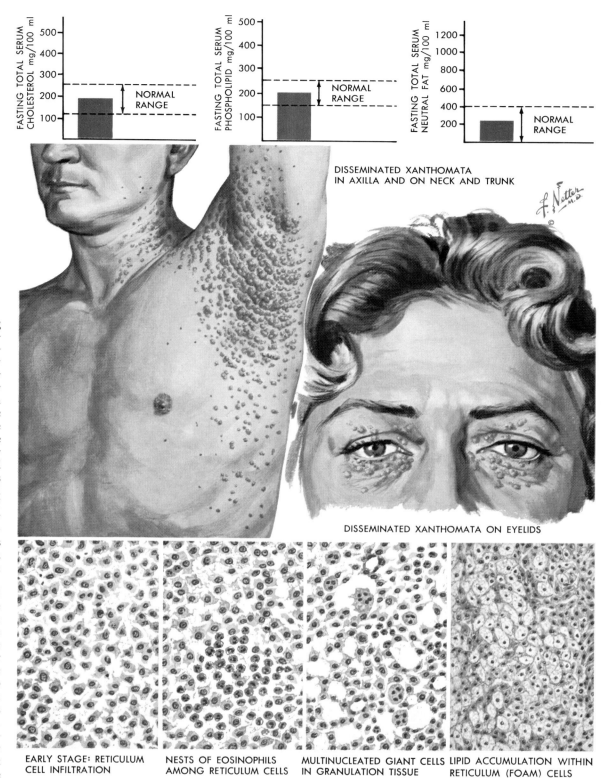

DISSEMINATED XANTHOMATA
IN AXILLA AND ON NECK AND TRUNK

F. Netter M.D.

DISSEMINATED XANTHOMATA ON EYELIDS

| EARLY STAGE: RETICULUM CELL INFILTRATION | NESTS OF EOSINOPHILS AMONG RETICULUM CELLS | MULTINUCLEATED GIANT CELLS IN GRANULATION TISSUE | LIPID ACCUMULATION WITHIN RETICULUM (FOAM) CELLS |

NORMOCHOLESTEROLEMIC EOSINOPHILIC XANTHOMATOUS GRANULOMA

(Continued from page 210)

The *skin lesions* show the following features, either singly or in various combinations: They are maroon or chamois-colored. Unlike the lesions of FHX, they are disseminated over the whole body (*xanthoma disseminatum*), especially around the *neck, axillae, trunk,* and in the *bends of the elbows. Xanthelasma of the eyelids* is found in both of these etiologically different diseases. The lesions, pinhead- to walnut-sized, may be discrete or clustered in ridges and furrows. A rare variety may occur as variolalike papules, also named isolated reticulosis of the skin. The papules of this variety may disappear completely or may degenerate into permanent xanthoma. In some juvenile and adult cases of *Hand-Schüller-Christian syndrome,* a seborrheic scaling lesion, especially on the scalp, is observed.

In xanthoma disseminatum small petechialike lesions are observed on the trunk. Histologically, the initial lesion of xanthoma disseminatum shows some hemorrhagic exudation in a conglomerate of adventitial cells derived from the outer wall of a small artery. In a later phase these adventitial reticulum cells develop into foam cells. A xanthomatous lesion may also develop in the visceral organs from the adventitial cells of blood vessels.

"Juvenile xanthoma", a pea-sized yellow or deep-orange lesion, may appear on the scalp, face, or trunk. It does not belong to the disseminated variety of the lipogranulomatous group, nor is it a lesion of the nevus group. It is a benign, wartlike xanthoma which disappears at maturity. It is important to recognize this harmless lesion and to distinguish it from the granulomatous group.

X-ray examination reveals *osteolytic lesions* which may involve every part of the skeleton. Since tooth sockets often show yellow, puslike lesions, the dentist is able to diagnose Hand-Schüller-Christian syndrome. Even isolated lesions of the ribs occur. The *skull* was erroneously considered the most frequently involved part of the skeleton. The lesions were named "eosinophilic granuloma", by Lichtenstein and Jaffe, because of the numerous eosinophils in the early phases. However, invasion of eosinophils in bone lesions is only a developmental stage.

The same is true for development of lipid granuloma of the lung and pleura, often called eosinophilic granuloma of the lung. Although the *lung lesions,* on X-ray, resemble those of miliary tuberculosis in the early stage, the apices of the lungs are not involved. Apparently, the fibrous stage develops in the lung faster than in other organs. Thus, in diffuse fibrosis of the lung of unknown etiology, lipid granuloma should be considered.

Letterer-Siwe syndrome, a systemic reticulosis of the *liver, spleen,* and lymph glands, is considered the reticulocytic phase of lipid granuloma.

Lipogranulomatous masses of the meninges may raise intracranial pressure and cause the *exophthalmos* in Hand-Schüller-Christian syndrome. Involvement of the brain substance itself is very rare. Lipid granuloma involving the cerebellum and long motor tracts in the pons starts as cufflike lesions of adventitial cells of the outer lining of the blood vessels, later forming yellow lipid granuloma of the pons. The clinical symptoms include disturbances of equilibrium, difficulty in speech, impairment of vision, weakness in limbs, with positive Babinski's sign, and, finally, spastic paresis. *Diabetes insipidus* is often found in Hand-Schüller-Christian syndrome, owing to lipid granuloma in the *pituitary* itself.

Gaucher's disease, a rare, familial disorder, occurs early in life and is characterized by splenomegaly, skin pigmentation, pingueculae, and various lytic bone lesions. Because of this symptomatology, it may, at first sight, be confused with normocholesterolemic xanthomatosis. Reticulum cells throughout are, however, filled with kerasin, not cholesterol. A bone marrow biopsy or splenic puncture will reveal the typically large reticulum cells filled by cytoplasm with numerous wavy fibrillae (see pages 208 and 209).

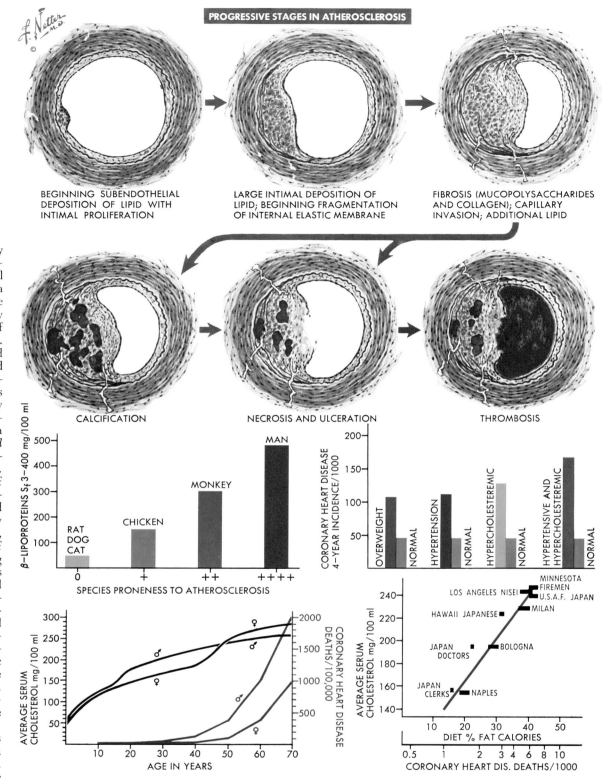

PROGRESSIVE STAGES IN ATHEROSCLEROSIS

BEGINNING SUBENDOTHELIAL DEPOSITION OF LIPID WITH INTIMAL PROLIFERATION

LARGE INTIMAL DEPOSITION OF LIPID; BEGINNING FRAGMENTATION OF INTERNAL ELASTIC MEMBRANE

FIBROSIS (MUCOPOLYSACCHARIDES AND COLLAGEN); CAPILLARY INVASION; ADDITIONAL LIPID

CALCIFICATION

NECROSIS AND ULCERATION

THROMBOSIS

ATHEROSCLEROSIS

Atherosclerosis is a disease which may lead to hardening, occlusion, or weakening of the arteries. The fundamental lesion of the disease is the atheroma (Greek: gruel), which is a discrete plaque arising in the intima of the artery and having a predilection for areas of tortuosity and turbulence of blood flow. The aorta is most frequently affected and then, in order, the coronary, cerebral, and peripheral arteries to the lower extremities. Interestingly, some arteries, such as the internal mammary artery, are rarely involved. Histologically, the lesion consists of focal *intimal thickening,* with various amounts of *subendothelial lipid deposition,* and deformation and *fragmentation* of the *internal elastic membrane.* The various stages in the development of an atheroma are shown in the illustration, which pictures subendothelial lipid deposition as a primary event followed by *endothelial proliferation.* Some authors, however, believe that a breakdown of the basement membrane is the initiating event in atherosclerosis. Scavenger cells and histiocytes appear in the intimal space, and the lesion takes on the appearance of a chronic granuloma with vascularization from the adventitia and *calcification.* The *ulceration* and hemorrhage may lead to *thrombosis* and occlusion, with the resulting galaxy of ischemic signs and symptoms. There is also some evidence that variable amounts of fibrin, deposited during the growth of the atheroma, become a further stimulus to the proliferating endothelial tissue.

Atherosclerosis and its complications are presently the leading cause of death in North America and Western Europe. The crude *death rate from arteriosclerotic (coronary) heart disease* is approximately 3 per 1000 in the United States. In countries such as Japan, China, and Central America, it is less than 0.5 per 1000. In men 55 to 59 years of age, the rates are generally 3 times those in the general population. The *incidence* of disease *rises with age,* being practically absent before puberty but moderate to high in persons reaching the age of 70. In *men,* atheromatosis begins early, as shown by the impressively high degree of involvement (40 per cent) by atherosclerosis of the coronary arteries of American soldiers, 20 to 30 years of age, killed in the Korean War. *Women* during the childbearing period are less susceptible than are men of that age group. Such diseases as diabetes mellitus and the hereditary

hyperlipidemias greatly increase the probabilities of clinical manifestations in both men and women.

Four major classes of lipoproteins exist in plasma. They are (1) the chylomicrons, (2) the *β-lipoproteins,* (3) the α-lipoproteins, and (4) nonesterified fatty acid–albumin complexes (see pages 198, 199, 202, and 203). The first three classes contain esterified lipid in various forms and amounts (triglycerides, phospholipids, *cholesterol,* and cholesterol ester), whereas the lipids associated with albumin are free fatty acids. Chylomicrons are synthesized in the intestine after absorption of dietary fat, NEFA is secreted by adipose tissue, and the α- and β-lipoproteins are produced in the liver. Of these four types of plasma lipoproteins, only the β-lipoproteins appear to bear any relationship to the incidence and prevalence of atheroma in both animals and man. This relationship to atheroma involves the two dimensions of concen-

tration and time. It appears, at present, that all molecules of the β-lipoprotein spectrum, if present in high concentration for a sufficient period of time, will promote atheroma in susceptible primates.

When the average plasma β-lipoprotein concentration for a number of species is plotted against the *species proneness to atherosclerosis,* it appears that the *dog, cat,* and *rat* are very resistant, and that the *chicken, monkey,* and *man* are more susceptible. Furthermore, if experimental atherosclerosis is to be induced in a resistant animal, the β-lipoprotein concentration must be increased. It also can be seen that the *serum cholesterol,* in given populations varying widely in *dietary habits,* correlates with the *mortality from coronary heart disease.* Total serum cholesterol is a fairly good index of β-lipoprotein concentration, over two thirds of plasma sterol being present in that form.

(Continued on page 213)

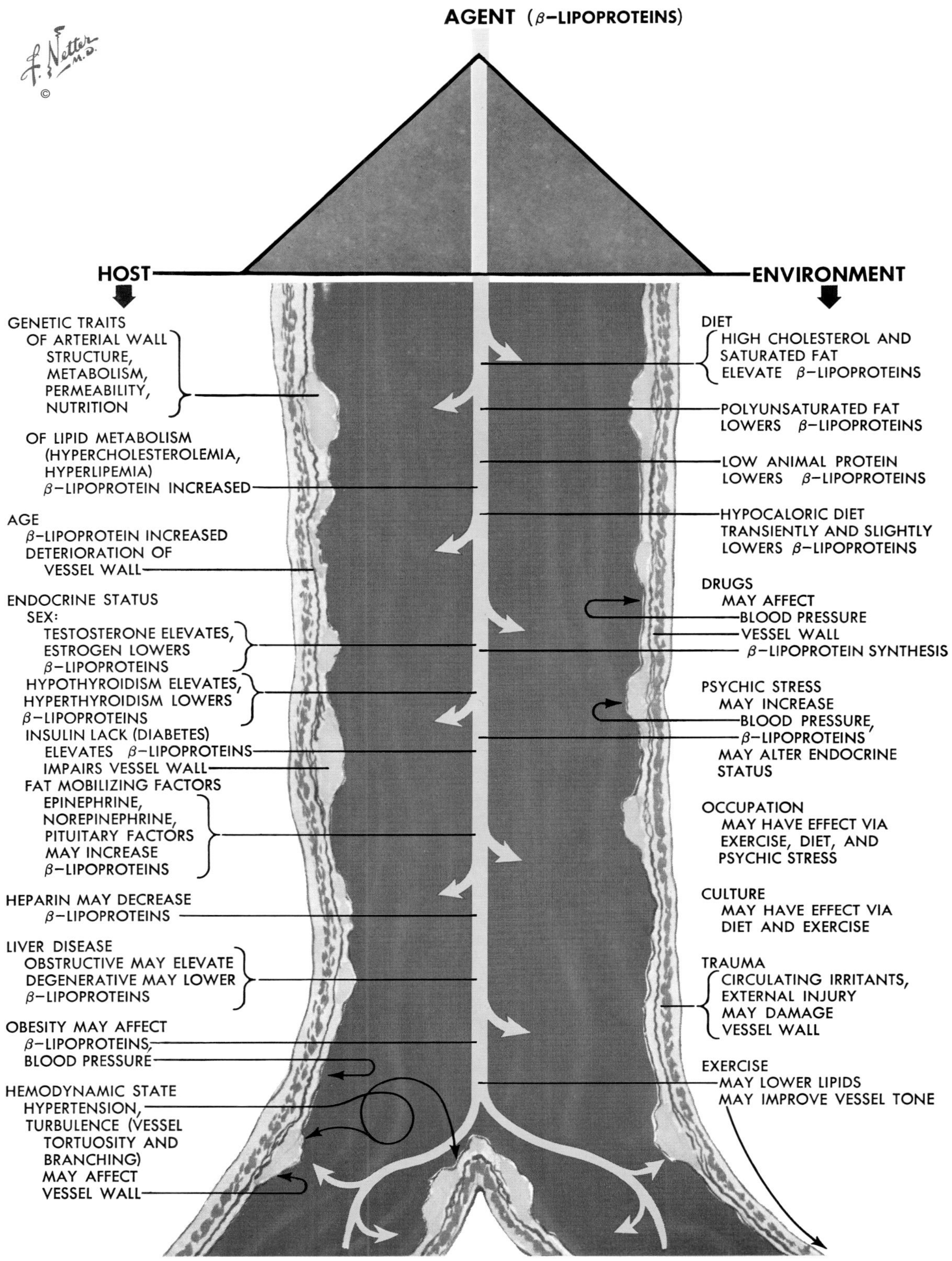

AGENT (β−LIPOPROTEINS)

HOST — **ENVIRONMENT**

GENETIC TRAITS
OF ARTERIAL WALL
STRUCTURE,
METABOLISM,
PERMEABILITY,
NUTRITION

OF LIPID METABOLISM
(HYPERCHOLESTEROLEMIA,
HYPERLIPEMIA)
β−LIPOPROTEIN INCREASED

AGE
β−LIPOPROTEIN INCREASED
DETERIORATION OF
VESSEL WALL

ENDOCRINE STATUS
SEX:
TESTOSTERONE ELEVATES,
ESTROGEN LOWERS
β−LIPOPROTEINS
HYPOTHYROIDISM ELEVATES,
HYPERTHYROIDISM LOWERS
β−LIPOPROTEINS
INSULIN LACK (DIABETES)
ELEVATES β−LIPOPROTEINS
IMPAIRS VESSEL WALL
FAT MOBILIZING FACTORS
EPINEPHRINE,
NOREPINEPHRINE,
PITUITARY FACTORS
MAY INCREASE
β−LIPOPROTEINS

HEPARIN MAY DECREASE
β−LIPOPROTEINS

LIVER DISEASE
OBSTRUCTIVE MAY ELEVATE
DEGENERATIVE MAY LOWER
β−LIPOPROTEINS

OBESITY MAY AFFECT
β−LIPOPROTEINS,
BLOOD PRESSURE

HEMODYNAMIC STATE
HYPERTENSION,
TURBULENCE (VESSEL
TORTUOSITY AND
BRANCHING)
MAY AFFECT
VESSEL WALL

DIET
HIGH CHOLESTEROL AND
SATURATED FAT
ELEVATE β−LIPOPROTEINS
POLYUNSATURATED FAT
LOWERS β−LIPOPROTEINS
LOW ANIMAL PROTEIN
LOWERS β−LIPOPROTEINS
HYPOCALORIC DIET
TRANSIENTLY AND SLIGHTLY
LOWERS β−LIPOPROTEINS

DRUGS
MAY AFFECT
BLOOD PRESSURE
VESSEL WALL
β−LIPOPROTEIN SYNTHESIS

PSYCHIC STRESS
MAY INCREASE
BLOOD PRESSURE,
β−LIPOPROTEINS
MAY ALTER ENDOCRINE
STATUS

OCCUPATION
MAY HAVE EFFECT VIA
EXERCISE, DIET, AND
PSYCHIC STRESS

CULTURE
MAY HAVE EFFECT VIA
DIET AND EXERCISE

TRAUMA
CIRCULATING IRRITANTS,
EXTERNAL INJURY
MAY DAMAGE
VESSEL WALL

EXERCISE
MAY LOWER LIPIDS
MAY IMPROVE VESSEL TONE

ATHEROSCLEROSIS

(Continued from page 212)

In addition to sex differences in cholesterol concentration, the *age-dependent change in serum cholesterol in men and women* is important. It may be shown that, in the United States, the serum cholesterol and β-lipoprotein concentration of *males* rises appreciably at *puberty*, whereas in *females* it remains *low during the childbearing period* but rises to approach the male slope after the menopause. *Mortality rates* for coronary heart disease are presented in the same diagram to show that, in general, *men* are more prone to coronary heart disease than are *women*.

Numerous hypotheses about the etiology of atherosclerosis have been proposed, from diet to degeneration of arterial tissue. No hypothesis proposing a single "cause" has gained acceptance. It seems clear that atherosclerosis is a disease of *multiple etiology,* in which a variety of factors, derived from both the host and his environment, contribute to the production of the lesion and the onset of vascular complications. What has been lacking for atherosclerosis, from the familiar *triad of host-agent-environment,* has been the agent. It seems, furthermore, that in this disease the agent arises within the host as a result of host-environment interaction and is, therefore, *endogenous* rather than exogenous, as are the more familiar disease agents of microbiological, chemical, or physical origin. If one accepts the view that an agent is an indispensable, but not necessarily sufficient, cause (satisfying Koch's postulates), then one may name the *β-lipoproteins* of plasma as the agents of atherosclerosis.

It is evident that local factors affecting the artery are important in the development of the disease. The lesion develops at the interphase of a two-phase system consisting of the arterial intima and the surrounding plasma. Local factors that determine the extent to which an artery can undergo change, in the presence of a given internal environment, include (1) *hemodynamic factors* relating to blood flow and *turbulence* and *pressure,* (2) *metabolic factors* intrinsic in the arterial tissue, (3) *structural factors* relating to differentiation of the internal elastic membrane and other components of the *arterial wall,* and (4) *traumatic factors* secondary to *injury,* ulceration, and repair.

Factors intrinsic to the host, which

may also modify the interplay of humoral and local factors, are *genetic constitution, age, sex, endocrine balance,* and *psychic state.* Finally, environmental factors operate to affect either the state of the artery or the concentration of the agent. Relevant environmental factors include *diet, drugs, exercise, occupation, culture,* and climate. Specific examples of host-environment interrelationship are presented in some detail in the accompanying illustration.

Worthy of special comment are the hyperlipidemias, *i.e.,* essential *hypercholesterolemia* (see pages 206 and 207) and essential *hyperlipemia* (see pages 204 and 205), which are hereditary disorders of lipoprotein synthesis, in which one or another portion of the β-lipoprotein spectrum is increased in the plasma, owing, primarily, to hypersynthesis of one or more components of the lipoprotein molecules in the liver. Such excess synthesis results in chronically and per-

sistently elevated concentrations of the agent. In both of these genetic disorders, atherosclerosis and, in particular, coronary artery disease are more prevalent.

Atherosclerosis is a notoriously silent, insidious disease. The clinician is generally confronted with complications which usually do not quantitatively measure the basic pathogenesis. Nonetheless, prospective studies of coronary morbidity in populations, such as that done at Framingham, Massachusetts, cast some light on the importance of such risk factors as high serum cholesterol, hypertension, and obesity. Such studies are in conformity with the hypotheses of etiology and pathogenesis presented here. The main corollary of these hypotheses, finally, is that this disease, usually a lifetime in the making, may be attenuated by suitable modification of the environment, particularly diet, exercise, and a constant surveillance of the host.

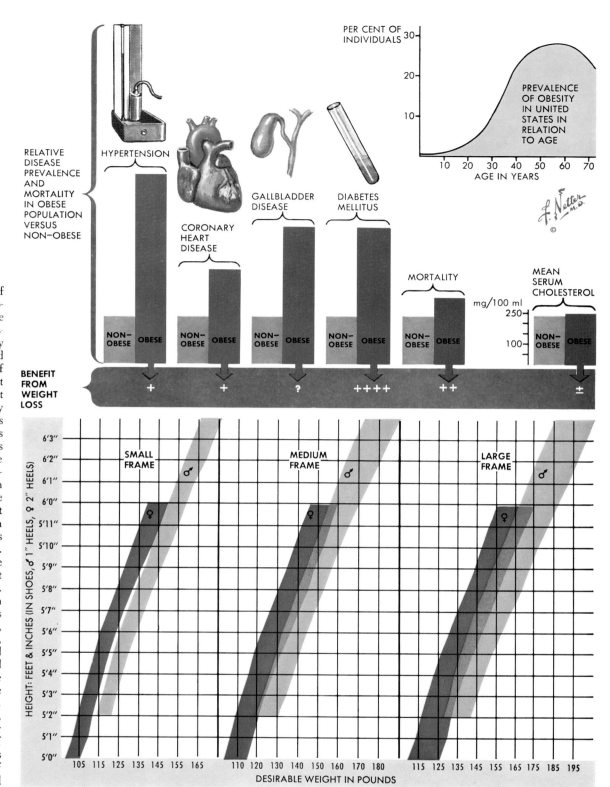

Obesity

Obesity may be defined as a state of excess fatness. Since depot fat is a physiological constituent, it is obvious that the clinical definition of obesity must, necessarily, be arbitrary. A study of the body composition of young adults in the third decade has revealed that 12 per cent of the body weight of men and 19 per cent of the body weight of women is depot fat. Although the distribution of body weights, in healthy adults of all ages, is skewed toward the high side, corrections can be made for the skew (which is minimal in the third decade) to arrive at a reasonable range of a normal distribution of body fat in men and women of this age group. Such calculations have indicated that an increase in body fat from 12 to 22 per cent in males and from 19 to 29 per cent in females constitutes a transition point to excessive fatness. This corresponds roughly to an increase in body weight which is 15 per cent above average at the age of 25 years. The average weight at age 25 is a norm called *desirable weight*. Desirable weights for men and women of *small, medium,* and *large frames* are shown on the chart, and, since the American population and populations in other well-nourished countries tend to become more obese with age, it is reasonable to use these curves as clinical norms for body weight.

Increases in other body constituents, such as extracellular water, muscle, or bone, may give falsely high estimates of the fat compartment, if body weight is relied on solely for the diagnosis of obesity. Clinical appraisal of skin-fold thickness and body contour can aid in estimating the size of the fat compartment.

The prevalence of *obesity rises markedly after the age of 25 years* and reaches a *peak* in the *sixth decade*. By the criterion proposed, 28 per cent of the middle-aged population in the United States is obese, which makes this our most prevalent health disorder. The *decline* in the *prevalence of obesity after the age of 60 years* is due to some spontaneous weight reduction plus the premature death of individuals who have been markedly obese. Several degenerative diseases are associated with obesity. *Hypertension, coronary heart disease, gallbladder disease,* and *diabetes mellitus* are associated with obesity; their *relative prevalence* is presented in the illustration. The majority of obese subjects will

eventually develop either a diabetic glucose tolerance test or frank diabetes, unless they reduce. Yet, early in obesity, there is an elevated insulin level in the serum, following glucose administration, which persists much longer than in normal subjects. It would appear that excessive insulin secretion over the years may critically decrease the insulin-synthesizing capacity of the pancreatic islets or may decrease the sensitivity of target organs to insulin, thus leading to frank diabetes in some subjects. Statistics collected by life-insurance companies show that, for those who are 25 per cent or more *overweight,* the *death rate* is about 1.7 times normal, and in those who are 40 per cent overweight, it increases to 2.2 times normal.

The etiology of obesity, in terms of altered biochemical pathways, is unknown. The often-repeated statement that obesity is caused by *ingestion of more calories* than are expended is true, but it does not give

us much insight into the basic cellular differences between persistently thin and fat individuals. Also, the clinical distinction which is often made between exogenous and endogenous obesity is meaningless, because, for the evolution of any kind of obesity, there must be a positive caloric balance as well as a derangement in the regulation of food intake.

Regulatory obesity is dependent on the *drive to eat,* a basic urge which arises within the *central nervous system.* Homeostatic mechanisms, which adjust the intake of food appropriately to the expenditure of energy, are not known with certainty, but they probably involve both neurological and biochemical *pathways* and signals which, if abnormal, may lead to *metabolic obesity.* The *hypothalamus* appears to be the coordinating center for both *afferent and efferent impulses* which adjust food intake to tissue

(Continued on page 215)

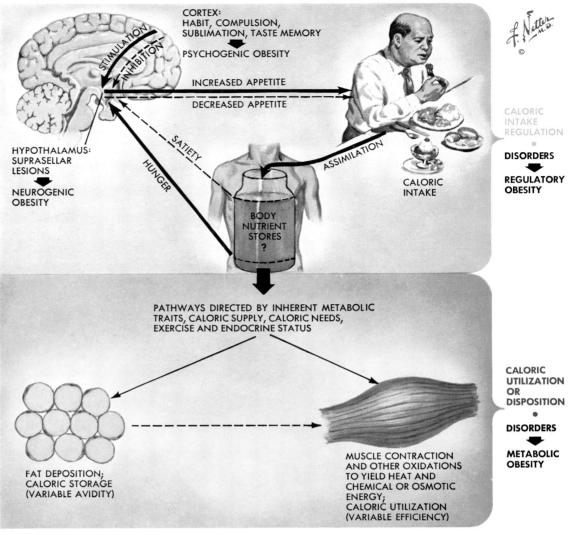

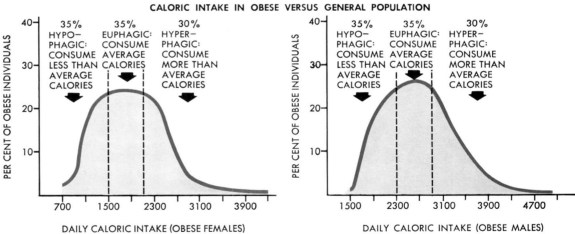

CALORIC INTAKE IN OBESE VERSUS GENERAL POPULATION

Obesity

(Continued from page 214)

needs (see CIBA COLLECTION, Vol. 3/1, pages 69 and 70). Neural pathways from the frontal lobes and other parts of the cerebral *cortex* to the hypothalamus provide the anatomic basis for the well-established relationship between psyche and appetite (see CIBA COLLECTION, Vol. 1, page 161). Regulatory disturbances in this axis account for *psychogenic obesity*. Frank neurological lesions in the midbrain may also abolish normal control and result in *neurogenic obesity*. The mobilization of fatty acids from fat depots depends on sympathetic *stimulation*, in part, so that the posterior hypothalamus may control fat mobilization.

The biochemical mechanisms which relate *hunger* and *appetite* to the fluctuating *body nutrient stores* are less well understood. Various theories have been proposed which postulate specific substrates or signals, but none, as yet, has been generally accepted. Glucostatic, lipostatic, and thermostatic mechanisms have been suggested. There is little doubt that biochemical mechanisms do exist to translate energy needs to hunger signals.

A primary determinant of food intake is *muscular contraction*. Since biochemical pathways are available which convert foodstuffs to a common intermediate, acetyl-coA, which either can go to *fat synthesis* and *deposition* or can provide *cellular energy* (ATP) through oxidation, food taken in excess of needs for energy expenditures is stored principally in the *fat depots*. It is of interest that rats or patients on isocaloric intakes will lay down more fat when consuming the calories all in one large meal than if they consume the same amount in six or more small helpings. Thus, "nibbling" would appear to reduce obesity. During fasting, the fat depots are mobilized to yield fatty acid for oxidation. Such fasting or chronic undernutrition will reduce the size of the fat stores. *Serum cholesterol levels* in obese persons are not appreciably different from those of individuals of normal weight.

Although gain in weight requires an input of calories in excess of expenditure, this positive caloric balance need not occur at high absolute caloric intakes. Recent studies have suggested that *dietary intakes of obese persons are normally distributed,* and some maintain obese weights at quite low dietary intakes. It

is suggested that a more useful classification of obesity (than that of exogenous versus endogenous) would, then, be based on the amount of food required to maintain the obese weight and, hence, a measure of energy expenditure. The terms *hypophagic, euphagic,* and *hyperphagic* obesity are suggested.

The treatment of obesity is based on the restriction of caloric intake below that required to maintain caloric balance and, if possible, the increase of energy expenditure through exercise. During early periods of weight loss, labile nonfatty tissue is mobilized, as well as fat; but, as weight reduction proceeds, the tissue loss is primarily that of adipose tissue. Salt and water balance may be erratic in reducing subjects, owing to endocrine adjustments to changing body composition. Dietary restriction of sodium to 1 to 2 gm per day will prevent the masking, by water retention, of adipose tissue loss.

The *benefits of weight reduction* are seen primarily in the reduction of glucose intolerance in diabetics, improvement of coronary disease (not so much in changes in serum lipid concentrations as in reduction of work load applied during exercise), and lessening of cardiorespiratory symptoms accompanying ambulation. In some patients, weight reduction leads to significant falls in blood pressure, and in others the effect is trivial. Insurance statistics suggest that weight reduction of an obese population will improve its longevity.

Obesity is a heterogeneous disorder, whose sufferers require serious individual study and treatment. A somatic trait may exist in a significant proportion of obese persons.

Its high prevalence and the signal lack of long-term success of weight-reduction programs make obesity a major health problem in the United States.

Section VIII

PROTEIN METABOLISM
GENETICS
GROWTH
HORMONES AND CANCER

by

FRANK H. NETTER, M.D.

in collaboration with

ALEXANDER G. BEARN, M.D.
Plates 3-6

PETER H. FORSHAM, M.D., M.A. (Cantab)
Plate 7

WALTER GILBERT, D. Phil.
Plates 1 and 2

ALBERT SEGALOFF, M.D.
Plates 13-15

HOWARD L. STEINBACH, M.D.
Plates 8 and 9

JUDSON J. VAN WYK, M.D.
Plates 10-12

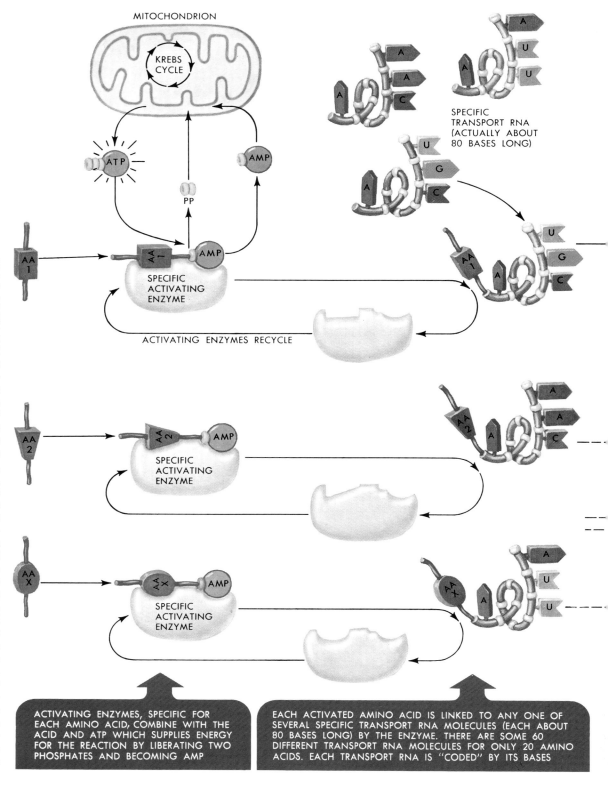

MITOCHONDRION

KREBS CYCLE

ATP

AMP

PP

SPECIFIC ACTIVATING ENZYME

ACTIVATING ENZYMES RECYCLE

SPECIFIC TRANSPORT RNA (ACTUALLY ABOUT 80 BASES LONG)

SPECIFIC ACTIVATING ENZYME

SPECIFIC ACTIVATING ENZYME

ACTIVATING ENZYMES, SPECIFIC FOR EACH AMINO ACID, COMBINE WITH THE ACID AND ATP WHICH SUPPLIES ENERGY FOR THE REACTION BY LIBERATING TWO PHOSPHATES AND BECOMING AMP

EACH ACTIVATED AMINO ACID IS LINKED TO ANY ONE OF SEVERAL SPECIFIC TRANSPORT RNA MOLECULES (EACH ABOUT 80 BASES LONG) BY THE ENZYME. THERE ARE SOME 60 DIFFERENT TRANSPORT RNA MOLECULES FOR ONLY 20 AMINO ACIDS. EACH TRANSPORT RNA IS "CODED" BY ITS BASES

Protein Metabolism

The mechanism of protein synthesis has been worked out by IN VITRO and IN VIVO studies in bacterial and mammalian cells. The problems are: what are the sources of specificity that yield a unique connection between a series of bases, strung along the deoxyribonucleic acid (DNA) molecule, and a series of amino acids inserted into a polypeptide chain; and how does the machinery — this nonspecific machinery that can be told to make any of ten thousand to several million different proteins — work?

The information which specifies the *order of amino acids in a protein* is carried from the DNA, *located in the nucleus,* to the final site of synthesis, the *ribosomes,* located in the cytoplasm, by a ribonucleic acid (RNA) molecule called *messenger RNA* (m-RNA). The m-RNA is a copy of the sequence of bases of one of the strands of the DNA molecule. The strands of the DNA molecule unwind, and a limited region is copied into a single strand of RNA by using the other strand of the DNA as a template for base pairing. The enzyme that does this is called RNA polymerase. (In RNA the base thymine, found in DNA, is replaced by uracil, which also pairs with adenine.)

The sequence of bases along the m-RNA molecule is read off in *groups of three,* starting at some fixed point. Almost every set of 3 bases (a triplet or "codon") stands for an amino acid. The code is degenerate; *i.e.,* there is more than one codon for an individual amino acid. The connection between the code carried on the nucleic acid and the amino acid is made by a "translator" molecule called *transport RNA* (t-RNA).

An amino acid is first recognized by a *specific activating enzyme* (one for each of the 20 amino acids) which binds to the amino acid and activates it with ATP. The amino acid linked to adenosine phosphate remains bound to the enzyme, which recognizes a specific t-RNA molecule and catalyzes the attachment of the amino acid to the t-RNA. The specificity of these two steps is guaranteed by the enzyme — first, in its recognition of the amino acid and, second, in the recognition by the amino acid enzyme complex of some appropriately shaped region on the t-RNA molecule.

The t-RNA molecules are small molecules of RNA, about 80 nucleotides long. At the 3' end of each of these chains, there is an adenylic acid to which the

carboxyl group of the amino acid is linked as an ester. At some place along the chain, the sequence of bases that match with the messenger is located.

The degeneracy of the code is reflected in that there often are different t-RNA's for the same amino acid (leucine, *e.g.,* has five). Each of these t-RNA's recognizes a different triplet on the messenger, but all of these possess regions which recognize a single amino acid activating enzyme complex.

Once the amino acid has been covalently linked to the t-RNA molecule, all the specificity is carried by the RNA moiety. The amino acid can be chemically modified, at this stage, to convert it into a different amino acid, but this will not affect the process of insertion. The altered amino acid will be inserted in the place in the polypeptide chain designated for the original one.

The formation of the polypeptide chain takes place

on, or inside, a ribosome. The ribosome has two parts, the larger one being twice the size of the smaller. The larger subunit contains an RNA molecule, about 3200 bases long (10,000 Å), and about 30 protein molecules. This whole complex folds up to be 150 Å across. The smaller subunit has half the RNA and half the number of proteins, and is about 150 Å × 70 Å. Thus, the entire structure is about 150 Å × 200 Å and has an aggregate molecular weight of about 3 million. The larger subunit holds the growing protein chain and has a site that binds t-RNA; the smaller subunit is known to have a site that binds m-RNA.

The protein chain grows from its amino-terminal amino acid. As shown in the illustration, the ribosome attaches to the m-RNA and binds the t-RNA that carries the first amino acid. This t-RNA forms specific base pairs with the m-RNA, matching a

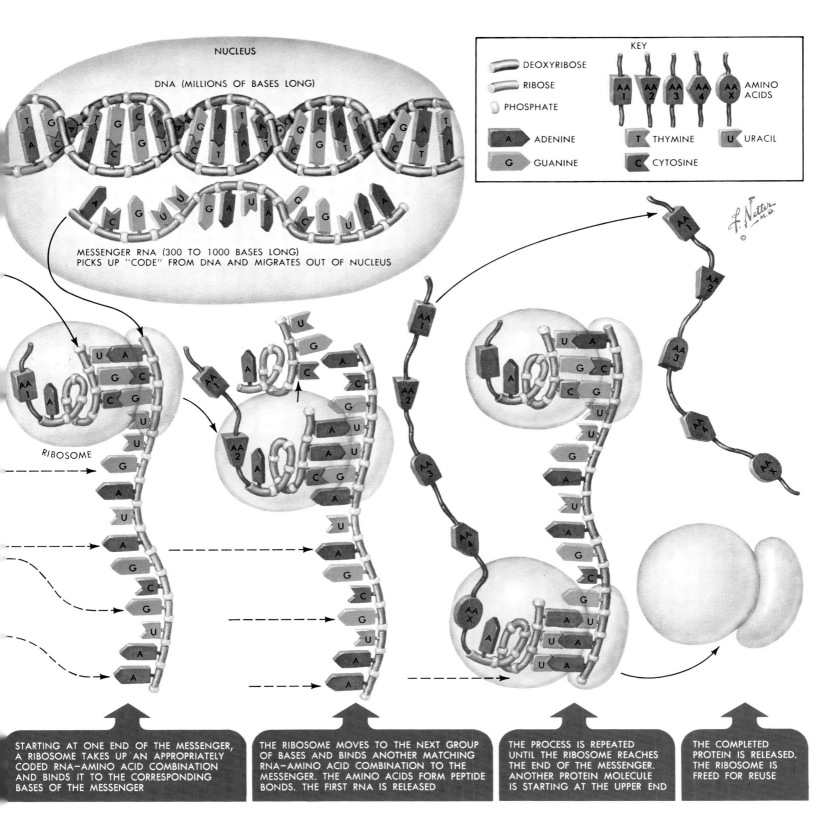

region of the t-RNA chain to the codon on the messenger. The ribosome holds the messenger and t-RNA together. The second amino acid to be inserted is carried up by its t-RNA; this t-RNA binds to a second site on the ribosome, in juxtaposition to the first, being selected, out of all the possible t-RNA's, by its specific bonding to the next codon along the messenger. The next step is the formation of a peptide bond between the two amino acids. The amino group on the second amino acid attacks the ester linkage between the carboxyl group of the first amino acid and its t-RNA, to split off the t-RNA and leave the amino acids linked together, still attached to the second t-RNA. The dipeptide t-RNA moves to the site in which the first amino acid t-RNA was held, pulling the m-RNA chain along with it. Now the structure is again in the initial state.

A t-RNA bearing the third amino acid can now be bound, the dipeptide transferred to the incoming amino acid to form a tripeptide attached to the last t-RNA to arrive. Again, movement of the messenger, with respect to the ribosome, will restore the initial configuration. The process continues, the ribosome moving along the messenger as the protein chain grows and folds toward its final configuration. How the chain is initiated or finished is not known.

The messenger molecule is long enough to handle many ribosomes simultaneously. Even for a small protein, at any one instant the m-RNA molecule would have several ribosomes traveling along it—one just beginning, one that has synthesized half the peptide chain, and one that could be nearly completed and be approaching the release signal. Such structures, called poly-

ribosomes or polysomes, are the peptide breeders.

The ribosome is not simply a passive bench on which the parts are assembled. It serves as part of the mechanism to guarantee specificity, by ensuring that only the correct fit between the messenger and the t-RNA is permitted.

The antibiotic streptomycin attacks at just this point, binding to the smaller subunit and altering the way in which the t-RNA and the messenger fit. This causes a high level of errors; t-RNA's for other amino acids can now bind to the ribosome by mistake. The mutation, in bacteria, causing a resistance to high levels of streptomycin, is, in fact, a change in the structure of the smaller subunit of the ribosome. Subsequently, the modified structure no longer allows streptomycin to alter the code so drastically.

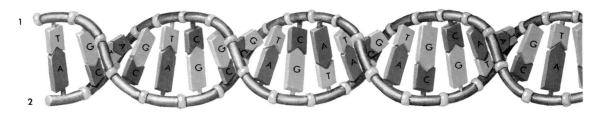

THE DNA MOLECULE CONSISTS OF TWO INTERTWINED HELICAL STRANDS OF DEOXYRIBOSE UNITS ALTERNATING WITH PHOSPHATE AND JOINED TOGETHER BY "RUNGS" OF PURINE AND PYRIMIDINE BASES; ADENINE ALWAYS JOINED TO THYMINE, AND GUANINE TO CYTOSINE. THE DNA MOLECULE HAS MILLIONS OF SUCH LINKAGES

DNA Replication

A schematic representation of a few turns of the *DNA molecule* is shown at the top of the plate. The molecule contains *two complementary strands,* bearing the same relation to each other as does a photographic negative to a positive print. The backbone of each strand consists of *deoxyribose sugar rings* linked together through phosphate diester bonds. To each of the sugars 1 of the 4 bases—*adenine, cytosine, guanine,* or *thymine*—is covalently linked to form nucleosides. These bases have the ability to form hydrogen bonds between each other: the pairs that occur in DNA are adenine (A) with thymine (T) and guanine (G) with cytosine (C). The Watson-Crick model for the spatial structure of DNA was based on the realization that these base pairings could form the basis of a complementary structure, the complementary strand carrying the other base of each pair. The specificity is guaranteed by the way in which the hydrogen bonds are placed, and by the constraint imposed by the backbone; the wrong base would be either too large or too small for the attached sugar to fit into the backbone. There is a direction defined along each backbone. The phosphate diester bonds are formed between the 3′ and the 5′ positions on the deoxyribose sugars, these positions carrying hydroxyl groups in the free sugar. For *chain 2,* a free end on the left is indicated; this would be the 3′ end. The first phosphate is linked between the 5′ position of this nucleoside and the 3′ position of the next. Thus, the 3′-to-5′ direction for chain 2 runs from left to right. The complementary chain has the opposite 3′-to-5′ direction; *chain 1* has its 5′ end on the left. The second strand carries the other base of each pair, in the reverse order, along the backbone.

Each full turn of the helix takes ten base pairs, about 34 Å, or 34×10^{-8} cm. The single molecules of DNA are very long: The DNA molecule in a bacteriophage has a length of the order of 30,000 to 50,000 Å, and the DNA molecule in the nucleus of the bacterium Escherichia coli is 1 mm long (3×10^6 base pairs). The total length of all DNA in a human cell is about 2 m, but this is not in a single molecule.

The strands are formed by the condensation of energy-rich nucleoside triphosphates (5′-triphosphates), which split off a pyrophosphate as they combine with the 3′-hydroxyl of another nucleotide. This process requires an enzyme, DNA polymerase, and uses a DNA strand as a template. The *two strands of the DNA molecule unwind.* The

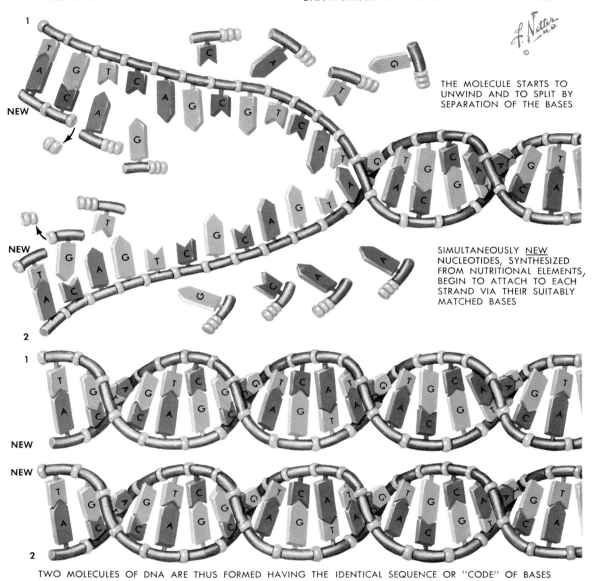

THE MOLECULE STARTS TO UNWIND AND TO SPLIT BY SEPARATION OF THE BASES

SIMULTANEOUSLY <u>NEW</u> NUCLEOTIDES, SYNTHESIZED FROM NUTRITIONAL ELEMENTS, BEGIN TO ATTACH TO EACH STRAND VIA THEIR SUITABLY MATCHED BASES

TWO MOLECULES OF DNA ARE THUS FORMED HAVING THE IDENTICAL SEQUENCE OR "CODE" OF BASES

KEY
DEOXYRIBOSE   PHOSPHATE   A ADENINE   G GUANINE   T THYMINE   C CYTOSINE

precursor nucleoside triphosphates approach their complementary mates, are held in place loosely by base pairing, and then are covalently linked into the growing backbone by the enzyme. The enzyme not only holds the template and the new nucleotide but also serves to guarantee the specificity of the insertion by requiring that the nucleotide fit correctly, so that the backbone of the growing chain is correctly formed. The two parental strands have unwound from the left. *On the lower strand* the *nucleoside triphosphates* are being *added to the growing 3′ end of a new chain,* and this is the way that the DNA polymerase acts IN VITRO. The other strand is being duplicated at the same time, but the exact mechanism is not known; either the strand grows in reverse, a new nucleotide being added using the 5′-triphosphate still on the end of the chain, or, possibly, the new chain is synthesized in short seg-

ments (which would run from right to left in the illustration) and then is fastened together by still another enzyme. Thus, two new helices form as the parent unwinds, a duplicate of strand 1 forming on strand 2 as a template, and a duplicate of strand 2 forming on strand 1.

The nature of the initiation step—how the replication begins and what controls it when it begins—is not known. Furthermore, the organization of the DNA into chromosomes, so that it can unwind and duplicate, is not understood. As an example of this problem, the 1-mm piece of DNA in E. coli is in the form of a circle, the ends are connected, and they remain connected during the duplication process. The structure that connects the ends, which is probably not DNA, embodies the characteristics of a swivel, for the long body of the molecule must rotate as the strands unwind.

INHERITANCE OF AUTOSOMAL DOMINANT TRAITS

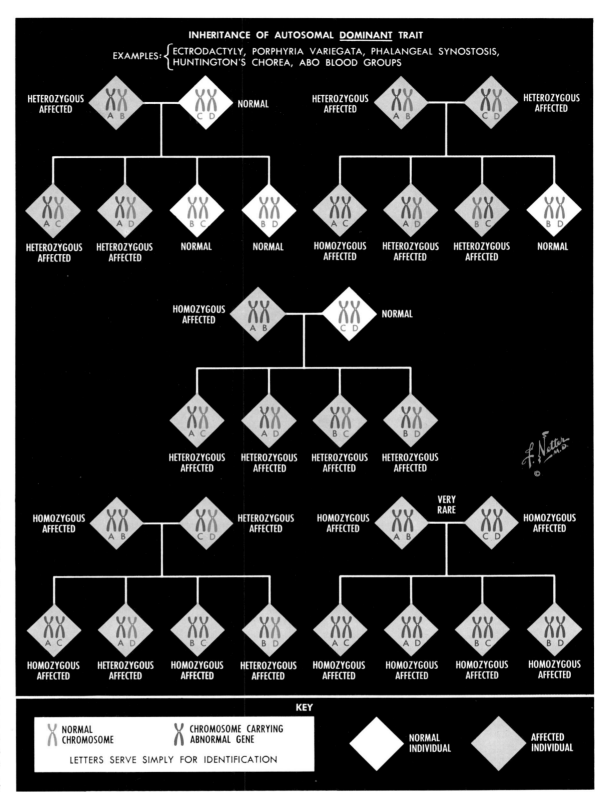

INHERITANCE OF AUTOSOMAL DOMINANT TRAIT

EXAMPLES: { ECTRODACTYLY, PORPHYRIA VARIEGATA, PHALANGEAL SYNOSTOSIS, HUNTINGTON'S CHOREA, ABO BLOOD GROUPS

KEY

X NORMAL CHROMOSOME — X CHROMOSOME CARRYING ABNORMAL GENE — NORMAL INDIVIDUAL — AFFECTED INDIVIDUAL

LETTERS SERVE SIMPLY FOR IDENTIFICATION

A trait is said to be dominant when the gene controlling it produces an effect in the heterozygous state. It should be emphasized that it is not strictly correct to speak of dominant genes. In recent years the terms dominant and recessive (see page 222) have been used less frequently, and now it is more common to state whether the gene is overtly manifest in the single dose (dominant) or only in the double dose (recessive).

Dominance is recognized in human pedigrees by the transmission of a trait through several generations. With the exception of mutation, a dominant trait is present in at least one biological parent. According to Mendelian laws, a heterozygous individual married to a normal homozygote will, on the average, pass on the trait to half his children, both sexes being equally affected. Dominant traits are usually mild and, frequently, are extremely variable in their expression. Variability may be expressed in terms of severity of symptoms or in age of onset. If the symptoms are mild, or there is a delay in their onset, an individual, even though he bears the abnormal gene, may be thought to be normal. If such an individual is fertile, approximately half of his offspring will be affected and half will be normal. "Apparent skipping" of a generation, in which a trait disappears from a pedigree only to reappear in subsequent generations, can frequently be explained in this way.

Several dominant skeletal defects are considered to be due to the effects of a single gene. Ectrodactyly (lobster-claw deformity) and interphalangeal synostosis, although both may have a variable expression, fit fairly well with a dominant trait. Interphalangeal synostosis is

of historical interest, since John Talbot, the first Earl of Shrewsbury, who was born about 1390, was known to have had this anomaly, and it has since been traced through 18 generations. Huntington's chorea is a good example of a dominant trait whose onset may not become apparent until middle age.

The mutation rate, expressed as the number of mutations per locus per generation, has been estimated for a number of dominant human traits. The estimated mutation rate for Huntington's chorea is 5×10^6 mutations per locus per generation. Other dominant traits have estimated mutation rates in the same range. In two dominant traits—acrocephalo-syndactyly and achondroplasia—the mutation rate is related to advancing paternal age.

The plate illustrates the possible mating patterns in a dominant trait. The most common pedigree is the marriage of an affected heterozygous individual with

a *normal heterozygote*, which will result in half the offspring being affected and half normal. If two affected heterozygous individuals marry, 1 out of 4 offspring will be homozygous for the abnormal gene. This type of mating is rare and, in some instances, it appears likely that the zygote with 2 abnormal genes does not survive. It is reasonable to assume that the homozygous individual, if viable, will be more severely affected than will be the heterozygote. A dominant trait may be manifested differently in the two sexes (sex-limited). Baldness in males is an example of such a trait. Environmentally determined conditions may simulate an incompletely dominant trait. In the past, pellagra and tuberculosis were erroneously ascribed to genetic causes on the basis of pedigree analysis. Chromosomal aberrations of the translocation type may also mimic a dominant trait, with variable expression.

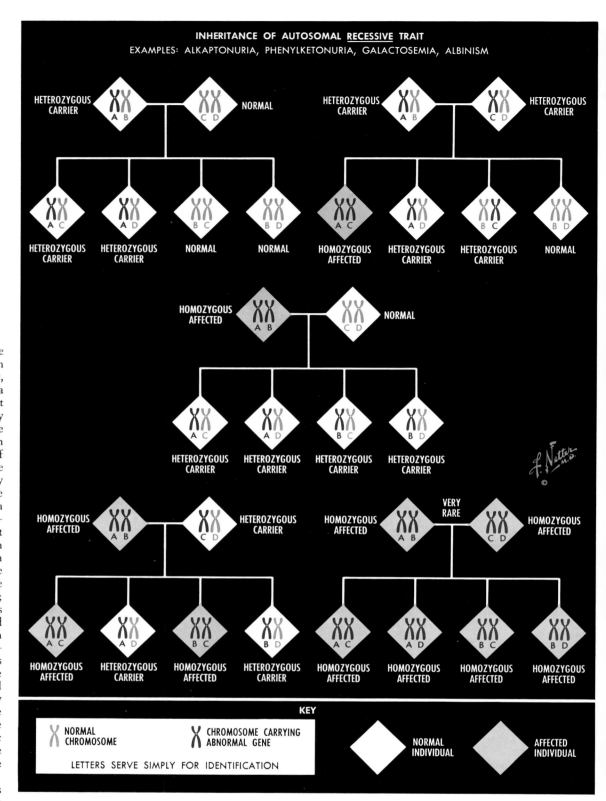

INHERITANCE OF AUTOSOMAL RECESSIVE TRAIT
EXAMPLES: ALKAPTONURIA, PHENYLKETONURIA, GALACTOSEMIA, ALBINISM

INHERITANCE OF AUTOSOMAL RECESSIVE TRAITS

A trait which depends on the presence of 2 identical genes, one derived from the father and the other from the mother, is called recessive. If the condition is a rare one, both parents, usually, exhibit no symptoms, although they both carry the gene in the heterozygous state. The probability that a rare gene is present in both parents is considerably increased if they have ancestors in common; the closer the relationship, the more likely it will be that the two parents will have genes in common. If one partner in a marriage is heterozygous for a rare recessive gene, the probability that a first cousin has the same gene is 1 chance in 8. If the individual were to marry an unrelated spouse, the chance of the spouse carrying the same gene is the frequency of the gene in the population; in most conditions, this would be less than 1 chance in 50. Thus, an increased consanguinity rate is extremely common in rare autosomal traits. The consanguinity rate, in most populations, does not exceed 0.1 per cent, but, among the parents of those affected with autosomal recessive conditions, the frequency may be as high as 30 per cent. It will be apparent that if an autosomal recessive condition is a common one, e.g., cystic fibrosis of the pancreas, no detectable increase in the consanguinity rate can be expected.

In most instances, affected individuals arise from the marriage of two clinically normal heterozygous carriers. From such a mating, 50 per cent of the offspring will be clinically normal carriers of the gene in a single dose (like their parents) and 25 per cent will be normal, but 25 per cent will inherit the abnormal gene from both parents and, thus, be affected; therefore, the probability of an affected child from the marriage of two heterozygotes is 1 in 4. If an affected individual marries a normal spouse, none of the children will be affected, but all of them will be carriers of the abnormal gene. If an affected individual marries a heterozygous carrier, half the offspring will be affected and half will be carriers. It is evident that, if two affected individuals, both homozygous for the same gene,

were to marry, all the offspring would be affected.

The proof that a condition is inherited in an autosomal recessive fashion can be established by demonstrating a 1:4 ratio of affected to unaffected children. Straightforward counting of affected and unaffected individuals in sibships will give a biased result and will overestimate the number of those affected. This is evident, since sibships of 1 affected person with 1 affected child will yield a proportion of 100 per cent affected, instead of the predicted 25 per cent. Simple arithmetic methods, designed to circumvent these difficulties, have been devised.

The detection of carriers of recessive genes represents one of the most important aspects of clinical genetics. Most recessive diseases in man are due to the absence of a gene product (or of a structurally altered gene product), frequently an enzyme. Since most heterozygous carriers of recessive traits are

clinically normal, it must be presumed that the single normal allele is sufficient for normal function. However, by the use of sensitive biochemical techniques, it has been possible to detect a decrease in the gene product of many clinically normal heterozygotes. One example will suffice: Galactosemia is a recessively inherited condition which is due to a deficiency of galactose-1-phosphate-uridyl transferase. Affected children have no detectable enzyme in their red cells. The clinically normal heterozygous parents have an enzyme level approximately 50 per cent of normal. It is clear that the detection of heterozygous carriers for an abnormal gene will have important consequences for genetic counseling. Calculations of the mutation rate for autosomal recessive traits are more unreliable than are similar calculations for dominant traits. The reported estimates suggest that the mutation rates are roughly comparable.

INHERITANCE OF SEX-LINKED (X-LINKED) TRAITS

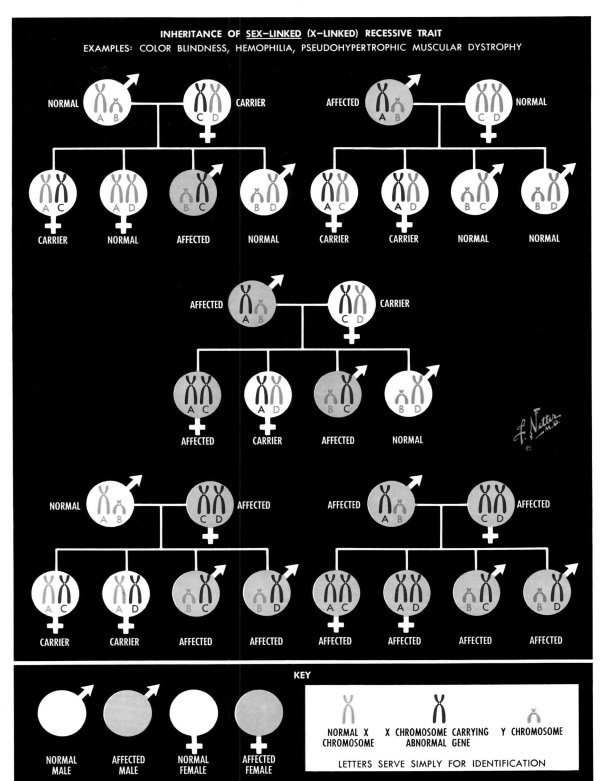

INHERITANCE OF SEX-LINKED (X-LINKED) RECESSIVE TRAIT
EXAMPLES: COLOR BLINDNESS, HEMOPHILIA, PSEUDOHYPERTROPHIC MUSCULAR DYSTROPHY

In females, 2 X chromosomes are found in addition to the 22 paired autosomes, whereas the male has 1 X chromosome and 1 Y chromosome. An X-linked dominant gene from the male is rare but can be easily recognized, for the gene will never be passed from father to son but will be transmitted to all daughters. An X-linked dominant gene from the mother will be transmitted to half the sons and half the daughters. Examples of X-linked dominant traits include glucose-6-phosphate dehydrogenase deficiency, which can give rise to hemolytic anemia, the Xg blood group, and vitamin-D-resistant rickets due to renal loss of phosphate.

X-linked recessive inheritance is more common, and a characteristic pattern of inheritance can be recognized from examination of pedigrees. In most outbred societies, males are almost exclusively affected. The rules for the recognition of rare X-linked recessive inheritance are summarized below and should be verified by reference to the plate.

Most pedigrees contain a normal male married to an unaffected carrier female. Half of the daughters will be carriers, and half of the sons will be affected. If an affected male marries a normal female, all the daughters will be carriers and all the sons will be normal. If an affected male marries a carrier female, half of the daughters will be affected and half will be carriers, and half of the sons will be affected. Other mating patterns are extremely uncommon; their consequences can be seen by examining the plate. It is sometimes necessary to distinguish an autosomal gene, which is only manifest in males, from an X-linked recessive. This distinction can be drawn if affected individuals are fertile. In the case of an autosomal gene, affected males

will be seen in the progeny; in X-linked genes, however, transmission from father to son is not ordinarily possible. It is of interest, in this regard, to recall that congenital agammaglobulinemia is properly considered a recessively controlled X-linked trait, yet few children with agammaglobulinemia have survived to reproductive age.

Color blindness occurs in approximately 8 per cent of males. To produce a color-blind female, there must be the coincidence of 2 affected X chromosomes; thus, the frequency in females should be 0.64 per cent. The observed frequency is slightly lower and has been ascribed to the existence of more than one locus for color blindness.

Hemophilia affects 1 in 25,000 males. The frequency in women is extremely rare. A chromosomal analysis is indicated where an affected female is observed with an X-linked recessive trait. In several

instances the affected "female" has had the chromosome constitution of a male. Detection of carriers of X-linked genes, such as hemophilia, would be of considerable importance. A tendency for female carriers of the hemophilic gene to have a slightly decreased antihemoglobin level has been reported. Unfortunately, this reduction is not always present. The frequency of an X-linked gene in the population is equivalent to the number of affected males. Thus, in the general population, the frequency of affected females will be equal to the square of the frequency of affected males. The mutation rates for several X-linked genes have been calculated. The estimate for hemophilia (3.2×10^5 mutations per locus per generation), made by Haldane, is probably too high, since the two conditions—hemophilia A and hemophilia B — had not been differentiated at the time his calculation was made.

GENETIC PATTERNS IN MONGOLISM

The malformation known as Mongolism was first recognized as a separate clinical entity by Langdon Down in 1866, and since that time there has been no shortage of etiological hypotheses. Although it had long been suspected that some chromosomal aberrations might be responsible, it was not until 1959 that a specific chromosomal aberration was discovered, viz., the presence of an additional autosomal chromosome, usually designated 21. It is assumed that this aberration is due to the consequences of nondisjunction during gametogenesis. The marked association of Mongolism with increasing maternal age indicates that the abnormal cell division occurs during oögenesis. The upper section of the accompanying plate illustrates the consequences of nondisjunction during oögenesis. For simplification, only 2 chromosomes, numbers 15 and 21, are depicted. As a result of nondisjunction during meiosis, an ovum is formed which contains 2 number-21 chromosomes. Fertilization of this ovum with a normal sperm will result in a zygote containing 3 number-21 chromosomes and a total chromosome count of 47. It is noteworthy that, as a result of disturbed segregation of chromosome 21, ova are formed which are deficient in this chromosome. When fertilized by a normal sperm, a zygote will be formed which will be monosomic for chromosome 21. Such individuals have not been observed, and it is assumed that the resulting zygote is lethal.

In another very important group, Mongolism is due to a translocation involving chromosome 21. A translocation occurs when two simultaneous breaks take place at or near the centromere of 2 chromosomes, and the wrong pair of ends are rejoined (see page 112). Most translocations occur between chromosome 21 and one of the members of the 13-to-15 group. As a result of the translocation, the greater part of a 21 is fused to a chromosome of the 13-to-15 group, usually a 15. The reciprocal of the translocation, comprising the short arms of both chromosomes, is usually lost after several cell divisions. The oöcyte with the translocation chromosome has only 45 chromosomes but contains virtually the normal amount of chromatin material. From a translocation, 8 possible types of ova can be obtained, only 4 of which are depicted in the plate. When those depicted are fertilized by normal sperm, the following offspring are possible: a completely normal individual; a

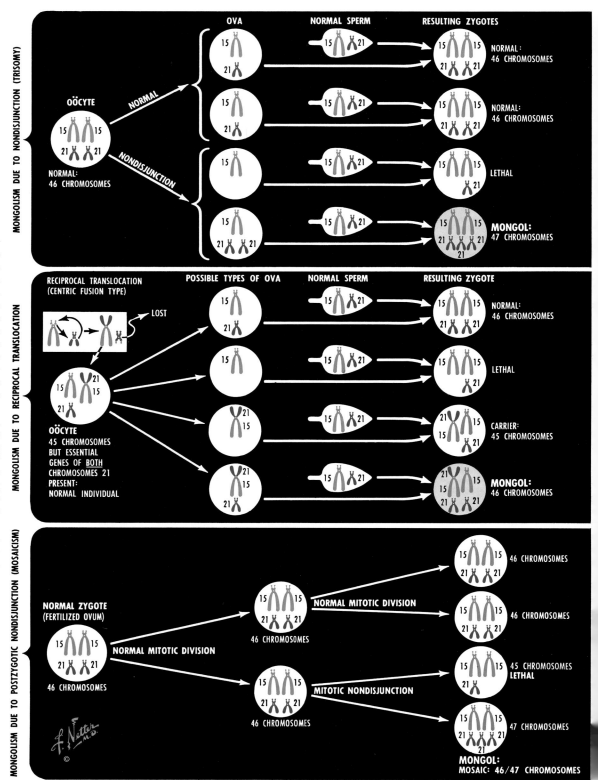

carrier of the translocation chromosome, who has 45 chromosomes; a Mongoloid individual with 46 chromosomes, who is carrying the translocated chromosome and, thus, is essentially trisomic for chromosome 21; and a zygote monosomic for chromosome 21. The monosomic 21 individual has not been observed, so the zygote is presumed to be lethal. The existence of translocation Mongoloids accounts for a number of instances of familial Mongolism. Transmission of the translocated chromosome varies in the two sexes. Female carriers of the translocated chromosome give rise to a relative excess of affected and carrier children, whereas, among the progeny of male translocations, there is a relative scarcity of affected children and an increase in the number of normal individuals carrying the translocation chromosome. It should be emphasized that probably not more than 25 per cent of familial Mongolism can be accounted for by translocations.

When nondisjunction occurs during the division of somatic cells, chromosomal mosaics may be formed. The most usual variation is that some of the somatic cells are trisomic for chromosome 21 and others are normal. The initial nondisjunction will give rise to 2 cells—one with 47 and one with 45 chromosomes. It seems probable that those cells with 45 chromosomes, which are monosomic for chromosome 21, are selected against and rapidly die out, leaving two classes of cells. The majority of cells will have 46 chromosomes, and a minority will have 47. Leukocyte cultures from mosaic Mongoloids frequently show a normal karyotype, and examination of more than one tissue is essential if Mongolism is suspected. A proportion of mosaic Mongoloids may be gonadal mosaics and give rise to Mongoloid offspring. In general, mosaic Mongoloids are less severely affected than are those in whom all the cells in the body are trisomic 21.

HORMONAL EFFECTS ON PROTEIN ANABOLISM AND CATABOLISM

Anabolism may be broadly defined as the building up of tissue, and *catabolism* as its breakdown. Given an adequate supply of essential foods, amino acids, vitamins, and trace elements, the over-all metabolism of an individual will depend on the balance between his intake and his energy output. However, certain hormones will affect both the distribution of amino acids (among various target organs and body tissues) and the metabolic pathways of any of the foodstuffs, *viz.*, carbohydrate, protein, and fat.

Amino acids may go either to *muscle, bone matrix,* or tissues of organs such as the *liver,* or to secondary sex organs, such as the penis, where they are integrated into the tissues in an anabolic process. Failing this, they are deaminated in the liver, and the remaining carbon skeleton is further broken down to CO_2 and water, while ammonia is transformed into *urea* and excreted as such by the *kidneys* in a catabolic process.

Among the *anabolic hormones,* the *pituitary,* providing *growth hormone* (STH), makes available one of the most potent anabolic agents. Typically, it enhances the entrance of amino acids into muscle, where they form protein; it also leads to the multiplication of nuclei of cells and, thus, to growth. Secretion of STH is inhibited by high levels of corticosteroids; a deficiency also occurs in states of malnutrition, whereas hypoglycemia enhances production. Lack of STH leads to small stature, but too much causes excessive height before puberty (see page 28).

Testosterone, one of the major androgens from the *testis,* is a strong anabolic agent which also is extremely androgenic. It, too, favors the penetration of amino acids into muscle cells, but, unlike STH, it leads to an increase in cell mass by augmenting cytoplasm (hypertrophy) rather than the number of nuclei (hyperplasia). It has relatively little effect on bone matrix; it acts mostly by depositing protein in muscles and being highly androgenic, specifically in the penis and clitoris. The *ingestion* of anabolic agents with little or no androgenic function, such as *methandrostenolone,* increases muscle mass without most of the androgenic side effects. The mechanism of action is that of weak androgens.

The *ovaries* contribute *estrogens* as mildly anabolic steroids. Their beneficial effect on postmenopausal osteoporosis may be attributed more to their renal calcium-retaining effect rather than to a direct anabolic action on the organic matrix of the bone.

The *pancreas* contributes *insulin,* which is anabolic, and the presence of which is essential for the action of STH. It enhances the penetration of both amino acids and glucose into muscle, as

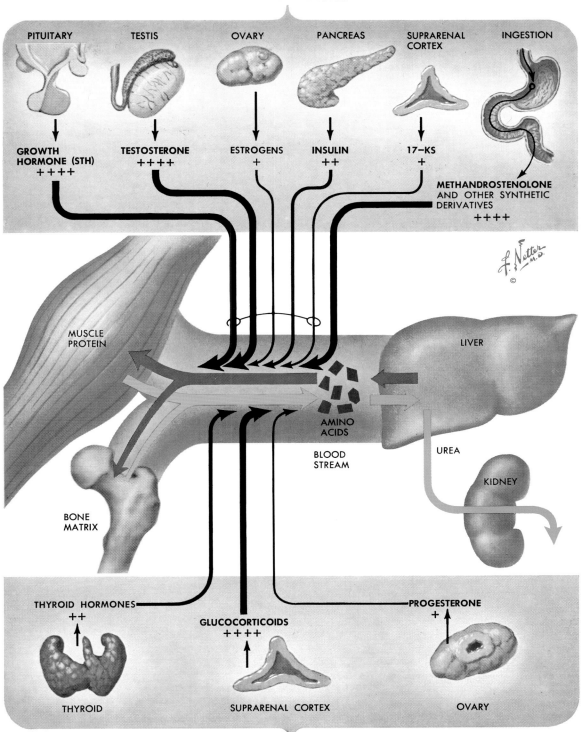

well as fat cells, against corticoid action.

The *adrenal cortex* contributes very weak androgens, collectively known as 17-ketosteroids (17-KS). Their anabolic effect is important in females, who obtain little androgen from their ovaries. Small amounts of testosterone and androsterone, both potent androgens and anabolic agents, are also secreted by the adrenal cortex.

The anabolic agents are opposed by only three frankly *catabolic hormones,* the most important being the *glucocorticoids of the suprarenal cortex.* With an excess of cortisol, as in Cushing's syndrome (see page 85), a negative nitrogen balance is established, and there is marked wasting of the muscles of the extremities and abdomen, accompanied by an abnormal redistribution of fat. A far weaker catabolic agent, *progesterone,* is secreted by the *corpus luteum of the ovary.* The *thyroid* contributes *thyroid*

hormones, notably thyroxine and tri-iodothyronine, which, in physiological amounts, are only mildly catabolic and are, in fact, anabolic in specific activities such as the maturation of the epiphysial plates of bone and growth of lymphoid tissue. Thyroid hormones direct amino acids from the muscle to the lymphoid tissue, which undergoes marked hyperplasia in hyperthyroidism. When in excess, as in this instance, thyroid hormones become frankly catabolic by increasing the turnover of all metabolic processes (by uncoupling the normal links between phosphorylating and oxidative reactions), thus wasting much energy because of excessive heat production. In hyperthyroidism, tissue wasting may be temporarily counteracted by an inordinately large intake of calories.

The body's balance between anabolic and catabolic hormones is normally anabolic in early life, gradually becoming more catabolic with advancing age.

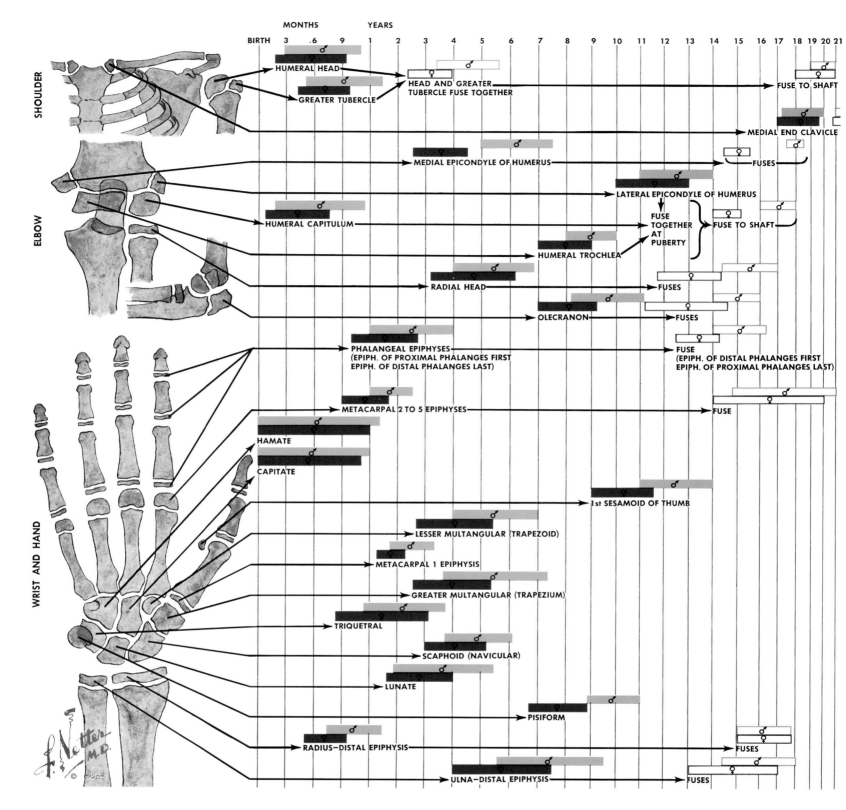

MONTHS **YEARS**

BIRTH 3 .6 9 1 2 3 4 5 6 7 8 9 10 11 12 13 14 15 16 17 18 19 20 21

SHOULDER
- HUMERAL HEAD
- GREATER TUBERCLE
- HEAD AND GREATER TUBERCLE FUSE TOGETHER — FUSE TO SHAFT
- MEDIAL END CLAVICLE

ELBOW
- MEDIAL EPICONDYLE OF HUMERUS — FUSES
- LATERAL EPICONDYLE OF HUMERUS
- HUMERAL CAPITULUM
- HUMERAL TROCHLEA
- FUSE TOGETHER AT PUBERTY — FUSE TO SHAFT
- RADIAL HEAD — FUSES
- OLECRANON — FUSES

WRIST AND HAND
- PHALANGEAL EPIPHYSES (EPIPH. OF PROXIMAL PHALANGES FIRST EPIPH. OF DISTAL PHALANGES LAST) — FUSE (EPIPH. OF DISTAL PHALANGES FIRST EPIPH. OF PROXIMAL PHALANGES LAST)
- METACARPAL 2 TO 5 EPIPHYSES — FUSE
- HAMATE
- CAPITATE
- 1st SESAMOID OF THUMB
- LESSER MULTANGULAR (TRAPEZOID)
- METACARPAL 1 EPIPHYSIS
- GREATER MULTANGULAR (TRAPEZIUM)
- TRIQUETRAL
- SCAPHOID (NAVICULAR)
- LUNATE
- PISIFORM
- RADIUS–DISTAL EPIPHYSIS — FUSES
- ULNA–DISTAL EPIPHYSIS — FUSES

SKELETAL MATURATION AND GROWTH

Human development, from fertilization of the ovum through birth and maturity, is achieved by two processes—GROWTH, an increase in mass and volume ordinarily measured by height and weight, and MATURATION, that state of developmental completion which denotes adulthood. In the skeleton, after initial ossification of pre-existing cartilage or mesenchyme, bones that originally were spherical or tubular change in shape, with the development of characteristic tuberosities, excrescences, and depressions. The degree of maturation is referred to as the *skeletal*, or *bone, age,* indicating the average age at which normal individuals possess the same degree of differentiation.

Skeletal maturation is most variable at the onset of ossification. As bones develop and approach their final stages of *epiphysial* and *diaphysial fusion,* the variability lessens. Assuming the same conditions of good nutrition and absence of disease for all children, the rate of maturation will be most rapid in warm regions, and more so in Negroes than in Caucasians. Skeletal development is more rapid in females than in males prior to birth, and it increases with advancing age. It is genetically determined, with the male Y chromosome exerting a retarding influence.

The appearance of primary or secondary centers in the early ages and the fusion of primary and secondary centers at puberty determine maturation. The change in the contour of the bones is the criterion used in the time between those two age groups. The times of onset and completion of various centers, for both sexes, are included in the accompanying tables. Also represented is the *age range* within which the ossification centers appear or fuse in most normal individuals. This range varies from 2 standard deviations to 75 per cent of normal, according to various authors.

When *deviations from normal* occur in different centers of the same individual, those *centers* that normally exhibit the *least variability* should be emphasized. This is represented on the charts as centers with the *least spread.* Also, the completion phase (fusion of epiphyses) is less

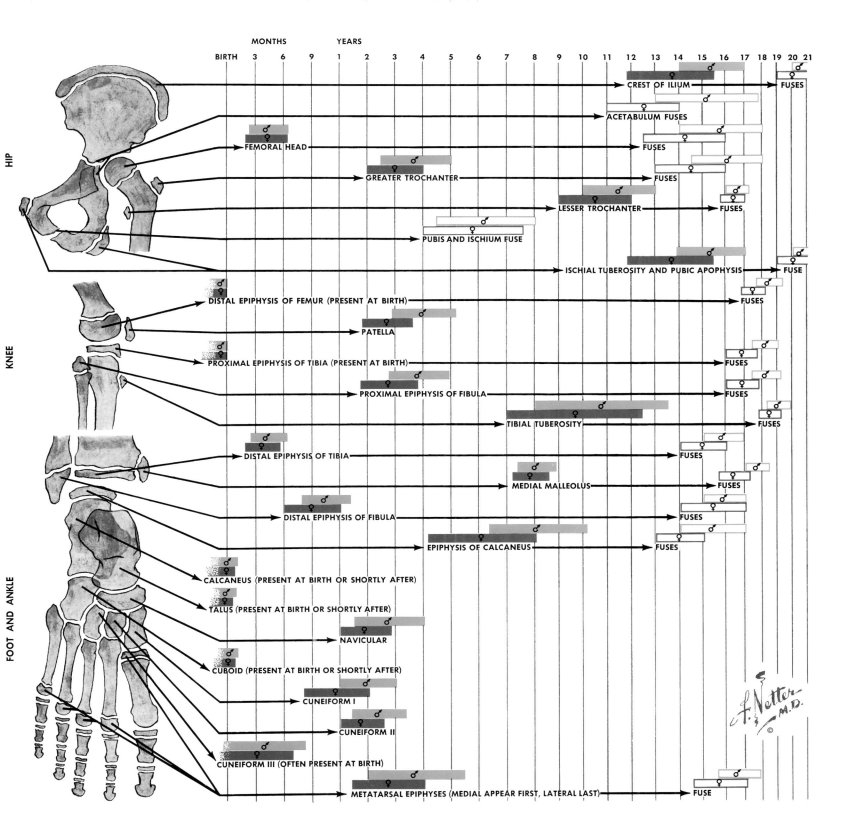

MONTHS | YEARS

BIRTH 3 6 9 1 2 3 4 5 6 7 8 9 10 11 12 13 14 15 16 17 18 19 20 21

HIP

CREST OF ILIUM → FUSES
ACETABULUM FUSES
FEMORAL HEAD → FUSES
GREATER TROCHANTER → FUSES
LESSER TROCHANTER → FUSES
PUBIS AND ISCHIUM FUSE
ISCHIAL TUBEROSITY AND PUBIC APOPHYSIS → FUSE

KNEE

DISTAL EPIPHYSIS OF FEMUR (PRESENT AT BIRTH) → FUSES
PATELLA
PROXIMAL EPIPHYSIS OF TIBIA (PRESENT AT BIRTH) → FUSES
PROXIMAL EPIPHYSIS OF FIBULA → FUSES
TIBIAL TUBEROSITY → FUSES

FOOT AND ANKLE

DISTAL EPIPHYSIS OF TIBIA → FUSES
MEDIAL MALLEOLUS → FUSES
DISTAL EPIPHYSIS OF FIBULA → FUSES
EPIPHYSIS OF CALCANEUS → FUSES
CALCANEUS (PRESENT AT BIRTH OR SHORTLY AFTER)
TALUS (PRESENT AT BIRTH OR SHORTLY AFTER)
NAVICULAR
CUBOID (PRESENT AT BIRTH OR SHORTLY AFTER)
CUNEIFORM I
CUNEIFORM II
CUNEIFORM III (OFTEN PRESENT AT BIRTH)
METATARSAL EPIPHYSES (MEDIAL APPEAR FIRST, LATERAL LAST) → FUSE

variable than the onset phase (first appearance of epiphyses).

Four ANABOLIC HORMONES, acting at different stages of development, influence growth and maturation. THYROID HORMONES are important prenatally and during the first years of life, when growth and development are rapid. They continue to influence maturation and (to a lesser extent) growth, throughout development. The PITUITARY GROWTH HORMONE (STH) (somatotropin) is essential for normal growth after the second year of life. Hypopituitary dwarfs and anencephalics are usually of normal size at birth, indicating that STH is not essential at this early age. Although human STH stimulates growth, it does not affect maturation, as is evidenced by the normal bone age in pituitary giants. ANDROGENS, produced by the adrenal cortex in both sexes, by the testes in the male, and, to a small extent, by the ovaries in the female, cause the growth spurt at puberty. Growth is stimulated more by androgens than is maturation. ESTROGENS in females are responsible for closure of the epiphyses, which is preceded by the usual growth spurt. However, recent evidence suggests that growth is due to androgens rather than to estrogens, which tend to affect growth less than maturation. In hypogonadal states the epiphyses fuse late, allowing growth to continue longer than in the normal individual.

The extent of skeletal maturation permits a certain degree of accuracy in predicting the onset of puberty. The adductor, or *first sesamoid,* of the thumb appears approximately 2 years before menarche in normal females. The *epiphyses* of the *distal phalanges* of the *second fingers* usually fuse a few months prior to menarche. The centers for the *crest of the ilium* and the *ischial tuberosity* usually appear within 6 months of the onset of menstruation.

Development and growth are retarded by febrile, nutritional, or chronic illness. Usually, growth is more affected than is maturation, and corresponding centers on the two sides of the body are more frequently asymmetrical. Ossification centers which are more retarded than others indicate illness just before they were due to ossify.

Variations in growth rates may be profitably compared with changes in the rate of maturation. In hypothyroid children, bone age is generally lower than length age, both being retarded. In hypopituitary and constitutional dwarfs and in children with delayed adolescence, length age is more retarded for lack of STH than is bone age.

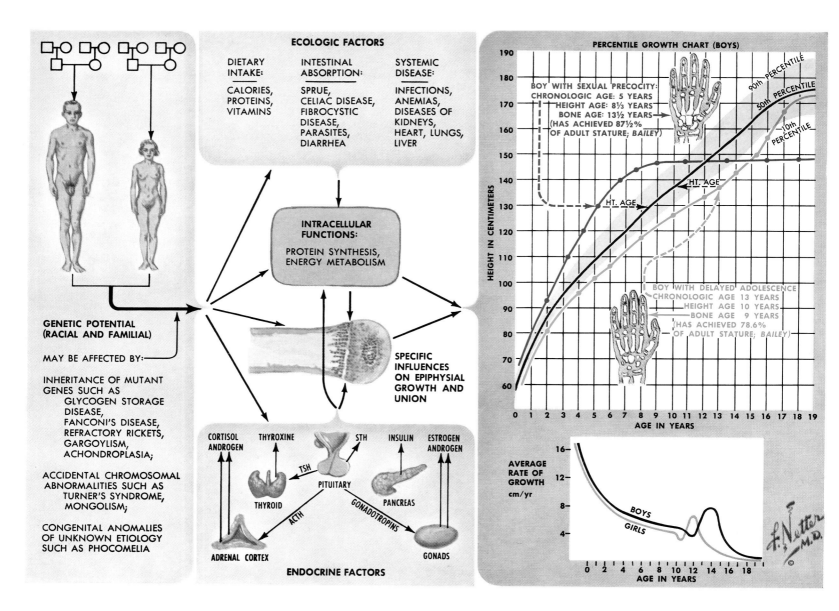

ECOLOGIC FACTORS

DIETARY INTAKE:	INTESTINAL ABSORPTION:	SYSTEMIC DISEASE:
CALORIES, PROTEINS, VITAMINS	SPRUE, CELIAC DISEASE, FIBROCYSTIC DISEASE, PARASITES, DIARRHEA	INFECTIONS, ANEMIAS, DISEASES OF KIDNEYS, HEART, LUNGS, LIVER

GENETIC POTENTIAL (RACIAL AND FAMILIAL)

MAY BE AFFECTED BY:—

INHERITANCE OF MUTANT GENES SUCH AS GLYCOGEN STORAGE DISEASE, FANCONI'S DISEASE, REFRACTORY RICKETS, GARGOYLISM, ACHONDROPLASIA;

ACCIDENTAL CHROMOSOMAL ABNORMALITIES SUCH AS TURNER'S SYNDROME, MONGOLISM;

CONGENITAL ANOMALIES OF UNKNOWN ETIOLOGY SUCH AS PHOCOMELIA

INTRACELLULAR FUNCTIONS: PROTEIN SYNTHESIS, ENERGY METABOLISM

SPECIFIC INFLUENCES ON EPIPHYSIAL GROWTH AND UNION

CORTISOL ANDROGEN — THYROXINE — STH — INSULIN — ESTROGEN ANDROGEN

TSH — PITUITARY — GONADOTROPINS

THYROID — ACTH — PANCREAS

ADRENAL CORTEX — GONADS

ENDOCRINE FACTORS

PERCENTILE GROWTH CHART (BOYS)

BOY WITH SEXUAL PRECOCITY: CHRONOLOGIC AGE: 5 YEARS HEIGHT AGE: 8⅓ YEARS BONE AGE: 13½ YEARS (HAS ACHIEVED 87½% OF ADULT STATURE; BAILEY)

BOY WITH DELAYED ADOLESCENCE CHRONOLOGIC AGE 13 YEARS HEIGHT AGE 10 YEARS BONE AGE 9 YEARS (HAS ACHIEVED 78.6% OF ADULT STATURE; BAILEY)

HT. AGE — 90th PERCENTILE — 50th PERCENTILE — 10th PERCENTILE

HEIGHT IN CENTIMETERS — AGE IN YEARS

AVERAGE RATE OF GROWTH cm/yr — BOYS — GIRLS — AGE IN YEARS

F. Netter M.D.

GROWTH AND DWARFISM

In a general sense, growth simply means the accretion of protoplasm, and it occurs whenever the generation of new cells exceeds the destruction of those already in existence. In short-term studies, growth is usually equated with a positive balance of such protoplasmic constituents as nitrogen, phosphorus, and potassium. The word "growth" is often restricted in its meaning to encompass only statural increments. The growth curves of individual tissues, however, often differ considerably from that of the whole body. Thus, half of the postnatal growth of the brain is accomplished during the first year of life, whereas sexual structures do not enlarge significantly until the second decade. In the discussion which follows, the term "growth" will be used in its restricted longitudinal sense.

Any influence which stimulates anabolism or retards catabolism, in the body as a whole, will normally result in linear growth as long as uncalcified cartilage remains at the junction between the epiphyses and metaphyses of the long bones.

Means of Assessing Growth

The stature ultimately attained is determined both by the rate of linear growth during childhood and by the duration of that growth before epiphysial fusion takes place. Since, in many growth disorders, the rate of *epiphysial maturation* diverges markedly from the rate of *growth*, it is essential that each be assessed independently. Indeed, most endocrine disorders make such a characteristic imprint on *linear growth* and *skeletal maturation* that a suggested diagnosis can often be confirmed or eliminated on these grounds alone.

Linear growth is most often plotted on *cumulative percentile growth charts*, as shown in the upper graph. From such charts the height of a given child can be compared with a standard distribution curve for stature, compiled from a "normal" population of children of similar age. Thus, a 7-year-old child in the tenth percentile ranks tenth in stature among a theoretical population of 100 "normal" children of the same age. His *height age* is that age at which the observed measurement coincides with the median or fiftieth percentile.

Adherence to a constant growth line on the periphery of the normal range is frequently an expression of genetic heritage, whereas a growth curve deviating across percentile channels is likely to have some pathologic basis.

Calculation of *growth rate in centimeters per year*, as shown in the lower graph, provides a more sensitive assessment of current growth performance than do the cumulative growth records. Serial measurements of growth rate are often used to assess the activity of a disease process or the response to a given form of treatment.

The *bone age* is usually determined from roentgenograms of hand, wrist, and other joints by comparing the presence and maturity of the various epiphysial centers with standards which have been compiled for each sex at the various ages. The final stature which a child will ultimately attain may be predicted with some accuracy from his bone age and attained stature.

Determinants of Ultimate Stature

Heredity Versus Environment. In a given child the relative importance of heredity versus environment is difficult to assess. The startling advances in stature exhibited by second-generation Japanese children reared on Western diets emphasize that genetic limitations should never be accepted as inevitable. Even when short stature is genetically determined, the modality of inheritance may be a biochemical error which may yield to appropriate therapy. Vitamin-D-resistant *rickets* and *Fanconi's disease* are such examples.

Endocrine Factors. PITUITARY GROWTH HORMONE (*STH*) is a powerful stimulant of protein anabolism and is the only hormone which increases the rate of growth without bringing about a net decrease in ultimate stature (see page 28). Growth hormone seems to work synergistically with *insulin* in bringing about growth.

THYROID HORMONE, likewise, is indispensable for both bone maturation and growth to take place. The dwarfism and skeletal retardation seen in congenital hypothyroidism are fully as profound as in panhypopituitarism. On the other hand, an excess of thyroid hormone in juvenile

(Continued on page 229)

GROWTH AND DWARFISM

(Continued from page 228)

thyrotoxicosis stimulates only a mild increase in stature and bone age. *Thyroxine,* thus, is not a true growth stimulant. Its rôle in growth and development, however, illustrates strikingly the "permissive" action which many hormones exert on physiologic functions.

ANDROGENS are potent growth stimulators and are responsible, at least in part, for the adolescent growth spurt in both boys and girls. Since androgens exert a relatively greater effect on skeletal maturation than they do on linear growth, they shorten the growing period by hastening epiphysial fusion. When pathologic virilization occurs in childhood, the net effect is to curtail ultimate stature.

Most of the so-called "protein anabolic stimulants" are, in reality, weak androgens which tend to accelerate bone age somewhat disproportionately to their effect on growth. This discrepancy is often obscured in short-term studies by a lag in the radiologic manifestations of epiphysial maturation.

ESTROGENS stimulate growth when administered to prepuberal girls, but it is not clear whether this is a primary effect or is due to the secondarily increased secretion of adrenal androgens. There is little doubt, however, that estrogens stimulate epiphysial maturation much more than they do growth. This accounts, at least in part, for the shorter stature of women when contrasted with that of men.

CORTISOL and similar glucocorticoids bring about a state of protein catabolism when present in excess and, hence, retard both growth and skeletal maturation. Following the withdrawal from corticosteroid excess, there is usually a compensatory growth spurt during which many of these deficiencies are made up.

Etiologic Factors of Growth Failure

In a broad sense, any child who fails to achieve his full genetic potential for growth may be considered to be dwarfed, even though his growth retardation does not lead to conspicuously short stature. In evaluating any short child, the physician must differentiate between intrinsic growth potential and extrinsic factors which may be limiting the attainment of this potential.

Dwarfism Due to Endocrine Disorders. Since the endocrine system plays such a dominant rôle in governing the rhythm of growth and the rate of maturation, endocrine disturbances are usually suspected first when a child fails to develop normally. In actuality, endocrine abnormalities are among the least common causes of dwarfism. HYPOTHYROIDISM (see page 61) and HYPOPITUITARISM (see page 20) are the most serious causes of endocrine dwarfism. Ultimate limitation of adult stature is also caused by sexual precocity of whatever cause (see pages 118 and 119).

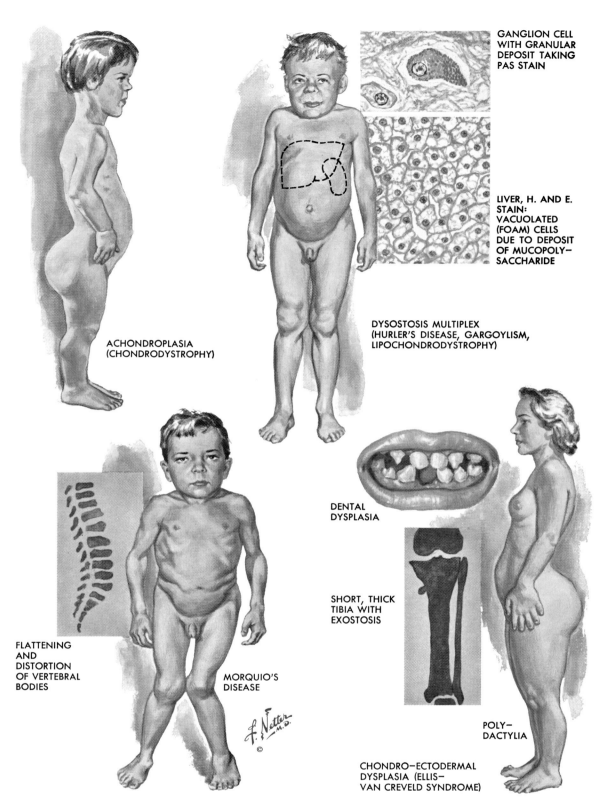

GANGLION CELL WITH GRANULAR DEPOSIT TAKING PAS STAIN

LIVER, H. AND E. STAIN: VACUOLATED (FOAM) CELLS DUE TO DEPOSIT OF MUCOPOLY- SACCHARIDE

ACHONDROPLASIA (CHONDRODYSTROPHY)

DYSOSTOSIS MULTIPLEX (HURLER'S DISEASE, GARGOYLISM, LIPOCHONDRODYSTROPHY)

FLATTENING AND DISTORTION OF VERTEBRAL BODIES

MORQUIO'S DISEASE

DENTAL DYSPLASIA

SHORT, THICK TIBIA WITH EXOSTOSIS

POLY- DACTYLIA

CHONDRO–ECTODERMAL DYSPLASIA (ELLIS– VAN CREVELD SYNDROME)

The short stature which occurs in the SYNDROMES OF GONADAL DYSGENESIS (see page 128) and PSEUDO-HYPOPARATHYROIDISM (see pages 187 and 188) cannot be accounted for by the endocrine disorders which are regularly present. In these conditions the apparent intrinsic limitation in growth potential is mediated, at least in the former case, through a faulty chromosomal make-up.

Dwarfism Due to Primary Bone Disease. Before *diets* were liberally supplemented with vitamin D, mild rickets affected many children in northern latitudes. The increase in stature of modern children over that of their parents may be due, in part, to the abolition of VITAMIN-D-DEFICIENT RICKETS. Most of the skeletal diseases which today cause dwarfism are due to inborn errors of metabolism or chromosomal anomalies.

VITAMIN-D-RESISTANT RICKETS (see page 192),

a hereditary disorder, is being recognized with increasing frequency as a cause of short stature. Mildly affected individuals often exhibit only a low serum phosphorus and short stature, with no obvious deformity of the extremities.

ACHONDROPLASIA is a hereditary disorder of cartilage which produces irregular and distorted calcification of the epiphyses and exceedingly short extremities. Afflicted individuals characteristically have a relatively elongated trunk, large head, and flat nose. Prominence of the buttocks is caused by an upward tilt of the sacrum.

OSTEOGENESIS IMPERFECTA results from an inborn error in the formation of collagen, both in the organic bone matrix and in connective tissue elsewhere, which explains the characteristic blue sclerae and the deafness often associated with the bone disease. The

(Continued on page 230)

GROWTH AND DWARFISM

(Continued from page 229)

severe osteoporosis causes many pathologic fractures, often unrecognized. The severe stunting of growth is brought about by almost literal "telescoping of the skeleton".

The mucopolysaccharide component of cartilage and the organic matrix of bone is abnormal in DYSOSTOSIS MULTIPLEX (HURLER'S DISEASE). In this hereditary disorder, abnormal collections of *mucopolysaccharide* accumulate in the skin, bones, brain, eyes, and visceral organs, including the heart, presenting as *foam cells*. The grotesque appearance of the face is responsible for the descriptive term, *gargoylism*.

OSTEOCHONDRODYSTROPHY (MORQUIO'S DISEASE) is a familial skeletal disorder in which the *vertebrae* are *flattened*, thus producing a spine which is shortened and greatly deformed. The epiphyses of the long bones are likewise distorted, giving rise to genu valgum and other deformities of the extremities.

CHONDRO-ECTODERMAL DYSPLASIA (ELLIS-VAN CREVELD SYNDROME) is similar to chondrodystrophy, but, in addition, there may be polydactylia, ectodermal dysplasia *such as a short tibia, dysplasia of the teeth,* and congenital malformations of the heart. The hair may be sparse, and some patients have difficulty with temperature regulation owing to involvement of their sweat glands.

Dwarfism Due to Systemic Disorders. Dwarfism may be caused by any disorder which limits the availability or *absorption* of food, hinders its transport to the periphery, or interferes with its utilization. Malabsorption syndromes may be due to *cystic fibrosis* of the pancreas, intolerance to wheat gluten (*celiac disease*), specific deficiencies in the intestinal saccharases, *parasitic infestations*, and many other causes.

In many diseases dwarfism may be produced by more than one mechanism. An example is that of *congenital heart disease,* where there is often a primary limitation in *caloric intake* as well as a vascular anomaly which deprives the tissues of both food and oxygen. In addition, however, there may be an underlying chromosomal anomaly responsible for both the heart lesion and the short stature. Such patients may fail to take their expected growth spurt after successful surgical correction of the heart lesion.

Although most systemic diseases severe enough to cause growth retardation can be readily detected by a careful history and physical examination, the presence of renal disease may be easily overlooked. Renal dwarfism may be caused either by malformation or obstruction of the urinary tract, or by an inherited disorder of tubular function, *e.g., renal tubular acidosis*.

Primordial Dwarfism. *Primordial dwarfism* is the rather unsatisfactory designation given those individuals who appear

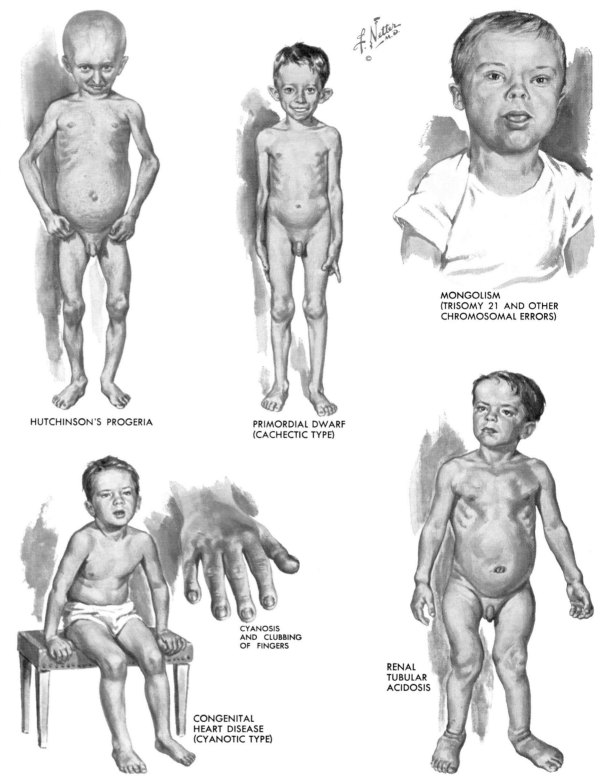

HUTCHINSON'S PROGERIA

PRIMORDIAL DWARF (CACHECTIC TYPE)

MONGOLISM (TRISOMY 21 AND OTHER CHROMOSOMAL ERRORS)

CYANOSIS AND CLUBBING OF FINGERS

CONGENITAL HEART DISEASE (CYANOTIC TYPE)

RENAL TUBULAR ACIDOSIS

to have some constitutional limitation in their growth potential not explainable on the basis of any known skeletal abnormality, endocrine disorder, or systemic ailment. It may occur as the result of either a *mutant gene,* an abnormal intra-uterine environment, or a gross *chromosomal anomaly. Mongolism* is typical of the latter category and is due either to trisomy of one of the small chromosomes (21 or 22) (see page 224) or to translocation of a small trisomic chromosome onto a larger chromosome in the 13-to-15 group. Frequently, such children are small at birth, even though born at term. Undoubtedly, many mechanisms are responsible for primordial dwarfism, and this category encompasses such dissimilar groups as pygmy tribes, patients with Mongolism, and otherwise normal individuals with familial short stature.

A number of distinctive syndromes have been described in which primordial dwarfism is associated with other characteristic congenital defects. *Progeria,* or the Hutchinson-Gilford syndrome, is characterized by *dwarfism,* premature senility, *alopecia,* atherosclerosis, and *atrophy of the subcutaneous fat* on the face and body. The weird *old-young appearance* of these children is strikingly similar in all cases.

Many primordial dwarfs have birdlike facial features and a cachectic appearance superficially resembling that in progeria. Mental deficiency is common, and numerous designations have been applied to subgroups which have various features in common.

The diagnosis of primordial dwarfism in a child with poor growth performance simply implies that the mechanism is poorly understood. No comfort should be derived from using this term unless all remediable causes of dwarfism have been fully explored and excluded.

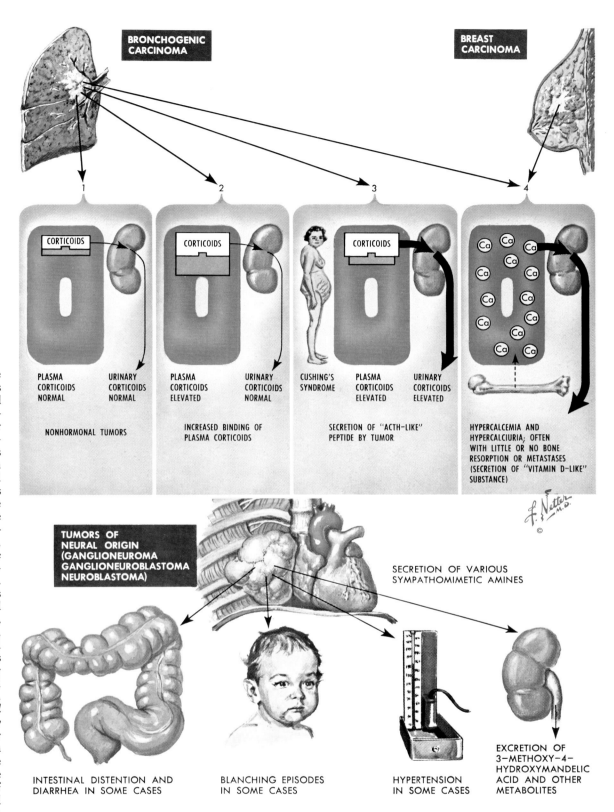

MALIGNANCIES WITH HORMONAL SECRETIONS

The sex difference in the incidence of *bronchogenic carcinoma* has always fascinated the endocrinologist interested in hormonal therapy of tumors. Unfortunately, to date, estrogen therapy for bronchogenic carcinoma has been disappointing. However, many patients with bronchogenic carcinomas have been found to have substantial hormonal abnormalities induced by products secreted into the blood stream by the tumor. Although many such tumors have no effect on the endocrine system, striking instances of *Cushing's syndrome,* caused by secretion of an *ACTH-like peptide* by the oat cell type of bronchogenic carcinoma, are occasionally seen. These patients have an enormous hyperplasia of the adrenals and marked hypersecretion of normal *corticoids,* which are then *elevated* in the *plasma,* spill over in the *urine,* and produce all the signs and symptoms of Cushing's syndrome. On the other hand, many pulmonary tumors produce a material capable of the *binding of plasma cortisol,* which results in greatly *elevated bound plasma corticoids* and *normal urinary corticoids,* as found characteristically in pregnancy or in patients on estrogen therapy. Many patients with this type of bronchogenic carcinoma are unable to respond adequately to the stress of thoracotomy because of the increased binding material which leaves inadequate amounts of physiologically active cortisol available. The surgical morbidity in such patients can be definitely reduced by preoperative preparation with cortisol or its derivatives. As a guide for the administration of these hormones, we employ a water-loading test, to which such patients give an Addisonianlike response. There are also patients who actually have Addison's disease (hypo-adrenalism) induced not by some secretion from the carcinoma but by metastatic destruction of the adrenals.

Pulmonary carcinoma, mammary carcinoma, and some other tumors apparently secrete a material physiologically similar to *vitamin D* or parathyroid hormone. If not adequately controlled, this produces *hypercalcemia, hypercalciuria,* and their accompanying difficulties. Fortunately, this abnormality can frequently be managed by the administration of liberal amounts of cortisol or its derivatives.

Rarely, a carcinoid syndrome is caused by a bronchogenic carcinoma.

Occasionally, patients with a bronchogenic carcinoma show hemodilution and edema due to excessive water retention through an inappropriate ADH (antidiuretic hormone) mechanism. An ADH-like peptide has, in fact, been isolated from such tumors. These are most of the inappropriate hormonal activities which can be ascribed to bronchogenic carcinoma.

Many *tumors of neural origin,* including *neuroblastoma,* pheochromocytoma, and *ganglioneuroma,* produce various *sympathomimetic amines.* Frequently, the physiologic consequences of such production are seen in the patient. These can be episodic or continuous, producing *diarrhea* or perhaps *episodes of blanching* accompanied by *hypertension* and perspiration, with *excretion of metabolites* of sympathomimetic amines in the urine. The most accurately measured, at present, is *3-methoxy-4-hydroxymandelic acid* (MHMA, vanyl mandelic acid, or VMA). This is a major metabolite excreted in much greater quantity and is much more stable than are the catecholamines (see page 105). Such symptoms, together with an elevation of the urinary excretion of catecholamines or of MHMA, should make one search vigorously for a tumor of neural origin.

The secretion of serotonin by carcinoid tumors is discussed in *Lower Digestive Tract* (see CIBA COLLECTION, Vol. 3/II, page 165). Tumors which produce a gastrinlike substance, causing the Zollinger-Ellison syndrome, may be found on page 159 of this volume.

HORMONAL TREATMENT OF CANCER OF THE BREAST

Although much has been written recently on the adequacy of simple mastectomy and massive radiation in the treatment of cancer of the breast, good clinical practice currently dictates radical mastectomy as the basic treatment for this disease. The cure rate depends on how early the primary lesion is extirpated. With tumors of a superficial organ like the breast, it is regrettable that most of them are not removed while they are still small and curable. On the other hand, it is fortunate that this common malignant lesion is frequently amenable to palliative therapy, because of a basic biologic difference between the tumor and the host, when radical extirpation has failed to halt the rapid growth of the tumor or when a known lesion has been neglected.

In *premenopausal women* who have *recurrences or metastatic spread,* the therapy of choice is *castration,* either surgically or by radiation. In *hormonally sensitive tumors, objective regression occurs. Hormonally insensitive tumors* should be treated with *oncolytic chemotherapy.* Probably among the best present choices are 5-fluoro-uracil or an alkylating agent such as nitrogen mustard. The first line of defense against local recurrences should be local irradiation. Furthermore, patients with painful osteolytic lesions, located in a position where fracture is threatened, often obtain permanent relief of pain and may be saved from sustaining fractures by the judicious use of local radiation.

In premenopausal patients or those with hormonally sensitive tumors in whom *renewed progression* of the disease follows objective improvement after castration, *androgen* is the therapy of choice. There is now evidence that the *objective regression* of metastatic or recurrent tumors, accomplished with androgens, is accompanied by a gratifying increase in longevity as well as subjective improvement. Indeed, more patients show substantial subjective improvement, and failure of the disease to progress, than show objective regression. After the androgen-induced objective regression has run its course, the patient should be given *other hormonal agents* effective against cancer of the breast, viz., estrogens, progestational agents, or different androgens.

Patients with hormonally sensitive tumors, who live in localities with adequate facilities for preoperative and postoperative care for their lifetime corticoid-maintenance needs, have an excellent chance of objective regression and prolongation of life following *hypophysectomy* or *adrenalectomy* requiring substitution therapy. If such facilities are not available, other hormonal agents or

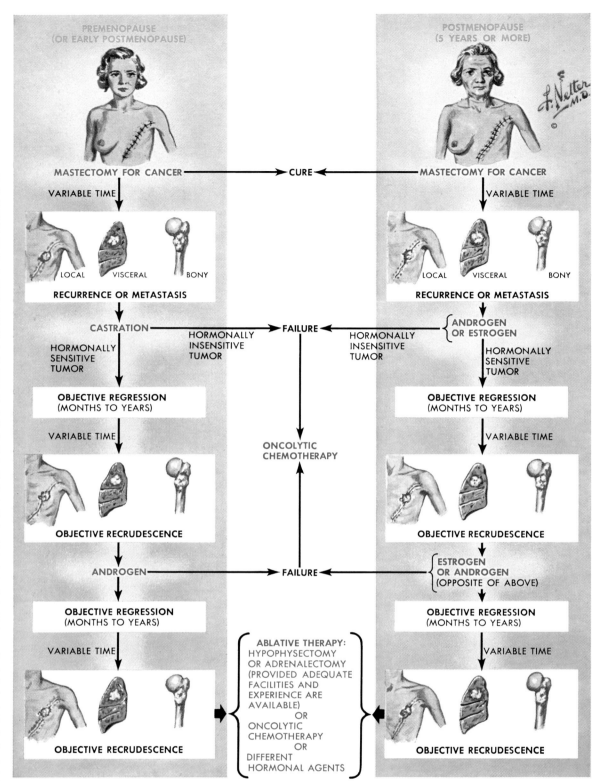

oncolytic chemotherapy may be employed.

In the *postmenopausal patient* (anyone who has menstruated within 1 year is considered premenopausal) who has a *recurrence,* castration is not sufficiently beneficial to be recommended. Therapy should immediately be started with *androgens or estrogens,* in order to determine whether the tumor is hormonally sensitive. For *insensitive* tumors *oncolytic chemotherapy* is indicated, as in the premenopausal patient. After the *sensitive* tumor no longer responds to the administration of one hormone, the *opposite sex hormone* should be tried. Thereafter, the plan is the same as for premenopausal patients. The demonstrated hormonally sensitive tumor may benefit further from other types of hormonal therapy or *ablative therapy* in the proper circumstances, and, finally, all tumors may respond favorably to judicious oncolytic chemotherapy.

Adrenal cortical hormones, as a primary means of hormonal therapy for advancing cancer of the breast, do not produce a high enough remission rate to warrant their use solely for this purpose. However, in certain situations they are the agents of choice. For example, late in the course of the advanced disease, after all hormonal and chemotherapeutic agents have been tried and when pain and anorexia are a major problem, corticoids often produce substantial subjective improvement.

Hypercalcemia is a frequent complication of cancer of the breast. Corticoids have proved successful, in a high percentage of patients, when administration of adequate fluids and ambulation (if possible) failed to lower the elevated serum calcium concentration. The dosage is frequently substantial, though it can be reduced as a decrease in the serum calcium concentration takes place.

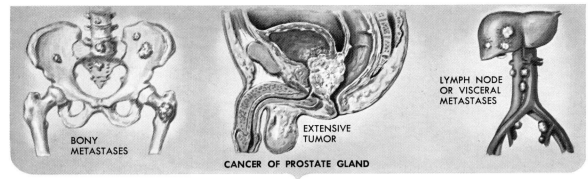

BONY METASTASES

EXTENSIVE TUMOR

LYMPH NODE OR VISCERAL METASTASES

CANCER OF PROSTATE GLAND

HORMONAL TREATMENT OF VARIOUS CANCERS

ANCILLARY THERAPY:

URINARY TRACT SURGERY TO MAINTAIN PASSAGEWAY

RADIATION THERAPY

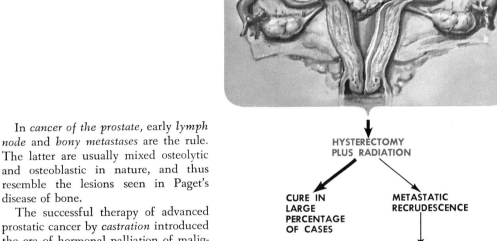

CASTRATION — ESTROGENS

FAILURE

REGRESSION (MONTHS TO YEARS)

VARIABLE TIME

RECRUDESCENCE

REGRESSION (MONTHS TO YEARS)

VARIABLE TIME

RECRUDESCENCE

FAILURE

OTHER TYPES OF HORMONAL THERAPY (OTHER ESTROGENS, ANDROGENS, ANABOLIC AGENTS, CORTICOIDS, PROGESTATIONAL AGENTS)
OR
ONCOLYTIC CHEMOTHERAPY IN CAUTIOUS DOSAGE BECAUSE OF REDUCED BONE MARROW RESERVE DUE TO INVOLVEMENT BY TUMOR

CANCER OF ENDOMETRIUM

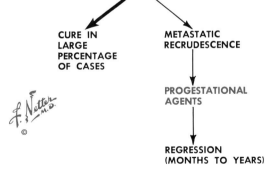

ACUTE LEUKEMIA

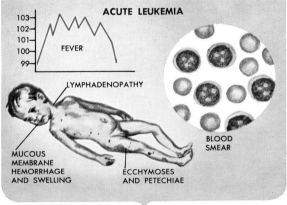

FEVER

LYMPHADENOPATHY

BLOOD SMEAR

MUCOUS MEMBRANE HEMORRHAGE AND SWELLING

ECCHYMOSES AND PETECHIAE

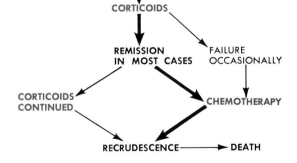

HYSTERECTOMY PLUS RADIATION

CURE IN LARGE PERCENTAGE OF CASES

METASTATIC RECRUDESCENCE

PROGESTATIONAL AGENTS

REGRESSION (MONTHS TO YEARS)

CORTICOIDS

REMISSION IN MOST CASES

FAILURE OCCASIONALLY

CORTICOIDS CONTINUED

CHEMOTHERAPY

RECRUDESCENCE → DEATH

In *cancer of the prostate*, early *lymph node* and *bony metastases* are the rule. The latter are usually mixed osteolytic and osteoblastic in nature, and thus resemble the lesions seen in Paget's disease of bone.

The successful therapy of advanced prostatic cancer by *castration* introduced the era of hormonal palliation of malignant disease. If castration cannot be carried out initially, *estrogen administration* is employed, even though the results do not appear to be as good as with castration and the inevitable recrudescence after castration cannot be countered with estrogen therapy, this being of value only when castration has been the initial treatment.

After one or both of these types of therapy, the physician can use *other hormonal agents* or cautious *oncolytic chemotherapy*. The dosage of oncolytic agents, which also produce marrow damage, is greatly limited in patients with prostatic carcinoma, because of the high percentage of invasion or destruction of the bone marrow by this tumor.

Although prostatic carcinoma is more common in older men, it is usually associated with substantial longevity. *Surgical correction of urinary obstruction,* local *radiation therapy* to bone, and orthopedic procedures to support impaired

bone are important adjuncts to hormonal therapy.

In *cancer of the endometrium*, metastases to the ovaries and lung occur relatively late. The Papanicolaou smear technique permits early recognition of the disease. The standard combination therapy of *surgical excision* and *radiation* has resulted in a gratifyingly *high percentage of cure* in endometrial cancer. There are still, however, an unfortunate number of these patients who have *metastases,* particularly to the lung. A wide variety of active *progestational agents,* ranging from progesterone preparations to 19-norsteroid derivatives, have now been shown to produce objective *regression* of these metastatic tumors in a reasonably high percentage of patients.

The *child with acute leukemia* is seriously ill and a pitiful sight, with *fever*, malaise, and general mor-

bidity. *Lymphadenopathy* is marked. Occasionally, infection accounts for the symptoms. A bleeding tendency leads to *mucous membrane hemorrhage, ecchymoses,* and *petechiae*. Terminally, massive gastro-intestinal hemorrhages may occur. Probably the commonest most severe and uncontrollable hemorrhage, leading to death in these individuals,. is intracranial. Administration of active *corticosteroids,* such as cortisol or one of its modern derivatives, or ACTH in fairly large amounts, produces a *high percentage* of complete *remissions* with relief of symptoms. In many of these patients, remission can be prolonged or another remission can be induced by the use of *chemotherapy,* either alone or with *corticoids,* particularly certain of the antimetabolites such as 6-mercaptopurine.

Section IX

INBORN ERRORS OF METABOLISM

by

FRANK H. NETTER, M.D.

in collaboration with

JOSEPH J. BUNIM, M.D.
Plates 1 and 2

ALEXANDER B. GUTMAN, M.D., Ph.D.
Plates 3-5

KURT J. ISSELBACHER, M.D.
Plates 10 and 11

FELIX O. KOLB, M.D.
and
LLOYD H. SMITH, M.D.
Plates 6 and 7

FRANK H. TYLER, M.D.
Plates 8 and 9

OCHRONOSIS

Alkaptonuria, an inherited metabolic disease, results from a deficiency of the enzyme *homogentisic acid oxidase;* it is characterized by *homogentisic acid* in the urine. Ochronosis is a later stage of alkaptonuria; in it, the connective tissue is stained brown-black as a result of deposits of melanin-like pigment, a polymer of homogentisic acid. Ochronotic spondylosis and arthropathy comprise a degenerative joint disease resulting from pigment deposits in cartilage and affecting, primarily, the intervertebral disks of the spine and the articular cartilage of large peripheral joints.

The basic lesion consists of *deposition of melanin-like pigment* in the connective tissue of various body structures, such as *sclera* and *cornea,* tympanic membrane and *pinna of ear,* cartilages of larynx and trachea, *valves of the heart* and *intima of the aorta,* interstitial tissue of prostate and kidneys and, most disabling of all, in *fibro-* and *hyaline cartilages of intervertebral disks* and *large peripheral joints.*

Degenerative joint disease in ochronosis, as in primary osteo-arthritis, originates in the articular cartilage. Pigment appears diffusely in the matrix, principally in the deeper (radial) zones of the cartilage, which becomes brittle, fibrillated, and fragmented. The gross appearance of the articular surface is striking. While the greater area of the surface is intact, glistening, and gray, a *black, deeper layer* is visible through it. At some points the cartilage is *ulcerated,* and the black layer is exposed. In more-advanced stages, white, smooth, *eburnated bone* appears at the base of the *chondral crater.* Sharp-edged pieces of cartilage break off and become embedded in synovial tissue. Synovial lining cells may then undergo metaplasia, become chondrocytes and proliferate. Masses of chondrocytes engulf fragments of displaced, pigmented cartilage and form a *synovial polyp.* Several polyps may appear in one joint, most commonly in the knee. A polyp may become vascularized, calcified, and ultimately ossified, presenting as an *osteochondroma.*

In the spine the *intervertebral disk* becomes first deeply *pigmented* and later *calcified, ossified,* or destroyed. The subchondral bone becomes sclerotic, and *adjacent vertebrae* may *fuse.* Calcific deposits in the intervertebral spaces are seen on *X-ray* as characteristic *radiopaque wafers.* Destruction of the disks may result in reduction of the patient's height by as much as 6 inches.

It has been demonstrated that, in the liver and kidneys of patients with alkaptonuria, homogentisic acid oxidase, the extremely specific enzyme that catalyzes the oxidative cleavage of the benzene ring in homogentisic acid, yielding *maleylaceto-acetic acid,* is totally absent. All other enzymes necessary for the catabolism of *phenylalanine* and *tyrosine* to *aceto-acetic acid* and *fumaric acid*

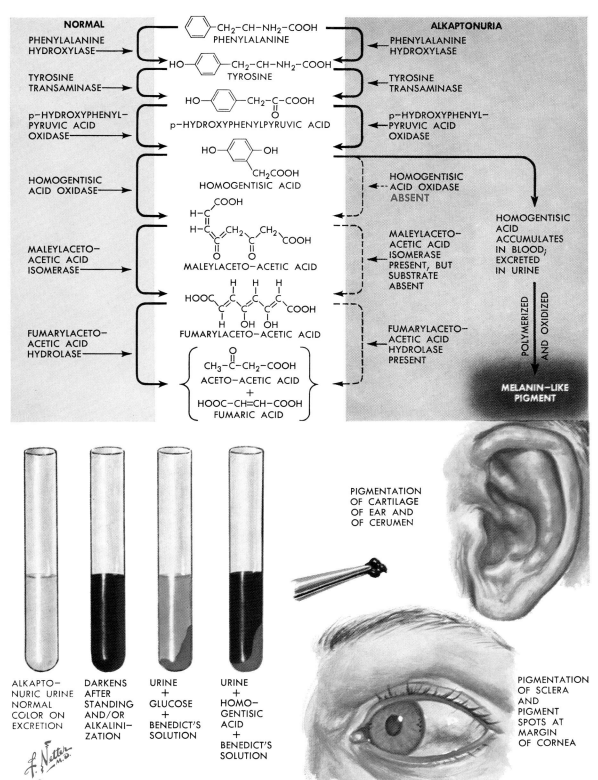

PIGMENTATION OF CARTILAGE OF EAR AND OF CERUMEN

PIGMENTATION OF SCLERA AND PIGMENT SPOTS AT MARGIN OF CORNEA

are present. As a result of this enzyme deficiency, oxidation of homogentisic acid is blocked, and this substance accumulates in the serum and tissues. Homogentisic acid has an unusually high affinity for skin and cartilage. Whereas this acid binds physically to proteins and collagen, the quinone form of homogentisic acid, *viz.,* benzoquinone-acetic acid (BOA) reacts chemically with homogenates of skin and cartilage in vitro. This product resembles the ochronotic pigmentation of connective tissue seen in patients with alkaptonuria. The melanin-like pigment deposited in ochronosis thus may very likely be a polymer of BOA bound chemically to macromolecules of connective tissue.

Alkaptonuria is transmitted as a single autosomal recessive gene. Historically, this disorder is one of the earliest classical illustrations of the correlation of a single gene to a single enzyme defect.

A child afflicted with alkaptonuria remains symptom-free until adult life, when he develops ochronosis. During this stage the diagnosis is suspected on the basis of a family history and a report that, in infancy, the patient's diaper or, later, his underwear was stained black. Freshly passed urine is of normal color but, *on standing,* gradually turns *brownish-black* as the homogentisic acid is oxidized. When, however, the *urine is alkalinized* with sodium hydroxide, it promptly turns *black.* When *Benedict's reagent* is used for routine testing of glucosuria, a *yellow-orange precipitate* (frequently mistaken for glucose) is formed, because the copper in Benedict's solution is reduced by the homogentisic acid. However, the *supernatant solution is black,* which is diagnostic of alkaptonuria.

The sites of relatively early ochronotic pigmenta-
(Continued on page 238)

OCHRONOSIS

(Continued from page 237)

tion which can be readily recognized clinically are the eye, ear, skin, and genito-urinary tract. In the sclera a small area of *brownish discoloration* first appears about midway between the *limbus* and *canthus* on either the nasal or temporal or on both sides of cornea. In the ear, cartilage in the pinna takes on a bluish discoloration, a thickened, stiff texture, and an opaque appearance, on transillumination, quite early in the course of ochronosis. The *cerumen* is densely black, and the ear drum and ossicles also may be discolored. Hearing is occasionally impaired, and some patients complain of tinnitus. A brownish hue may be noted in the malar areas of the face, as well as in the axilla and genital regions where sweat glands are numerous. The sweat is discolored and stains clothing brown. In the genito-urinary tract, stones may form in the prostate and, less frequently, in the kidneys of both men and women. Soft, black prostatic calculi can be felt by rectal examination and, when calcified, can be seen by abdominal X-ray or intravenous pyelogram.

Ochronotic arthropathy, usually more severe in males, occurs in the spine and large peripheral joints; the knees, shoulders, and hips are most commonly affected and begin to present symptoms, in that sequence, at about the fourth decade of life. The course of spondylosis and arthropathy is chronic and progressive; many patients become totally disabled when they reach the age of 60 years.

In about 20 per cent of male patients with spondylosis, the onset occurs with acute herniation of the intervertebral disks, giving rise to symptoms that are indistinguishable from the common acute disk syndrome. In most patients the onset is gradual, with dull aching pain in the lower back. First, the lumbar and, later, the thoracic spine becomes stiff; range of motion is reduced and, eventually, lost. The normal lumbar lordosis is obliterated and, indeed, mild *kyphosis* may develop in this region. The stance and gait of the patient are quite typical and resemble those of patients with ankylosing spondylitis. The patient *stands on a broad base*, his *knees and hips flexed* and his *trunk stooped forward*. He walks slowly and stiffly, without flexing or rotating his lower spine. Roentgenograms reveal a characteristic calcification of the intervertebral disks, with narrowing of these spaces, later sclerosis and eburnation at the borders of vertebral bodies and, finally, in some cases bony fusion.

The peripheral joints become involved several years after spondylosis has developed. The knees, shoulders, and hips are affected, in descending order of frequency. It is noteworthy that the small joints of the hands and feet escape involvement. Symptoms in the affected joints usually develop gradually and con-

TYPICAL NARROWING AND CALCIFICATION OF INTERVERTEBRAL DISKS, WITHOUT INVOLVEMENT OF SACRO—ILIAC JOINTS

PIGMENTATION, CALCIFICATION AND OSSIFICATION OF INTERVERTEBRAL DISKS, AND FUSION OF VERTEBRAE

OCHRONOTIC PIGMENTATION OF CARTILAGE ON FEMORAL HEAD; UNDERLYING BONE NORMAL

FEMORAL CONDYLE

PATELLA

EBURNATION

OSTEOCHONDROMA

SEMILUNAR CARTILAGE

ULCERATION

EXPOSURE OF KNEE JOINT: PIGMENTATION, EBURNATION AND ULCERATION OF CARTILAGES; OSTEOCHONDROMA WITH PEDICLE TO SYNOVIAL LINING

CHARACTERISTIC POSTURE IN ADVANCED OCHRONOTIC SPONDYLITIS: KYPHOSIS, RIGID SPINE, FLEXED KNEES, WIDE BASE

PIGMENTATION OF ENDOCARDIUM

sist of pain, stiffness, and restricted range of motion. Synovial effusions in the knees occur frequently, and the fluid contains homogentisic acid. Free or *pedunculated osteochondral bodies* may develop in the knees. They are easily palpable, quite movable and may present at any border or surface of the joint.

The diagnosis of alkaptonuria or ochronosis is missed initially in about 1 of 3 cases. A specific enzymatic method for quantitative determination of homogentisic acid in urine and plasma has recently been developed. Homogentisic acid is not normally present in plasma, urine, or synovial fluid. Calcification of the intervertebral disks of the lumbar vertebrae, seen on roentgenogram, is typical of ochronotic spondylosis. The *sacro-iliac joints appear normal*, and calcification of the spinal ligaments is absent. Changes, seen by X-ray, of affected peripheral joints are not diagnostic. The presence of homogentisic

acid in synovial fluid clinches the diagnosis.

The differential diagnosis must take into consideration that porphyria, myoglobulinuria, hemoglobulinuria, and melaninuria are associated with dark-colored urine, but homogentisic acid is not present in the urine in these cases. Spondylitis of Marie-Strümpell type (ankylosing spondylitis) is readily distinguishable from the ochronotic type by the absence of calcified intervertebral disks and by the presence of calcified vertebral ligaments and the fusion of sacro-iliac joints. Rheumatoid arthritis is characterized by a positive serological test for rheumatoid factor, frequent involvement of small joints of the hands and feet and an absence of homogentisic acid from synovial fluid and urine.

No effective means of correcting or overcoming the inherited enzyme deficiency of this disease is known at present.

Uric Acid Metabolism, Gout

Gout is conveniently defined as a metabolic disorder characterized by hyperuricemia, recurrent attacks of acute arthritis and a tendency to *deposition of urate* in predisposed tissues (*tophi*) and in the urinary tract (*calculi*). In primary (classical) gout the metabolic error is inborn and is presumed, as in other inborn errors of metabolism, to reflect a genetically transmitted enzyme deficiency, resulting in hyperuricemia. Gout occasionally may be acquired (secondary gout) as a complication of some underlying, usually hematopoietic, disorder in which there are augmented formation and degradation of nucleic acids and hence of purines, including uric acid.

The uric acid of the body is derived, in part, from preformed *nucleoproteins* taken in the diet, particularly *liver, pancreas,* and *kidney;* the protein moieties are split off by the gastric juice; in the small intestine the ribo- and deoxyribonucleic acids (*RNA* and *DNA*) thus liberated are hydrolyzed by pancreatic nucleases to nucleotides, which are then dephosphorylated by intestinal nucleotidases to nucleosides, for absorption as *exogenous purines.* The major part of the body's uric acid, however, except when the intake of preformed purines is excessive, derives from de novo purine biosynthesis, probably chiefly in the liver. This formation of *endogenous purines* ordinarily is particularly dependent on the amount of *protein ingested,* since, except for high-purine meals, a high-protein intake most markedly increases uric acid formation. In the sequential enzymatic reactions leading to creation of the purine molecule, *glycine* contributes atoms C-4, C-5, and N-7; the amide nitrogen of *glutamine,* N-3 and N-9; *aspartic acid,* N-1; *carbon dioxide,* C-6; and the *"formyl"* of a tetrahydrofolic acid derivative, C-2 and C-8. The first purine thus synthesized is inosinic acid, which is converted to other nucleotides, containing *adenine* and *guanine,* in the formation of polynucleotides such as the endogenous nucleic acids. Uric acid, a nitrogenous waste, is produced via *xanthine* and *hypoxanthine* by xanthine oxidase. Because human tissues lack uricase (unlike the tissues of most other mammals), the rather insoluble uric acid cannot be transformed into the highly soluble allantoin. Turnover studies with isotopically labeled uric acid indicate that normal man, taking a moderately restricted diet, elaborates, on the average, about 750 mg of uric acid a day. Of this quantity, about 500 mg of uric acid are *excreted in the urine,* by a process

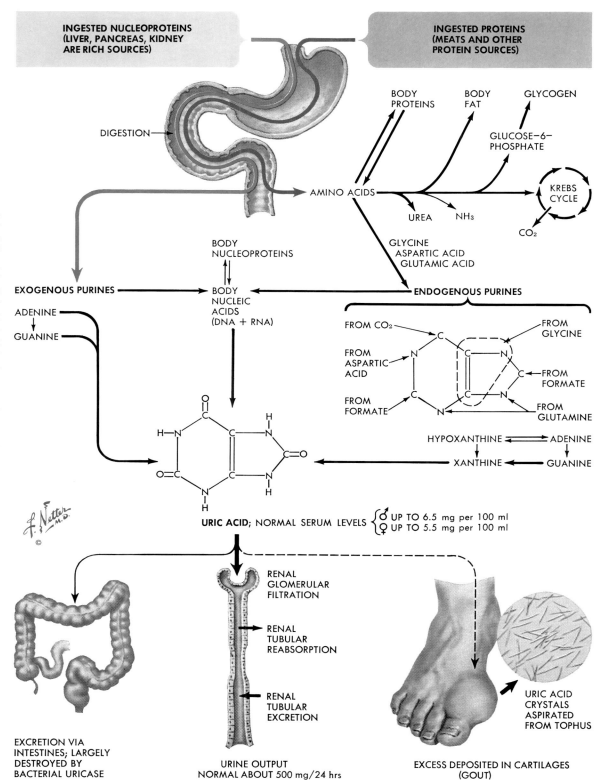

INGESTED NUCLEOPROTEINS (LIVER, PANCREAS, KIDNEY ARE RICH SOURCES)

INGESTED PROTEINS (MEATS AND OTHER PROTEIN SOURCES)

DIGESTION

BODY PROTEINS   BODY FAT   GLYCOGEN

GLUCOSE–6–PHOSPHATE

AMINO ACIDS   KREBS CYCLE

UREA NH_3 CO_2

GLYCINE ASPARTIC ACID GLUTAMIC ACID

BODY NUCLEOPROTEINS

EXOGENOUS PURINES

BODY NUCLEIC ACIDS (DNA + RNA)

ENDOGENOUS PURINES

ADENINE

GUANINE

FROM CO_2 FROM GLYCINE

FROM ASPARTIC ACID

FROM FORMATE

FROM FORMATE   FROM GLUTAMINE

HYPOXANTHINE ⇌ ADENINE

XANTHINE ← GUANINE

URIC ACID; NORMAL SERUM LEVELS { ♂ UP TO 6.5 mg per 100 ml / ♀ UP TO 5.5 mg per 100 ml

RENAL GLOMERULAR FILTRATION

RENAL TUBULAR REABSORPTION

RENAL TUBULAR EXCRETION

EXCRETION VIA INTESTINES; LARGELY DESTROYED BY BACTERIAL URICASE

URINE OUTPUT NORMAL ABOUT 500 mg/24 hrs

URIC ACID CRYSTALS ASPIRATED FROM TOPHUS

EXCESS DEPOSITED IN CARTILAGES (GOUT)

involving *filtration at the glomerulus,* active *tubular reabsorption* of the filtered uric acid, and active *tubular secretion;* the remainder is chiefly eliminated by way of the gut, where it is degraded by the *uricase* of the intestinal bacteria. The rates of formation and elimination of uric acid normally are so adjusted that the *serum uric acid,* as determined spectrophotometrically, does not exceed 6.0 to 6.5 mg per 100 ml in men or 5.0 to 5.5 mg per 100 ml in women. By following the dilution of labeled uric acid in the body, the so-called miscible pool of uric acid has been determined. It amounts to approximately 1 gm in the normal adult, but 3 or 4 gm or more in gouty subjects.

The hyperuricemia and augmented uric acid pool of gouty subjects are attributable chiefly to overproduction of uric acid, which, in most cases, is demonstrable by isotopic methods and other means; in some instances, however, overproduction is not demonstrable, and there may be an innate defect in renal tubular transport, with retention, specifically, of uric acid. The derangement of metabolic pathways responsible for the overproduction of uric acid in primary gout is not known. It has been suggested that the error may lie in the initiating reaction of de novo purine biosynthesis, in which 5-phosphoribosyl-1-amine is formed from 5-phosphoribosyl-1-pyrophosphate and glutamine, purines being synthesized in excess because either the specific amidotransferase involved is superabundant or feedback control of the reaction is defective. Perhaps more consistent with the isotope data is the view that augmentation of purine biosynthesis is secondary to a block in an alternative pathway for the disposition of certain amino acids. A defect in the utilization of glutamine for renal formation of ammonia has recently been implicated as one of the biochemical defects in gout.

CLINICAL ASPECTS OF GOUT

A familial history of gouty arthritis is obtainable, in the United States, in only 10 to 30 per cent of cases of primary gout. If, in such a genealogy, *hyperuricemia* is used as a discriminant to identify the genotype, the familial segregation of the trait, both in successive generations and in siblings, clearly implies inheritance by an autosomal dominant gene. Penetrance is variably incomplete, with a marked predilection for *overt disease* in males; clinically inapparent bearers of the trait (hyperuricemia) are far more common, particularly in females, than are those afflicted. When overt, the expression varies from late emergence of mild and occasional symptoms to fulminant disease, erupting relatively early in life. Environmental factors, notably dietary, affect the clinical course.

The natural history of gout, for centuries considered so bizarre as to verge on the supernatural, is now recognized to conform to the pattern of an *inborn error of metabolism*. Although present in the *infant* at birth, there is no symptom or sign of gout until *asymptomatic hyperuricemia* develops, at *puberty* in *males*, later in life and less pronounced in females. Except for occasional instances of explosive juvenile gout, the persistent hyperuricemia is unaccompanied by any symptoms until (most often between the ages of *30 and 50 years in males,* usually later in females) the disease finally becomes abruptly manifest as fulminating arthritis of a peripheral joint or, less often, as renal colic due to uric acid urolithiasis. The initial attack of *acute gouty arthritis,* ordinarily monarticular, most often involves the feet, classically the metatarsophalangeal joint of the *great toe.* Frequently, however, the ankle or instep is the site, occasionally the knee (or prepatellar bursa), elbow (or olecranon bursa), wrist, or a metacarpophalangeal joint. The attack subsides in 1 or 2 weeks, with complete recovery of the affected part. There ensues a symptom-free interval (intercritical gout) of variable duration; in 75 per cent this lasts less than 2 years, but it may persist for many years. Then there is a recurrence, affecting the initial joint or another one. In about half of the cases, the symptom-free intervals tend to shorten over the years; the attacks become more severe and prolonged, spread to other peripheral joints and are apt to be polyarticular. In severe cases there may be incapacitation for many months.

About 95 per cent of recurrent acute gouty arthritis occurs in men, middle-aged and sthenic. The affected area is acutely *inflamed, swollen,* hot, *red,* and excruciatingly tender and *painful,* simulating acute infection or traumatic injury. Often, there are accompanying fever, leukocytosis, and an increased erythrocyte sedimentation rate. The attack may be incited by minor trauma to the affected joint, dietary or alcoholic indiscretions (occasionally, a particular food or drink),

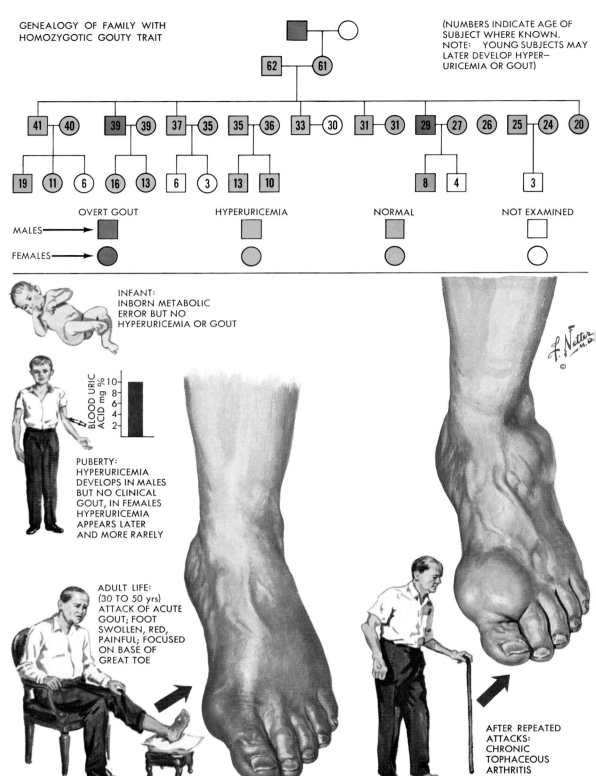

GENEALOGY OF FAMILY WITH HOMOZYGOTIC GOUTY TRAIT

(NUMBERS INDICATE AGE OF SUBJECT WHERE KNOWN. NOTE: YOUNG SUBJECTS MAY LATER DEVELOP HYPER-URICEMIA OR GOUT)

OVERT GOUT — MALES / FEMALES
HYPERURICEMIA
NORMAL
NOT EXAMINED

INFANT: INBORN METABOLIC ERROR BUT NO HYPERURICEMIA OR GOUT

BLOOD URIC ACID mg %

PUBERTY: HYPERURICEMIA DEVELOPS IN MALES BUT NO CLINICAL GOUT, IN FEMALES HYPERURICEMIA APPEARS LATER AND MORE RARELY

ADULT LIFE: (30 TO 50 yrs) ATTACK OF ACUTE GOUT; FOOT SWOLLEN, RED, PAINFUL; FOCUSED ON BASE OF GREAT TOE

AFTER REPEATED ATTACKS: CHRONIC TOPHACEOUS ARTHRITIS

intercurrent illnesses, surgical procedures, or emotional upsets, or it may be regularly seasonal or drug-induced. Often, there is no obvious association with any incitant. A prompt symptomatological response to colchicine, provided no other analgesic is given simultaneously, is practically diagnostic of gout.

The crisis of acute gouty arthritis, occurring, as it does, sporadically in the steady course of persistent hyperuricemia, has long been attributed to an occasional sudden precipitation of urate crystals in articular tissues. This view is supported by the presence of urate crystals in the joint fluid and synovial membranes of affected joints, and by provocation of similar, but usually milder, inflammatory responses to intra-articular injection of urate microcrystals. Nevertheless, most tophaceous deposits form painlessly. Moreover, hyperuricemia is present in a variety of diseases without acute arthritis (including the

gouty trait), and acute attacks may occur in gout after the serum uric acid has been reduced to normal. Colchicine, which terminates acute gouty seizures, has no known effect on uric acid metabolism, whereas uricosuric drugs, which reduce the uric acid pool, do not abolish acute gouty arthritis. There is, therefore, no clearly established pathogenesis of the acute attack, nor is it known why peripheral joints, notably the great toe, are selectively affected, or why they respond to colchicine therapy and prophylaxis.

Early recurrences of acute gouty arthritis resolve with complete restitution of the affected joint. In milder cases this holds throughout life, but, when the disease is more severe, eventually there is residual swelling due to the accumulation of urate. In such instances tophi form also (in fact, much more frequently) without antecedent inflammation. Some 40

(Continued on page 241)

CLINICAL ASPECTS OF GOUT

(Continued from page 240)

per cent of gouty subjects thus pass insidiously into the stage of tophaceous gout, and, if joint function is significantly compromised (which occurs only in a minority of cases), *chronic tophaceous arthritis* develops, with stiffness and chronic pain. The progressive deposition of urate in the tophaceous stage of gout indicates positive uric acid balance and expansion of the body store. Production of uric acid, whether due to inordinate endogenous purine biosynthesis or excessive exogenous purine intake, surpasses elimination by the kidneys, which may become impaired by disease or aging. Man's lack of tissue uricase and the meager solubility of urate facilitate tophaceous deposits. This process is, in every essential, comparable to accumulation in other inborn errors of metabolism, characterized as "storage" diseases, when excretion and degradation of one or another compound cannot keep pace with biosynthesis and gastro-intestinal absorption.

The articular structures most vulnerable to *tophaceous deposit* are those of the feet (particularly at the base of the *great toe*), ankles, knees, *elbows, hands,* and *wrists,* with their adjoining tendinous and subcutaneous tissues; the cartilaginous *pinna,* a characteristic site; and the *olecranon* and patellar bursae. In advanced tophaceous gout the *extremities* may become grotesquely misshapen, with incapacitating crippling. In subcutaneous tissues *tophi* may *ulcerate* through the distended skin and discharge a grumose material, which, on microscopic examination, is found to be rich in urate crystals. Surgical removal of tophi may be necessary when they cause troublesome limitation of motion. This, somewhat surprisingly, is followed by prompt healing, as a rule.

Even if multiple and extensive, tophaceous deposits are discrete and thus differ in appearance from the diffuse joint swellings of rheumatoid arthritis. The urate aggregates invoke a chronic inflammatory and granulomatous response in surrounding connective tissues and are erosive in cartilage and bone; in the *roentgenogram* these urate granulomas present as typical, but not pathognomonic, "punched-out" areas, sometimes grossly destructive of the contiguous bony parts, and surrounded by soft tissue tumescences. Not infrequently, calcium flecks can be discerned within these masses.

Of the viscera, the most frequently involved are the *kidney* and urinary tract. In gout, 50 to 100 per cent more than the normal 5 to 10 gm of uric acid is filtered daily at the glomeruli, but then is largely or virtually completely reabsorbed by active tubular transport. (This latter process is inhibited, usually by approximately 20 per cent, by *uricosuric agents,* thus increasing the renal elimination of uric acid, with consequent lowering of serum uric acid and depletion of the body stores of uric acid, including

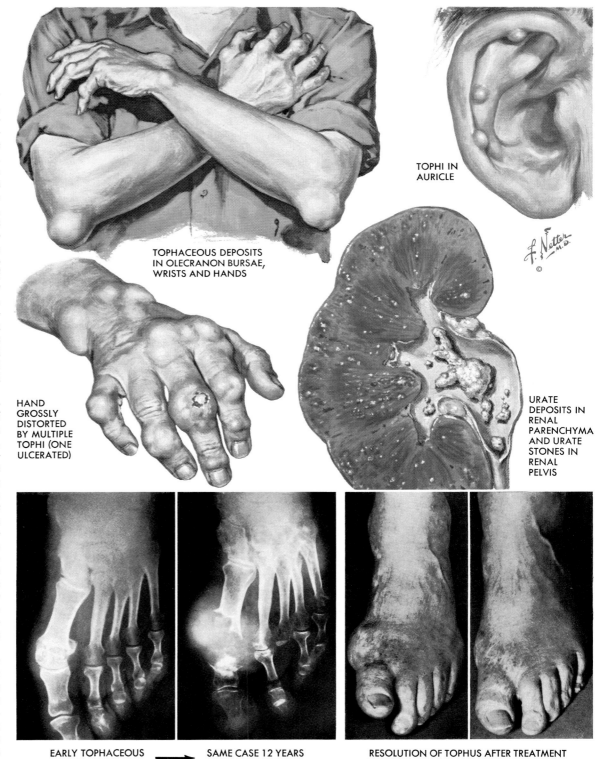

TOPHI IN AURICLE

TOPHACEOUS DEPOSITS IN OLECRANON BURSAE, WRISTS AND HANDS

HAND GROSSLY DISTORTED BY MULTIPLE TOPHI (ONE ULCERATED)

URATE DEPOSITS IN RENAL PARENCHYMA AND URATE STONES IN RENAL PELVIS

EARLY TOPHACEOUS GOUTY ARTHRITIS → SAME CASE 12 YEARS LATER; UNTREATED

RESOLUTION OF TOPHUS AFTER TREATMENT WITH URICOSURIC AGENTS (27 MONTHS)

tophaceous deposits.) The uric acid excreted in urine, apparently derived almost entirely from active tubular secretion, is within the broad limits of normal in most gouty subjects but is habitually excessive in about 30 per cent (gouty "overexcretors"). When urinary uric acid is increased, or the urinary volume is unduly contracted, or its pH is lowered, precipitation of uric acid is facilitated. Uric acid urolithiasis (*uric acid stones*) occurs in 10 to 20 per cent of gouty subjects, sometimes antedating the onset of acute arthritis. Uric acid stones are not radiopaque and thus are not visualized on a flat film of the abdomen.

The enhanced transtubular fluxes of uric acid in gout also favor *deposition within the kidney substance.* Here, as elsewhere, the urate crystals incite a chronic inflammatory and granulomatous response, particularly in the medullary interstitium, with tubular degeneration. These changes (often with

pyelonephritis as a complication of stone formation) and the vascular and parenchymal damage of aging and hypertension (frequently present in gout) together make up the "gouty kidney". Marked renal insufficiency is rare in gout, however, and gout usually does not seem to hasten death.

Gout is thus a disease with protean manifestations, based on an heritable abnormality in uric acid metabolism. Although it cannot be prevented, the manifestations of the acute attacks are amenable to specific therapy with colchicine, and the gradual accumulation of uric acid in the body can be prevented by uricosuric agents or with a recently developed inhibitor of uric acid synthesis, 4-hydroxypyrazalopyridin (allopurinol). Tophaceous deposits, once established, may be gradually reduced by their use, together with a high fluid intake to prevent formation of uric acid stones.

OXALATE STONES, PRIMARY HYPEROXALURIA, OXALOSIS

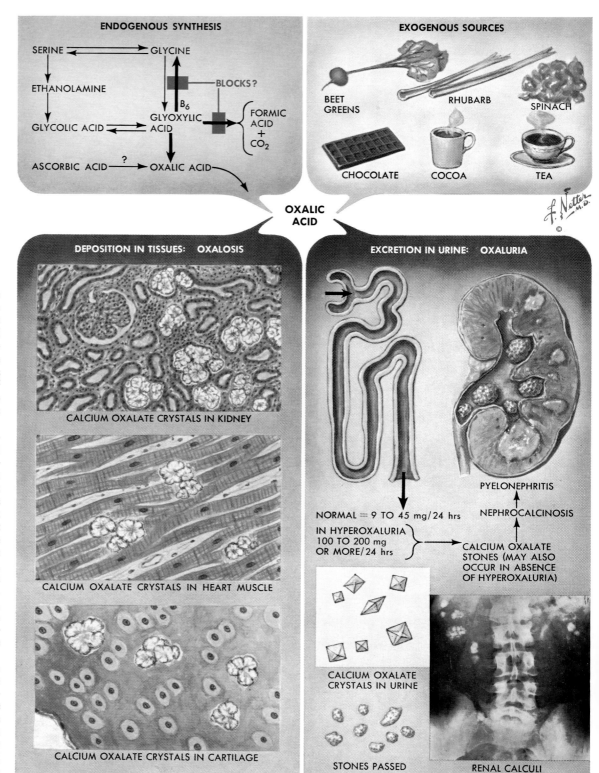

ENDOGENOUS SYNTHESIS

SERINE ⇄ GLYCINE

ETHANOLAMINE

GLYCOLIC ACID ⇄ GLYOXYLIC ACID

B_6

BLOCKS?

FORMIC ACID + CO_2

ASCORBIC ACID —?→ OXALIC ACID

EXOGENOUS SOURCES

BEET GREENS   RHUBARB   SPINACH
CHOCOLATE   COCOA   TEA

OXALIC ACID

DEPOSITION IN TISSUES: OXALOSIS

CALCIUM OXALATE CRYSTALS IN KIDNEY

CALCIUM OXALATE CRYSTALS IN HEART MUSCLE

CALCIUM OXALATE CRYSTALS IN CARTILAGE

EXCRETION IN URINE: OXALURIA

NORMAL = 9 TO 45 mg/24 hrs

IN HYPEROXALURIA 100 TO 200 mg OR MORE/24 hrs

PYELONEPHRITIS

NEPHROCALCINOSIS

CALCIUM OXALATE STONES (MAY ALSO OCCUR IN ABSENCE OF HYPEROXALURIA)

CALCIUM OXALATE CRYSTALS IN URINE

STONES PASSED

RENAL CALCULI

Two disorders result from excessive deposition of oxalates in the system. The common condition of *calcium oxalate stones* is usually associated with normal amounts of oxalic acid in urine and tissues. The much rarer hereditary, recessive disease, *primary hyperoxaluria,* involves excessive production and *excretion of oxalic acid in the urine,* and there also may be *deposition of calcium oxalate in tissues,* a state called *oxalosis.*

Calcium oxalate stones (which comprise roughly 60 to 70 per cent of all calcium stones passed) occur most commonly in the absence of hyperoxaluria or of any demonstrable defect in calcium or oxalate metabolism. They may be due to the fact that calcium oxalate, even in small amounts, is extremely insoluble at the pH ranges of the urinary tract. The only complications are those of recurrent *renal stones,* which are often multiple, or, more rarely, a diffuse calcification of renal parenchyma (*nephrocalcinosis*). Even in the absence of hyperoxaluria, any type of hypercalciuria, as, *e.g.,* in hyperparathyroidism or idiopathic hypercalciuria, may be associated with the formation of calcium oxalate stones.

Oxalic acid is derived principally from *endogenous sources,* primarily *glycine* and also *ascorbic acid.* Ordinarily, glycine is reversibly changed to *glyoxylic acid* which may form *oxalic acid* but is normally nearly completely *converted to formic acid and CO_2.* Another precursor of glyoxylic acid is *glycolic acid* derived from *serine* and *ethanolamine.* Various types of *metabolic blocks* have been postulated in hyperoxaluria. Pyridoxine (vitamin B_6) has been demonstrated as a cofactor in the transamination reaction from glyoxylic acid to glycine. Pyridoxine deficiency in animals has been shown to lead to excessive oxalic acid production and oxalate stones. A similar enzymatic block in converting glyoxylic acid to glycine may be present in primary hyperoxaluria. Alternatively, there may be a *block* in the catabolism of glyoxylic acid to formic acid and CO_2. Either block would lead to an accumulation of glyoxylic acid and, hence, also of oxalic acid. A high intake of glycine has been shown to cause a small increase of oxalic acid production. The principal *dietary sources* of oxalic acid are *beet greens, rhubarb, spinach, chocolate, cocoa,* and

black tea. There have been instances of oxalic acid poisoning from excessive ingestion of rhubarb stalks and from accidental ingestion of ethylene glycol.

The *urinary oxalic acid* excretion, *normally* up to 50 mg per 24 hours, may rise to *100 to 500 mg* in *hyperoxaluria.* Since calcium oxalate is extremely insoluble in the urinary tract, renal stones are formed. The severe form of the disease is associated with hematuria and passage of sand and gravel or nephrocalcinosis from early childhood. With renal damage due to obstruction and *pyelonephritis,* progressive renal failure ensues.

In oxalosis as a complication of primary hyperoxaluria, *calcium oxalate crystals* may appear in many tissues such as *kidney* and *heart muscle,* bone marrow, and *cartilage.* Milder forms of the disease, which may occur in other members of a family, seem to be associated only with recurrent calcium oxalate

stones. The urines of these patients show consistent *calcium oxalate crystals,* and *passage* of *renal stones* is frequent. A rare form of familial glycinuria, associated with calcium oxalate stones, has been reported.

Treatment with a diet low in oxalic acid has been far from satisfactory. Attempts to reduce oxalic acid excretion, by using low-glycine diets, sodium benzoate (which uses up glycine in its detoxification to hippuric acid), or pyridoxine, have had only limited success. Most recently, administration of excessive amounts of neutral phosphates has seemed to decrease the tendency for calcium oxalate stone formation. Certain ions, especially magnesium and possibly zinc, may, in some way, prevent calcium oxalate stone formation. As in the management of all patients with calcium-containing kidney stones, dietary restriction of calcium and the maintenance of a large urine volume have been the most successful measures to date.

CYSTINURIA AND CYSTINE STONE DISEASE, CYSTINOSIS (FANCONI-LIGNAC SYNDROME)

Two disorders are associated with the amino acid cystine, *viz.*, cystinuria and cystinosis. However, they have an entirely different physiologic and metabolic background, and there is *no evidence that cystinuria ever progresses to cystine storage disease, or cystinosis.*

Cystinuria and Cystine Stone Disease

Cystinuria is a congenital or hereditary renal tubular defect, which occurs, roughly, in 1 in 600 of the population. It is either recessive or incompletely recessive and is primarily a *failure of reabsorption,* by the renal tubule, of several amino acids, specifically *cystine, lysine, arginine,* and *ornithine.* A gut-absorptive defect for some of these amino acids has been found as well. Recently, an excessive excretion of the asymmetric disulfide of cysteine and homocysteine has also been demonstrated. The sources of urinary cystine are primarily endogenous or dietary *methionine* and *cysteine.* Cystine itself is not an important dietary precursor, since its sources are usually not edible. The *plasma levels* of all amino acids involved in this disorder are *normal* or *low.* Although normal subjects excrete up to 80 mg of cystine per 24 hours, cystinuric individuals may excrete many times that amount. Losses of lysine (and arginine) may exceed those of cystine, but cystine is the only amino acid which is insoluble at the acid pH range of the urinary tract and, therefore, crystallizes out and forms renal stones. *Cystine crystals,* shaped like *benzene rings,* can be demonstrated by adding *glacial acetic acid* to a freshly voided urine and refrigerating it overnight. In severe cystinuria, crystals may be demonstrated in fresh urine. The qualitative *"nitroprusside" test* for cystine is outlined in the illustration. Quantitative measurements require paper or column chromatography.

The principal complication of the excessive cystine excretion is the appearance of *cystine calculi,* which may progress to the formation of *stag-horn stones,* visible on plain X-ray film. Stones may cause obstruction and, at times, urinary *infection.* Only about 1 per cent of all renal stones result from cystinuria; however, it is a prominent cause of urinary calculi in children. Treatment by forcing fluids and alkalinization is usually successful. In severe cases, dietary restriction of methionine- and cysteine-containing foods is valuable. Recently, D-penicillamine has been used effectively.

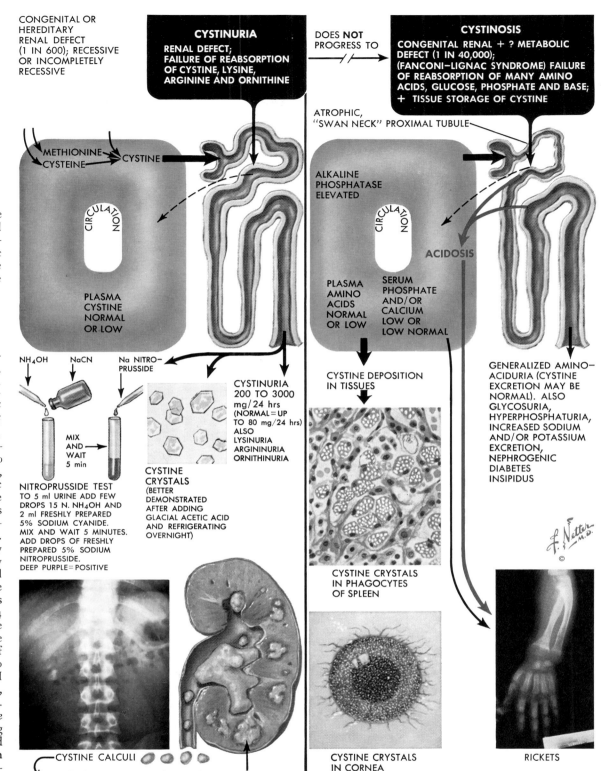

Cystinosis (Fanconi-Lignac Syndrome)

Cystinosis, by contrast, is far more serious. It consists of a *congenital renal tubular defect* and an associated *metabolic defect* in cystine metabolism. It is quite rare, occurring, roughly, in 1 in 40,000 of the population. The renal component, the de Toni-Fanconi syndrome (see also page 191), is associated with excessive renal tubular *losses of glucose,* of most *amino acids* (including cystine), of *phosphate,* and of uric acid, with *low levels in the blood.* Renal tubular acidosis and *nephrogenic diabetes insipidus* may also occur. A metabolic defect causes excessive *storage of cystine,* with *deposition in* various *tissues* (Lignac's disease), including the *reticuloendothelial system* of *spleen,* liver, and bone marrow, in the *cornea,* and in the conjunctiva. The clinical picture is that of severe vitamin-D-resistant *renal rickets* (see page 191) with a *low serum phosphate level* (at times also *low serum calcium*), the presence of an *elevated alkaline phosphatase* and systemic *acidosis.* The X-ray appearance is that of any form of *rickets,* with typical epiphysial changes (see page 192). Recently, biopsy specimens of the kidney have shown structural changes in the *proximal tubule,* the so-called *"swan neck" tubule,* which is shortened and deformed. Cystine renal stones do not occur, as a rule, in this form of cystine storage disease. The loss of amino acids in this syndrome and in cystinuria has little metabolic importance, except, perhaps, for some stunting of growth and for anemia. This disease has a bad prognosis as it progresses to a chronic interstitial *pyelonephritis.* Milder or partial forms, the so-called "adult Fanconi syndrome", have recently been described.

PHENYLKETONURIA

(Phenylpyruvic Oligophrenia)

Phenylalanine is one of the essential amino acids. It is the substrate for a number of substances (*e.g., melanin* and *epinephrine*) formed by the body for special purposes. Excess amounts of phenylalanine normally are disposed of by conversion to *tyrosine* in the *liver.*

A number of genetically determined enzyme deficiencies of the phenylalanine-tyrosine system result in human disease. One of the more serious is *phenylketonuria*. In this disorder the hepatic enzyme system, which converts phenylalanine to tyrosine, is absent. As a result, phenylalanine, which is present in *plasma* normally in only small amounts (1 mg per 100 ml), accumulates and is excreted in the *urine* in greater than normal quantities.

At the increased plasma and tissue levels, other processes for the disposition of excess phenylalanine by metabolic modification become important. Deamination and oxidation result in the formation of *phenyl-lactic, phenylpyruvic* and *phenylacetic acids*. Phenylpyruvic acid is a major excretion product and is easily identified by *testing* of the *urine with ferric chloride*. A transient *green color* is produced when excess amounts of phenylpyruvic acid are present. This is the basis of a routine screening test for the disease. The accumulation of phenylalanine and its metabolites interferes with a number of normal body processes and accounts for most, if not all, of the manifestations of the disease.

The most striking and distressing manifestation of phenylketonuria is retardation of mental development. Wide variation in the severity of the mental defect has now been observed. Although an occasional individual has dull normal intelligence, most of the affected subjects are unable to learn to care for themselves.

At birth, such children appear to be normal, as would be expected from the fact that they must derive their phenylalanine supply from the maternal circulation. Indeed, the small load of phenylalanine thus presented to a normal fetus fails to enhance development of the phenylalanine hydroxylase system, and some degree of "phenylketonuria" may result on phenylalanine loading of normal infants during the first days of life. However, the adaptive enzymes rapidly increase in the liver of normal infants as they take in phenylalanine orally, but this is impossible in the phenylketonuric child.

This defect appears to result from the abnormality of a *single autosomal gene.* When both of the genes present in an individual are of the abnormal type, phenylketonuria results. The parents of such children appear to be normal, except in the rare instance of reproduction by an individual who has the disease. However, each parent must carry the

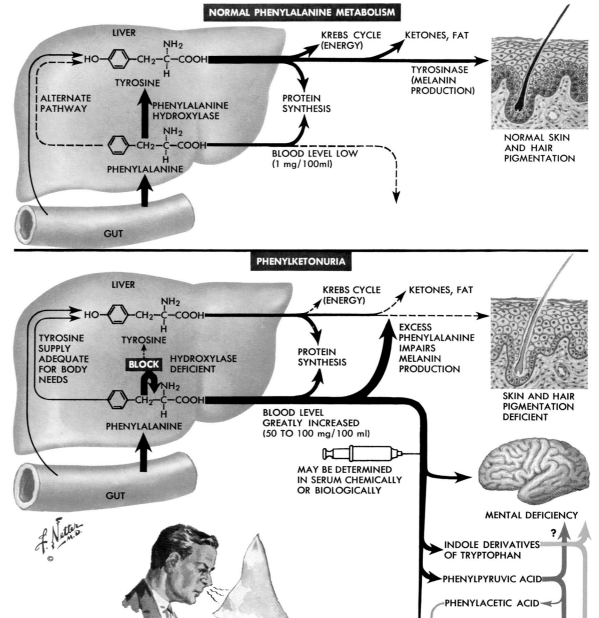

NORMAL PHENYLALANINE METABOLISM

LIVER

TYROSINE

HO—⬡—CH₂—C—COOH (with NH₂)

ALTERNATE PATHWAY

PHENYLALANINE HYDROXYLASE

⬡—CH₂—C—COOH (with NH₂)

PHENYLALANINE

GUT

KREBS CYCLE (ENERGY) → KETONES, FAT

TYROSINASE (MELANIN PRODUCTION)

PROTEIN SYNTHESIS

BLOOD LEVEL LOW (1 mg/100ml)

NORMAL SKIN AND HAIR PIGMENTATION

PHENYLKETONURIA

LIVER

TYROSINE SUPPLY ADEQUATE FOR BODY NEEDS

BLOCK — HYDROXYLASE DEFICIENT

PHENYLALANINE

GUT

KREBS CYCLE (ENERGY) → KETONES, FAT

PROTEIN SYNTHESIS

EXCESS PHENYLALANINE IMPAIRS MELANIN PRODUCTION

SKIN AND HAIR PIGMENTATION DEFICIENT

BLOOD LEVEL GREATLY INCREASED (50 TO 100 mg/100 ml)

MAY BE DETERMINED IN SERUM CHEMICALLY OR BIOLOGICALLY

MENTAL DEFICIENCY

?

INDOLE DERIVATIVES OF TRYPTOPHAN

PHENYLPYRUVIC ACID

PHENYLACETIC ACID

PHENYL—LACTIC ACID

CHARACTERISTIC DIAPER ODOR

FERRIC CHLORIDE

DETERMINED IN ACIDIFIED URINE BY ADDING FERRIC CHLORIDE

EXCRETION IN URINE

KIDNEY

abnormal gene, but if heterozygous, *i.e.,* with one normal and one abnormal gene, no clinical abnormality results from the presence of the gene. Studies of known *carriers* (heterozygous individuals) have shown that, as a group, they have a statistically significant elevation of the plasma phenylalanine level on a normal diet, although the difference is so small that considerable overlap occurs between the values found in normal and in heterozygous individuals. Phenylalanine loading tests exaggerate the abnormality in many heterozygous individuals. It may be expected that a mating of two *heterozygotes* has a risk of 25 per cent (1:4) that any individual pregnancy will produce a phenylketonuric, and that two thirds of the apparently normal children will be carriers.

A few weeks after birth the typical biochemical anomaly becomes evident, if tests are made. The child appears normal, although *pigmentation of skin* and

hair is *less* than should be present if the phenylalanine accumulation had not occurred. Many of the children are blond but offspring from more darkly pigmented families may be *red-haired* or *brunet*. In addition, because most of the patients are of Northern European extraction, the occurrence of blond children does not attract undue attention. The defect in pigmentation appears to result from interference by the high phenylalanine level itself with the *tyrosine oxidase reaction*, which initiates the conversion of tyrosine to dopa and melanin.

Simultaneously with the appearance of the biochemical abnormality and excretion of large amounts of phenylketones in the urine, an aromatic *musty odor* may begin to pervade the child and his surroundings. In high concentration it is penetrating and unpleasant. The odor is that of phenylacetic acid,

(*Continued on page 245*)

PHENYLKETONURIA

(Phenylpyruvic Oligophrenia)

(Continued from page 244)

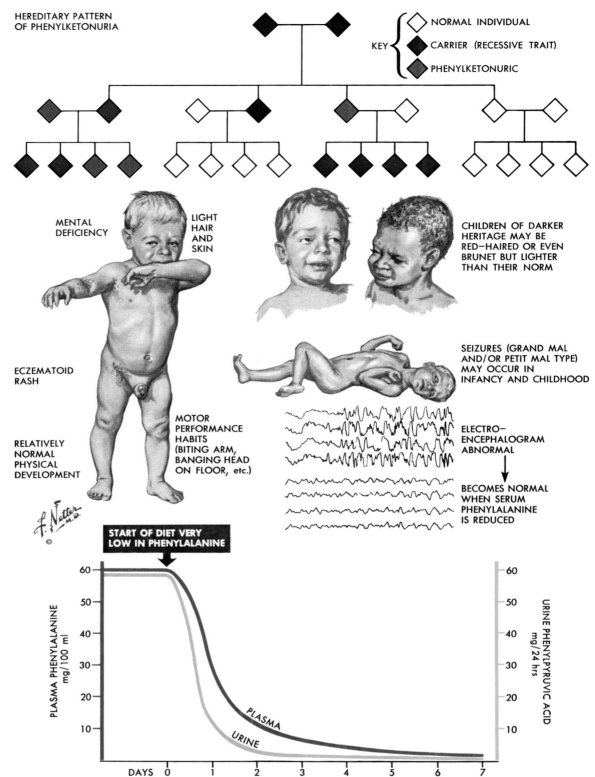

which is formed largely by bacterial action on phenylpyruvic acid. Unless the opportunity for bacterial growth in urine is present, the odor may not be obvious.

Many of the infants develop an *eczematoid dermatitis*, in the body folds and diaper area, which may be quite intractable to ordinary therapy. Its relation to the metabolic error is unknown.

Evidence of mental retardation begins in the first few months of life, but it is extremely difficult to evaluate because of the poor mechanisms available for testing during this period and the wide range of normal variation. It is specifically to be noted that the dull, vacant appearance and structural abnormalities, frequent in some other types of mental deficiency, are absent here. *Body growth is normal.*

The first gross clinical abnormality may be *seizures. Grand mal* or *petit mal* may occur. Overt seizure activity is uncommon; abnormalities of the *electro-encephalogram* (EEG) are nearly universal. Frequently, severe and nearly continuous dysrhythmia occurs in the absence of overt seizures. Seizure activity, observed both clinically and by EEG, tends to disappear with advancing age.

As these children grow older, mental deficiency becomes evident. The children are hyperactive and have adequate physical strength. They are particularly prone to develop severe *motor performance habits* such as *chewing on an arm* or banging the head on the floor, and to carry them on with some violence. Neurologic examination usually yields no specific abnormalities. Sometimes, a little spasticity may be evident without corticospinal signs; under unfamiliar circumstances, tremulousness, which may become severe, is common. Temper tantrums and other evidence of delayed maturity are also frequent.

The cause of the mental deficiency is still somewhat obscure. Both the results of therapy and theoretical considerations suggest that it must be related to the fundamental biochemical defect. It would appear that interference with structural development of the brain, rather than a direct effect on performance, is present. When patients with phenylketonuria are provided with a *diet very low in phenylalanine,* rapid disappearance of *phenylalanine* and *phenylpyruvic acid from the urine* occurs. Somewhat more slowly, the *plasma phenylalanine level returns to normal,* and, indeed, all biochemical abnormalities disappear. If amounts of phenylalanine only sufficient to supply needs for growth and replacement of other essential needs are given with sufficient tyrosine and other amino acids to supply body needs, biochemical normality can be maintained. Unfortunately, phenylalanine is ubiquitously present (about 6 per cent of total amino acids in all food

proteins). This far exceeds the approximate value of 15 mg per kilogram of body weight each day, which is the maximum beyond which phenylketonuria recurs in patients with the disease. Therefore, either synthetic diets, which are prohibitively expensive and unpalatable, or diets of protein from which phenylalanine has been removed must be given. Satisfactory preparations of the latter type are now available commercially. The effectiveness of phenylalanine restriction must be monitored by repeated testing, preferably of phenylalanine levels in plasma, which should be below 2 mg per 100 ml. On such a regimen, seizures and *EEG abnormalities disappear,* pigmentation becomes normal, and skin rashes disappear. The change in intellectual performance is slight in the early weeks of therapy. Only a modest improvement in behavior, with less violence and more tractability, has been observed. Relatively prolonged

restriction seems not to result in acceleration of mental maturation and intelligence in older children. In very young children who still appear quite normal or in whom seizures or other features of the disease have RECENTLY appeared, regression of the biochemical features is especially good, and, when maintained at normal phenylalanine levels, the children appear to develop mentally at a normal rate. The duration of therapy required to ensure development of maximal intellectual capability is uncertain at present but may involve only the first years of life (3 to 6). It seems probable that some abnormality in the formation of normal central nervous system tissue occurs, during these first years, in the presence of phenylalanine excess, which would appear to have no ill effects on the central nervous system function in later years. Thus, the dietary restrictions need not be carried on indefinitely.

GLYCOGEN STORAGE DISEASES

Currently, seven different forms of glycogen storage disease have been recognized and described. Glycogen, a complex polymer of glucose found in liver and muscle, is synthesized by one biochemical pathway and degraded by another metabolic route (see page 149). Normally, *glucose* is phosphorylated to *glucose-6-phosphate* and then converted to *glucose-1-phosphate*. After interacting with *uridine triphosphate (UTP)* to form *UDP-glucose,* glucose molecules are donated from this uridine nucleotide and react with small "primers" of glycogen to yield progressively larger units. A *branching enzyme* is necessary in order to form the typical *treelike structure of glycogen,* with its branches. In the breakdown of glycogen, the enzyme *phosphorylase,* in either *muscle* or *liver,* is involved. This enzyme is able to break down the straight chains of glycogen but is not able to go beyond a branch point. In order to hydrolyze this bond, a specific enzyme, known as *debranching enzyme,* is required. The product liberated is glucose-1-phosphate.

The most common of the seven disorders is *Type I,* or *von Gierke's disease.* In this condition there is a deficiency of the enzyme *glucose-6-phosphatase,* which prevents the liberation of glucose into the blood stream owing to the failure of glucose-6-phosphate to be hydrolyzed. Thus, glycogen in the liver can be broken down only as far as glucose-6-phosphate, and, as a consequence, glycogen accumulates in the liver in large amounts, leading to *hepatomegaly* and an *enlarged abdomen,* and *hypoglycemia* occurs (see page 157). These children show *growth retardation* but usually eat frequently in order to compensate for the hypoglycemia and, as a result, tend to become *obese.* As would be expected, *epinephrine* and *glucagon,* which normally catalyze the production of glucose from glycogen, are ineffective owing to the deficiency of glucose-6-phosphatase. In biopsy specimens of liver, a glycogen stain (*e.g., Best's carmine stain*) may be obtained in specimens left at room temperature, a procedure which would normally lead to its disappearance.

Because of the inadequate supply of glucose to the adipose tissue and the consequent reduction in glycerophosphate, an increased mobilization of fatty acids from adipose tissue takes place (see page 153). There is an increased fatty acid oxidation which, in turn, leads to ketosis (see page 161). Other lipid changes consist of elevated levels of plasma triglycerides and cholesterol with *xanthoma,* and, in the liver, an increase in fat takes place. Rarely, hyperuricemia and gout accompany glycogen storage disease.

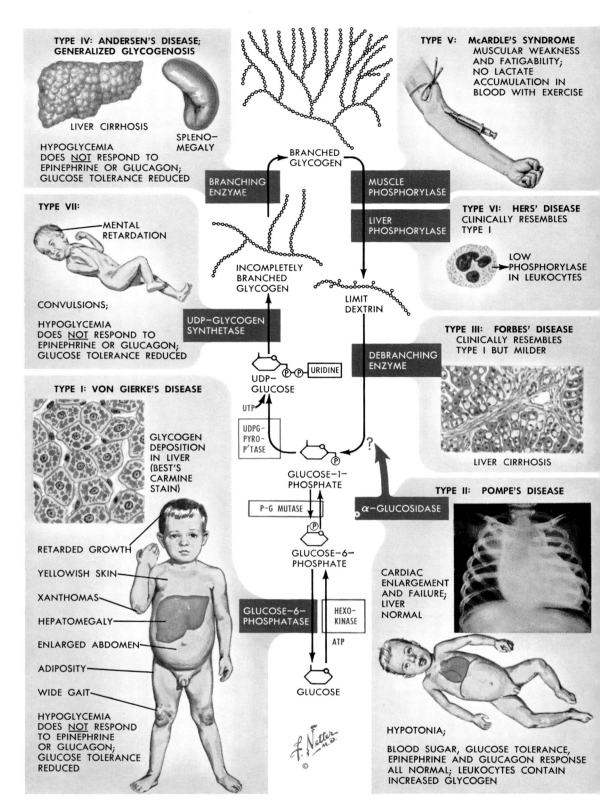

Type II, known as *Pompe's disease,* is a disorder found in infants. It is associated with *marked cardiac enlargement* and *congestive failure,* and usually leads to death within the first year of life. The enzyme deficit has not been completely elucidated, but there may be a deficiency of α-glucosidase, an enzyme which normally splits off glucose (not glucose-1-phosphate) molecules from glycogen.

Types III and *IV, Forbes' disease* and *Andersen's disease,* respectively, are rather rare disorders associated with *cirrhosis* and believed to be associated with deficiencies of debranching and branching enzymes, respectively. As a result, abnormal structural forms of glycogen accumulate in the tissues, and this may be the basis for the cirrhosis.

Type V, or *McArdle's syndrome,* is due to a phosphorylase deficiency in muscle. This disease may be found in children as well as in adults. There is a

failure of glycogen breakdown (*i.e.,* glycogenolysis) and, as a result, excess amounts of glycogen are found in muscle. Pain, *weakness,* and *fatigability* occur in the extremities (in association with *exercise*) owing to inadequate breakdown of glycogen to glucose.

Type VI, or *Hers' disease,* is the counterpart of phosphorylase deficiency in liver and very much *resembles von Gierke's disease.* This enzyme deficiency can be diagnosed by finding *low phosphorylase levels in leukocytes.*

Type VII is a rare disorder in which there is a deficiency in the synthetic enzyme UDP-glycogen synthetase. In the few cases described, *convulsions* and *hypoglycemia* occur, which, again, *do not respond to epinephrine or glucagon.* In contrast to many of the other disorders with large accumulations of glycogen, there is a deficit of glycogen in the tissues in this genetic disease.

GALACTOSEMIA

Galactose is an important constituent of *galactolipids* and *mucopolysaccharides* (see pages 208 and 209), but, normally, most of the ingested galactose is converted to *glucose*. Conversely, much of the endogenous galactose, in compounds such as galactolipids, is derived endogenously by the conversion of glucose to galactose.

Galactosemia is an inborn error of metabolism, transmitted as an autosomal recessive which involves an enzymatic defect in the conversion of galactose to glucose derivatives. The disease tends to manifest itself shortly after birth when the infant is exposed to large amounts of galactose, since this sugar is a component of *lactose,* the disaccharide which is the main source of carbohydrate in *milk.* Normally, as indicated in the accompanying diagram, lactose is split into glucose and galactose within the epithelial cells of the intestine. The galactose is then transported to the liver, where it is phosphorylated by *galactokinase* to *galactose-1-phosphate.* In galactosemia, there is a *block* in the subsequent step, whereby galactose-1-phosphate reacts with *uridine diphosphate glucose* (*UDP-glucose*) to form *UDP-galactose,* which may then be transformed to glucose-1-phosphate by an *epimerase.* As a consequence, galactose-1-phosphate accumulates in the tissues, and it is believed that the toxic manifestations are a consequence of this accumulation.

The exact incidence of the disease is unknown, but the gene frequency in the population is currently estimated at 1 in 18,000. It is important to make the diagnosis at birth, on cord blood, if a previous sibling is known to have had the disease. It is not clear whether the toxic manifestations may occur in utero, but, on the basis of current information, women pregnant with a potentially homozygous offspring should avoid lactose ingestion and alcohol, since alcohol inhibits galactose utilization by the liver.

The main clinical features, which occur in infancy when the patient is exposed to galactose, consist of *cataract formation, hepatosplenomegaly, nutritional failure* and *mental retardation.* The hepatosplenomegaly is associated with an underlying *cirrhosis of the liver,* if galactose ingestion continues for a prolonged period. All these features are reversible, if the offending carbohydrate is removed, except for mental retardation which, unfortunately, leaves its mark for the rest of the patient's life. Jaundice may occur if the liver involvement is progressive.

Hypoglucosemia may occur if the blood galactose levels are high, and, if the drop in blood sugar is significant, convulsions will be seen.

The diagnosis is usually suspected in

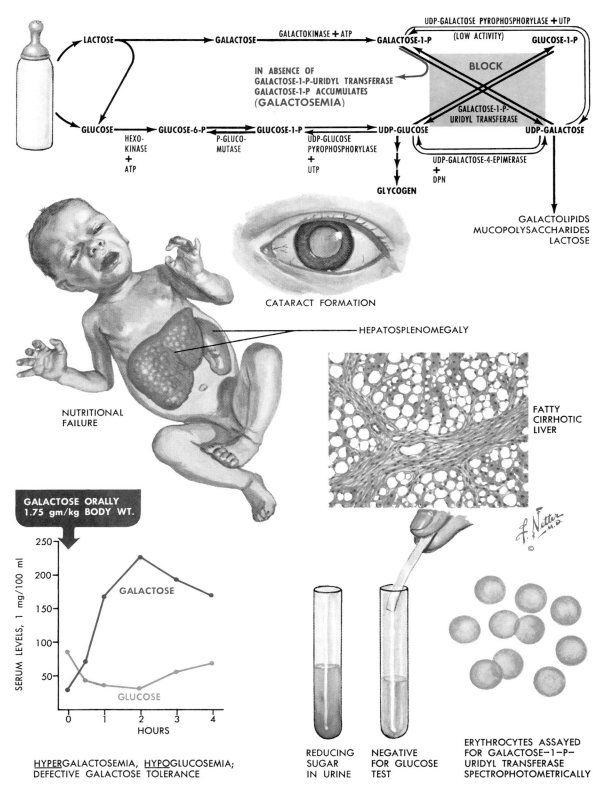

CATARACT FORMATION

HEPATOSPLENOMEGALY

NUTRITIONAL FAILURE

FATTY CIRRHOTIC LIVER

GALACTOSE ORALLY 1.75 gm/kg BODY WT.

HYPERGALACTOSEMIA, HYPOGLUCOSEMIA; DEFECTIVE GALACTOSE TOLERANCE

REDUCING SUGAR IN URINE

NEGATIVE FOR GLUCOSE TEST

ERYTHROCYTES ASSAYED FOR GALACTOSE-1-P- URIDYL TRANSFERASE SPECTROPHOTOMETRICALLY

an infant with nutritional failure, who develops jaundice and hepatosplenomegaly with a reducing sugar in the urine. The sugar in the urine gives a positive Benedict test for *reducing sugar* but does not react with glucose-specific glucose oxidase. The sugar can be identified as galactose by the formation of the characteristic osazone. The *galactose tolerance test* may be performed, but it is somewhat risky because of the potential of aggravating central nervous system damage and also leading to low blood glucose levels. The currently used test, which is specific for this disease, consists of the demonstration, spectrophotometrically, of the absence or *deficiency of galactose-1-phosphate-uridyl transferase* in the *erythrocytes* of these patients.

Treatment consists of placing infants on a galactose-free diet, which is achieved by nutrients such as Dextri-Maltose® or Nutramigen®. On this program,

if the diagnosis is made early enough, either no symptoms will develop or no progression of symptoms will occur, and, in fact, as stated above, many of the toxic manifestations will be reversed.

Another biochemically rather similar disorder, hereditary fructosemia, or fructose intolerance, is due to a deficiency of fructose-1-phosphate splitting aldolase. This leads to an accumulation of fructose-1-phosphate in the tissues, where it inhibits normal glucose metabolism. In the liver it prevents glycogenolysis and thus produces hypoglycemia. These patients cannot tolerate fructose ingested in fruits and fruit juices, which make them nauseated and produce intestinal colic. Just as in galactosemia, hypoglycemia and hepatosplenomegaly are common, but mental retardation has not, as yet, been described in this condition, which is inherited as an autosomal recessive.

Section X

SELECTED VITAMIN DEFICIENCIES

by

FRANK H. NETTER, M.D.

in collaboration with

BENJAMIN M. KAGAN, M.D.
Plate 8

ROBERT E. OLSON, Ph.D., M.D.
Plates 1-7

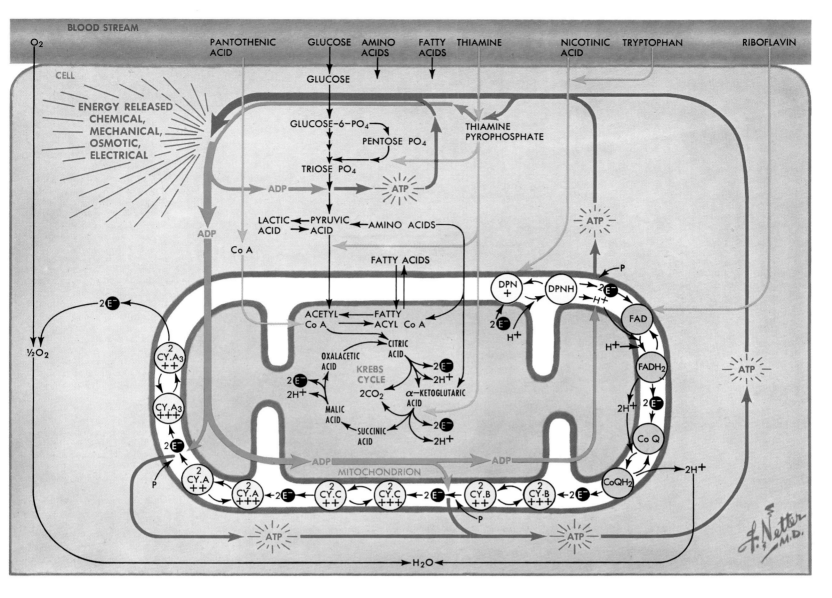

METABOLIC RÔLE OF VITAMIN B COMPLEX

Thiamine, Riboflavin, Nicotinic Acid, Pantothenic Acid

Metabolism deals with the transformation of matter and the production and utilization of *energy* by living cells through (1) *energy liberation,* (2) energy conservation, and (3) energy utilization.

The phase of ENERGY LIBERATION includes the biochemical reactions by which substrates such as *glucose, amino acids,* and *fatty acids* undergo oxidation to *carbon dioxide* and *water,* with the liberation of free energy. The processes of glycolysis, *pyruvate oxidation, fatty acid oxidation,* and the terminal oxidative reactions of the *Krebs tricarboxylic acid cycle* occur in this phase. In energy liberation, there is a division of chemical labor among the various components of the cell. The reactions of glycolysis, *i.e.,* the conversion of glucose to pyruvate and lactate (see page 148), occur in the cytoplasm, or cell sap; pyruvate oxidation, fatty acid oxidation, and the dehydrogenations of the Krebs tricarboxylic acid cycle occur in the *mitochondria,* tiny elliptical bodies about 0.3 by 1 micron in their major axes. They are composed of a pair of *membranes,* the *outer* one of which forms a simple envelope for the *inner* one, which is highly *folded* and invaginated in projections, or cristae. Terminal respiration of all tissues occurs in their mitochondria, and the magnitude of the respiration of any given tissue is a function of the size and number of local mitochondria.

The enzymes carrying out the initial reactions of pyruvate and fatty acid oxidation and of the tricarboxylic acid cycle transformations are in the matrix, or central juice, of the mitochondrion. The result of the action of these enzymes is to effect the near-quantitative conversion of the bond energy of their substrates into the free energy of hydrogen. Released by dehydrogenases, hydrogen is then introduced into the *hydrogen or electron transport chain* of enzymes, principally via *diphosphopyridine nucleotide* (*DPN*), which is the cofactor for most of the mitochondrial dehydrogenases, and thence to *flavin adenine dinucleotide* (*FAD*), *coenzyme Q* (*CoQ*), and the *cytochromes,* as shown. The enzymes of the electron transport chain are spatially fixed in a primary transport particle located on the inner mitochondrial membrane. Since hydrogen consists of a *proton* (H^+) plus an *electron* ($\textcircled{E}$), and since the energy of the atom available to the cell resides in the electron, it makes little difference whether the hydrogen atom or its electron is transported along the respiratory chain. In fact (as is shown in the figure), in some instances ($FADH_2$, $CoQH_2$), 2 hydrogen atoms are carried; in one instance ($DPNH$), 1 electron and 1 hydrogen atom are carried; and, in other instances (the cytochromes), only 1 electron is carried. Protons thus enter or leave the chain as needed. Protons combine with reduced oxygen at the terminus of the chain (*cytochrome A*) to form water. The enzymes of the transport chain are arranged in order of their oxidation-reduction potential, and thus electrons can flow smoothly, with a steady stepwise release of energy during the transport process.

ENERGY CONSERVATION lies in the production of *adenosine triphosphate* (*ATP*) from energy released by electron transport. The latter is thus coupled to phosphorylation, a step commonly referred to as oxidative phosphorylation. The cell recognizes only ATP as a useful form of energy, and, thus, ATP is the "currency of the cell". It is formed, as depicted, at three steps in electron transport and conserves about 60 per cent of the free energy of hydrogen liberated in its oxidation. Small amounts of ATP are also formed in glycolysis.

ENERGY UTILIZATION, the third phase of cellular energetics, is concerned with the use of *ATP.* The energy stored in the terminal phosphate bonds of ATP is transformed into other chemical bonds or is used for biological work.

The *vitamins* depicted are crucial to the reactions of energy production. *Thiamine* is synthesized into *thiamine pyrophosphate,* which is required in keto acid oxidation. *Pantothenic acid* is converted to coenzyme A, which is the acyl-transferring cofactor for fatty acid and pyruvate oxidation and for *citric acid* formation. *Nicotinic acid* and *riboflavin* are precursors, respectively, of DPN and FAD and, hence, are vital for the electron transport process.

THIAMINE DEFICIENCY (BERIBERI)

Beriberi is a nutritional-*deficiency disease caused* by thiamine lack. It may occur in *infants on breast milk* low in thiamine (because of borderline thiamine deficiency in their mothers), in children and adults subsisting on *polished rice,* or in *alcoholics.* The principal food sources of thiamine include *whole wheat bread, brown rice, whole grain cereals, yeast, many vegetables,* and *fresh meats.*

The clinical manifestations of thiamine deficiency are variable, depending on the severity of the deprivation, but they principally involve muscle and nervous tissue. In infant beriberi, central nervous system disability and cardiac disease with sudden death are mainly noted. In adult beriberi the manifestations are primarily those of peripheral neuropathy and muscular disease affecting both skeletal and cardiac muscle. The term *dry beriberi* is applied to that form of the disease in which the nervous manifestations predominate. In these cases the onset is gradual, with increased fatigability, irritability, *muscle tenderness* and *weakness,* appearance of *paresthesia, loss of sensation,* and diminution of *deep tendon reflexes.* In more advanced cases there may be *flaccid paralysis, foot drop, wrist drop,* and muscle wasting with creatinuria. Generally, peripheral neuritis appears first in the lower extremities and may later involve the upper extremities. Weakness may be so extreme that the patient takes to his bed.

The degree of salt retention plays an important rôle in the development of *wet beriberi* and its often-accompanying *cardiac failure.* Observers in the Orient have been impressed with the extent to which the sudden onset of hot weather, which is known to cause a rise in blood volume initially, often precedes a wave of wet beriberi cases. The pathogenesis of cardiac failure in wet beriberi is related to an increased venous supply, coupled with decreased cardiac contractility. The latter, furthermore, appears to be the result of failure of the thiamine-deficient heart to generate energy at an appropriate rate. The *ATP levels* of such a deficient heart muscle fall as *keto acid oxidation* is reduced owing to *lack of thiamine pyrophosphate,* the *coenzyme* form of the vitamin. Because of peripheral vasodilatation, cardiac failure of beriberi classically occurs at cardiac outputs higher than those usually found at rest. This high-output failure is the result of the thiamine-deficient heart

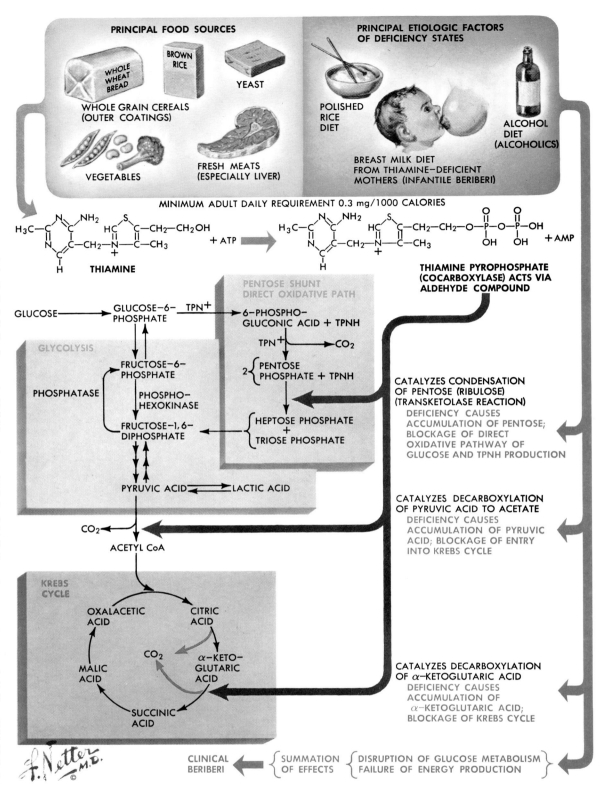

PRINCIPAL FOOD SOURCES

WHOLE WHEAT BREAD
BROWN RICE
YEAST
WHOLE GRAIN CEREALS (OUTER COATINGS)
VEGETABLES
FRESH MEATS (ESPECIALLY LIVER)

PRINCIPAL ETIOLOGIC FACTORS OF DEFICIENCY STATES

POLISHED RICE DIET
BREAST MILK DIET FROM THIAMINE–DEFICIENT MOTHERS (INFANTILE BERIBERI)
ALCOHOL DIET (ALCOHOLICS)

MINIMUM ADULT DAILY REQUIREMENT 0.3 mg/1000 CALORIES

THIAMINE + ATP → THIAMINE PYROPHOSPHATE (COCARBOXYLASE) ACTS VIA ALDEHYDE COMPOUND + AMP

GLUCOSE → GLUCOSE-6-PHOSPHATE → TPN^+

PENTOSE SHUNT DIRECT OXIDATIVE PATH

6-PHOSPHO-GLUCONIC ACID + TPNH

TPN^+ → CO_2

2 { PENTOSE PHOSPHATE + TPNH

GLYCOLYSIS

FRUCTOSE-6-PHOSPHATE

PHOSPHATASE

PHOSPHO-HEXOKINASE

FRUCTOSE-1,6-DIPHOSPHATE

HEPTOSE PHOSPHATE + TRIOSE PHOSPHATE

CATALYZES CONDENSATION OF PENTOSE (RIBULOSE) (TRANSKETOLASE REACTION)
DEFICIENCY CAUSES ACCUMULATION OF PENTOSE; BLOCKAGE OF DIRECT OXIDATIVE PATHWAY OF GLUCOSE AND TPNH PRODUCTION

PYRUVIC ACID ⇌ LACTIC ACID

CO_2

ACETYL CoA

CATALYZES DECARBOXYLATION OF PYRUVIC ACID TO ACETATE
DEFICIENCY CAUSES ACCUMULATION OF PYRUVIC ACID; BLOCKAGE OF ENTRY INTO KREBS CYCLE

KREBS CYCLE

OXALACETIC ACID
CITRIC ACID
CO_2
α-KETO-GLUTARIC ACID
MALIC ACID
SUCCINIC ACID

CATALYZES DECARBOXYLATION OF α-KETOGLUTARIC ACID
DEFICIENCY CAUSES ACCUMULATION OF α-KETOGLUTARIC ACID; BLOCKAGE OF KREBS CYCLE

CLINICAL BERIBERI ← { SUMMATION OF EFFECTS { DISRUPTION OF GLUCOSE METABOLISM FAILURE OF ENERGY PRODUCTION

F. Netter, M.D.

being unable to meet the increased circulatory load imposed.

The most extreme form of thiamine deficiency in the adult is *Wernicke's syndrome.* This serious disorder is characterized by *ophthalmoplegia* (*6th nerve palsy*), ataxia, *confusion,* and *coma.* It frequently terminates in *death.* It may be associated with other manifestations of beriberi, but it is a distinct syndrome with a prognosis so grave that it must be quickly recognized and vigorously treated if the patient is to survive. It is seen mainly in alcoholics who have been exhaustively depleted of thiamine through prolonged drinking bouts. It resembles, to a certain extent, the central nervous system syndrome seen in thiamine-deficient infants.

The *biochemical function of thiamine* is well understood. The *vitamin* is first converted to its *pyrophosphate* through the action of *ATP. Thiamine*

pyrophosphate (TPP) functions as a coenzyme for at least three enzyme systems. Its chemical function as a coenzyme is that of aldehyde group transfer from a donor molecule to a recipient molecule. The aldehyde moiety forms a covalent chemical compound with TPP. For example, acetaldehyde, which is produced from *pyruvic acid* with loss of CO_2, is transferred to oxidized lipoic acid in the pyruvic oxidase system via hydroxyethyl-TPP as a short-lived intermediate. With transfer of acetaldehyde, the oxidized lipoic acid is reduced, and the resulting acetyl lipoic acid transfers an acetyl group to coenzyme A, forming acetyl coenzyme A. Thiamine pyrophosphate performs an analogous function in the α-ketoglutarate oxidase system. The net result of this latter reaction is the oxidation of α-*ketoglutaric acid* to succinyl coenzyme A, and ultimately to *succinate.*

(Continued on page 253)

THIAMINE DEFICIENCY (BERIBERI)

(Continued from page 252)

In addition to these two keto acid oxidases, TPP serves as a *coenzyme for transketolase,* an enzyme that transfers the glycolaldehyde moiety from one pentose phosphate to another. The first 2-carbon atoms with their functional groups are transferred from xylulose-5-phosphate to ribose-5-phosphate to yield a *heptose* (a 7-carbon sedoheptulose-7-phosphate) and a *triose* (a 3-carbon glyceraldehyde-3-phosphate). This reaction is part of the *pentose shunt* in mammalian tissues, which accomplishes, in a cyclic manner, the oxidation of 6 molecules of glucose-6-phosphate to 6 molecules of CO_2 and 6 molecules of glucose-6-phosphate. Incidental to this cycle is the generation of *TPNH,* which is important in many biochemical syntheses requiring the addition of hydrogen. The transketolase enzyme is present in most animal tissues, including the red blood cell. In the absence of thiamine, transketolase activity decreases because of the lack of TPP, which results in the *accumulation of pentose* in cells and the lack of TPNH for many synthetic reactions.

The function of TPP in the above-mentioned three strategic reactions (*i.e.,* the oxidative decarboxylation of 2 keto acids, one at the gateway of entry of carbohydrate metabolites into the *Krebs cycle,* the other within the Krebs cycle itself, and the transketolase reaction which *blocks formation of TPNH* for synthetic reactions) is vital to energy production and certain syntheses which are thus blocked in beriberi and other thiamine-deficient states. This leads to a general *failure of energetic reactions,* loss of ATP energy from the cell, and reduced cell function, all of which are particularly noteworthy in nervous and muscular tissue.

Microscopic examination of tissue from thiamine-deficient animals and man has shown evidence of vacuolization and hyalinization of myofibrils, followed by total necrosis in the heart. An inflammatory reaction then occurs. The necrosis may be focal or diffuse. Grossly, this change is revealed by marked *dilatation of the myocardium,* with failure of contractility, as noted earlier. Electrocardiographic changes are also seen in thiamine-deficient animals and in man. In Wernicke's disease, many small petechial hemorrhages are found in the hypothalamus and gray matter of the upper part of the brain stem. The corpora mamillaria are constantly involved, and, frequently, there is a zone of congestion in the gray matter surrounding the third ventricle. In the peripheral nerves, noninflammatory atrophic degeneration is seen, as well as chromatolysis and clumping of cellular elements in the neurons of the spinal cord and brain stem.

The diagnosis of beriberi is made on both clinical and biochemical grounds. As the TPP concentration in tissues falls, the concentrations of pyruvate, lactate, and α-ketoglutarate rise in the blood in both animals and man. In addition, the transketolase activity in red blood cells has proved to be a useful early sign of thiamine deficiency in both man and animals. The excretion of thiamine in the urine is also markedly reduced in thiamine deficiency. On a normal intake of 0.8 to 1.5 mg of thiamine per day, the excretion ranges from 70 to 150 μg per gram of creatinine. When the intake drops below 0.3 mg per day, the excretion of thiamine falls to levels less than 30 μg per gram of creatinine and then may essentially disappear from the urine. The reduced coenzyme (TPP) content of tissues remains at levels of the order of 20 to 30 per cent of normal until death.

When diets devoid of thiamine are fed to human beings, a marked deficiency, with clinical manifestations, may occur in as short a time as 1 to 2 weeks, whereas on intakes associated with endemic beriberi, the induction period may range from 3 to 6 weeks.

The treatment of thiamine deficiency involves the administration of nutritious food and of thiamine (5 to 15 mg daily) as well as other B-complex vitamins. Since other vitamins may have been limited in the patient's previous dietary, all the B-complex vitamins should be administered to be sure that ancillary deficiencies are not produced by treatment with thiamine alone. Man's *daily requirement* for thiamine is of the order of 0.3 mg per 1000 calories.

COMMON EARLY MANIFESTATIONS

LOSS OF TENDON REFLEXES

PARESTHESIA

PAINFUL, TENDER MUSCLES (PAIN ON COMPRESSING CALF)

NUMBNESS OF FEET

FOOT DROP

DYSPNEA, ORTHOPNEA

SLIGHT CYANOSIS

EDEMA

WET BERIBERI

DRY BERIBERI

EMACIATION

APHONIA MAY APPEAR (POOR PROGNOSIS; VAGUS NERVE INVOLVED)

WRIST DROP

GREAT WEAKNESS

DILATATION OF RIGHT HEART; HEART FAILURE

3.0   4.8

20.8

15.1

7.4

29.7

WERNICKE'S SYNDROME

OPHTHALMOPLEGIA (6th NERVE PALSY)
↓
CONFUSION
↓
COMA
↓
DEATH

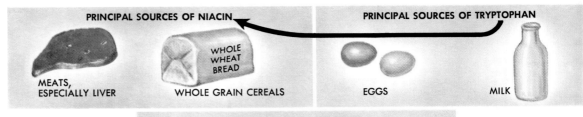

PRINCIPAL SOURCES OF NIACIN

MEATS, ESPECIALLY LIVER

WHOLE WHEAT BREAD

WHOLE GRAIN CEREALS

PRINCIPAL SOURCES OF TRYPTOPHAN

EGGS

MILK

PRINCIPAL CAUSES OF PELLAGRA

CORN AND MOLASSES DIET

ALCOHOL DIET

DEFICIENCY OF **BOTH** NIACIN AND TRYPTOPHAN

Pellagra

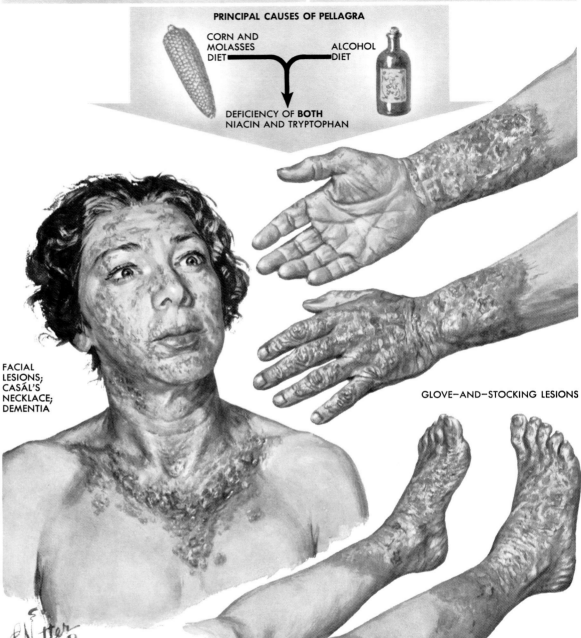

FACIAL LESIONS; CASÁL'S NECKLACE; DEMENTIA

GLOVE–AND–STOCKING LESIONS

Pellagra is a nutritional-deficiency disease caused by insufficient intake of the vitamin *nicotinic acid* or its precursor *tryptophan*. Clinical pellagra may be complicated by marginal intakes of other B-complex vitamins.

Pellagra was first observed by Casál, in Spanish peasants eating maize diets, in the eighteenth century. Since then it has been found in many other parts of the world where *corn* or maize is the principal source of food. Prior to 1930, in the southern part of the United States where the diet of farmers consisted principally of maize, *molasses,* and sowbelly, pellagra was very prevalent. It has been found that the nicotinic acid content is low in maize, and its proteins are deficient in tryptophan. Pellagra is also seen, occasionally, in chronic alcoholics if their *alcohol* intake during drinking bouts is prolonged long enough, and if their dietary restoration of nicotinic acid between drinking bouts is insufficient. This disease is rarely seen in populations subsisting on mixed diets, particularly any containing animal protein (and hence tryptophan) or whole grain cereals, which are good sources of nicotinic acid.

Pellagra is characterized by *dermatitis, stomatitis,* gastritis, *diarrhea,* encephalopathy, and, not infrequently, anemia and peripheral neuropathy. The oft-quoted 3-d's—dermatitis, diarrhea, and *dementia*—aptly describe most cases. The dermatitis is characterized by photosensitivity, appearing, oftentimes, with the first intense sunlight in the spring. The lesions are symmetrical and occur with a sharp line of demarcation between involved and uninvolved skin. These lesions are likely to be found on the extensor surfaces of the *hands, arms,* and *feet.* Another favorite site is the exposed area of the *neck,* where the circumferential lesion is called *Casál's necklace.* Lesions on the *face* tend to be distributed over the alae of the *nose* and on the *forehead.* Intertriginous folds and areas of skin, such as the *perineum* and sites

beneath the breast, are typical for pellagral lesions. Dermatitis begins with an erythema resembling sunburn, which then becomes reddish-brown, roughened, and scaly. Desquamation usually starts in the center of the lesion and reveals an underlying skin which is red and thickened. With exacerbations and remissions of the disease, the skin tends to become permanently roughened and pigmented. Microscopically, the skin lesions begin with dilatation of blood vessels to the superficial portion of the corium, followed by hyperkeratosis of the epithelium. The epithelium then separates from the corium, producing vesicles filled with red blood cells, fibrin, and melanin pigment. With rupture of the vesicles, capillary proliferation occurs. Skin over bony prominences shows particularly marked hyperkeratosis.

The patients usually complain of a sore mouth and indigestion. The *tongue* is bright red, with flattened

papillae. The mucous membranes of the mouth and the epithelium of the whole gastro-intestinal tract may be involved. Small ulcers may be seen in the esophagus and stomach. The small intestine does not reveal much, either grossly or microscopically, but the colon shows many small ulcers, with abscesses in the submucosa. Cystic dilatations of the mucous glands are prominent. The *diarrhea,* which occurs in over half of the pellagrins, is *watery* in nature and, not infrequently, contains blood and pus. The liver usually shows some degree of fatty infiltration. Vaginitis and urethritis are also found.

The encephalopathy of pellagra may simulate any mental disease, although depression with suicidal tendency usually predominates. Disorientation, hallucinosis, delirium, and confusion, terminating in coma, may be observed. The peripheral manifestations

(Continued on page 255)

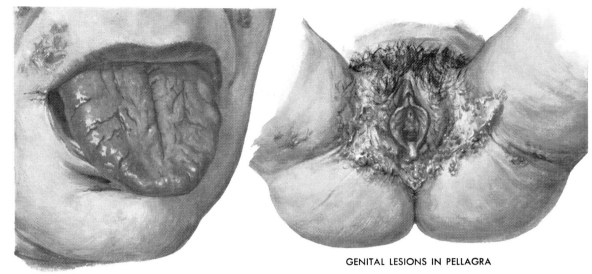

PELLAGRA TONGUE

GENITAL LESIONS IN PELLAGRA

PELLAGRA

(Continued from page 254)

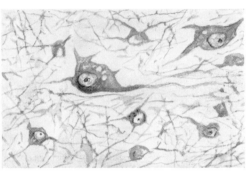

DEGENERATION OF CELLS OF CEREBRAL CORTEX

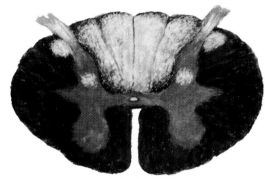

DEGENERATION IN SPINAL CORD

of diminished sensory perception, paresthesias, and reflex changes are less constant. Clinically, hyperactive tendon reflexes are seen, as a result of pyramidal tract involvement, before their final diminution in a typical combined systemic disease. Microscopically, the brain is diffusely involved in severe pellagra. *Cortical nerve cells* show *degeneration*, with an increase in pigment and fat in their cytoplasm and with displacement of their nuclei to the periphery; dendrites may swell and break. Nerve tracts in the cord and periphery may undergo demyelination, particularly in the *posterior columns of the cord*. Chromatolysis and pigmentary degeneration have also been noted in the cells of the cord.

Pellagrous human beings and animals deficient in nicotinic acid show a reduction of total nicotinic acid and, hence, of the coenzymes DPN and TPN (see page 251) in some tissues (liver, skeletal muscle, intestine, and brain) but not in others (lung, heart, or kidney). In human beings, the skin, where the classical lesions occur, has not been sufficiently studied, and the biochemical pathogenesis of the dermatitis is obscure. The urinary excretion of nicotinic acid and the metabolic end products of nicotinamide liberated from pyridine nucleotides decrease to low levels.

The ordinary daily diet in the United States contains about 10 mg of nicotinic acid and approximately 1 gm of tryptophan. It has been found that 1 to 2 per cent of the dietary tryptophan is converted to nicotinic acid via anthranilic acid, as shown below. This means that 10 to 20 mg of nicotinic acid can be derived from dietary protein. Thus, the usual intake of total nicotinic acid is of the order of 25 mg daily in the adult. When the total available nicotinic acid is less than 8 mg daily, clinical pellagra will result in 2 to 4 months. On adequate diets the excretion of N-methyl nicotinamide in adult humans varies from 5 to 15 mg per day. In pellagrins it falls to

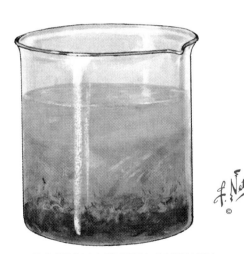

AQUEOUS STOOL IN DIARRHEA OF PELLAGRA

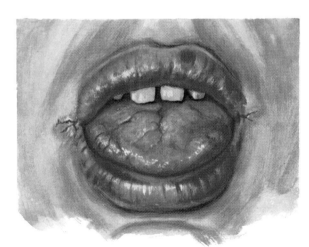

CHEILOSIS, ANGULAR STOMATITIS AND MAGENTA TONGUE IN ARIBOFLAVINOSIS

values less than 2 mg per day. This metabolite thus serves as a useful chemical index of a deficiency in nicotinic acid.

$$\underset{\text{Tryptophan}}{\overset{}{\boxed{}}} \longrightarrow \underset{\text{Anthranilic Acid}}{\overset{\text{COOH}}{\boxed{}}} \longrightarrow \underset{\text{Nicotinic Acid}}{\overset{\text{COOH}}{\boxed{}}}$$

Ariboflavinosis, which is due to reduced riboflavin intake, may complicate pellagra or may be seen as a distinct entity. Many of its specific manifestations are part of the pellagra syndrome, *viz.*, dermatitis (particularly in the nasolabial and scrotal areas), *glossitis* (of *magenta hue*), *stomatitis*, and *cheilosis*. In experimentally induced riboflavin deficiency, the dermatitis seems to be seborrheic in nature. Corneal vascularization has been observed in riboflavin-deficient animals

but not in man. Severe riboflavin deficiency in animals and riboflavin-antagonist-induced deficiency in man have been shown to arrest red cell maturation at an undetermined stage and to induce normocytic anemia.

In riboflavin deficiency, flavin adenine dinucleotide (FAD) coenzyme levels decrease. This is particularly true of the liver, heart, and red blood cells. The excretion of riboflavin in the urine also falls markedly. In human beings on a normal intake of 1 to 2 mg daily, the excretion ranges from 100 to 300 μg per gram of creatinine. Values below 30 μg per gram of creatinine, occurring when the intake drops below 0.5 mg per day, are diagnostic of ariboflavinosis.

Since most of the cereals and breads are now enriched with vitamins of the B complex, deficiencies have become rare in the United States except in a limited group of chronic alcoholics.

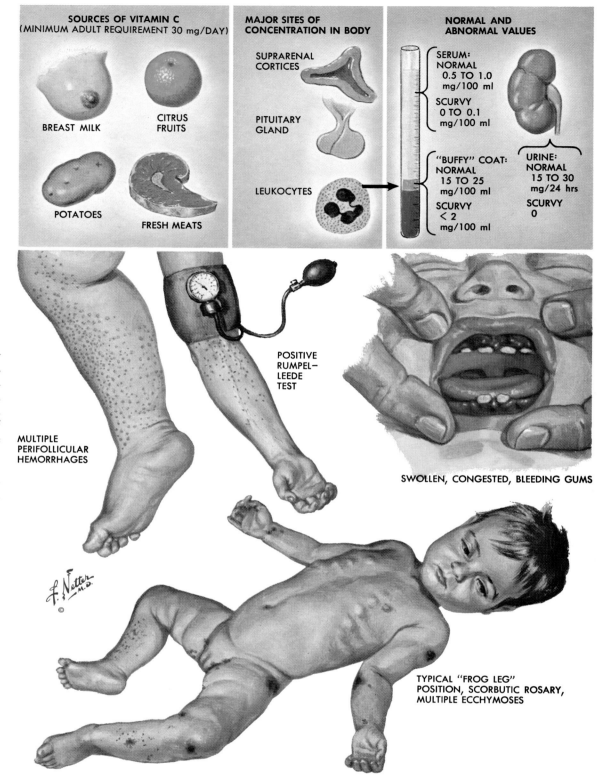

SOURCES OF VITAMIN C
(MINIMUM ADULT REQUIREMENT 30 mg/DAY)

BREAST MILK

CITRUS FRUITS

POTATOES

FRESH MEATS

MAJOR SITES OF CONCENTRATION IN BODY

SUPRARENAL CORTICES

PITUITARY GLAND

LEUKOCYTES

NORMAL AND ABNORMAL VALUES

SERUM:
NORMAL
0.5 TO 1.0
mg/100 ml

SCURVY
0 TO 0.1
mg/100 ml

"BUFFY" COAT:
NORMAL
15 TO 25
mg/100 ml

SCURVY
< 2
mg/100 ml

URINE:
NORMAL
15 TO 30
mg/24 hrs

SCURVY
0

MULTIPLE PERIFOLLICULAR HEMORRHAGES

POSITIVE RUMPEL-LEEDE TEST

SWOLLEN, CONGESTED, BLEEDING GUMS

TYPICAL "FROG LEG" POSITION, SCORBUTIC ROSARY, MULTIPLE ECCHYMOSES

VITAMIN C DEFICIENCY (SCURVY)

Scurvy is a nutritional-deficiency disease resulting from a lack of *vitamin C,* or ascorbic acid. Scurvy has been known since antiquity and, during the fifteenth and sixteenth centuries, became well recognized as an important malady of seafaring men. It was realized that the illness was in some way connected with the lack of fresh foods on prolonged journeys. It was not until 1754, however, that James Lind, a British ship's surgeon, declared that the consumption of oranges or lemons could prevent this dreaded illness. In 1907, it was found that scurvy could be produced experimentally in guinea pigs. This marked the beginning of advances in the understanding of the etiology of scurvy and culminated in the discovery of ascorbic acid, in 1928, and in its synthesis soon thereafter.

Man and other primates, as well as the guinea pig, are particularly vulnerable to dietary ascorbic acid deficiency, because they lack an enzyme, present in the tissues of many mammals, required for the synthesis of L-ascorbic acid from glucose. The only significant *dietary sources* of ascorbic acid are *fruits,* vegetables, and *fresh meat.* In the United States, *citrus fruits,* tomatoes, and *potatoes* are the chief sources. *Breast milk* contributes sufficient amounts of ascorbic acid for the suckling infant, but cow's milk is essentially devoid of the vitamin. All tissues normally contain some ascorbic acid, but endocrine tissue, such as the *pituitary* and the *adrenal cortex,* is very rich in it. The *leukocyte* also has appreciable amounts and can be sampled as an aid in the diagnosis of the disease. The so-called *"buffy" coat* of white cells contains ascorbic acid in the amount of 15 to 25 mg per 100 ml. In scurvy this drops to less than 2 mg per 100 ml. *Normal serum* contains 0.5 to 1 mg per 100 ml but, in scurvy, is generally devoid of ascorbic acid.

Scurvy usually develops with an insidious onset of weakness, fatigability, and shortness of breath, with aching in the bones, joints, and muscles. The skin becomes dry, rough, and dingy in color, followed by the appearance of hyperkeratotic papules and *perifollicular hemorrhages.* Clinical findings generally do not appear until the ascorbic acid is absent from the plasma and *urine,* and the "buffy" coat concentration has dropped to less than 4 mg per 100 ml. Petechial hemorrhages appear in the lower extremities, which are under higher hydrostatic pressure, and then spread upward, involving the skin around the joints or along other irritated areas. The *Rumpel-Leede test* for abnormal capillary fragility is positive. After inflating the cuff to between diastolic and systolic pressure for 1 minute, numerous pete-

chial hemorrhages will appear in scurvy, whereas only an occasional one arises in the normal subject. Massive hemorrhages *with ecchymoses* and, rarely, *proptosis* due to *retrobulbar hemorrhage* may occur. *"Splinter" hemorrhages* may be seen under the nails in adult cases. *Gums* become *swollen, reddish-blue,* spongy, and friable, and the *teeth loosen* and *bleed* and may fall out. Hemorrhages into joints cause much local heat, swelling, pain, and immobility. Because of subperiosteal hemorrhages, infants with scurvy adopt a typical *"frog leg"* position, this being the least painful for them. Also noted in severe infantile scurvy is the prominence of the *costochondral junctions,* a condition which has been termed the *scorbutic rosary.*

(Continued on page 257)

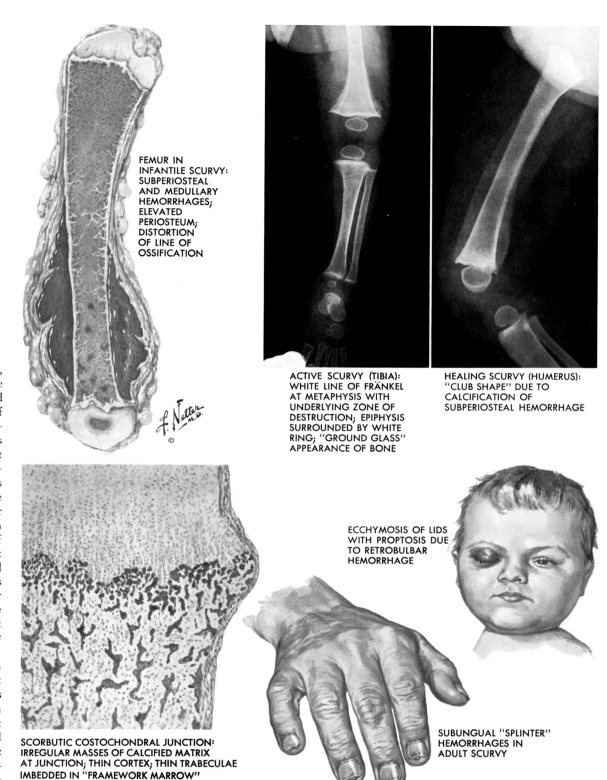

FEMUR IN INFANTILE SCURVY: SUBPERIOSTEAL AND MEDULLARY HEMORRHAGES; ELEVATED PERIOSTEUM; DISTORTION OF LINE OF OSSIFICATION

ACTIVE SCURVY (TIBIA): WHITE LINE OF FRÄNKEL AT METAPHYSIS WITH UNDERLYING ZONE OF DESTRUCTION; EPIPHYSIS SURROUNDED BY WHITE RING; "GROUND GLASS" APPEARANCE OF BONE

HEALING SCURVY (HUMERUS): "CLUB SHAPE" DUE TO CALCIFICATION OF SUBPERIOSTEAL HEMORRHAGE

ECCHYMOSIS OF LIDS WITH PROPTOSIS DUE TO RETROBULBAR HEMORRHAGE

SCORBUTIC COSTOCHONDRAL JUNCTION: IRREGULAR MASSES OF CALCIFIED MATRIX AT JUNCTION; THIN CORTEX; THIN TRABECULAE IMBEDDED IN "FRAMEWORK MARROW"

SUBUNGUAL "SPLINTER" HEMORRHAGES IN ADULT SCURVY

VITAMIN C DEFICIENCY (SCURVY)

(*Continued from page 256*)

Ascorbic acid catalyzes, in some way, the formation of the connective tissue constituents — collagen, osteoid, and dentine. The pathologic physiology of scurvy stems entirely from this biochemical defect. The bleeding in scurvy is due to a lack of the intercellular cement substance which holds together the endothelial cells of the capillary. There is very poor wound healing owing to failure of the fibroblasts to secrete intracellular matrix. The failure of bone growth in scorbutic children is due to the lack of elaboration of osteoid, with consequent osteoporosis. This lack causes marked changes in the development of the bones in children, including weakness, corner fractures (minute fractures into the zones of rarefaction, seen best at the wrist and ankle), and scorbutic rosary at the costal margin.

One of the classic X-ray findings in scurvy is the *white line of Fränkel* at the epiphysial-diaphysial juncture. This results from the excessive calcification of cartilage cells, which are then not replaced in the usual way by osteoid and calcified osteoid (bone). The *cortex* of the bone is *thin*, producing a *ground-glass appearance* and making the white line of Fränkel more prominent. *Subperiosteal hemorrhage* is common in children. The periosteum is ballooned out by this hemorrhage and may be revealed by *calcification* of the subperiosteal hemorrhage after treatment.

Although water-soluble, ascorbic acid does not have a classic coenzyme function. The biochemical mechanism by which it catalyzes the formation of collagen and osteoid is unknown. It has been suggested that it may promote the hydroxylation of proline to hydroxyproline, a reaction essential in the formation of collagen. In vitro, iron plus ascorbic acid is an effective hydroxylating mixture for simple aromatic compounds. In vivo, ascorbic acid catalyzes the oxidation of phenolic amino acids, such as tyrosine, by protecting *p*-hydroxyphenylpyruvic oxidase from substrate inhibition. Ascorbic acid plays some rôle in adrenal physiology, since its concentration in the gland falls markedly after stimulation with ACTH, although its precise local action is unknown.

The anemia sometimes seen in scurvy tends to be macrocytic and may represent a form of folic acid deficiency. It has been shown that, in scurvy, the rate of formation of tetrahydrofolic acid from folic acid is retarded, and the lack of this folate coenzyme may induce a macrocytic anemia.

Persons most likely to get scurvy are those infants who are improperly fed (because they do not receive orange juice in addition to breast milk, through either the ignorance or the neglect of the mother) or old people who are indigent and unable to feed themselves adequately. Boiled soup and milk make a potent scorbutigenic diet. Death may occur in scurvy because of petechial hemorrhages in the brain, with hyperpyrexia accompanied by tachycardia, cyanosis, hypotension, and Cheyne-Stokes respirations.

The treatment of scurvy is the administration of 300 to 500 mg of ascorbic acid daily for 10 days. With complete desaturation of tissues, the average adult will need 3 to 4 gm to replenish stores.

The daily requirement of ascorbic acid is probably of the order of 10 mg for infants and 30 mg for adults, although the Nutritional Research Council allowance provides about 25 mg for children and 70 mg for adults. One orange supplies 50 to 75 mg of ascorbic acid.

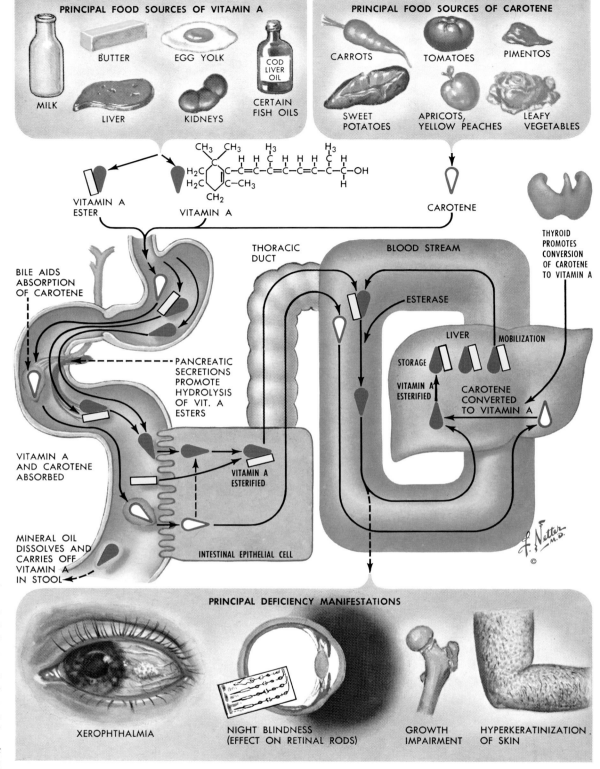

PRINCIPAL FOOD SOURCES OF VITAMIN A

MILK · BUTTER · EGG YOLK · COD LIVER OIL · CERTAIN FISH OILS · LIVER · KIDNEYS

PRINCIPAL FOOD SOURCES OF CAROTENE

CARROTS · TOMATOES · PIMENTOS · SWEET POTATOES · APRICOTS, YELLOW PEACHES · LEAFY VEGETABLES

VITAMIN A ESTER · VITAMIN A · CAROTENE

THYROID PROMOTES CONVERSION OF CAROTENE TO VITAMIN A

BILE AIDS ABSORPTION OF CAROTENE

THORACIC DUCT · BLOOD STREAM

ESTERASE · LIVER · MOBILIZATION · STORAGE · VITAMIN A ESTERIFIED · CAROTENE CONVERTED TO VITAMIN A

PANCREATIC SECRETIONS PROMOTE HYDROLYSIS OF VIT. A ESTERS

VITAMIN A AND CAROTENE ABSORBED

VITAMIN A ESTERIFIED

MINERAL OIL DISSOLVES AND CARRIES OFF VITAMIN A IN STOOL

INTESTINAL EPITHELIAL CELL

PRINCIPAL DEFICIENCY MANIFESTATIONS

XEROPHTHALMIA · NIGHT BLINDNESS (EFFECT ON RETINAL RODS) · GROWTH IMPAIRMENT · HYPERKERATINIZATION OF SKIN

VITAMIN A DEFICIENCY

All the sources of vitamin A in animals probably are certain plant pigments known as *carotenes,* or carotenoid pigments; these are the provitamins A, which are synthesized by all plants except parasites and saprophytes. The provitamins A are transformed into vitamin A in the animal body. *Vitamin A,* an alcohol, is thus *found only in the animal kingdom.* One form, vitamin A_1, is found in mammals and saltwater fish; another, vitamin A_2, is found in freshwater fish. Vitamin A_1 is derived from β-carotene by hydrolytic cleavage at the midpoint in the *polyene chain* connecting the two β-ionone rings. The β-carotene yields 2 molecules of vitamin A, whereas the α- and γ-carotenes yield only 1 molecule each, since they are not symmetrical. In the diet of man, carotene has one half or less of the biological value of an equal quantity of vitamin A. The potency of vitamin A_1 is 100 times greater than that of vitamin A_2, from which it differs in the structure of the side chain. Vitamin A occurs, mainly as an *ester* of higher fatty acids, in the liver, kidney, lung, and fat depots. The *conversion of carotenes to vitamin A* occurs largely in the *intestinal wall,* and perhaps also in the liver, in rats, pigs, goats, rabbits, sheep, and chickens; in man, however, the *liver* is thought to be the only organ, or the principal organ, capable of accomplishing this transformation. Thyroid speeds up this reaction, and carotenemia may appear in hypothyroidism, with resultant yellow skin.

Many factors affect the efficiency of *absorption* and utilization of preformed vitamin A and carotene. Small amounts of *mineral oil* in the diet interfere with absorption of both vitamin A and carotene.

Sources of vitamin A and carotene are all yellow vegetables and fruits (*e.g., sweet potatoes, apricots,* and *yellow peaches*), and the *leafy green vegetables,* supplying provitamin A in the diet; preformed vitamin A is supplied by *milk,* fat, *liver,* and *kidney.*

The recommended daily requirement is 5000 international units per day for an adult, 6000 during the second half of pregnancy, and 8000 during lactation. It is 1500 for infants 2 to 12 months of age. For children, it is 2000 from 1 to 3 years old; 2500, 4 to 6 years; 3500, 7 to 9 years; 4500, 10 to 12 years; and

5000, 13 to 20 years. One international unit is equivalent to the activity of 0.3 μg of crystalline vitamin A alcohol, 0.344 μg of crystalline vitamin A acetate, or 0.6 μg of β-carotene.

Vitamin A deficiency can occur not only from inadequate intake but also because of poor intestinal absorption (as in malabsorption syndromes), since the fat-soluble vitamins are poorly absorbed from the intestine in the absence of bile or pancreatic enzymes, or with inadequate conversion of provitamin A (as in liver disease).

Maintenance of the integrity of epithelial tissue is an important function of vitamin A. In its absence, normal secretory epithelium is replaced by a dry, *keratinized epithelium,* which is more susceptible to invasion by infectious organisms. Vitamin A is a constituent of *visual purple,* the pigment involved in *rod vision* in the retina. *Night blindness,* which is

caused by a disturbance of rod vision, is a manifestation of vitamin A deficiency. *Xerophthalmia, i.e.,* keratinization of ocular tissue, which may progress to blindness, is a late result of vitamin A deficiency.

In the absence of vitamin A, the *growth* of experimental animals does not progress normally. The skeleton is affected first, then the soft tissues. Mechanical damage to the brain and cord occurs when these structures attempt to grow within the arrested limits of the surrounding bony framework.

Hypervitaminosis A may result from the administration of large amounts of vitamin A (usually in the form of concentrates) to infants and small children. The principal manifestations are painful joints, periosteal thickening of the long bones, and loss of hair.

Calciferol, or vitamin D_2, another clinically significant fat-soluble vitamin, is discussed on page 192.

GLOSSARY OF ABBREVIATIONS

ACTH — adrenocorticotropic hormone; *also called* adrenocorticotropin; adrenal cortical hormone

ADH — antidiuretic hormone

ADP — adenosine diphosphate

AFI — amaurotic familial idiocy

AMP — adenosine monophosphate

A.T. 10 — dihydrotachysterol

ATP — adenosine triphosphate

BAAF — Bensley's acid aniline fuchsin

BBT — basal body temperature

B.E.I. — butanol-extractable radioactive iodine; *also called* butanol-extractable iodine

BM — basement membrane

B.M.R. — basal metabolic rate

BOA — benzoquinone-acetic acid

B.U. — Bodansky unit

BUN — blood urea nitrogen

CBG — corticosterone-binding globulin; *also called* transcortin

CNS — central nervous system

CoA — coenzyme A

COMT — catechol-O-methyl transferase

CoQ — coenzyme Q

CPIB — ethyl-*p*-chlorophenoxyisobutyrate

CRF — corticotropin-releasing factor

CY — cytochrome

CY.A — cytochrome A

DEA — dehydroepiandrosterone

DHA-P — dihydroxyacetone phosphate

DNA — deoxyribonucleic acid

DOPA — dihydroxyphenylalanine

DPN — diphosphopyridine nucleotide

DPNH — reduced diphosphopyridine nucleotide

(E) — electron

EEG — electro-encephalogram

FAD — flavin adenine dinucleotide

FFA — free fatty acid; *also abbreviated* NEFA, UFA, *which see*

FHX — familial hypercholesterolemic xanthomatosis

FSH — follicle-stimulating hormone

G ald-P — glyceraldehyde phosphate

GH — growth hormone; *also abbreviated* STH, *which see*

G.I. — gastro-intestinal

H. and E. stain — hematoxylin and eosin stain

HDL — high-density lipoproteins

HIOMT — hydroxyindole-O-methyl transferase

ICSH — interstitial-cell-stimulating hormone; *also called* luteinizing hormone (LH)

ILA — insulinlike activity

17-KS — 17-ketosteroids

LATS — long-acting thyroid stimulator

LDL — low-density lipoprotein

LH — luteinizing hormone; *also called* interstitial-cell-stimulating hormone (ICSH)

LTH — luteotropic hormone; *also called* prolactin

MAO — mono-amine oxidase

MHMA — 3-methoxy-4-hydroxymandelic acid; *also called* vanyl mandelic acid (VMA)

m-RNA — messenger RNA

MSH — melanocyte-stimulating hormone

NEFA — free, or nonesterified, fatty acid; *also abbreviated* FFA, UFA, *which see*

NPN — nonprotein nitrogen

PAS — periodic acid Schiff reagent

P.B.I. — protein-bound radioactive iodine; *also called* protein-bound iodine; serum protein-bound iodine

P-G mutase — phosphoglucomutase

P-triol — pregnanetriol

RNA — ribonucleic acid

S_f values — flotation constants

STH — somatotropin; *also called* somatotropic hormone; growth hormone of the pituitary

T_3 — tri-iodothyronine

T_4 — thyroxine

TBG — thyroxine-binding globulin

TPN — triphosphopyridine nucleotide

TPNH — reduced triphosphopyridine nucleotide

TPP — thiamine pyrophosphate

t-RNA — transport RNA

TRP — tubular reabsorption of phosphate

TSH — thyrotropic hormone; *also called* thyrotropin; thyroid-stimulating hormone

UDPG — uridine diphosphoglucose

UDP-galactose — uridine diphosphogalactose

UDP-glucose — same as UDPG

UDP-glycogen — uridine diphosphoglycogen

UDPG-p'tase — uridine diphosphoglucose pyrophosphatase

UFA — unesterified fatty acids; *also abbreviated* FFA, NEFA, *which see*

UTP — uridine triphosphate

VMA — vanyl mandelic acid; *also called* 3-methoxy-4-hydroxymandelic acid (MHMA)

SELECTED REFERENCES

Section I

	PLATE NUMBER

ALBERT, A.: *Human urinary gonadotropin*, Recent Progr. Hormone Res., 12:227, 1956. — 10

BAILEY, P.: *Tumors involving the hypothalamus and their clinical manifestations*, in *The Hypothalamus*, Vol. XX, Williams & Wilkins Company, Baltimore, 1940. — 13

BARCHAS, J. D., AND LERNER: *Localization of melatonin in the nervous system*, J. Neurochem., 11:489, 1964. — 35

BARLOW, E. D., AND DE WARDENER: *Compulsive water drinking*, Quart. J. Med., 28:235, 1959. — 32

BOGDANOVE, E. M.: *Local actions of target gland hormones on the rat adenohypophysis*, in *Cytologie de l'Adenohypophyse* (Editions du Centre National de la Recherche Scientifique), ed. by Benoit, J., Paris, 1963. — 8, 9

BUSTON, C. L., KASE AND VAN ORDEN: *The effect of FSH and HCG on the anovulatory ovary*, Amer. J. Obstet. Gynec., 87:773, 1963. — 7

CARTER, A. C., AND ROBBINS: *The use of hypertonic saline infusions in the differential diagnosis of diabetes insipidus and psychogenic polydipsia*, J. clin. Endocr., 7:753, 1947. — 23

CUSHING, H.: *The basophil adenoma of the pituitary body and their clinical manifestations (pituitary basophilism)*, Bull. Johns Hopk. Hosp., 50:137, 1932. — 29

——: *The Pituitary Body and Its Disorders*, J. B. Lippincott Co., Philadelphia and London, 1912. — 7

DANIEL, P. M., PRICHARD AND TREIP: *Traumatic infarction of anterior lobe of the pituitary gland*, Lancet, 2:927, 1959. — 17

DAUGHADAY, W. H., AND PARKER: *Human pituitary growth hormone*, Ann. Rev. Med., 16:47, 1965. — 25

DINGMAN, J. F., AND HAUGER-KLEVENE: *Treatment of diabetes insipidus: Synthetic lysine vasopressin nasal solution*, J. clin. Endocr., 24:550, 1964. — 32

DOMINGUEZ, J. M., AND PEARSON: *Immunologic measurement of growth hormone in human sera*, J. clin. Endocr., 22:865, 1962. — 28

EARLEY, L. E., AND ORLOFF: *The mechanism of antidiuresis associated with the administration of hydrochlorothiazide to patient with vasopressin-resistant diabetes insipidus*, J. clin. Invest., 41:1988, 1962. — 32

EZRIN, C., AND MURRAY: *The cells of the human adenohypophysis in pregnancy, thyroid disease and adrenal cortical disorders*, in *Cytologie de l'Adenohypophyse* (Editions du Centre National de la Recherche Scientifique), ed. by Benoit, J., Paris, 1963. — 8, 9

FARQUHARSON, R. F.: *Simmonds' disease; extreme insufficiency of the adenohypophysis*, in *American Lecture Series*, No. 34, Charles C Thomas, Springfield, Ill., 1950. — 28

FRANTZ, A. G., AND RABKIN: *Human growth hormone: Clinical measurement, response*

Section I (continued)

	PLATE NUMBER

to hypoglycemia and suppression by corticosteroids, New Engl. J. Med., 271:1375, 1964. — 28

FRASER, R., AND JOPLIN: *Discussion on the assessment of endocrine function after hypophysectomy or pituitary destruction*, Proc. Roy. Soc. Med., 53:81, 1960. — 31

FERGUSON, J. K. W.: *A study of the motility of the intact uterus at term*, Surg. Gyn. & Obstet., 73:359, 1941. — 30

FISKE, V. M.: *Serotonin rhythm in the pineal organ: Control by the sympathetic nervous system*, Science, 146:253, 1964. — 35

FRIESEN, H., AND ASTWOOD: *Hormones of the anterior pituitary body*, New Engl. J. Med., 272:1216, 1272, 1328, 1965. — 7

FROHLICH, A.: *A case of tumor of the hypophysis cerebri without acromegaly*, in *Classic Descriptions of Disease*, Major, R. H., Charles C Thomas, Springfield, Ill., 1939. — 14

GOLDBERG, M.: *Hyponatremia and the inappropriate secretion of antidiuretic hormone*, Amer. J. Med., 35:293, 1963. — 31

GORDON, D. A., HILL AND EZRIN: *Acromegaly: A review of 100 cases*, Canad. med. Ass. J., 87:1106, 1962. — 27

HERLANT, M.: *The cells of the adenohypophysis and their functional significance*, Int. Rev. Cytol., 17:299, 1964. — 8, 9

HERTZ, D. P.: *Ueber die akute Wirkung von synthetischem Oxytocin auf die Nierenhämodynamik und renale Elektrolytabsscheidung beim Menschen*, Naunyn-Schmiedeberg's Arch. exp. Path. Pharmak., 239:410, 1960. — 30

HIRSCH, O., AND HAMLIN: *Symptomatology and treatment of hypophyseal duct tumors (craniopharyngiomas)*, Confin. Neurol. (Basel), 19:153, 1959. — 15

HOLLINSHEAD, W. H.: *Interphase of diabetes insipidus*, Proc. Mayo Clin., 39:92, 1964. — 32

HOYT, W. F.: *Neuro-ophthalmology, annual review*, Arch. Ophthal., 72:679, 1964. — 16

KAHANA, L., LEBOVITZ, LUSK, McPHERSON, DAVIDSON, OPPENHEIMER, ENGEL, WOODHALL AND ODOM: *Endocrine manifestations of intracranial extrasellar lesions*, J. clin. Endocr., 22:304, 1962. — 13

KAPPERS, A. J.: *The development, topographical relations and innervation of the epiphysis cerebri in the albino rat*, Z. Zellforsch., 52:163, 1960. — 34

KELLY, D. E.: *Pineal organs*, Amer. Scientist, 50:597, 1962. — 34, 35

KLINEFELTER, H. F., JR., ALBRIGHT AND GRISWOLD: *Experience with quantitative test for normal or decreased amounts of follicle-stimulating hormone in urine in endocrinological diagnosis*, J. clin. Endocr., 3:529, 1943. — 10

KRACHT, J., AND TAMM: *Invasiv-gewachsenes basophiles Adenom des Hypophysenvorderlappens bei Cushing-Syndrom*, Acta endocr. (Kbh.), 43:330, 1963. — 29

LEVINGER, E. L., AND ESCAMILLA: *Heredi-*

Section I (continued)

	PLATE NUMBER

tary diabetes insipidus: Report of 20 cases in seven generations, J. clin. Endocr., 15:547, 1955. — 32

LOHRENZ, F. N., RAFAEL-FERNANDEZ AND DOE: *Isolated thyrotropin deficiency. Review and report of three cases*, Ann. intern. Med., 60:990, 1964. — 19

LORAINE, J. A.: *Bioassay of pituitary and placental gonadotropins in relation to clinical problems in man*, Vitam. and Horm., 14:305, 1956. — 10

McCANN, S. M.: *Recent studies on the regulation of hypophysial luteinizing hormone secretion*, Amer. J. Med., 34:379, 1963. — 11

NURNBERGER, J. I., AND KOREY: *Pituitary Chromophobe Adenomas*, Springer Publishing Company, New York, 1953. — 22

OWMAN, C.: *Evidence for a functional significance of the fetal pineal gland of the rat*, Gen. comp. Endocr., 3:723, 1963. — 34, 35

PURNELL, D. C., RANDALL AND RYNEARSON: *Postpartum pituitary insufficiency*, Proc. Mayo Clin., 39:321, 1964. — 23

QUAY, W. B.: *Cytologic and metabolic parametus of pineal inhibition by continuous light in the rat*, Z. Zellforsch., 60:479, 1963. — 34

RASMUSSEN, A. T.: *The proportions of the various subdivisions of the normal adult human hypophysis cerebri*, in *The Pituitary Gland* (Ass. Res. nerv. Dis. Proc.), Vol. XVII, Waverly Press, Inc., Baltimore, 1938. — 2

RICHARDSON, H. B.: *Simmonds' disease and anorexia nervosa*, Arch. intern. Med., 63:1, 1939. — 24

ROSS, G. T., AND BAHN: *Hormonal activities of an eosinophilic adenoma associated with acromegaly*, Proc. Mayo Clin., 35:400, 1960. — 7

ROTH, J., GLICK, YALOW AND BERSON: *Hypoglycemia: a potent stimulus to secretion of growth hormone*, Science, 140:987, 1963. — 25

SHEALY, C. N., KAHANA, ENGEL AND McPHERSON: *Hypothalamic-pituitary sarcoidosis*, Amer. J. Med., 30:46, 1961. — 17

SHEEHAN, H. L.: *Atypical hypopituitarism*, Proc. roy. Soc. Med., 54:43, 1961. — 23

—— AND SUMMERS: *The syndrome of hypopituitarism*, Quart. J. Med., 18:319, 1949. — 21

SHELINE, G. E., BOLDREY AND PHILLIPS: *Chromophobe adenomas of the pituitary gland*, Amer. J. Roentgenol., 92:160, 1964. — 22

SILVERMAN, F. N.: *Roentgen standards for size of the pituitary fossa, from infancy through adolescence*, Amer. J. Roentgenol., 78:451, 1957. — 6

THOMAS, W. C.: *Diabetes insipidus. Review of clinical, experimental, and physiologic aspects*, J. clin. Endocr., 17:565, 1957. — 32

TOBIAS, C. A., LAWRENCE, BORN, McCOMBS, ROBERTS, ANGER, LOW-BEER AND HUGGINS: *Pituitary irradiation with high-energy proton beams*, Cancer Res., 18:121, 1958. — 27

Section I (continued)

PLATE NUMBER

TRAFFORD, J. A., AND LILLICRAP: *Human growth hormone in pituitary infantilism,* Lancet, I:1128, 1963. — 18

VAN DYKE, H. B., ADAMSONS, JR., AND ENGEL: *Aspects of biochemistry and physiology of the neurohypophyseal hormones,* Recent Progr. Hormone Res., 11:1, 1955. — 30, 31

WALCH, F. B.: *Clinical Neuro-ophthalmology,* 2nd ed., Williams & Wilkins, Baltimore, 1957. — 16

WIDE, L., AND GEMZELL: *Immunological determination of pituitary luteinizing hormone in urine of fertile and post-menopausal women and adult men,* Acta Endocr. (Kbh.), 39:539, 1962. — 10

WURTMAN, R. J., AND AXELROD: *The pineal gland,* Scientific American (page 50), July, 1965. — 34, 35

——, —— AND CHU: *The relation between melatonin and the effects of light on the rat gonad,* Ann. N. Y. Acad. Sci., 117:228, 1964. — 35

YOUNG, D. G., BAHN AND RANDALL: *Pituitary tumors associated with acromegaly,* J. clin. Endocr., 25:249, 1965. — 27

Section II

General References

MEANS, J. H., DE GROOT AND STANBURY: *The Thyroid and Its Diseases,* McGraw-Hill, Inc., New York, 1963.

PITT-RIVERS, R., EDITOR: *The Thyroid Gland,* Butterworth & Co., Ltd., London, 1964.

WAYNE, E. J., KONTRAS AND ALEXANDER: *Clinical Aspects of Iodine Metabolism,* Blackwell Scientific Publications, Oxford, 1964.

———

ADAMS, D. D., AND KENNEDY: *Evidence of a normally functioning pituitary TSH secretion mechanism in a patient with a high blood level of long-acting thyroid stimulator,* J. clin. Endocr., 25:571, 1965. — 9–12

AREY, L. B.: *Developmental Anatomy,* W. B. Saunders Company, Philadelphia, 1954. — 3, 4, 5

——: *Human Histology,* W. B. Saunders Company, Philadelphia, 1957. — 3, 4, 5

BADILLO, J., SHIMAOKA, LESSMANN, MARCHETTA AND SOKAL: *Treatment of non-toxic goiter with sodium liothyronine. A double-blind study,* J. Amer. med. Ass., 184:29, 1963. — 20

BARKER, S. B., AND SHIMADA: *Metabolism of thyroxine and analogues,* Proc. Mayo Clin., 39:609, 1964. — 7

BECKER, F. O., ECONOMON AND SCHWARTZ: *The occurrence of carcinoma in "hot" thyroid nodules. Report of two cases,* Ann. intern. Med., 58:877, 1963. — 16, 17

BECKERS, C., DE CROMBRUGGHE AND VISSCHER: *Dynamic disturbances of intrathyroid iodine in sporadic nontoxic goiter,* J. clin. Endocr., 24:327, 1964. — 24

BLIZZARD, R. M., CHANDLER, LANDING, PETTIT AND WEST: *Maternal autoimmunization to thyroid as a probable cause of athyrotic cretinism,* New Engl. J. Med., 263:327, 1960. — 21

Section II (continued)

PLATE NUMBER

BRAVERMAN, L. E., AND INGBAR: *Anomalous effects of certain preparations of desiccated thyroid on serum protein-bound iodine,* New Engl. J. Med., 270:439, 1964. — 8

CATZ, B., GINSBURG AND SALENGER: *Clinically inactive thyroid U.S.P.,* New Engl. J. Med., 266:136, 1962. — 8

CLARK, F., AND HORN: *Assessment of thyroid function by the combined use of the serum protein-bound iodine and the resin uptake of I¹³¹-triiodothyronine,* J. clin. Endocr., 25:39, 1965. — 8

CRILE, G., JR.: *Survival of patients with papillary carcinoma of the thyroid after conservative operations,* Amer. J. Surg., 108:862, 1964. — 28

CRISPELL, K. R., EDITOR: *Hypothyroidism,* MacMillan Company, New York, 1963. — 58–60

DE GROOT, L. J.: *Current views on formation of thyroid hormones,* New Engl. J. Med., 272:243, 297, 355, 1965. — 47

——, HALL, McDERMOTT AND DAVIS: *Hashimoto's thyroiditis: A genetically conditioned disease,* New Engl. J. Med., 267:267, 1962. — 27

DIMITRIADOU, A., FRASER AND TURNER: *Iodotyrosine-like substances in human serum,* Nature (Lond.), 201:575, 1964. — 7

DONIACH, D., AND ROITT: *Auto-antibodies in disease,* Ann. Rev. Med., 13:213, 1962. — 26, 27

DUNN, J. T., AND CHAPMAN: *Rising incidence of hypothyroidism after radioactive iodine therapy in thyrotoxicosis,* New Engl. J. Med., 271:1037, 1964. — 14, 15

FORESTER, C. F.: *Coma in myxedema,* Arch. intern. Med., 111:734, 1963. — 18–20

FRIES, T., AND HAHNEMANN: *Latent parathyroid insufficiency following thyroidectomy,* Acta med. scand., 176:711, 1965. — 14, 15

GREENSPAN, F. S., LOWENSTEIN, SPILLSER AND CRAIG: *Abnormal iodoprotein in plasma of patients with non-toxic goiter,* New Engl. J. Med., 269:830, 1963. — 24

GREER, M. A.: *Graves' disease,* Ann. Rev. Med., 15:65, 1964. — 13

HAMOLSKY, M. W., GOLODETZ AND FREEDBERG: *The plasma protein-thyroid hormone complex in man. III. Further studies on the use of the in vitro red blood cell uptake of I¹³¹-L-triiodothyronine as a diagnostic test of thyroid function,* J. clin. Endocr., 19:103, 1959. — 8

HAYNIE, T. P., NOFAL AND BLIERWALTER: *Treatment of thyroid carcinoma with I¹³¹. Results at fourteen years,* J. Amer. med. Ass., 183:303, 1963. — 28–33

HAYS, M. T., AND SOLOMON: *Influence of the gastrointestinal iodide cycle on the early distribution of radioactive iodide in man,* J. clin. Invest., 44:117, 1965. — 7

HOCH, F. L.: *Thyrotoxicosis as a disease of mitochondria,* New Engl. J. Med., 266:446, 498, 1962. — 9–12

HOLLANDER, C. S., GARCIA, STURGIS AND SELENKOW: *Effect of an ovulatory suppressant on the serum protein-bound iodine and the red-cell uptake of radioactive triiodothyronine,* New Engl. J. Med., 269:501, 1963. — 8

JORGENSEN, E. C.: *Stereochemistry of thy-*

Section II (continued)

PLATE NUMBER

roxine and analogues, Proc. Mayo Clin., 39:560, 1964. — 7

KENDALL, E. C.: *Isolation of thyroxine,* Proc. Mayo Clin., 39:548, 1964. — 7

KOGUT, M. D., KAPLAN, COLLIPP, TIAMSIC AND BOYLE: *Treatment of hyperthyroidism in children; analysis of forty-five patients,* New Engl. J. Med., 272:217, 1965. — 14, 15

KRISS, J. P., PLESHAKOV AND CHIEN: *Isolation and identification of the long-acting thyroid stimulator and its relation to hyperthyroidism and circumscribed pretibial myxedema,* J. clin. Endocr., 24:1005, 1964. — 9, 12

KUSAKABE, T., AND MUJAKE: *Defective deiodination of I¹³¹-labeled L-diiodotyrosine in patients with simple goiter,* J. clin. Endocr., 23:132, 1963. — 22

LANGMAN, J.: *Medical Embryology,* Williams & Wilkins Company, Baltimore, 1963. — 1–5

LEADING ARTICLE: *Thyrotoxic myopathy,* Lancet, II:25, 1963. — 9–12

LINDSAY, S., AND CHAIKOFF: *The effects of irradiation on the thyroid gland with particular reference to the induction of thyroid neoplasm: A review,* Cancer Res., 24:1099, 1964. — 14, 15

LOHRENZ, F. N., FERNANDEZ AND DOE: *Isolated thyrotropin deficiency. Review and report of three cases,* Ann. intern. Med., 60:990, 1964. — 6

McADAMS, G. B., AND REINFRANK: *Resin sponge modification of the I¹³¹ T3 test,* J. nucl. Med., 5:112, 1964. — 8

McKENZIE, J. M.: *Neonatal Graves' disease,* J. clin. Endocr., 24:660, 1964. — 9–12

——: Review: *Pathogenesis of Graves' disease: Role of the long-acting thyroid stimulator,* J. clin. Endocr., 25:424, 1965. — 9–12

MECK, J. C., JONES, LEWIS AND VANDERLAAN: *Characterization of the long-acting thyroid stimulator of Graves' disease,* Proc. nat. Acad. Sci. (Wash.), 52:342, 1964. — 9–12

MICHEL, R., RALL, ROCHE AND TUBIANA: *Thyroidal iodoproteins in patients with goitrous hypothyroidism,* J. clin. Endocr., 24:352, 1964. — 24

MORRIS, H.: *Morris' Human Anatomy,* ed. by Schaeffer, Blakiston Company, New York, 1953. — 1–5

PATTEN, B. M.: *Human Embryology,* Blakiston Company, New York, 1953. — 1–5

PERLMUTTER, M., AND COHN: *Myxedema crisis of pituitary or thyroid origin,* Amer. J. Med., 36:883, 1964. — 18–20

PINCHERA, A., PINCHERA AND STANBURY: *Thyrotropin and long-acting thyroid stimulator assays in thyroid disease,* J. clin. Endocr., 25:189, 1965. — 6, 9

PITT-RIVERS, R.: *Structure of thyroxine,* Proc. Mayo Clin., 39:553, 1964. — 7

RAWSON, R. W.: *Physiologic effects of thyroxine in man,* Proc. Mayo Clin., 39:637, 1964. — 7

SATOYOSHI, E., MURAKAMI, KOWA, KINOSHITA AND NISHIYAMA: *Periodic paralysis in hyperthyroidism,* Neurology, 13:746, 1963. — 9–12

SHIMAOKA, K., BADILLO, SOKAL AND MARCHETTA: *Clinical differentiation between*

Section II (continued)

PLATE NUMBER

thyroid cancer and benign goiter, J. Amer. med. Ass., 181:179, 1962. 22, 23

—— AND JASANI: *The application of two-dimensional paper chromatography and low-level counting to the study of triiodothyronine in plasma*, J. Endocr., 32:59, 1965. 8

SILLIPHANT, W. M., KLINCK AND LEVITIN: *Thyroid carcinoma and death. A clinico-pathological study of 193 autopsies*, Cancer (Philad.), 17:513, 1964. 28

SOLOMON, N., CARPENTER, BENNET AND McGEHRE: *Schmidt's syndrome (thyroid and adrenal insufficiency) and coexistent diabetes mellitus*, Diabetes, 14:300, 1965. 18–20

STANBURY, J. B., RICCABONA AND JANSSEN: *Iodotyrosyl coupling defect in congenital hypothyroidism with goitre*, Lancet, I:917, 1963. 24

STERLING, K.: *Thyroxine in blood*, Proc. Mayo Clin., 39:586, 1964. 7

TAPLEY, D. F.: *Mode of action of thyroxine*, Proc. Mayo Clin., 39:626, 1964. 7

TAUROG, A.: *Biosynthesis of thyroxine*, Proc. Mayo Clin., 39:569, 1964. 7

VEITH, F. J., BROOKS, GRIGSBY AND SELENKOW: *The nodular thyroid gland and cancer. A practical approach to the problem*, New Engl. J. Med., 270:431, 1964. 25

VOLPE, R., ROW, WEBSTER, JOHNSTON AND EZRIN: *Studies of iodine metabolism in Hashimoto's thyroiditis*, J. clin. Endocr., 25:593, 1965. 27

WERNER, S. C., EDITOR: *Thyrotropin*, Charles C Thomas, Springfield, Ill., 1963. 6

WHITE, R. G., BASS AND WILLIAMS: *Lymphadenoid goitre and the syndrome of systemic lupus*, Lancet, I:368, 1961. 26

WILLIAMS, E. D., ENGEL AND FORBES: *Thyroiditis and gonadal dysgenesis*, New Engl. J. Med., 270:805, 1964. 27

WINSHIP, T., AND ROSVOLL: *Childhood thyroid carcinoma*, Cancer (Philad.), 14:734, 1961. 28–33

WOLFF, J., THOMPSON AND ROBBINS: *Congenital goitrous cretinism due to absence of iodide-concentrating ability*, J. clin. Endocr., 24:699, 1964. 21

WOODBURNE, R. T.: *Essentials of Human Anatomy*, Oxford University Press, New York, 1961. 1–5

Section III

General References

FORSHAM, P. H.: *The Adrenals*; page 282 in *Textbook of Endocrinology*, ed. by Williams, W. B. Saunders Company, Philadelphia and London, 3rd edition, 1962.

PRUNTY, F. T. G.: *Chemistry and Treatment of Adrenocortical Diseases*, Charles C Thomas, Springfield, Ill., 1964.

——, EDITOR: *The adrenal cortex*, Brit. med. Bull., 18:89, 1962.

SHERWIN, R. P.: *Histopathology of pheochromocytoma*, Cancer (Philad.), 12:861, 1959.

SOFFER, L. J., DORFMAN AND GABRILOVE: *The Human Adrenal Gland*, Lea and Febiger, Philadelphia, 1961.

Section III (continued)

PLATE NUMBER

ADDISON, T.: *On the Constitutional and Local Effects of Disease of the Suprarenal Capsules*, D. Highley, London, 1855. 22

AREY, L. B.: *Developmental Anatomy*, W. B. Saunders Company, Philadelphia, 1954. 1

——: *Human Histology*, W. B. Saunders Company, Philadelphia, 1957. 5

AXELROD, J.: *Metabolism of epinephrine and other sympathomimetic amines*, Physiol. Rev., 39:751, 1959. 26

BAGGETT, B., ENGEL, BALDERAS AND LANMAN: *Conversion of C^{14}-testosterone to C^{14}-estrogenic steroids by endocrine tissues*, Endocrinology, 64:600, 1959. 82, 83

BLAIR, R. G.: *Pheochromocytoma and pregnancy. Report of a case and review of 51 cases*, J. Obstet. Gynaec. Brit. Cwlth., 70:110, 1963. 27

BLIZZARD, R. M., AND KYLE: *Studies of the adrenal antigens and antibodies in Addison's disease*, J. clin. Invest., 42:1653, 1963. 22, 23

BOLAND, E. W.: *Clinical comparison of the newer anti-inflammatory corticosteroids*, Ann. rheum. Dis., 21:176, 1962. PAGE 108

BONGIOVANNI, A. M., AND ROOT: *The adrenogenital syndrome*, New Engl. J. Med., 268:1283, 1342, 1391, 1963. 13–15

BROOKS, R. V., DUPRÉ, GOGATE, MILLS AND PRUNTY: *Appraisal of adrenocortical hyperfunction: Patients with Cushing's syndrome or "non-endocrine" tumors*, J. clin. Endocr., 23:725, 1963. 9

BRUNJES, S., JOHNS AND CRANE: *Pheochromocytoma—Postoperative shock and blood volume*, New Engl. J. Med., 262:393, 1960. 27

CARPENTER, C. C. J., SOLOMON, SILVERBERG, BLEDSOE, NORTHCUTT, KLINENBERG, BENNETT AND HARVEY: *Schmidt's syndrome (thyroid and adrenal insufficiency): A review of the literature and a report of fifteen new cases including ten instances of coexistent diabetes mellitus*, Medicine (Baltimore), 43:153, 1964. 22

CONN, J. W., COHEN, ROVNER AND NESBIT: *Normokalemic primary aldosteronism*, J. Amer. med. Ass., 193:200, 1965. 17, 18

——, KNOPF AND NESBIT: *Clinical characteristics of primary aldosteronism from analysis of 145 cases*, Amer. J. Surg., 107:159, 1964. 17, 18

COUPLAND, R. E.: *The innervation of the rat adrenal medulla*, J. Anat. (Lond.), 96:141, 1962. 4

CREWS, S. L.: *Posterior subcapsular lens opacities in patients on long-term corticosteroid therapy*, Brit. med. J., 1:1644, 1963. PAGE 108

CROUT, J. R., AND SJOERDSMA: *Turnover and metabolism of catecholamines in patients with pheochromocytoma*, J. clin. Invest., 43:94, 1964. 27

CURRIE, A. R., SYMINGTON AND GRANT: *The morphology and zoning of the human adrenal cortex*, in *The Human Adrenal Cortex*, by Currie, A. R., E. and S. Livingstone, Edinburgh, 1962. 4

DELLER, J. J., WEGIENKA, CONTE, ROSNER AND FORSHAM: *Testosterone metabolism*

Section III (continued)

PLATE NUMBER

in idiopathic hirsutism, Ann. intern. Med., in press. 15

DE MOOR, P., STEENO, MEULEPAS, HENDRIKX, DELAERE AND OSTYN: *Influence of body size and of sex on urinary corticoid excretion in a group of normal young men and females*, J. clin. Endocr., 23:677, 1963. 82, 83

DI RAIMONDO, V. C., AND FORSHAM: *Pharmacophysiologic principles in the use of corticoids and adrenocorticotropin*, Metabolism, 7:5, 1958. PAGE 108

DOE, R. P., LOHRENZ AND SEAL: *Familial decrease in corticosteroid-binding globulin*, Metabolism, 14:940, 1965. 6

EDELMAN, I., BOGOROCH AND PORTER: *On the mechanism of action of aldosterone on sodium transport: The role of protein synthesis*, Proc. nat. Acad. Sci. (Wash.), 50:1169, 1963. 16

EDITORIAL: *Mechanism of aldosterone action*, New Engl. J. Med., 270:1124, 1964. 16

ENGLEMAN, K., MUELLER AND SJOERDSMA: *Elevated plasma free fatty acid concentrations in patients with pheochromocytoma: Changes with therapy and correlations with the basal metabolic rate*, New Engl. J. Med., 270:865, 1964. 26

—— AND SJOERDSMA: *Chronic medical therapy for pheochromocytoma. A report of four cases*, Ann. intern. Med., 61:229, 1964. 27

GABRILOVE, J. L., SHARMA, WOTIZ AND DORFMAN: *Feminizing adrenocortical tumors in the male: A review of 52 cases including a case report*, Medicine (Baltimore), 44:37, 1965. 15

GIFFORD, R. W., KVALE, MAHER, ROTH AND PRIESTLY: *Clinical features, diagnosis and treatment of pheochromocytoma: A review of 76 cases*, Proc. Mayo Clin., 39:281, 1964. 26–28

GLICKMAN, P. B., PALMER AND KAPPAS: *Steroid fever and inflammation*, Arch. intern. Med., 114:46, 1964. 12

GLUSHIEN, A. S., MANSUY AND LITTMAN: *Pheochromocytoma. Its relationship to neurocutaneous syndromes*, Amer. J. Med., 14:318, 1953. 27

GOLD, E. M., KENT AND FORSHAM: *Clinical use of a new diagnostic agent methapyrapone (SU-4885) in pituitary and adrenocortical disorders*, Ann. intern. Med., 54:175, 1961. 10, 25

GRABER, A. L., NEY, NICHOLSON, ISLAND AND LIDDLE: *Natural history of pituitary-adrenal recovery following long-term suppression with corticosteroids*, J. clin. Endocr., 25:11, 1965. PAGE 108

HARTOG, M., GAAFAR AND FRASER: *Effect of corticosteroids on serum growth hormone*, Lancet, II:376, 1964. 7

HILTON, J. G., WESTERMAN, BERGEN AND CRAMPTON: *Syndrome of mineralocorticoid excess due to bilateral adrenocortical hyperplasia*, New Engl. J. Med., 260:202, 1959. 18

HOLLINSHEAD, W. H.: *The innervation of the adrenal glands*, J. comp. Neurol., 64:449, 1936. 4

HUNG, W., MIGEON AND PARROTT: *A pos-*

sible autoimmune basis for Addison's disease in three siblings, one with idiopathic hypoparathyroidism, pernicious anemia and superficial moniliasis, New Engl. J. Med., 269:658, 1963.   22

JENKINS, D., FORSHAM, LAIDLAW, REDDY AND THORN: *Use of ACTH in the diagnosis of adrenal cortical insufficiency*, Amer. J. Med., 18:3, 1955.   24

JOHNSTON, C. I., AND JOSÉ: *Reduced vascular response to angiotensin II in secondary hyperaldosteronism*, J. clin. Invest., 42:1411, 1963.   18, 20

KAPLAN, N. M.: *Assessment of pituitary ACTH secretory capacity with metopirone: I. Interpretation, II. Comparison with other tests*, J. clin. Endocr., 23:945, 1963.   10, 25

KISS, T.: *Experimentell-morphologische Analyse der Nebenniereninnervation*, Acta anat. (Basel), 13:81, 1951.   4

KREINES, K., PERIN AND SALZER: *Pregnancy in Cushing's syndrome*, J. clin. Endocr., 24:75, 1964.   8, 9

KURÉ, K., WADA AND OKINAKA: *The spinal parasympathetic: the nerve supply of the suprarenal gland*, Quart. J. exp. Physiol., 21:227, 1931.   4

LANGMAN, J.: *Medical Embryology*, Williams & Wilkins Company, Baltimore, 1963.   1

LEVER, J. D.: *Nerve fibres in the adrenal cortex of the rat*, Nature (Lond.), 171:882, 1953.   4

LIDDLE, G. W.: *Tests of pituitary-adrenal suppressibility in the diagnosis of Cushing's syndrome*, J. clin. Endocr., 20:1539, 1960.   10

——, ESTEP, KENDALL, WILLIAMS, JR., AND TOWNES: *Clinical applications of a new test of pituitary reserve*, J. clin. Endocr., 19:875, 1959.   10

LINFOOT, J. A., LAWRENCE, BORN AND TOBIAS: *The alpha particle or proton beam in radiosurgery of the pituitary gland for Cushing's disease*, New Engl. J. Med., 269:597, 1963.   8

LIPSETT, M. B., HERTZ AND ROSS: *Clinical and pathophysiologic aspects of adrenocortical carcinoma*, Amer. J. Med., 35:374, 1963.   8, 15

LUETSCHER, J. A.: *Primary aldosteronism. Observations in six cases and review of diagnostic procedures*, Medicine (Baltimore), 43:437, 1964.   17

MALMEJAC, J.: *Activity of the adrenal medulla and its regulation*, Physiol. Rev., 44:196, 1964.   26

MASON, A. S., AND GREENBAUM: *Cushing's syndrome and skin pigmentation*, Brit. med. J., 2:445, 1962.   11

MASON, H. L.: *Steroid nomenclature*, J. clin. Endocr., 8:190, 1948.   6

MEADOR, C. K., LIDDLE, ISLAND, NICHOLSON, LUCAS, NUCKTON AND LUETSCHER: *Cause of Cushing's syndrome in patients with tumors arising from "non-endocrine" tissue*, J. clin. Endocr., 22:693, 1962.   9

MITCHELL, G. A. G.: *The Anatomy of the Autonomic Nervous System*, E. and S. Livingstone, Edinburgh, 1953.   4

MONTALBANO, F. P., BARONOFSKY AND BALL: *Hyperplasia of the adrenal medulla: Clinical entity*, J. Amer. med. Ass., 182:267, 1962.   27

MORRIS, H.: *Morris' Human Anatomy*, ed. by Schaeffer, Blakiston Company, New York, 1953.   2, 3

NELSON, D. H., MEAKIN AND THORN: *ACTH-producing pituitary tumors following adrenalectomy for Cushing's syndrome*, Ann. intern. Med., 52:560, 1960.   11

OKUDA, S.: *Non-existence of the direct nervous connection between the vagal nerves and the suprarenal glands in dogs*, Tohoku J. exper. Med., 50:363, 1949.   4

PASQUALINI, J. R., AND JAYLE: *Structure and Metabolism of Corticosteroids*, Academic Press, London and New York, 1964.   6, 7

PATTEN, B. M.: *Human Embryology*, Blakiston Company, New York, 1953.   1

POSNER, J. B., AND JACOBS: *Isolated analdosteronism. I. Clinical entity, with manifestations of persistent hyperkalemia, periodic paralysis, salt-losing tendency, and acidosis*, Metabolism, 13:513, 1964.   19

ROOK, A. J.: *Endocrine influences on hair growth*, Brit. med. J., 1:609, 1965.   12

SLATON, P. E., AND BIGLIERI: *Hypertension and hyperaldosteronism of renal and adrenal origin*, Amer. J. Med., 38:324, 1965.   18

SOFFER, L. J., IANNACONNE AND GABRILOVE: *Cushing's syndrome*, Amer. J. Med., 30:129, 1961.   9

SWEAT, M. L.: *The Nomenclature of the Steroid Hormones*, University of Utah Press, Salt Lake City, 1959.   6

SWINYARD, C. A.: *The innervation of the suprarenal glands*, Anat. Rec., 68:417, 1937.   4

TEITELBAUM, H. A.: *The innervation of the adrenal gland*, Quart. Rev. Biol., 17:135, 1942.   4

TISHERMAN, S. E., GREGG AND DANOWSKI: *Familial pheochromocytoma*, J. Amer. med. Ass., 182:152, 1962.   26

WILKINS, L.: *The Diagnosis and Treatment of Endocrine Disorders in Childhood and Adolescence*, Charles C Thomas, Springfield, Ill., 1960.   14

WILKINSON, I. M. S.: *The intrinsic innervation of the suprarenal gland*, Acta Anat. (Basel), 46:127, 1961.   4

WILSON, D., AND GOETZ: *Selective hypoaldosteronism after prolonged heparin administration*, Amer. J. Med., 36:635, 1964.   21

WOODBURNE, R. T.: *Essentials of Human Anatomy*, Oxford University Press, New York, 1961.   2, 3

Section IV

ALBRIGHT, F., SMITH AND FRASER: *A syndrome characterized by primary ovarian insufficiency and decreased stature. Report of 11 cases with a digression on hormonal control of axillary and pubic hair*, Amer. J. med. Sci., 204:625, 1942.   17

AMELAR, R. D., AND HOTCHKISS: *Congenital aplasia of the epididymides and vasa deferentia: Effects on semen*, Fertil. and Steril., 14:44, 1963.   25

ARGONZ, J., AND DEL CASTILLO: *A syndrome characterized by estrogenic insufficiency, galactorrhea and decreased urinary gonadotropin*, J. clin. Endocr., 13:79, 1953.   27

ARRONET, G. H.: *Studies on ovulation in the normal menstrual cycle*, Fertil. and Steril., 8:301, 1957.   21

BARR, M. L., CARR, POZSONY, WILSON, DUNN, JACOBSON, MILLER, LEWIS AND CHOWN: *The XXXXY sex chromosome abnormality*, Canad. med. Ass. J., 87:891, 1962.   1

BURGER, H. G., KENT AND KELLIE: *Determination of testosterone in human peripheral and adrenal venous plasma*, J. clin. Endocr., 24:432, 1964.   7, 20

BUXTON, C. L., AND SOUTHAM: *Human Infertility*, Hoeber-Harper, New York, 1958.   24, 25

COHEN, M. R., AND HANKIN: *Detecting ovulation*, Fertil. and Steril., 11:497, 1960.   24

——, STEIN, SR., AND KAYE: *Spinnbarkeit: A characteristic of cervical mucus. Significance at ovulation time*, Fertil. and Steril., 3:201, 1952.   24

COWIE, A. T., AND FOLLEY: *The mammary gland and lactation*, in *Sex and Internal Secretions*, ed. by Young, Williams & Wilkins Company, Baltimore, 1961.   26

DAVIDSON, W. M., AND FLUTE: *Sex dimorphism in polymorphonuclear neutrophil leucocytes*, Acta cytol. (Philad.), 6:13, 1962.   15

DE ALLENDE, I. L. C., AND ORIAS: *Cytology of the Human Vagina*, Paul B. Hoeber, New York, 1950.   22

DECKER, A.: *Culdoscopy*, W. B. Saunders Company, Philadelphia, 1952.   24

DELLER, J. J., WEGIENKA, CONTE, ROSNER AND FORSHAM: *Testosterone metabolism in idiopathic hirsutism*, Ann. intern. Med., in press.   7, 20

DOWLING, J. T., RICHARDS, FREINKEL AND INGBAR: *Nonpuerperal galactorrhea. Eleven cases without enlargement of the sella turcica*, Arch. intern. Med., 107:885, 1961.   27

EDITORIAL: *Incidence and significance of gynecomastia*, J. Amer. med. Ass., 184:233, 1963.   26

EDMONDSON, H. A., GLASS AND SOLL: *Gynecomastia associated with cirrhosis of the liver*, Proc. Soc. exper. Biol. (N. Y.), 42:97, 1939.   26

ENGLE, E. T.: *Endometrial interpretation*, in Buxton, C. L., and Southam: *Human Infertility*, Hoeber-Harper, New York, 1958.   24

FERGUSON-SMITH, M. A., AND JOHNSTON: *Chromosome abnormalities in certain diseases of man*, Ann. intern. Med., 53:359, 1960.   3

FOLLEY, S. J.: *Disorders of mammary development and lactation*, in *Clinical Endocrinology*, ed. by Astwood, Grune & Stratton, Inc., New York, 1960.   26, 27

FONTANA, A. L., AND SIMPSON: *Arrhenoblastoma: Review of the literature and report of a case*, Obstet. and Gynec., 23:730, 1964.   20

FORBES, A. P., HENNEMAN, GRISWOLD AND ALBRIGHT: *Syndrome characterized by galactorrhea, amenorrhea and low urinary*

FSH: *Comparison with acromegaly and normal lactation,* J. clin. Endocr., 14:265, 1954.   27

Foss, G. L.: *Abnormalities of form and function of the human breast,* J. Endocr., 14:VI, 1956.   26, 27

—— AND SHORT: *Abnormal lactation,* J. Obstet. Gynaec. Brit. Emp., 58:35, 1951.   27

GARCIA, C. R., AND ROCK: *Ovulation,* in *Essentials of Human Reproduction,* ed. by Velardo, J. T., Oxford University Press, New York, 1958.   21

GENTILE, L. A.: *Galactorrhea following extirpation of the uterus and both ovaries,* N. Y. St. J. Med., 60:3468, 1960.   27

GREENBLATT, R. B.: *The Hirsute Female,* Charles C Thomas, Springfield, Ill., 1963.   20

——, CARMONA AND HAGLER: *Chiari-Frommel syndrome: A syndrome characterized by galactorrhea, amenorrhea, and pituitary dysfunction; Report of two cases,* Obstet. and Gynec., 7:165, 1956.   27

GRUMBACH, M. M., AND BARR: *Nuclear sex in sexual anomalies,* Recent Progr. Hormone Res., 14:225, 1958.   1, 2, 3, 15

—— AND ——: *Cytologic tests of chromosomal sex in relation to sexual anomalies in man,* Recent Progr. Hormone Res., 14:255, 1958.   2

GUMPEL, R. C.: *Pituitary tumor, postpartum amenorrhea, and galactorrhea, with comments on Chiari-Frommel syndrome,* N. Y. St. J. Med., 60:3304, 1960.   27

HALL, P. F.: *Gynecomastia,* in *Clinical Endocrinology,* ed. by Astwood, Grune & Stratton, Inc., New York, 1960.   26

HAMBLEN, E. C.: *A rational approach to the management of the infertile couple,* in *Sterility, Office Management of the Infertile Couple,* ed. by Tyler, McGraw-Hill Book Company, New York, 1961.   24, 25

HARDY, J. P.: *Gynecomastia associated with lung cancer,* J. Amer. med. Ass., 173:1462, 1960.   26

HOOPER, J. H., JR., WELCH AND SHACKELFORD: *Abnormal lactation associated with tranquilizing drug therapy,* J. Amer. med. Ass., 178:506, 1961.   27

JACOBS, P. A., HARNDEN, BUCKTON, BROWN, KING, MCBRIDE, MACGREGOR, MACLEAN, FOTHERINGHAM AND ISDALE: *Cytogenetic studies in primary amenorrhea,* Lancet, I:1183, 1961.   24

JOHNSON, H. W., POSHYACHINDA, MCCORMICK AND HAMBLEN: *Lactation with a phenothiazine derivative (Temaril),* Amer. J. Obstet. Gynec., 80:124, 1960.   27

KISTNER, R. W.: *Infertility, diagnosis and treatment,* Med. Science, 11:161, 1961.   24, 25

KLINEFELTER, H. F., JR., REIFENSTEIN, JR., AND ALBRIGHT: *Syndrome characterized by gynecomastia, aspermatogenesis without A-Leydigism and increased excretion of follicle-stimulating hormone,* J. clin. Endocr., 2:615, 1942.   16

LEVINE, H. J., BERGENSTAL AND THOMAS: *Persistent lactation: Endocrine and histologic studies in 5 cases,* Amer. J. med. Sci., 243:118, 1962.   27

LEWINN, E. B.: *Gynecomastia during digitalis therapy. Report of eight additional cases with liver-function studies,* New Engl. J. Med., 248:316, 1953.   26

LJUNBERG, T.: *Hereditary gynecomastia,* Acta med. scand., 168:371, 1960.   26

MACLEAN, N.: *The drumsticks of polymorphonuclear leucocytes in sex-chromosome abnormalities,* Lancet, I:1154, 1962.   2

MACLEOD, J.: *The male factor in fertility and infertility,* Fertil. and Steril., 8:387, 1956.   25

—— AND GOLD: *The male factor in fertility and infertility. II. Spermatozoan counts in 1000 men of known fertility and in 1000 cases of infertile marriages,* J. Urol. (Baltimore), 66:436, 1951.   25

——, —— AND MCLANE: *Correlation of the male and female factors in human infertility,* Fertil. and Steril., 6:112, 1955.   24, 25

—— AND TIETZE: *Control of reproductive capacity,* Ann. Rev. Med., 15:299, 1965.   24, 25

MAHESH, V. B.: *Urinary steroid excretion patterns in hirsutism. I. Use of adrenal and ovarian suppression tests in the study of hirsutism,* J. clin. Endocr., 24:1283, 1964.   20

——, GREENBLATT, AYDER AND ROY: *Secretion of androgens by the polycystic ovary and its significance,* Fertil. and Steril., 13:513, 1962.   7

MASTROIANNI, L.: *Clinical concepts of infertility,* in *Essentials of Human Reproduction,* ed. by Velardo, Oxford University Press, New York, 1958.   24, 25

MCCULLAGH, E. P., ALIVISATOS AND SCHAFFENBURG: *Pituitary tumor with gynecomastia and lactation. Case report,* J. clin. Endocr., 16:397, 1956.   26, 27

MCKUSICK, V. A.: *On the X chromosome of man,* Quart. Rev. Biol., 37:69, 1962.   15

MOORE, K. L., AND BARR: *Smears from the oral mucosa in the detection of chromosomal sex,* Lancet, II:57, 1955.   2

——, GRAHAM AND BARR: *The detection of chromosomal sex in hermaphrodites from a skin biopsy,* Surg. Gynec. Obstet., 96:641, 1953.   2

MORRIS, J. M.: *The syndrome of testicular feminization in male pseudohermaphrodites,* Amer. J. Obstet. Gynec., 65:1192, 1953.   12

—— AND MAHESH: *Further observations on the syndrome of "testicular feminization",* Amer. J. Obstet. Gynec., 87:731, 1963.   12

NELSON, W. O.: *Interpretation of testicular biopsy,* J. Amer. med. Ass., 151:449, 1953.   25

NYDICK, M., BUSTOS, DALE, JR., AND RAWSON: *Gynecomastia in adolescent boys,* J. Amer. med. Ass., 178:449, 1961.   26

PAPANICOLAOU, G. N.: *Sexual cycle in the human female as revealed by vaginal smears,* Amer. J. Anat., 52:519, 1933.   22

PINCUS, G., ROMANOFF AND CARLO: *The excretion of urinary steroids by men and women of various ages,* J. Geront., 9:113, 1954.   21

REECE, R. P.: *Mammary gland development and function,* in *The Endocrinology of Reproduction,* ed. by Velardo, Oxford University Press, New York, 1958.   26, 27

REICHLIN, S.: *Neuroendocrinology,* New Engl. J. Med., 269:1182, 1246, 1296, 1963.   21

ROBINSON, A.: *Nomenclature of human mitotic chromosomes,* J. Amer. med. Ass., 174:159, 1960.   2

ROGERS, J.: *Endocrine and Metabolic Aspects of Gynecology,* W. B. Saunders Company, Philadelphia, 1963.   21

——: *The menopause,* New Engl. J. Med., 254:697, 750, 1956.   21

ROSS, G. T., AND TIJO: *Cytogenetics in clinical endocrinology,* J. Amer. med. Ass., 192:977, 1965.   15

SEGRE, E. J., KLAIBER, LOBETSKY AND LLOYD: *Hirsutism and virilizing syndromes,* Ann. Rev. Med., 15:315, 1964.   20

SHORR, E.: *An evaluation of the clinical applications of the vaginal smear method,* J. Mt. Sinai Hosp., 12:667, 1945.   22

SHUSTER, S., AND BROWN: *Gynaecomastia and urinary oestrogens in patients with generalized skin disease,* Lancet, II:1358, 1962.   26

SOHVAL, A. R.: *Chromosomes and sex chromatin in normal and anomalous sexual development,* Physiol. Rev., 43:306, 1963.   1, 2, 3, 15

——: *Recent progress in human chromosome analysis and its relation to the sex chromatin,* Amer. J. Med., 31:397, 1961.   1, 2, 3, 15

—— AND CASSELMAN: *Alteration in size of nuclear sex-chromatin mass (Barr body) induced by antibiotics,* Lancet, II:1386, 1961.   15

SOMLYO, A. P., AND WAYE: *Abnormal lactation. Report of a case induced by reserpine and a brief review of the subject,* J. Mt. Sinai Hosp., 27:5, 1960.   27

STARR, P.: *Gynecomastia during hyperthyroidism,* J. Amer. med. Ass., 104:1988, 1935.   26

STEIN, I. F., SR.: *Eight years experience with roentgen diagnosis in gynecology; pneumoperitoneum and lipiodol in pelvic diagnosis,* Amer. J. Obst. Gynec., 21:671, 1931.   24

TAYLOR, A. I.: *Ambiguous sex and sex chromatin in the newborn,* Lancet, II:1059, 1962.   2, 3, 15

TILLINGER, K. A.: *Testicular morphology. A histo-pathologic study with special reference to biopsy findings in hypogonadism with mainly endocrine disorders and in gynecomastia,* Acta Endocr. (Kbh.), 24: (Suppl. 30), 1957.   26

TINDAL, J. S., AND MCNAUGHT: *Hormonal factors in breast development and milk secretion,* in *Modern Trends in Endocrinology,* ed. by Gardiner-Hill, Paul B. Hoeber, Inc., New York, 1958.   26, 27

TREVES, N.: *Gynecomastia: The origins of mammary swelling in the male: an analysis of 406 patients with breast hypertrophy, 525 with testicular tumors, and 13 with adrenal neoplasms,* Cancer, 11:1083, 1958.   26

TURNER, H. H.: *A syndrome of infantilism, congenital webbed neck and cubitus valgus,* Endocrinology, 23:566, 1938.   17

TYLER, E. T.: *Evaluation of male fertility,* in *Sterility, Office Management of the Infertile Couple,* McGraw-Hill Book Company, New York, 1961.   25

——: *Postcoital tests,* in *Sterility, Office Management of the Infertile Couple,* ed. by

Section IV (continued)	PLATE NUMBER

Tyler, McGraw-Hill Book Company, New York, 1961. — 25

Van Wyk, J. J., and Grumbach: *Syndrome of precocious menstruation and galactorrhea in juvenile hypothyroidism: An example of hormonal overlap in pituitary feedback*, J. Pediat., 57:416, 1960. — 27

Warburg, E.: *A fertile patient with Klinefelter's syndrome*, Acta Endocr. (Kbh.), 43:12, 1963. — 16

White, M. J. D.: *The Chromosomes, Methuen's Monographs*, John Wiley & Sons, Inc., New York, 1961. — 1

Whitelaw, M. J.: *Hormonal control of the basal body temperature pattern*, Fertil. and Steril., 3:230, 1952. — 24

Williams, M. J.: *Gynecomastia. Its incidence, recognition and host characterization in 447 autopsy cases*, Amer. J. Med., 34:103, 1963. — 26

—— and Sommer: *Endocrine and certain other changes in men with carcinoma of the lung*, Cancer, 15:109, 1962. — 26

Section V

General References

Danowski, T. S., Editor: *Diabetes Mellitus. Diagnosis and Treatment*, American Diabetes Association, Inc., New York, 1964.

Joslin, E. P., Root, White and Marble: *The Treatment of Diabetes Mellitus*, Lea & Febiger, Philadelphia, 1959.

Marble, A., and Cahill: *The Chemistry and Chemotherapy of Diabetes Mellitus*, Charles C Thomas, Springfield, Ill., 1962.

White, P., Editor: *Diabetes*, Med. Clin. N. Amer., 49:855, 1965.

Williams, R. H., Editor: *Diabetes*, Paul B. Hoeber, Inc., New York, 1960.

Albrink, M. J., Lavietes and Man: *Vascular disease and serum lipids in diabetes mellitus*, Ann. intern. Med., 58:305, 1963. — 27, 28

Amatuzio, D. S., Rames and Nesbitt: *The practical application of the rapid intravenous glucose tolerance test in various disease states affecting glucose metabolism*, J. Lab. clin. Med., 48:714, 1956. — 29

Antoniades, H. N., Bougas and Pyle: *Studies on the state of insulin in blood. Examination of splenic, portal and peripheral blood serum of diabetic and nondiabetic subjects for "free" insulin and insulin complexes*, New Engl. J. Med., 267:218, 1962. — 18

Ashton, N.: *Studies of the retinal capillaries in relation to diabetic and other retinopathies*, Brit. J. Ophthal., 47:521, 1963. — 23

Beck, P., Koumans, Winterling, Stein, Daughaday and Kipnis: *Studies of insulin and growth hormone secretion in human obesity*, J. Lab. clin. Med., 64:654, 1964. — 21

Beetham, W. P.: *Visual prognosis of proliferating diabetic retinopathy*, Brit. J. Ophthal., 47:611, 1963. — 23

Section V (continued)	PLATE NUMBER

Bernhard, H.: *Long term observations on oral hypoglycemic agents in diabetes. The effect of carbutamide and tolbutamide*, Diabetes, 14:59, 1965. — 31

Boshell, B. R.: *Diabetic acidosis*, GP (Kansas), 30:112, 1964. — 19

——, Barret, Wilensky and Patton: *Insulin resistance. Response to insulin from various animal sources, including human*, Diabetes, 13:144, 1964. — 18

Cogan, D. G., and Kuwabara: *Capillary shunts in the pathogenesis of diabetic retinopathy*, Diabetes, 12:293, 1963. — 23

Cushman, P., Jr., Dubois, Dwyer and Izzo: *Protracted tolbutamide hypoglycemia*, Amer. J. Med., 35:196, 1963. — 31

Danowski, T. S.: Editorial: *Lactic acidosis in diabetes mellitus*, J. Amer. med. Ass., 184:47, 1963. — 31

Dible, J. H.: *Some pathological adaptations in the peripheral circulation*, Lancet, I(7029):1031, 1958. — 28

Ellenberg, M.: *Clinical concepts of prediabetes*, N. Y. St. J. Med., 64:1885, 1964. — 29

——: *Diabetic neuropathy*, in *Clinical Diabetes Mellitus*, ed. by Ellenberg, McGraw-Hill Book Company, New York, 1962. — 26

Engelhardt, H. T., and Vecchio: *The long-term effect of tolbutamide on glucose in adult, asymptomatic, latent diabetics*, Metabolism, 14:885, 1965. — 31

Fajans, S. S.: *Current concepts: Leucine induced hypoglycemia*, New Engl. J. Med., 272:1224, 1965. — 16

Field, J. B., Keen, Johnson and Herring: *Insulinlike activity of nonpancreatic tumors associated with hypoglycemia*, J. clin. Endocr., 23:1229, 1963. — 16

Floyd, J. C., Jr., Fajans, Knopf and Conn: *Plasma insulin in organic hyperinsulinism: Comparative effects of tolbutamide, leucine and glucose*, J. clin. Endocr., 24:747, 1964. — 16

Foa, P. P., and Galansino: *Glucagon*, Charles C Thomas, Springfield, Ill., 1962. — 4, 17

Freinkel, N., Singer, Arky, Bleicher, Anderson and Silbert: *Alcohol hypoglycemia. I. Carbohydrate metabolism of patients with clinical alcohol hypoglycemia and the experimental reproduction of the syndrome with pure ethanol*, J. clin. Invest., 42:1112, 1963. — 15

Grodsky, G. M., and Forsham: *An immunochemical assay of total extractable insulin in man*, J. clin. Invest., 39:1070, 1960. — 23

Hansen, R. O.: *Bacteriuria in diabetic and non-diabetic out-patients*, Acta med. scand., 176:721, 1965. — 25

Hardy, J. D.: *Surgery of islet cell tumors*, Amer. J. med. Sci., 246:218, 1963. — 16, 17

Harper, H. A.: *Review of Physiological Chemistry*, Lange Medical Publications, Los Altos, 1965. — 6–15, 19

Heuizenga, K. A., Goodnick and Summerskill: *Peptic ulcer with islet cell tumor. A reappraisal*, Amer. J. Med., 37:564, 1964. — 17

Section V (continued)	PLATE NUMBER

Karam, J. H.: *Critical factors in excessive serum insulin response to glucose*, Lancet, I:286, 1965. — 21

——, Grodsky and Forsham: *Excessive insulin response to glucose in obese subjects as measured by immunochemical assay*, Diabetes, 12:197, 1963. — 21

Krall, L. P., and Bradley: *Long term phenformin therapy for diabetes—with emphasis on the older patient*, Geriatrics, 17:337, 1962. — 31

Kvane, D. O., and Stanton: *Studies on diazoxide hyperglycemia*, Diabetes, 13:639, 1964. — 16

Lawrence, R. D.: *Treatment of 90 severe diabetics with soluble insulin for 20-40 years*, Brit. med. J., 2(5373):1624, 1963. — 31

Levine, R.: *On some biochemical aspects of diabetes mellitus*, Amer. J. Med., 31:901, 1961. — 6–15, 19

—— and Mahler: *Production, secretion and availability of insulin*, Ann. Rev. Med., 15:413, 1964. — 2, 3

Lukens, F. D. W.: *Insulin and protein metabolism*, Diabetes, 13:451, 1964. — 12, 14

——: *The rediscovery of regular insulin*, New Engl. J. Med., 272:130, 1965. — 31

Maccario, M., Massis and Vastola: *Focal seizures as a manifestation of hyperglycemia without ketoacidosis: A report of seven cases with review of the literature*, Neurology, 15:195, 1965. — 15

Marble, A.: *Diabetic nephropathy*, in *Diseases of the Kidney*, ed. by Strauss, Little Brown & Company, Boston, 1963. — 25

Moorhouse, J. A., Steinberg and Tessler: *Effect of glucose dose upon intravenous glucose tolerance in health and in diabetes*, J. clin. Endocr., 23:1074, 1963. — 29

Narva, W. M., Benoit and Ringrose: *Necrobiosis lipoidica diabeticorum*, Arch. intern. Med., 115:718, 1965. — 22

Nilsson, S. E.: *Genetic and constitutional aspects of diabetes mellitus*, Acta med. scand., 171: (Suppl.) 375, 1962. — 29

Palumbo, P. J., Molnar and Tauxe: *Adrenal steroid therapy in insulin resistance*, Proc. Mayo Clin., 39:161, 1964. — 31

Power, L., Lucas and Conn: *Further studies on insulin augmentation capacities of various serum proteins*, Metabolism, 14:845, 1965. — 30

Randle, P. J., Hales, Garland and Newsholme: *The glucose fatty-acid cycle. Its role in insulin sensitivity and the metabolic disturbances of diabetes mellitus*, Lancet, II:7285, 1963. — 5

Remein, O. R., and Wilkerson: *Efficiency of screening method for diabetes mellitus*, J. chron. Dis., 13:6, 1961. — 29

Renold, A. E., Martin, Dagenais, Steinke, Nickerson and Sheps: *Measurement of small quantities of insulin-like activity using rat adipose tissue*, J. clin. Invest., 39:1487, 1960. — 30

Roth, J., Glick, Yalow and Berson: *Hypoglycemia: A potent stimulus to secretion of growth hormone*, Science, 140:987, 1963. — 15

SIPERSTEIN, M. D., COLWELL AND MEYER: *Small Blood Vessel Involvement in Diabetes Mellitus,* American Institute of Biological Sciences, Washington, D. C., 1964.   22

SPRAGUE, R. G.: *Impotence in male diabetics,* Diabetes, 12:559, 1963.   26

STEINBERG, A. G.: *The genetics of diabetes. A review,* Ann. N. Y. Acad. Sci., 82:197, 1959.   29

STEINKE, J., SOELDNER, CAMERINI-DAVALOS AND RENOLD: *Studies on serum insulin-like activity (ILA) in prediabetes and early overt diabetes,* Diabetes, 12:502, 1963.   30

STRANDNESS, D. E., PRIEST AND GIBBINS: *Combined clinical and pathologic study of diabetic and nondiabetic peripheral arterial disease,* Diabetes, 13:366, 1964.   27, 28

UNGER, R. H., AND MADISON: *Comparison of response to intravenously administered sodium tolbutamide in mild diabetic and nondiabetic subjects,* J. clin. Invest., 37:627, 1958.   29

—— AND EISENTRAUT: *Studies of the physiological role of glucagon,* Diabetes, 13:563, 1964.   4

VALLANCE, O. J., DARMANDY, NELIGAM AND LLOYD: *Hypoglycemia in childhood,* Proc. roy. soc. Med., 57:1055, 1964.   17

VALLENCE-OWEN, J.: *Insulin antagonists,* Brit. med. Bull., 16:214, 1960.   18

——, HURLOCK AND PLEASE: *Plasma insulin activity in diabetes mellitus measured by the rat diaphragm technic,* Lancet, II:583, 1955.   30

WARREN, S., AND LE COMPTE: *The Pathology of Diabetes Mellitus,* Lea & Febiger, Philadelphia, 1952.   21

WATERS, W. C., HALL AND SCHWARTZ: *Spontaneous lactic acidosis,* Amer. J. Med., 35:781, 1963.   31

WERNER, P.: *Endocrine adenomatosis and peptic ulcer in a large kindred. Inherited multiple tumors and mosaic pleistropism in man,* Amer. J. Med., 35:205, 1963.   17

WEST, K. M., AND JOHNSON: *Comparative pharmacology of tolbutamide, carbutamide, chlorpropamide and metahexamide in man,* Metabolism, 8:596, 1959.   31

WILKERSON, H. L. C., HYMAN, KAUFMAN, McCUISTION AND FRANCIS: *Diagnostic evaluation of oral glucose tolerance tests in nondiabetic subjects after various levels of carbohydrate intake,* New Engl. J. Med., 262:1047, 1960.   29

YALOW, R. S., AND BERSON: *Immunoassay of endogenous plasma insulin in man,* J. clin. Invest., 39:1157, 1960.   30

—— AND ——: *Reaction of fish insulins with human insulin antiserums: Potential value in the treatment of insulin resistance,* New Engl. J. Med., 270:1171, 1964.   18

ZIERLER, K. L., AND RABINOWITZ: *Roles of insulin and growth hormone based on studies of forearm metabolism in man,* Medicine (Baltimore), 42:385, 1963.   12

ZOLLINGER, R., AND ELLISON: *Primary peptic ulcerations of the jejunum associated with islet cell tumors of the pancreas,* Ann. Surg., 142:709, 1955.   17

Section VI

General References

ALBRIGHT, F.: *The Parathyroid Glands and Metabolic Bone Disease,* Williams & Wilkins Company, Baltimore, 1948.

AVERY, M. E., McAFEE AND GUILD: *The course and prognosis of reticulo-endotheliosis (eosinophilic granuloma, Schüller-Christian disease and Letterer-Siwe disease); a study of forty cases,* Amer. J. Med., 22:636, 1957.

BARTTER, F. C.: *Osteoporosis,* Amer. J. Med., 22:797, 1957.

COPP, D. H.: *Calcium and phosphorus metabolism,* Amer. J. Med., 22:275, 1957.

FOLLES, R. H., JR.: *A survey of bone disease,* Amer. J. Med., 22:469, 1957.

GOLDMAN, L., AND GREENSPAN: *Applied physiology of the thyroid and parathyroid glands,* Surg. Clin. N. Amer., 45:317, 1965.

NEUMAN, W. F., AND NEUMAN: *Emerging concepts of the structure and metabolic functions of bone,* Amer. J. Med., 22:123, 1957.

RASMUSSEN, H., AND REIFENSTEIN, JR.: *The Parathyroid Glands,* page 731 in *Textbook of Endocrinology,* ed. by Williams, W. B. Saunders Company, Philadelphia and London, 3rd edition, 1962.

RAY, R. D.: *Metabolic diseases of bone,* Med. Clin. N. Amer., 49:241, 1965.

SNAPPER, I., AND NATHAN: *Rickets and osteomalacia,* Amer. J. Med., 22:939, 1957.

PLATE NUMBER

AEGERTER, E.: *The possible relationship of neurofibromatosis, congenital pseudarthrosis and fibrous dysplasia,* J. Bone Jt Surg., 32A:618, 1950.   19

ALBRIGHT, F., BURNETT, PARSON, REIFENSTEIN, JR., AND ROOS: *Osteomalacia and late rickets,* Medicine (Baltimore), 25:399, 1946.   14, 15

BALOGH, K., JR., AND COHEN: *Oxidative enzymes in the epithelial cells of normal and pathological human parathyroid glands. A histochemical study,* Lab. Invest., 10:354, 1961.   1, 2

BARNES, B. A., AND COPE: *Carcinoma of the parathyroid glands,* J. Amer. med. Ass., 178:556, 1961.   7

BELL, N. H., GERARD AND BARTTER: *Pseudohypoparathyroidism with osteitis fibrosa cystica and impaired absorption of calcium,* J. clin. Endocr., 23:759, 1963.   11, 12

BENEDICT, P. H.: *Endocrine features in Albright's syndrome (fibrous dysplasia of bone),* Metabolism, 11:30, 1962.   19

BETHUNE, J. E.: *The recognition and management of hypercalcemia,* GP (Kansas), 28:114, 1963.   5

BLACK, B. M.: *Difficulties in the treatment of hyperparathyroidism,* Surg. Clin. N. Amer., 43:1115, 1963.   4

——: *Hyperparathyroidism,* Charles C Thomas, Springfield, Ill., 1953.   3–7

BRONSKY, D., KUSHNER, DUBIN AND SNAPPER: *Idiopathic hypoparathyroidism and pseudohypoparathyroidism: case reports and review of the literature,* Medicine (Baltimore), 37:317, 1958.   10–12

CASTLEMAN, B.: *Tumors of the parathyroid gland,* Sec. IV, Fasc. 15, *Atlas of Tumor Pathology* (pages 1–74), Armed Forces Institute of Pathology, Washington, D. C., 1952.   7

—— AND MALLORY: *Parathyroid hyperplasia in chronic renal insufficiency,* Amer. J. Path., 13:553, 1937.   6, 7

CHAMBERS, E. L., GORDAN, GOLDMAN AND REIFENSTEIN: *Tests for hyperparathyroidism: tubular reabsorption of phosphate, phosphate deprivation and calcium infusion,* J. clin. Endocr., 16:1507, 1956.   5

COSTELLO, J. M., AND DENT: *Hypo-hyperparathyroidism,* Arch. Dis. Childh., 38:397, 1963.   15

DE DEUXCHAISNES, C. N., AND KRANE: *Paget's disease of bone: clinical and metabolic observations,* Medicine (Baltimore), 43:233, 1964.   18

DENT, C. E.: *Some problems of hyperparathyroidism,* Brit. med. J., 2(5317):1419 and 1495, 1962.   3, 4

FOSTER, G. V.: *Calcitonin (Thyrocalcitonin),* New Engl. J. Med., 279:349, 1968.   2

HAAS, H. G., CANARY, KYLE, MEYER AND SCHAAF: *Skeletal calcium retention in osteoporosis and in osteomalacia,* J. clin. Endocr., 23:605, 1963.   14–17

HAMPERL, H.: *Onkocytes and the so-called Hürthle-cell tumor,* Arch. Path., 49:563, 1950.   1, 7

HENNEMAN, P. H., AND WALLACH: *The use of androgens and estrogens and their metabolic effects. Symposium: A review of the prolonged use of estrogens and androgens in postmenopausal and senile osteoporosis,* Arch. intern. Med., 100:715, 1957.   17

HERMANS, P. E., GORMAN, MARTIN AND KELLY: *Pseudopseudohypoparathyroidism (Albright's hereditary osteodystrophy),* Proc. Mayo Clin., 39:81, 1964.   11, 12

HOLZMANN, K., AND LANGE: *Zur Zytologic der Glandula parathyreoidea des Menschen, Weitere Untersuchungen an Epithelkorperadenomen,* Z. f. Zellforsch., 58:759, 1963.   1

HUNG, W., MIGEON AND PARROTT: *A possible autoimmune basis for Addison's disease in three siblings, one with idiopathic hypoparathyroidism, pernicious anemia and superficial moniliasis,* New Engl. J. Med., 269:658, 1963.   8

JONES, K. H., AND FOURMAN: *Prevalence of parathyroid insufficiency after thyroidectomy,* Lancet, II:121, 1963.   9

KOLB, F. O.: *Paget's disease; changes occurring following treatment with newer hormonal agents,* Calif. Med., 91:245, 1959.   18

—— AND STEINBACH: *Pseudohypoparathyroidism with secondary hyperparathyroidism and osteitis fibrosa,* J. clin. Endocr., 22:59, 1962.   11

KRANE, S. M.: *Selected features of the clinical course of hypoparathyroidism,* J. Amer. med. Ass., 178:472, 1961.   9, 10

LAFFERTY, F. W., SPENCER AND PEARSON: *Effects of androgens, estrogens and high*

Section VI (continued)

PLATE NUMBER

calcium intakes on bone formation and resorption in osteoporosis, Amer. J. Med., 36:514, 1964. — 17

LANGE, R.: *Zur Histologie und Zytologic der Glandula parathyreoidea des Menschen, Licht-und Elektronemikroskopische Untersuchungen an Epithelkorperadenomen,* Z. f. Zellforsch., 53:765, 1961. — 1

LUTWAK, L., AND WHEDON: *Osteoporosis.* Disease-A-Month. Year Book, April, 1963. — 17

McCARROLL, H. R.: *Clinical manifestations of congenital neurofibromatosis,* J. Bone Jt Surg., 32A:601, 1950. — 19

MUNGER, B. L., AND ROTH: *The cytology of the normal parathyroid glands of man and Virginia deer. A light and electron microscopic study with morphologic evidence of secretory activity,* J. Cell Biol., 16:379, 1963. — 1

NORDIN, B. E. C.: *Tests for parathyroid function,* Postgrad. Med., 35:A-42, 1964. — 5

RICH, C., ENSINCK AND IVANOVICH: *The effects of sodium fluoride on calcium metabolism of subjects with metabolic bone diseases,* J. clin. Invest., 43:545, 1964. — 17

ROTH, S. I.: *Pathology of the parathyroids in hyperparathyroidism. Discussion of recent advances in anatomy and pathology of the parathyroid glands,* Arch. Path., 73:495, 1962. — 7

—— AND MUNGER: *The cytology of the adenomatous, atrophic, and hyperplastic parathyroid glands of man. A light and electron microscopic study,* Virchows Arch. path. Anat., 335:389, 1962. — 7

——, OLEN AND HANSEN: *The eosinophilic cells of the parathyroid (oxyphil cells), salivary (oncocytes), and thyroid (Hürthle cells) glands. Light and electron microscopic observations,* Lab. Invest., 11:933, 1962. — 7

STANBURY, S. W., AND LUMB: *Metabolic studies of renal osteodystrophy. I. Calcium, phosphorus and nitrogen metabolism in rickets, osteomalacia and hyperparathyroidism complicating chronic uremia and in the osteomalacia of the adult Fanconi syndrome,* Medicine (Baltimore), 41:1, 1962. — 15

STEINBACH, H. L., GORDAN, EISENBERG, CRANE, SILVERMAN AND GOLDMAN: *Primary hyperparathyroidism: a correlation of roentgen, clinical and pathologic features,* Amer. J. Roentgenol., 86:329, 1961. — 4

——, KOLB AND CRANE: *Unusual roentgen manifestations of osteomalacia,* Amer. J. Roentgenol., 82:875, 1959. — 14, 15

—— AND NOETZLI: *Roentgen appearance of the skeleton in osteomalacia and rickets,* Amer. J. Roentgenol., 91:955, 1964. — 14, 15

THOMAS, W. C., JR., CONNOR AND MORGAN: *Diagnostic considerations in hypercalcemia,* New Engl. J. Med., 260:591, 1959. — 5

WEYMOUTH, R. J., AND BAKER: *The presence of argyrophilic granules in the parenchymal cells of the parathyroid glands,* Anat. Rec., 119:519, 1954. — 1

Section VII

General References

HARPER, H. A.: *Review of Physiological Chemistry,* Lange Medical Publications, Los Altos, 1965.

STANBURY, J. B., WYNGAARDEN AND FREDRICKSON, EDITORS: *The Metabolic Basis of Inherited Disease,* McGraw-Hill Book Company, Inc., 1960.

PLATE NUMBER

ADDISON, T., AND GULL: *On a certain affection of the skin, vitiligoidea—(a) plana: (b) tuberosa, with remarks,* Guy's Hosp. Rep., 7:265, 1851. — 7, 8

AHRENS, E. H., JR., HIRSH, OETTE, FARQUHAR AND STEIN: *Carbohydrate-induced and fat-induced hyperlipemia,* Trans. Ass. Amer. Phycns, 74:134, 1961. — 5, 6

ALBRINK, M. J.: *Triglycerides, lipoproteins and coronary artery disease,* Arch. intern. Med., 109:345, 1962. — 12, 13

ALVORD, R. M.: *Coronary heart disease and xanthoma tuberosum associated with hereditary hyperlipemia, study of 30 affected persons in family,* Arch. intern. Med., 84:1002, 1949. — 7, 8

ARONSON, S. M., AND VOLK, EDITORS: *Cerebral Sphingolipidoses,* Academic Press, New York, 1962. — 9

BLOCH, K. E., EDITOR: *Lipide Metabolism,* John Wiley and Sons, Inc., New York, 1960. — 1, 4

BURWELL, C. S., ROBIN, WHALEY AND BICKELMANN: *Extreme obesity associated with alveolar hypoventilation; a Pickwickian syndrome,* Amer. J. Med., 21:811, 1956. — 14, 15

DOLE, V. P., AND HAMLIN: *Particulate fat in lymph and blood,* Physiol. Rev., 42:674, 1962. — 1, 5, 6

ENGELBROTH-HOLM, J., TEILUM AND CHRISTENSEN: *Eosinophil granuloma of bone—Schüller-Christian's,* Acta med. scand., 118:292, 1944. — 10, 11

EPSTEIN, F. H., BLOCK, HAND AND FRANCIS, JR.: *Familial hypercholesterolemia, xanthomatosis and coronary heart disease,* Amer. J. Med., 26:39, 1959. — 7, 8

FREDRICKSON, D. S.: *The inheritance of high density lipoprotein deficiency (Tangier's disease),* J. clin. Invest., 43:228, 1964. — 2

——, ONO AND DAVIS: *Lipolytic activity of post heparin plasma in hyperglyceridemia,* J. Lipid Res., 4:24, 1963. — 5, 6

GOFMAN, J. W.: *Coronary Heart Disease,* Charles C Thomas, Springfield, Ill., 1959. — 12, 13

GORDON, E. S., GOLDBERG AND CHOSY: *A new concept in the treatment of obesity,* J. Amer. med. Ass., 186:50, 1963. — 14, 15

HARRIS-JONES, J. N., JONES AND WELLS: *Xanthomatosis and essential hypercholesterolemia,* Lancet, I:855, 1957. — 7, 8

HAVEL, R. J., EDER AND BRAGDON: *The distribution and chemical composition of ultracentrifugally separated lipoproteins in human serum,* J. clin. Invest., 34:1345, 1955. — 1, 4

—— AND GORDON, JR.: *Idiopathic hyperlipemia: Metabolic studies in an affected family,* J. clin. Invest., 39:1777, 1960. — 5, 6

HEALD, F. P., MUELLER AND DRUGELA: *Glucose and free fatty acid metabolism in*

Section VII (continued)

PLATE NUMBER

obese adolescents, Amer. J. clin. Nutr., 16:256, 1965. — 14, 15

HIRSCHHORN, K., AND WILKINSON: *The mode of inheritance in essential familial hypercholesterolemia,* Amer. J. Med., 26:60, 1959. — 7, 8

HOLT, L. E., JR., AYLWARD AND TIMRES: *Idiopathic familial lipemia,* Bull. Johns Hopk. Hosp., 64:279, 1939. — 5, 6

JEANRENAUD, B.: *Dynamic aspects of adipose tissue metabolism: A review,* Metabolism, 10:535, 1961. — 4

KANE, J. P., LONGCOPE, PAVLATOS AND GRODSKY: *Studies of carbohydrate metabolism in idiopathic hypertriglyceridemia,* Metabolism, 14:471, 1965. — 5, 6

KEKWICK, A., AND PAWAN: *Metabolic study in human obesity with isocaloric diets high in fats, protein and carbohydrate,* Metabolism, 6:447, 1957. — 14, 15

KENNEDY, E. P.: *The metabolism and function of complex lipids,* Harvey Lect., 57:143, 1961-62. — 9-11

KRITCHEVSKY, D.: *Cholesterol,* John Wiley and Sons, Inc., New York, 1958. — 3

KUNKEL, H. G., AND AHRENS: *The relationship between serum lipids and the electrophoretic pattern with particular reference to patients with primary biliary cirrhosis,* J. clin. Invest., 28:1575, 1949. — 5, 6

LICHENSTEIN, L., AND JAFFEE: *Eosinophilic granuloma of bone,* Amer. J. Path., 16:595, 1940. — 10, 11

MAYER, J.: *Obesity: diagnosis and Obesity: etiology and pathogenesis,* Postgrad. Med., 25:469 and 623, 1959. — 14, 15

MOORE, F. D.: *Metabolic Care of the Surgical Patient,* W. B. Saunders Company, Philadelphia, 1959. — 14, 15

NEWBURGH, L. H.: *Obesity: energy metabolism,* Physiol. Rev., 24:18, 1944. — 14, 15

OLSON, R. E., AND VESTER: *Nutrition-endocrine interrelationships in the control of fat transport in man,* Physiol. Rev., 40:677, 1960. — 1

PAWAN, G.: *Final Report on the Symposium on Obesity,* William R. Warren and Co., Ltd., Eastleigh (England), 1962. — 14, 15

PINCUS, G., EDITOR: *Hormones and Atherosclerosis,* Academic Press, New York, 1959. — 12, 13

PORTMAN, O. W., AND STARE: *Dietary regulation of serum cholesterol levels,* Physiol. Rev., 39:407, 1959. — 3

RENOLD, A. E., AND CAHILL, JR., EDITORS: *Handbook of Physiology, Section 5: Adipose Tissue,* American Physiological Society, Washington, D. C., 1965. — 4

SALT, H. B., WOLFF, LLOYD, FOSBROOKE, CAMERON AND HUBBLE: *On having no beta-lipoprotein. A syndrome comprising A-beta-lipoproteinaemia, acanthocytosis and steatorrhea,* Lancet, II:325, 1960. — 2

SANDLER, M., AND BOURNE: *Atherosclerosis and Its Origin,* Academic Press, New York, 1963. — 12, 13

SHERLOCK, S.: *Primary biliary cirrhosis (chronic intrahepatic obstructive jaundice),* Gastroenterology, 37:574, 1959. — 5-8

STEFANIK, P. A., HEALD AND MAYER: *Caloric intake in relation to energy output of obese and non-obese adolescent boys,* Amer. J. clin. Nutr., 7:55, 1959.   14, 15

THANNHAUSER, S. J.: *Diseases of the nervous system associated with disturbances of lipid metabolism,* Ass. Res. nerv. Dis. Proc., 32:238, 1953.   5–11

——: *Lipidoses, Diseases of the Intracellular Lipid Metabolism,* Grune & Stratton, Inc., New York, 1959.   1–12

—— AND MAGENDANTZ: *The different clinical groups of xanthomatous diseases: a clinical physiological study of 22 cases,* Ann. intern. Med., 11:1662, 1938.   5–11

VAN BOGAERT, L., CHAIRMAN: *Cerebral Lipidosis, A Symposium,* ed. by Cumings, J. N., and Lowenthal, Blackwell Scientific Publications, Oxford, 1957.   9

VAN ITALLIE, T. B.: *Physiologic aspects of hunger and satiety,* Diabetes, 8:226, 1959.   14, 15

YUDKIN, J.: *The cause and cure of obesity,* Lancet, II:1135, 1959.   14, 15

Section VIII

ARLINGHAUS, R., SHAEFFER AND SCHWEET: *Mechanism of peptide bond formation in polypeptide synthesis,* Proc. nat. Acad. Sci. (Wash.), 51:1291, 1964.   1, 2

BAYLEY, N.: *Tables for predicting adult height from skeletal age and present height,* J. Pediat., 28:49, 1946.   8, 9

BOWER, B. F., AND GORDAN: *Hormonal effects of nonendocrine tumors,* Ann. Rev. Med., 16:83, 1965.   13

BOYER, S. H., EDITOR: *Papers on Human Genetics,* Prentice-Hall, Inc., Englewood Cliffs, N. J., 1963.   3–6

CAFFEY, J.: *Pediatric X-ray Diagnosis,* Year Book Medical Publishers, Chicago, 1961.   8, 9

CAIRNS, J.: *The bacterial chromosome and its manner of replication as seen by autoradiography,* J. molec. Biol., 6:208, 1963.   2

CHAPEVILLE, F., LIPMANN, VON EHRENSTEIN, WEISBLUM, RAY, JR., AND BENZER: *On the role of soluble ribonucleic acid in coding for amino acids,* Proc. nat. Acad. Sci. (Wash.), 48:1086, 1962.   1, 2

CLARKE, C. A.: *Genetics for the Clinician,* F. A. Davis Company, Philadelphia, 1964.   3–6

DAVIES, J., GILBERT AND GORINI: *Streptomycin suppression and the code,* Proc. nat. Acad. Sci. (Wash.), 51:883, 1964.   1, 2

DREIZEN, S., SNODGRASSE, WEBB-PEPLOE AND SPIES: *The retarding effect of protracted undernutrition on the appearance of the postnatal ossification centers in the hand and wrist,* Hum. Biol., 30:253, 1958.   8, 9

ELGENMARK, O.: *The normal development of the ossific centres during infancy and childhood,* Acta Paediat. (Uppsala), (Suppl. 1), 33:1, 1946.   8, 9

GARN, S. M., AND ROHMANN: *Variability in the order of ossification of the bony centers of the hand and wrist,* Amer. J. Phys. Anthrop., 18:219, 1960.   8, 9

GILBERT, W.: *Polypeptide synthesis in E. coli. I. Ribosomes and the active complex,* J. molec. Biol., 6:389, 1963.   1, 2

GOLDSCHMIDT, R. B.: *Understanding Hered-*

ity. An Introduction to Genetics, John Wiley & Sons, Inc., New York, 1952.   3–6

GREULICH, W. W., AND PYLE: *Radiographic Atlas of Skeletal Development of the Hand and Wrist,* Stanford University Press, Stanford, 1959.   8–9

HAMERTON, J. L., EDITOR: *Chromosomes in Medicine,* Grune & Stratton, Inc., New York, 1963.   2

HARPER, H. A.: *Review of Physiological Chemistry,* Lange Medical Publications, Los Altos, 1965.   7

HODGES, P. C.: *An epiphyseal chart,* Amer. J. Roentgenol., 30:809, 1933.   8, 9

HOERR, N. L., PYLE AND FRANCIS: *Radiographic Atlas of Skeletal Development of Foot and Ankle, a Standard of Reference,* Charles C Thomas, Springfield, Ill., 1962.   8, 9

HUGGINS, C., AND HODGES: *Studies on prostatic cancer. I. The effect of castration, of estrogen and of androgen injection on serum phosphatases in metastatic carcinoma of the prostate,* Cancer Res., 1:293, 1941.   15

KELLEY, R. M., AND BAKER: *Progestational agents in the treatment of carcinoma of the endometrium,* New Engl. J. Med., 264:216, 1961.   15

KORNBERG, A.: *Biologic synthesis of deoxyribonucleic acid,* Science, 131:1503, 1960.   2

LEDERBERG, J.: *A view of genetics,* Science, 131:269, 1960.   2

McKUSICK, V. A.: *Human Genetics,* Prentice-Hall, Inc., Englewood Cliffs, N. J., 1964.   2–6

MONTAGU, M. F. A., EDITOR: *Genetic Mechanisms in Human Disease: Chromosomal Aberrations,* Charles C Thomas, Springfield, Ill., 1961.   2–6

PINCUS, G., AND VOOMER: *Biological Activities of Steroids in Relation to Cancer,* Academic Press, New York, 1960.   14, 15

PYLE, S. I., AND HOERR: *Radiographic Atlas of Skeletal Development of the Knee: a Standard of Reference,* Charles C Thomas, Springfield, Ill., 1955.   8, 9

——, STUART, CORONI AND REED: *Onsets, Completions, and Spans of the Osseous Stage of Development in Representative Bone Growth Centers of the Extremities,* Child Development Publications, Purdue University, Lafayette, Indiana, 1961.   8, 9

SEGALOFF, A.: *The endocrinologic effects of tumors,* J. chron. Dis., 16:727, 1963.   13

—— (GROUP CHAIRMAN): *Progress report: Results of studies by the Cooperative Breast Cancer Group, 1956-1960.* Cancer Chemother. Rep., 11:109, 1961.   14, 15

——: *Antitumor activity of endocrine agents in tumors in humans,* Cancer Chemother. Rep., 16:49, 1962.   14, 15

——: *Alterations in hormonal balance as cancer therapy,* Proc. National Cancer Conf., 4:195, 1960.   14, 15

——, HATCH AND RONGONE: *Elevated plasma corticoids associated with lung cancer,* Cancer Chemother. Rep., 16:343, 1962.   13

STERN, C.: *Principles of Human Genetics,* W. H. Freeman & Company, San Francisco, 1960.   2–6

STRAUSS, B. S.: *An Outline of Chemical*

Genetics, W. B. Saunders Company, Philadelphia and London, 1960.   2–6

TANNER, J. M., PRADER, HABICH AND FERGUSON-SMITH: *Genes on the Y chromosome influencing rate of maturation in man; skeletal age studies in children with Klinefelter's (XXY) and Turner's (XO) syndromes,* Lancet, II:141, 1959.   8, 9

TAYLOR, S. G., TYLER AND VOLK (COOPERATIVE BREAST CANCER GROUP): *Testosterone propionate therapy of breast cancer—a progress report,* Cancer Chemother. Rep., 16:273, 1962.   14, 15

WATSON, J. D., AND CRICK: *Molecular structure of nucleic acids,* Nature (Lond.), 171:737, 1953.   1, 2

WILKINS, M. H. F.: *Physical studies of the molecular structure of deoxyribose nucleic acid and nucleoprotein,* Cold Spring Harbor Symposia on Quantitative Biology, 21:75, 1956.   1, 2

Section IX

General References

GARROD, A. E.: *Inborn Errors of Metabolism.* (Reprinted with a supplement by Harry Harris.) Oxford University Press, London, 1963.

HARPER, H. A.: *Review of Physiological Chemistry,* Lange Medical Publications, Los Altos, 1965.

STANBURY, J. B., WYNGAARDEN AND FREDERICKSON, EDITORS: *The Metabolic Basis of Inherited Disease,* McGraw-Hill Book Company, New York, 1960.

———

BARTER, F. C., LOTZ, THIER, ROSENBERG AND POTTS, JR.: *Cystinuria. Combined Clinical Staff Conference at the National Institutes of Health,* Ann. intern. Med., 62:796, 1965.   7

BICKEL, H., BAAR, ASTLEY, DOUGLAS, FINCH, HARRIS, HARVEY, HICKMANS, PHILPOTT, SMALLWOOD, SMELLIE AND TEALL: *Cystine storage disease with aminoaciduria and dwarfism (Lignac-Fanconi disease),* Acta paediat. (Uppsala), (Suppl. 90), 42:9, 1952.   7

BUCHANAN, J. M.: *The enzymatic synthesis of the purine nucleotides,* Harvey Lectures, 54:104, 1960.   3

CRAWHALL, J. C., SCOWEN AND WATTS: *Further observations on use of D-Penicillamine in cystinuria,* Brit. med. J., 1(5395):1411, 1964.   7

DENT, C. E., FRIEDMAN, GREEN AND WATSON: *Treatment of cystinuria,* Brit. med. J., 1(5432):403, 1965.   7

DE TONI, G., DURAND AND ROSSO: *Oxalosis: A new metabolic disease of the "storage" type,* Minerva pediat., 9:623, 1957 (in Italian, Turin, Italy) and J. Amer. med. Ass., 165:1341, 1957.   6

DONNELL, G. N., COLLADO AND KOCH: *Growth and development of children with galactosemia,* J. Pediat., 58:836, 1961.   11

ELDER, T. D., AND WYNGAARDEN: *The biosynthesis and turnover of oxalate in normal and hyperoxaluric subjects,* J. clin. Invest., 39:1337, 1960.   6

FROESCH, E. R., WOLF, BAITSCH, PRADER

Section IX (continued)	PLATE NUMBER

AND LABHART: *Hereditary fructose intolerance, an inborn defect of hepatic fructose. I. Phosphate-splitting aldolase,* Amer. J. Med., 34:151, 1963. — 11

GARROD, A. E.: *A Treatise on Gout and Rheumatic Gout,* Longmans, Green & Company, London, 1876. — 3–5

GUTMAN, A. B., AND YÜ: *Gout, a derangement of purine metabolism,* Advanc. intern. Med., 5:227, 1952. — 3

—— AND ——: *Uric acid metabolism in normal man and in primary gout,* New Engl. J. Med., 273:252, 1965. — 3–5

——, ——, ADLER AND JAVITT: *Intramolecular distribution of uric acid-N^{15} after administration of glycine-N^{15} and ammonium-N^{15} chloride to gouty and nongouty subjects,* J. clin. Invest., 41:623, 1962. — 3–5

HOCKADAY, T. D. R., CLAYTON, FREDERICK AND SMITH, JR.: *Primary hyperoxaluria,* Medicine (Baltimore), 43:315, 1964. — 6

HSIA, D. Y. Y., AND WALKER: *Variability in the clinical manifestation of galactosemia,* J. Pediat., 59:872, 1961. — 11

ILLINGWORTH, B.: *Glycogen storage disease,* Amer. J. clin. Nutr., 9:683, 1961. — 10

ISSELBACHER, K. J.: *Galactose metabolism and galactosemia,* Amer. J. Med., 26:715, 1959. — 11

LEWIS, G. M., SPENCER-PEET AND STEWARD: *Infantile hypoglycemia due to inherited deficiency of glycogen synthetase in liver,* Arch. Dis. Childh., 38:40, 1963. — 10

MILCH, R. A.: *Studies of alcaptonuria: a genetic study of 58 cases occurring in eight generations of seven interrelated Dominican kindreds,* Arthr. & Rheum., 4:131, 1961. — 1, 2

——: *Studies of alcaptonuria: mechanisms of swelling of homogentisic acid-collagen preparations,* Arthr. & Rheum., 4:253, 1961. — 1, 2

O'BRIEN, W. M., BANFIELD AND SOKOLOFF: *Studies on the pathogenesis of ochronotic arthropathy,* Arthr. & Rheum., 4:137, 1961. — 1, 2

——, LA DU AND BUNIM: *Biochemical, pathologic and clinical aspects of alcaptonuria, ochronosis and ochronotic arthropathy. Review of world literature (1584–1962),* Amer. J. Med., 34:813, 1963. — 1, 2

PARKER, W. S., PRADER AND FANCONI: *Further observations on cystine storage disease,* Pediatrics, 16:228, 1955. — 7

SEEGMILLER, J. E., GRAYZEL, LASTER AND LIDDLE: *Uric acid production in gout,* J. clin. Invest., 40:1304, 1961. — 3

SOKAL, J. E., LOWE, SARCIONE, MOSOVICH AND DORAY: *Studies of glycogen metabolism in liver glycogen disease (von Gierke's*

Section IX (continued)	PLATE NUMBER

disease): six cases with similar metabolic abnormalities and responses to glucagon, J. clin. Invest., 40:364, 1961. — 10

TALBOTT, J. H.: *Gout,* Grune & Stratton, Inc., New York, 1957. — 4, 5

WEINBERG, A. N.: *Detection of congenital galactosemia and the carrier state using galactose C-14 and blood cells,* Metabolism, 10:728, 1961. — 11

WILLIAMS, H. E., AND FIELD: *Low leukocyte phosphorylase in hepatic phosphorylase deficient glycogen storage disease,* J. clin. Invest., 40:1841, 1961. — 10

WYNGAARDEN, J. B., AND JONES: *The pathogenesis of gout,* Med. Clin. N. Amer., 45:1241, 1961. — 3–5

YÜ, T. F., BERGER AND GUTMAN: *Renal function in gout. II. Effect of uric acid loading on renal excretion of uric acid,* Amer. J. Med., 33:829, 1962. — 4, 5

ZANNONI, V. G., SEEGMILLER AND LA DU: *Nature of the defect in alcaptonuria,* Nature (Lond.), 193:952, 1962. — 1, 2

Section X

General References

HARPER, H. A.: *Review of Physiological Chemistry,* Lange Medical Publications, Los Altos, 1965.

———

ALTSCHUL, R.: *Niacin in Vascular Disorders and Hyperlipemia,* Charles C Thomas, Springfield, Ill., 1964. — 1, 4, 5

BHUVANESWARAN, C., AND SREENIVASAN: *Problems of thiamine deficiency states and their amelioration,* Ann. N. Y. Acad. Sci., 98:576, 1962. — 2, 3

BRO-RASMUSSEN, F.: *The riboflavin requirement of animals and man and associated metabolic relations. Part II: Relation of requirement to the metabolism of protein and energy,* Nutr. Abstr. Rev., 28:369, 1958. — 1

BURNS, J. J., AND CONNEY: *Water-soluble vitamins, Part I. (Ascorbic acid, nicotinic acid, vitamin B_6, biotin, inositol),* Ann. Rev. Biochem., 29:413, 1960. — 1–7

DINNING, J. S.: *Water-soluble vitamins, II. Vitamin B_{12}, folic acid, thiamine, riboflavin, pantothenic acid,* Ann. Rev. Biochem., 29:437, 1960. — 1–7

DOWLING, J. E., AND WALD: *The role of vitamin A acid,* Vitam. and Horm., 18:515, 1960. — 8

EDITORIAL: *Relation of pantothenic acid to adrenal cortical function,* Nutr. Rev., 19:79, 1961. — 1

Section X (continued)	PLATE NUMBER

EMERSON, G. A.: *Summary and comment on tissue changes in vitamin B_6 deficiency,* Vitam. and Horm., 22:655, 1964. — 4, 5

GANGULY, J.: *Absorption, transport, and storage of vitamin A,* Vitam. and Horm., 18:387, 1960. — 8

GLOVER, J.: *The conversion of β-carotene into vitamin A,* Vitam. and Horm., 18:371, 1960. — 8

HARRIS, P. L.: *Bioassay of vitamin A compounds,* Vitam. and Horm., 18:341, 1960. — 8

HORWITT, M. K.: *Water-soluble vitamins, Part I,* Ann. Rev. Biochem., 28:411, 1959. — 1–7

ISLER, O., RÜEGG, SCHWIETER AND WÜRSCH: *The synthesis and labeling of vitamin A and related compounds,* Vitam. and Horm., 18:295, 1960. — 8

JOHNSON, B. C., AND WOLF: *The function of vitamin A in carbohydrate metabolism; its role in adrenocorticoid production,* Vitam. and Horm., 18:457, 1960. — 8

KNOX, W. E., AND GOSWAMI: *Ascorbic acid in man and animals,* Advanc. clin. Chem., 4:121, 1961. — 6, 7

KOFLER, M., AND RUBIN: *Physicochemical assay of vitamin A and related compounds,* Vitam. and Horm., 18:315, 1960. — 8

MOORE, T.: *Vitamin A and proteins,* Vitam. and Horm., 18:431, 1960. — 8

——: *The pathology of vitamin A deficiency,* Vitam. and Horm., 18:499, 1960. — 8

STARE, F., EDITOR: *Intestinal conversion of C^{14} carotene to vitamin A,* Nutr. Rev., 19:334, 1961. — 8

——: *The conversion of beta-carotene to vitamin A ester by rat liver,* Nutr. Rev., 21:238, 1963. — 8

STOKSTAD, E. L. R.: *Biochemistry of the water-soluble vitamins,* Ann. Rev. Biochem., 31:451, 1962. — 1–7

SZORADY, I.: *Pantothenic acid: experimental results and clinical observations,* Acta paediat. Acad. Sci. hung., 4:73, 1963. — 1

VARIAVA, N. S.: *Vitamin C in clinical practice,* Curr. med. Pract., 2:292, 1958. — 6, 7

WAGNER, A. F., AND FOLKERS: *Vitamins and Coenzymes,* Interscience Publishers, New York, 1964. — 1–7

WALD, G.: *The visual function of the vitamins A,* Vitam. and Horm., 18:417, 1960. — 8

WISS, O., AND GLOOR: *Vitamin A and lipid metabolism,* Vitam. and Horm., 18:485, 1960. — 8

WOLF, G., AND JOHNSON: *Metabolic transformations of vitamin A,* Vitam. and Horm., 18:403, 1960. — 8

—— AND ——: *Vitamin A and mucopolysaccharide biosynthesis,* Vitam. and Horm., 18:439, 1960. — 8

SUBJECT INDEX

(Numerals refer to pages, *not* plates. Boldface numerals indicate major
emphasis. Meanings of abbreviations may be found in the glossary.)

273

277

279

285

286

THE NETTER COLLECTION OF MEDICAL ILLUSTRATIONS

The NETTER COLLECTION OF MEDICAL ILLUSTRATIONS has enjoyed an enthusiastic reception from the medical community since the publication of its first volume. The remarkable illustrations by Frank H. Netter, M.D., and text by leading specialists make these books unprecedented in their educational and clinical value.

Copies of all NETTER COLLECTION books may be purchased from Icon Learning Systems, 295 North Street, Teterboro, N.J. 07608. Call 201-727-9123 or visit us at www.netterart.com.

DATE DUE
